Paediatric
Handbook

Paediatric Handbook

TENTH EDITION

Edited by

Kate Harding
The Royal Children's Hospital, Melbourne
Victoria, Australia

Daniel S. Mason
The Royal Children's Hospital, Melbourne
Victoria, Australia

Daryl Efron
Associate Professor
The Royal Children's Hospital, Melbourne
Victoria, Australia

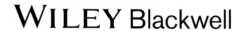

This edition first published 2021
© 2021 John Wiley & Sons Ltd

Edition History
Wiley-Blackwell (9e, 2015)

The right of Kate Harding, Daniel S. Mason and Daryl Efron to be identified as the authors of the editorial material in this work has been asserted in accordance with law.

Registered Office(s)
John Wiley & Sons, Inc., 111 River Street, Hoboken, NJ 07030, USA
John Wiley & Sons Ltd, The Atrium, Southern Gate, Chichester, West Sussex, PO19 8SQ, UK

Editorial Office
9600 Garsington Road, Oxford, OX4 2DQ, UK

For details of our global editorial offices, customer services, and more information about Wiley products visit us at www.wiley.com.

Wiley also publishes its books in a variety of electronic formats and by print-on-demand. Some content that appears in standard print versions of this book may not be available in other formats.

Library of Congress Cataloging-in-Publication Data
Names: Harding, Kate, 1973– editor. | Mason, Daniel S. (Pediatrician),
    editor. | Efron, Daryl, editor.
Title: Paediatric handbook / edited by Kate Harding, Daniel S. Mason,
    Daryl Efron.
Other titles: Paediatric handbook (Royal Children's Hospital)
Description: Tenth edition. | Hoboken, NJ : Wiley-Blackwell, 2021. |
    Includes index.
Identifiers: LCCN 2020025484 (print) | LCCN 2020025485 (ebook) |
    ISBN 9781119647072 (paperback) | ISBN 9781119647164 (adobe pdf) |
    ISBN 9781119647386 (epub)
Subjects: MESH: Pediatrics | Handbook
Classification: LCC RJ61 (print) | LCC RJ61 (ebook) | NLM WS 39 | DDC
    618.92–dc23
LC record available at https://lccn.loc.gov/2020025484
LC ebook record available at https://lccn.loc.gov/2020025485

Cover Design: The Royal Children's Hospital, Melbourne
Cover Illustration: Jane Reiseger

Set in 7.5/9.5pt Frutiger Light Condensed by SPi Global, Pondicherry, India
Printed and bound in Singapore by Markono Print Media Pte Ltd

10 9 8 7 6 5 4 3 2 1

Contents

Contents

List of Contributors

RCH is The Royal Children's Hospital, Melbourne
UoM is The University of Melbourne
MON is Monash University
MCRI is Murdoch Children's Research Institute

Giuliana Antolovich BSc (Hons) PhD MBBS FRACP
Paediatrician
Stream Leader Physical Disability, Department of
Neurodevelopment and Disability, RCH
Senior Fellow, Department of Paediatrics, UoM
Honorary Fellow, MCRI

Peter Archer MBBS FACEM
Emergency Physician
Emergency Department, RCH

Ruth Armstrong BSc MBChB MRCPCH FRACP
Neonatologist
Department of Neonatal Medicine, RCH

Gordon Baikie MD MBBS BMedSci Grd Dip Hlth Econ
FRACP FRCP
Paediatrician
Department of Neurodevelopment and Disability, RCH
Honorary Clinical Senior lecturer, Department of
Paediatrics, UoM
Honorary Fellow, MCRI

Liz Bannister MBBS FRACP PhD
Paediatric Gastroenterologist
Department of Gastroenterology & Clinical Nutrition,
RCH

Julie E. Bines MBBS FRACP MD
Paediatric Gastroenterologist
Head of Clinical Nutrition, Department of
Gastroenterology & Clinical Nutrition, RCH
Victor & Loti Smorgon Professor of Paediatrics,
Department of Paediatrics, UoM
Leader, RV3 Vaccine Program, Intestinal Failure &
Clinical Nutrition Group, MCRI

Antun Bogovic BPharm MSHP
Deputy Director
Pharmacy Department, RCH

Aurore Bouty MD
Paediatric Urologist
Department of Urology, RCH
Reproductive Biology, MCRI

Natasha J. Brown MBBS FRACP PhD
Clinical Geneticist
Victorian Clinical Genetics Service, RCH
Honorary Fellow, UoM
Honorary Fellow, MCRI

Fergus Cameron BMedSci MBBS DipRACOG FRACP MD
Paediatric Endocrinologist
Director, Department of Endocrinology and Diabetes,
RCH
Honorary Professorial Fellow, Department of
Paediatrics, UoM
Head, Diabetes Research Group, MCRI

Sally Campbell MBBS FRACP FRCPA
Paediatric Haematologist
Department of Clinical Haematology, RCH

George Chalkiadis MBBS DA (Lon) F ANZCA
FFPMANZCA
Paediatric Anaesthetist and Pain Management
Specialist
Head, Children's Pain Management Service,
Department of Paediatric Anaesthesia and Pain
Management, RCH
Honorary Clinical Associate Professor, Department of
Paediatrics, UoM
Honorary Fellow, MCRI

Daryl Cheng MBBS MPH FRACP AFAIDH CHIA
Paediatrician
Department of General Medicine, RCH
Honorary Fellow, Department of Paediatrics, UoM
Clinical Research Fellow, SAEFVIC, MCRI

Michael Cheung Bsc (Hons) MBChB MRCP MD FRACP
Paediatric Cardiologist
Director, Department of Cardiology, RCH
Principal Fellow, UoM
Heart Research Group Leader, MCRI

Sharon Choo MBBS FRACP FRCPA
Paediatric Allergist, Immunologist and
Immunopathologist
Immunology Laboratory, Laboratory Services
Department of Allergy & Immunology, RCH

Michael Clifford MBBS (Hons) FCICM FANZCA
Paediatric Intensivist & Anaesthetist
Paediatric Intensive Care Unit, Department of
Anaesthesia and Pain Management, RCH

Luisa Clucas MBBS (Hons) BMedSci DCH
Haematology Fellow
Department of Clinical Haematology, RCH

Rachel Conyers MBBS (Hons) FRACP PhD
Consultant Oncologist
Clinical Lead, Bone Marrow transplant, Children's
Cancer Centre, RCH
Clinical Associate Professor, Department of
Paediatrics, UoM
Clinician Scientist Fellow, Cardiac Regeneration
Laboratory, MCRI

Noel Cranswick MBBS BmedSc LLB FRACP
Paediatrician
Director, Clinical Pharmacology, Department of
General Medicine, RCH
Director, Australian Paediatric Pharmacology
Research Unit, RCH
Associate Professor, UoM
Associate Director Melbourne Children's Trials
Centre, MCRI

Nigel Crawford MBBS MPH PhD FRACP
Paediatrician
Medical Head Immunisation Services, Department of
General Medicine, RCH
Associate Professor, Department of Paediatrics, UoM
Director and Group leader, SAEFVIC, MCRI

Gemma Crighton MBChB FRACP FRCPA
Paediatric Haematologist
Department of Clinical Haematology, RCH

Nigel Curtis MA MBBS DTM&H FRCPCH PhD
Paediatric Infectious Diseases Physician

Head of Infectious Diseases, Department of General
Medicine, RCH
Professor of Paediatric Infectious Diseases,
Department of Paediatrics, UoM
Leader of Infectious Diseases Group, Infectious
diseases, MCRI

Clare Delany PhD M Hlth&Med Law M Physio BAppSci
(Physio)
Clinical Ethicist
Children's Bioethics Centre, RCH
Professor of Health Professions Education,
Department of Medical Education, UoM

Leo Donnan MBBS FRACS
Orthopaedic Surgeon
Department of Orthopaedics, RCH
Associate Professor, UoM

Trevor Duke MD FRACP FJFICM
Paediatric Intensivist
Clinical Director, General Intensive Care Unit,
Paediatric Intensive Care Unit, RCH
Professor, Department of Paediatrics, UoM

Daryl Efron MBBS FRACP MD
Paediatrician
Department of General Medicine, RCH
Associate Professor, Department of Paediatrics, UoM
Senior Research Fellow, MCRI

Charlotte V. Elder MBBS BMEDSCI FRANZCOG IFEPAG
Paediatric Gynaecologist
Department of Gynaecology, RCH
Honorary Clinical Fellow, Department of Paediatrics,
UoM

Victoria Evans BSc (Hons)
Clinical Nutrition Nurse Consultant
Department of Gastroenterology & Clinical Nutrition,
RCH

Mike Forrester MBBS FRACP
Paediatrician
University Hospital Geelong
Senior Clinical Lecturer, Deakin University

Tali Gadish MD FCICM
Paediatric Intensivist
Department of Paediatric Intensive Care, RCH
Honorary Clinical Lecturer, Department of Paediatrics,
UoM
Honorary Fellow, MCRI

List of Contributors

Susan Gibb MBBS FRACP
Paediatrician,
Medical Lead Complex Care Hub, Department of
Neurodevelopmental and Disability &
Department of General Medicine, RCH
Honorary Fellow, Infection and Immunity Theme,
MCRI

Lynn Gillam BA (Hons) MA PhD
Clinical Ethicist
Academic Director, Children's Bioethics Centre, RCH
Professor, Melbourne School of Population and
Global Health, UoM

Anthea Greenway MBBS (Hons) FRACP FRCPA
Paediatric Haematologist
Director of Clinical Haematology, Clinical Lead
Apheresis, Sickle Cell Anaemia, Department of
Clinical Haematology and Laboratory services, RCH
Honorary Fellow, MCRI

Amanda Griffiths MBBS BmedSc FRACP
Respiratory and Sleep Physician
Head of Sleep Medicine, Department of Respiratory
Medicine, RCH
Senior Clinical Fellow, UoM
Honorary Fellow, MCRI

Joanne Grindlay MBBS FACEM FRACGP FARGP DA (UK)
Grad Dip (Rural GP) EMDM HOSM
Paediatric Emergency physician
Deputy Director, Emergency Department, RCH
Clinical Associate Professor, UoM
Research Associate, MCRI

Sonia R. Grover MBBS FRANZCOG MD FFPMANZCA
Paediatric and Adolescent Gynaecologist, Pain
Medicine Specialist
Department of Gynaecology, RCH
Clinical Professor, Department of Paediatrics, UoM
Honorary Fellow, MCRI

Kerrod Hallett MDSc MPH FRACDS FICD
Paediatric Dentist
Director, Department of Dentistry, RCH
Clinical Associate Professor, UoM
Research Fellow, Clinical Sciences, MCRI

Diane Hanna MBBS (Hon) FRACP
Paediatric Oncologist (Leukaemia and Bone Marrow
Transplantation)
Children's Cancer Centre, RCH

Winita Hardikar MBBS FRACP PhD AM
Paediatric Gastroenterologist
Head of Liver and Intestinal Transplantation
Director, Department of Gastroenterology and
Clinical Nutrition, RCH

Lynne Harrison BAppSc (Sp.Path) MBA (UWA)
Speech Pathologist
Speech Pathology Department, Allied Health, RCH

Ric Haslam MSc AKC FRACP CertChildPsych
Child Psychiatrist
Director, Department of Mental Health, RCH
Honorary Clinical Senior Lecturer, UoM

Leah Hickey MB BCh BAO (Hons) MRCPI FRACP MD
Neonatologist
Department of Neonatal Medicine, RCH
Clinical Senior Lecturer, Department of Paediatrics,
UoM
Honorary Fellow, Neonatal Research Group, MCRI

Harriet Hiscock MBBS FRACP MD
Paediatrician
Director, Health Services Research Unit, RCH
Professorial Fellow, Department of Paediatrics, UoM
Group Leader, Health Services, Centre for Community
Child Health, MCRI

Jenny Hynson MBBS FRACP FAChPM PhD
Consultant Paediatrician
Head, Victorian Paediatric Palliative Care Program, RCH
Clinical Associate Professor, UoM

Michael B. Johnson MBBS FRACS FAOA
Paediatric Orthopaedic Surgeon,
Head, Department of Orthopaedics, RCH

Bryn Jones MBBS FRACP FCSANZ
Paediatric Cardiologist
Deputy Director, Department of Cardiology, RCH
Clinical Senior Fellow, Department of Paediatrics, UoM
Honorary Fellow, MCRI

Jeff Kao MBChB FRACP DMedSc
Paediatric Endocrinologist
Department of Endocrinology and Diabetes, RCH
Diabetes Research Associate, MCRI

Joshua Kausman MBBS FRACP PhD
Paediatric Nephrologist
Director, Department of Nephrology, RCH
Honorary Senior Fellow, Department of Paediatrics, UoM
Honorary Fellow, MCRI

Andrew Kornberg MBBS (Hons) DipTA (ATTA) ACCAM FRACP
Senior Paediatric Neurologist
Department of Neurology, RCH
Associate professor, Department of Paediatrics, UoM
Associate professor, Neuromuscular disorders, MCRI

Remi Kowalski MBBS (Hons) FRACP FCSANZ PhD
Paediatric Cardiologist
Department of Cardiology, RCH
Clinical Senior Lecturer, Department of Paediatrics, UoM
Honorary Fellow, Heart Research Group, MCRI

Joy Lee MD FRACP
Metabolic Consultant
Department of Metabolic Medicine, RCH
Clinical Senior Lecturer, Department of Paediatrics, UoM
Honorary Fellow, MCRI

Mark Mackay MBBS PhD FRACP
Paediatric Neurologist
Department of Neurology, RCH
Associate Professor & Principal Fellow, UoM
Clinician Scientist, Fellow & Paediatric Stroke Research Team Leader, MCRI

Deborah Marks MBBS BMedSci FRACP CertChildPsych
Paediatrician (Specialist Autism Team)
Department of Mental Health, RCH

Catherine Marraffa MBBS FRACP FRCPCH
Paediatrician
Deputy Director & Stream Leader Intellectual Disability and Autism, Department of Neurodevelopment and Disability, RCH
Clinical Lecturer, Department of Paediatrics, UoM
Honorary Fellow, MCRI

John Massie MBBS FRACP PhD
Paediatric Respiratory Physician
Department of Respiratory and Sleep Medicine, Clinical lead of The Children's Bioethics Centre, RCH
Professorial Fellow, Department of Paediatrics, UoM
Honorary Fellow MCRI

Anu Mathew MBChB MD FRANZCO
Ophthalmologist
Department of Ophthalmology, RCH

Zoe McCallum MBBS FRACP
Paediatrician
Department of Neurodevelopment and Disability, Department of Gastroentrology and Clinical Nutrition, RCH
Senior Lecturer, Department of Paediatrics, UoM

Ian McKenzie MBBS DipRACOG FANZCA
Anaesthetist
Director, Department of Anaesthesia and Pain Management, RCH

Sarah McNab MBBS (Hon) FRACP PhD
General Paediatrician
Director, Department of General Medicine, RCH
Honorary Senior Fellow (Clinical), Department of Paediatrics, UoM
Honorary Fellow, MCRI

David Metz MBBS FRACP
Paediatric Nephrologist & Clinical Pharmacologist
Department of Nephrology, RCH

Paul Monagle MBBS MSc MD FRACP FRCPA FCCP
Paediatric Haematologist
Department of Clinical Haematology, RCH
Professor, Department of Paediatrics, UoM
Group Leader, Haematology Research, MCRI

Jane Munro MBBS FRACP MPH MHMS
Paediatric Rheumatologist
Head of Rheumatology Unit, Department of General Medicine, RCH
Associate Professor, Department of Paediatrics, UoM
Group Leader, Arthritis and Rheumatology, MCRI

Michael Nightingale FRACS
Paediatric Surgeon
Department of Paediatric Surgery, RCH
Honorary senior lecturer, UoM
Research Associate, MCRI

Michele O'Connell MRCPI FRACP MD
Paediatric Endocrinologist
Department of Endocrinology & Diabetes and Adolescent Gender service, RCH
Honorary fellow, Centre for Hormone Research, MCRI

David Orchard MBBS FACD
Paediatric Dermatologist
Director of Dermatology, RCH
Associate Professor (Clinical), UoM

List of Contributors

Josh Osowicki MBBS BMedSci FRACP
Paediatric Infectious Diseases physician
Infectious Diseases unit, Department of General
Medicine, RCH
Department of Paediatrics, UoM
Tropical Diseases Research Group, MCRI

Greta Palmer MBBS FANZCA FFPMANZCA
Paediatric Anaesthetist and Specialist Pain Medicine
Physician
Deputy Head, Children's Pain Management Service,
Department of Anaesthesia and Pain Management,
RCH
Clinical Associate Professor, Department of
Paediatrics, UoM
Research Associate, MCRI

Ken Pang MBBS (Hons) BMedSc FRACP PhD
Paediatrician
Department of Adolescent Medicine, RCH
Honorary Associate Professor, Department of
Paediatrics, UoM
Team Leader and Clinician Scientist Fellow, MCRI

Georgia Paxton MBBS (Hons) BMedSci MPH FRACP OAM
Paediatrician
Head of Immigrant Health, Department of General
Medicine, RCH
Associate Professor, Department of Paediatrics, RCH
Research Fellow, Infection and Immunity, MCRI

Heidi Peters MBBS FRACP PhD HGSA MClinMed (L&Mgt)
Metabolic Consultant
Department of Metabolic Medicine, RCH
Senior lecturer, Department of Paediatrics, UoM
Honorary Fellow, MCRI

Rod Phillips BSc MBBS PhD FRACP AOM
Paediatric Dermatologist
Department of General Medicine, RCH
Associate Professor, Department of Paediatrics, MON
Honorary Fellow, MCRI

Chidambaram Prakash MBBS FRANZCP Cert Child
Psychiatry (RANZCP)
Authorised Psychiatrist
Principal Hospital Pyschiatrist, Department of Mental
Health, RCH

Lochana Ramalingam BDS Dip Clin Dent MDSc FRACDS
(Gen) FRACDS (Paed)
Dentist
Director of Clinical Services, Department of Dentistry, RCH
Research Associate, Facial Sciences, MCRI

Sarath Ranganathan MBCHB MRCPCH MRCP FRACP
PhD ATSF
Paediatric Respiratory Physician
Department of Respiratory and Sleep Medicine, RCH
Stevenson Chair & Head, Department of Paediatrics, UoM

Colette Reveley MBChB BSc FRACP AYAM
Paediatrician
Department of Adolescent Medicine, RCH

Gehan Roberts MB BS MPH PhD FRACP
Developmental-Behavioural Paediatrician
Associate Director, Centre for Community Child
Health, RCH
Associate Professor, Department of Paediatrics, UoM
Honorary Fellow, Population Health, MCRI

Liz Rogers BAppsci MND
Clinical Specialist Dietitian
Department of Gastroenterology and Clinical
Nutrition, RCH

Elizabeth Rose MBBS FRACS
Otolaryngologist
Department Otolaryngology, RCH
Senior Lecturer, Department of Otolaryngology, UoM
Honorary Fellow, MCRI

Kathy Rowe MBBS MD FRACP MPH Dip Ed (Lond)
Grad Dip Int Health
Paediatrician
Department of General Medicine, RCH
Research Fellow, MCRI

Bronwyn Sacks MBBS FRACP FAChPM MBioethics
Paediatric Palliative Care Physician
Victorian Paediatric Palliative Care Program, RCH

Helen Savoia MBBS FRCPA
Haematologist
Director, Laboratory services, RCH

Susan Sawyer MBBS MD FRACP
Paediatrician
Centre for Adolescent Health, RCH
Geoff and Helen Handbury Chair of Adolescent
Health, Department of Paediatrics, UoM
Group Leader, Adolescent Health, MCRI

Adam Scheinberg MBBS DCH FRACP FAFRM MMED
Consultant in Paediatric Rehabilitation
Director, Victorian Paediatric Rehabilitation Service
Clinical Associate Professor, Faculty of Medicine,
Dentistry and Health Sciences, UoM
Honorary Fellow, Manager, MCRI

Peter Simm MBBS (Hons) MD FRACP
Paediatric Endocrinologist
Department of Endocrinology and Diabetes, RCH
Honorary Senior Fellow, Department of Paediatrics, UoM
Honorary Fellow, MCRI

Joanne Smart Bsc MBBS PhD FRACP
Paediatric Allergist and Immunologist
Director, Department of Allergy and Immunology, RCH

Anne Smith MBBS FRACP MForensMed FFCFM (RCPA)
Forensic Paediatrician
Director, Victorian Forensic Paediatric Medical
Service, RCH
Clinical Associate Professor, Department of
Paediatrics, UoM
Senior Lecturer, MON

Jane Standish MBBS FRACP
Paediatrician
Department of General Medicine, Department of
Gastroenterology and Clinical Nutrition, RCH
Honorary Fellow, MCRI

Mike Starr MBBS FRACP
Paediatrician, Infectious Diseases Physician,
Consultant in Emergency Medicine
Director of Paediatric Education
Departments of General Medicine, Infectious
Diseases and Emergency Medicine, RCH
Honorary Clinical Associate Professor, UoM

Valerie Sung MBBS (Hons) FRACP MPH PhD
Paediatrician
Department of General Medicine
Centre for Community Child Health, RCH
Honorary Clinical Associate Professor, Department of
Paediatrics, UoM
Team Leader and Senior Research Officer, Prevention
Innovation Group, Population Health, MCRI

Christos Symeonides Bsc MBCHB MRCPCH FRACP
General and Developmental Paediatrician
Centre for Community Child Health, RCH
Postgraduate Research Scholar, MCRI

Daniella Tassoni
Clinical Specialist Dietitian
Weight Management Service, RCH

Warwick Teague MBBS DPhil (Oxford) FRACS
Paediatric Surgeon
Department of Paediatric Surgery, RCH
Associate Professor, Department of Paediatrics, UoM
Co-group Leader, MCRI

Michelle Telfer MBBS (Hons) FRACP
Paediatrician and Adolescent Physician
Director, Department of Adolescent Medicine, RCH
Honorary Associate Professor, UoM
Honorary Fellow, MCRI

Dean Tey MBBS FRACP
Paediatric Allergist & Immunologist
Department of Allergy & Immunology, RCH
Honorary Fellow, MCRI

James Tibballs BMedSc (Hon) MBBS Med MBA MD
MHlth&MedLaw PGDipArts (Fr) DALF FANZCA FICICM FACLM
Paediatric Intensivist
Paediatric Intensive Care Unit, RCH
Associate Professor, Principal Fellow, Departments of
Pharmacology and Paediatrics, UoM

Georgina Tiller MBBS BSc FRACP
Paediatric Rheumatologist, General Paediatrician
Rheumatology Unit, Department of General
Medicine, RCH

Joanna Tully BSc MBBS MD FRACP
Forensic Paediatrician
Deputy Director, Victorian Forensic Paediatric Medical
Service, RCH

Sidharth Vemuri MBBS FRACP FAChPM
Paediatrician and Palliative Care Physician
Victorian Paediatric Palliative Care Program, RCH

Evelyn Volders AdvAPD
Dietitian
Department Nutrition and Food Services, RCH

Mary White MB BAO BCH MRCP FRACP MD
Paediatric Endocrinologist
Department of Endocrinology & Diabetes, RCH
Honorary Senior Fellow, Department of Paediatrics,
UoM
Research Officer, Health Services Research Unit,
MCRI

Molly Williams MBBS FRACP FAChPM
Paediatric Palliative Care Physician and Oncologist
Victorian Paediatric Palliative Care Program
Children's Cancer Centre, RCH

Neil Wimalasundera MBBS MRCPCH MSc
FRACP FAFRM
Consultant in Paediatric Rehabilitation
Victorian Paediatric Rehabilitation Service, RCH

List of Contributors

Alison Wray MBChB FRACS
Paediatric Neurosurgeon
Director, Department of Neurosurgery, RCH
Honorary Fellow, MCRI

Danielle Wurzel MBBS (Hons) PhD FRACP
Paediatric Respiratory Physician
Department of Respiratory and Sleep Medicine, RCH
Honorary Senior Fellow, Department of Paediatrics,
UoM
Research Clinician, MCRI

Margaret Zacharin MBBS D Med Sci FRACP
Paediatric Endocrinologist
Department of Endocrinology, RCH
Professor, Department of Paediatrics, UoM
Honorary Fellow, MCRI

Acknowledgements

We greatly appreciate and acknowledge the contributions of the following people:

Editorial team of the tenth edition: Mike Forrester, Susan Gibb, Amy Gray, Amanda Gwee, Sebastian King, Jane Munro, Romi Rimer, Mike Starr.

The Royal Children's Hospital Foundation for funding support.

Kirsten Noakes, Department of General Medicine, for project planning and management support.

The Royal Children's Hospital, Melbourne Creative Services; James Watson, Tom Marriott, Anne Hunt, Bhavya Boopathi and Mary Malin (Copyeditor) at Wiley for their assistance with handbook design.

Previous edition authors:

George Alex
Roger Allen
David Amor
Peter Barnett
Tom Clarnette
Tom Connell
Margot Davey
James Elder
Ralf Heine

Yves Heloury
Rod Hunt
John Hutson
Julian Kelly
Lionel Lubitz
Wirginia Maixner
Francoise Mechinaud
Michele Meehan
Ed Oakley

Mike O'Brien
Dinah Reddihough
Sheena Reilly
Matthew Sabin
Russell Taylor
Amanda Walker
George Werther

Foreword

It is 55 years since the Royal Children's Hospital Paediatric Handbook was established, and its growth from a small number of pages in a vinyl ring binder to its current form has been a marker of the modern era of paediatrics, which was more or less coincident with the relocation of the Royal Children's Hospital in Melbourne from Carlton to its current location in Parkville in the early 1960s. First, there was consolidation of paediatrics itself as a subspecialty, and then the many and various subspecialties in medicine and surgery as they emerged. The associated knowledge explosion was fuelled by a progressively more scientific approach to research-led clinical care and its evidence base, and by an increasing emphasis on quality and safety in the care of children and adolescents.

The first edition was released in 1964 as the Resident Medical Officers' Handbook, and the 2nd edition and its revision in 1975 and 1982 respectively (as the Residents' Handbook). For several years, their renewal and production lapsed. After returning from my doctoral studies at McGill and Montreal Children's Hospital in the late 1980s, I was asked whether we should resurrect the Handbook, and modernise it. My enthusiastic positive response was shared by my colleagues, senior and junior, and so we embarked on its renewal.

Resisting the temptation to grow it into a textbook, we were keen to maintain its niche as definitive and clear guidance for the commonest clinical problems that confronted junior doctors, and as a resource for the most senior doctors for clinical issues outside their area of sub-specialty.

We established the model of a senior clinician providing steerage and oversight (myself for the 3rd to 6th editions; Dr Michael Marks 7th to 9th editions; Associate Professor Daryl Efron for this new 10th edition), and one or two advanced trainees or clinical fellows acting as the editors. All were assisted by a larger editorial committee to ensure that a multi-speciality and generalist breadth of input and oversight was provided. Chapter authors were often a mix of junior and senior clinicians. This proved enormously helpful in resolving, or at least recognising, differing sub-specialty perspectives on the same clinical problem, evidence of health professional rivalries always motivated by a belief in what was best for the child, and sometimes by the evidence base underpinning that position!

A distinguished lineage of fellows as editors ensued, all of whom have gone on to become leaders in their various fields within paediatrics: Dr Lindsay Smith (3rd edition, 1989), Dr Michael Marks (4th edition, 1992 – Blackwells), Dr Daryl Efron (5th edition, 1995), Dr Joanne Smart (6th edition, 2000), Dr Georgia Paxton and Dr Jane Munro (7th edition, 2003; supervision taken over by Dr Michael Marks), Dr Kate Thomson and Dr Dean Tey (8th edition, 2009), Dr Amanda Gwee and Dr Romi Rimer (9th edition, 2015).

For the 4th edition in 1992, we initiated and then concluded a deal with international publisher Blackwells (now Wiley Blackwell) to take the Handbook to a new level of professional production and marketing to the world. Since then, there have been significant internationals sales in the United Kingdom, Europe, USA and Canada, India, Malaysia, Singapore, China (including Hong Kong), and New Zealand.

Whether in the RCH itself, or in other urban, regional and rural hospitals and in primary care settings and now overseas, it is one of the key resources that has guided many thousands of doctors (and nurses) over more than half a century. The common (and even trivial) in a specialist paediatric setting can seem exotic and occasionally bizarre in general and other non-specialist settings. The Handbook has cemented its position as a key clinician resource, and this is because it is the product of the highest clinical standards, underpinned by a sustained commitment to evidence-based quality of care.

The 10th edition, edited by Dr Kate Harding and Dr Daniel Mason, with editorial oversight provided by Associate Professor Daryl Efron, lives up to the tradition of excellence established by its predecessors. It has retained its pragmatic and sharp focus, and has been brought up to date in many areas, and expanded particularly in relation to clinical conditions often managed in community settings. Although it began its life as a 'Resident Medical Officers' Handbook', the Paediatric Handbook is an essential resource for all clinicians involved in the care of children and adolescents.

Professor Terry Nolan, AO FRACP FAHMS
Melbourne, September 2020

RCH Handbook List

1st edition (1964). *Resident Medical Officers' Handbook*, Lawson JS, ed. (Foreword: Sloan LEG). 100 p. Snap-lock ring binder.

2nd edition (1975–1976). *Residents Handbook*, Roy N, Vance J, eds. (Foreword: Sloan LEG). 203 p. Snap-lock ring binder.

2nd edition, revised (1982–1983). *Residents Handbook*, Roy N, Vance J, eds. (Foreword: Westwood G). 228 p. Snap-lock ring binder.

3rd edition (1989). *Paediatric Handbook*, Smith LJ, ed. (Preface: Phelan PD). xiv, 287 p. Paperback. ISBN 0-7316-2463-7.

3rd edition (1990). *Paediatric Handbook Supplement*, 1989 Edition. 12 p. Paperback. ISBN 0-9590-6187-8.

4th edition (1992). *Paediatric Handbook*, Marks MK, ed. (Preface: Phelan PD). xiv, 234 p. Paperback. ISBN 0-86793-217-1.

5th edition (1995). *Paediatric Handbook*, Efron D, Nolan T, eds. (Foreword: Phelan PD). xv, 520 p. Paperback. ISBN 0-86793-337-2.

6th edition (2000). *Paediatric Handbook*, Smart J, Nolan T, eds. (Foreword: Smith PJ). xviii, 630 p. Paperback. ISBN 0-86793-011-X.

7th edition (2003). *Paediatric Handbook*, Paxton G, Munro J, Marks M, eds. (Foreword: Bowes G). xviii, 709 p. Paperback. ISBN 0-86793-431-X.

8th edition (2009). *Paediatric Handbook*, Thomson K, Tey D, Marks M, eds. (Foreword: Bines J). xv, 640 p. Paperback. ISBN 978-1-4051-7400-8.

9th edition (2015). *Paediatric Handbook*, Gwee A, Rimer R, Marks M, eds. (Foreward: Shann F). xv, 526 p. Paperback. ISBN 978-1-11877748-0.

10th edition (2021). *Paediatric Handbook*, Kate Harding, Daniel S. Mason, Daryl Efron, eds. (Foreward: Terry Nolan). xviii, 608 p. Paperback. ISBN 978-1-1196-4707-2.

Preface

Since the first edition in 1964, the RCH Paediatic Handbook has brought together the collective knowledge and experience of our specialist clinicians to present current best practice in the assessment and management of common paediatric medical and surgical problems. The Handbook has always been popular with medical students, paediatricians, general practitioners, emergency physicians and other child health professionals who value its practical, easily accessible and high quality information.

The 10th edition happily coincides with the 150th anniversary of the RCH. This is a moment to celebrate our past, and also to look to the future in the ever-evolving field of neonatal, child and adolescent health care. Since the 9th edition we have seen the formation of the Melbourne Children's Campus, bringing together four interlinked organisations at a single site: The Royal Children's Hospital, Melbourne, the Murdoch Children's Research Institute, the University of Melbourne, Department of Paediatrics and The Royal Children's Hospital Foundation. Our research, teaching and clinical practice are fully integrated with the goal of delivering consistent excellence in paediatric care, education and training.

This edition is a comprehensive revision and update of the Handbook, broadened to include conditions often managed in community settings. This is aligned with one of the key principals of the RCH strategic plan for 2019–21 *Great Care, Everywhere*.

New chapters in this edition include:
- Communication skills
- Ethics
- Trans and gender diverse health
- Gynaecology
- Rehabilitation medicine

Many of the chapters have been expanded or extensively revised, including Neonatal medicine, Palliative care, Haematology, Allergy, Genetics, Immunisation and Dentistry. All chapters in the 10th edition include easy to access Key points and Clinical Pearls.

We would like to thank all the authors for giving their time and expertise to contribute to the Handbook. We acknowledge the contributions and teaching of authors in previous editions; the 10th edition of the Handbook stands upon the solid foundations they built. We would also like to thank the dedicated editorial committee for bringing great enthusiasm and commitment to this project.

The RCH has a proud tradition, much loved by both the public and the staff. The Handbook represents the breadth of excellence we strive for across all clinical areas. We trust that the reader finds it a valuable resource to support the provision of high quality paediatric care everywhere.

Kate Harding
Daniel S. Mason
Daryl Efron

CHAPTER 1

Communication in the paediatric consultation

Mike Forrester
Daryl Efron

Key Points
- Elicit the family's main concerns, ideas about the problem, and how they think you can help.
- Involve children in the consultation according to their developmental level and interest.
- Learn to use a range of structural models and communication 'microskills' to enhance consultation efficiency and achieve shared decision making.
- Be alert to verbal and non-verbal cues and use a range of techniques to respond to emotion.
- Conscious communication skill practice will improve the child and family's experience, increase adherence, decrease errors, health care costs and litigation and also improve clinician well-being or 'joy in work.'

Effective communication is fundamental to effective clinical medicine. Flexibly employing a range of communication skills is key to eliciting accurate diagnostic information and understanding the child/family context, which is necessary for shared decision making. Yet clinical communication skills are not innate, nor do they necessarily improve with clinical experience alone. They require learning and conscious practice. Good communication skills improve patient experience, increase adherence, decrease errors, decrease health care costs and litigation and also improve clinician well-being or 'joy in work'.

The triadic consultation of paediatrics (doctor–parent–child) poses extra challenges. The child and all carers present need to be encouraged to engage and share their agendas. This requires flexibility in approach, allowing for differing educational, cultural, and religious backgrounds, and levels of social connectedness and advantage. The possibility of trauma or adverse childhood experiences may need to be considered as they will influence the best approach to communication and building trust (See Chapter 14, Behaviour and mental health). Connection with the child and family will be enhanced if the clinician embodies empathy, patience, a non-judgmental approach and conveys curiosity and enthusiasm.

It is professionally satisfying to complete the consultation knowing that clinician and family have both met their agendas in the available time and also enjoyed a human connection. However, all clinicians will have moments when they feel there is a disconnect with the child and the family one is trying to help. Sometimes it can be difficult to pinpoint why the disconnect has occurred. Breaking down the elements of the consultation structure can help (Figure 1.1).

Clinicians employ a range of communication skills to build the relationship, allow a consultation to flow or to recognise the need for repair. These 'Microskills' are the elements of effective communication. They include techniques such as asking open questions, use of silence, responding to verbal and non-verbal cues, responding to emotion, chunking and checking, microsummaries, and signposting (Table 1.1). This chapter introduces the reader to some of these core communication skills.

Paediatric Handbook, Tenth Edition. Edited by Kate Harding, Daniel S. Mason and Daryl Efron.
© 2021 John Wiley & Sons Ltd. Published 2021 by John Wiley & Sons Ltd.

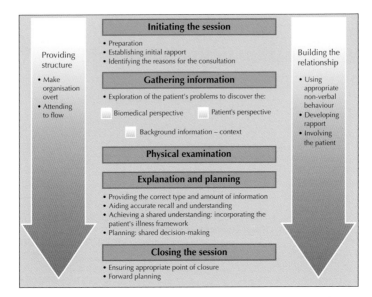

Figure 1.1 The Calgary Cambridge process. *Sources: Skills for Communicating with Patients.* 3rd Ed. Jonathan Silverman, Suzanne Kurtz, Juliet Draper. CRC Press, Published September 2013 and Kurtz S, Silverman J, Benson J, Draper J. Marrying content and process in clinical method teaching: enhancing the Calgary–Cambridge guides. *Acad Med.* 2003; 78:802–9. Reprinted with permission.

Table 1.1 Micro-skills to enhance communication effectiveness.

Micro-skills to enhance communication effectiveness.
Explore shared agenda 'What do we want to achieve today?'
Open to closed cone questions (start open, then move to more directive questions) and screening questions, 'is there anything else that's troubling you'
Listen actively, avoid interrupting
Encourage more information 'Tell me more', use of silence
Facilitate by encouragement, paraphrasing, interpretation
Identify and explore cues to underlying concerns, verbal and non-verbal e.g. eye contact, facial expressions, posture, vocal rate/volume/intonation
Use explicit empathy e.g. 'I'm sorry to hear that', 'That sounds really tough', 'I can't imagine how this might feel for you, but I wonder…'
Demonstrate confidence with your assessment/differentials/plan (e.g. with regards to what you find reassuring and why)
Explain rationale for suggested investigations and management plan
Avoid jargon: Use concise and easily understood language
Progress using Signposting: explicitly sharing the structure/plan e.g. 'would it be ok if we first talked about… and then…' or 'There are three important things I'd like to discuss, first…'
Use visual methods for conveying information where useful
Chunk and check: Provide information in assimilable chunks, check for understanding, use child's response as guide to how to proceed with providing information. 'Just to make sure we're on the same page'
Teach Back: Invite the child/family to restate the agreed plan
Final check: 'Have we covered everything we needed to sort out today?'

The consultation

Preparation

- Ensure you have the information and time that you need; invite relevant family and staff (and interpreter if needed).
- Find an appropriate space (privacy/toys/books/seating).
- Consider handing your phone or pager to a colleague for particularly high-stakes consultations.
- Offer to phone a non-present carer into the consultation where appropriate.

Specific Initiation and Engagement Tips

- **Babies <12m**: Usually a calm voice and gentle approach is all that is required if the baby is in the mood!
- **Toddlers aged 1–3 years**: Stranger awareness generally develops late in the first year. Chat to parents to show that you can be trusted, trade toys, smile, allow the toddler to come to you. Avoid intense focus and eye contact initially.
- **Children 3–6 years:** Try to establish a playful relationship with a child to reduce apprehension. This facilitates assessment and treatment. Give the child space and let them warm to you. Sitting on the floor or low chair is less threatening to small children than towering over them. Remember that the child is likely listening to all that is being said.
- **Children 7–11 years:** Research shows that children of this age want to be involved in discussions about their diagnosis and treatment. Introduce yourself to the child first. Explain that you are a doctor for kids so you will be very interested in what they have to say. Ask the child to introduce their family or carers to you. Start a conversation about everyday topics, e.g. who lives at home, what they like doing for fun, school, friends.
- **Teenagers:** Teenagers respond to an authentic, non-judgemental approach. Start by treating them like an adult and modify if this is resisted. Allow the young person to educate you, as *experts* on teen culture, about what is going on in their world. Bring the young person back into the conversation if they are sidelined by the parents/carers.

Gathering information

The three critical questions for child and carers are:

- What is the family/carer's key concern? (Concerns) *'What are you most worried about?'*
- What does the family/carer think is wrong? (Ideas) *'You've obviously given this some thought, what were you thinking it might be?'*
- How do they hope the clinician can help? (Expectations) *'How are you hoping I/we might be able to help with this?'*

Note that wording and order of these questions should be modified to suit clinician and child/family.

Children

- Ask the child who will start the story, so the child has the option of initiating the history or deferring to their parents. Child involvement is improved if parents are also encouraged to voice their concerns early on in the consultation and the child is then invited to speak further.
- If the child is shy or hesitant, start by talking to the parents/carers, and tell the child that you would like them to add their thoughts and corrections along the way.
- Ask an open question about the problem or concern. Listen attentively, try to avoid interrupting, and tolerate silence. Most of the valuable information will be here. You will understand the concerns up front and avoid missing key cues.
- Use mini summaries to clarify what you have understood along the way.
- Closed questions with choices work better for younger children and open-ended questions allowing for free, or narrative, responses with older children.
- Be alert to non-verbal cues which often reveal important information.
- If the opening statement from the parent is negative about the child and their problem, e.g. in emotional/behavioural issues, you may need to help them reframe this. Ask the parent to describe how the child is at their best, or when they are happy, and when things are difficult for the child. Then ask the child to contribute to the discussion to have a sense of control.

- Recognise good parenting and convey a belief in family competence. Identify and work with strengths in the family system.
- Model respect for the child. Let the child know you are open to hearing any questions from them about their health.
- Check what the child has understood and if they have any questions.

Adolescents

- Support the transition to independence by including time alone with adolescents. This builds the adolescent's health literacy skills relevant to self-management, e.g. self-efficacy and self-advocacy.
- Explain to the family and young person that it is part of your routine practice to spend some portion of the consultation without the family. One good method is to set an agenda together, then spend time with the young person alone (where trust permits and/or age appropriate) and then conclude by coming back together to develop a negotiated plan.
- It is important to explain confidentiality and the relevant exceptions to both the young person and the family. (See Chapter 12, Adolescent medicine).
- Praise the young person for any efforts after they present their needs or complaints. This helps build autonomy and an evolving relationship as the young person transitions towards independence.
- Once the young person signals that they have exhausted their list, re-direct the same questions to the family.

Explanation and Planning

Provide an appropriate amount and type of information for both the child and family to understand. This will be easier to organise if you understand their Concerns, Ideas, Expectations (see above) and health literacy. Key communication skills for giving information are microsummaries during longer explanations and 'chunking and checking' (Table 1.1) breaking information into manageable 'chunks' and checking what has been understood.

Shared decision-making

This involves both the child and family in the decision-making process. There is some confusion about what shared decision-making looks like, but it is essentially a middle way between the 'Paternalistic' model and the 'Informed' model (Table 1.2).

- 'Paternalistic' model: Physician informs and decides. Few people seek this when asked about their desired level of involvement in decision making.
- 'Informed' model: Shifts the burden of the decision to child/family, 'Here are the options. What would you like us to do?'
- 'Shared decision-making' (the middle-way): Doctor gathers the information i.e. concerns, fears, values, goals, to then offer specific advice informed by the above.

Table 1.2 Models of treatment decision making.

	Paternalistic	Shared decision-making	Informed
Information transfer	One way: from doctor to patient, minimum necessary for informed consent	Two way: doctor provides all medical information needed for decision- aking. patient provides information about her preferences	One way: from doctor to patient, all medical information needed for decision-making
Deliberation	Physician alone, or with other physicians	Physician and Patient (plus potential others)	Patient (plus potential others)
Decision about implementing treatment	Physician	Physician and Patient	Patient

Source: Murray, E, Charles, C and Gafni, A. 'Shared decision-making in primary care: tailoring the Charles et al. model to fit the context of general practice.' *Patient education and counselling* 62.2 (2006): 205–211. Reprinted with permission of Elsevier.

Clinical Pearl: Consultation efficiency
- Once you have understood the child's and family's agenda, help them prioritise what is most important to cover today and signpost what might be needed to be covered in subsequent consultations.
- When seeing a child who has been seen by other clinicians prior, after introduction and establishing initial rapport, say 'It would be helpful for me to know what you already understand about your/child's condition and what you would like to know or talk about today'.
- If you can sit down on a ward round the perception will be that you have spent significantly more time.
- Many examination findings can be elicited by observing the child while taking the history e.g. colour, respiratory pattern, gait, speech, play skills.

Challenging communication scenarios
Responding to intense emotion
When you feel the heat rise in the consultation, try to pause, avoid being reactive, and ask yourself what is the child or family's *underlying emotion*? Often it is worry, fear, or being overwhelmed. We need to respond to the underlying emotion first, before we can move onto further information gathering, explanation or shared decision making. The mnemonic 'NURSE' can be helpful in this situation:
- **Name the underlying emotion** *'You look pretty worried.'*. Naming the underlying emotion is much more likely to be effective than naming the surface emotion i.e. *'You seem angry / frustrated…'*
- **Understand** *'If I understand properly, you are most concerned about…'*
- **Respect and praise** e.g. *'You are the expert on your child'*
- **Support and silence** e.g. supports such as offering to involve social work, write to workplace etc
- **Empathy and explore**. We do not need to 'fix' the issues that come out of this exploration but to hear and guide if possible.

Not all of these skills need be used in a given exchange but choose those which are likely to be most helpful in the context. Once the emotion has settled, the child or family will signal that they are ready to proceed. You may need to revisit the child/family's main concerns or ideas at this point.

Identifying and repairing mismatches
A mismatched expectation is where the clinician and child/family agenda are not aligned. Mismatches can be identified by observing body language (non-verbal cues), circular conversations, anger, dismissal, and your own feelings of discomfort.
- Consider the need for repair 'I'm sorry but could we pause for a moment? I'm wondering if I may have misunderstood/missed something important?'.
- Respond to the emotion ('NURSE' mnemonic above), allow space for child/family to settle.
- Then return to exploring child/family's agenda.
- The goal is to identify your shared agenda with the child/family (what you are both wanting to achieve) and work from there.

Breaking bad news
Consider whether to discuss with the child/family initially together or separately. The family will usually have a preference. There are sound ethical principles for telling pre-adolescent children the truth, even before the 'mature minor' stage.
Key Steps
1. Check how much the child/family already knows (or understands about what is going on).
2. Find out how much the child/family wants to know (this may or may not be relevant to the situation).
3. Prepare the child/family: give a warning shot e.g. Do you remember the test we discussed? I'm afraid the news is not what we had hoped.
4. Give the news in a stepwise manner to enable you to continuously monitor 1 and 2 and the reaction (5).
5. Allow time for reaction.
6. Allow the child's emotions to be expressed.
7. Be prepared to repeat and clarify.
8. Give a clear plan for the next steps of care.
9. Arrange further contact.

USEFUL RESOURCES

- Jonathan Silverman, Suzanne Kurtz, Juliet Draper. Skills for Communicating with Patients. 3rd Ed. CRC Press, Published September 2013
- University of Cambridge School of Medicine Pack: Clinical and Communicating Skills Theme, Stage 2: Interviewing Children and Parents
- Thinking Ahead Communication Guide www2.health.vic.gov.au/about/publications/policiesandguidelines/thinking-ahead-resources
- Thinking Ahead Framework www2.health.vic.gov.au/about/publications/policiesandguidelines/thinking-ahead-resources

CHAPTER 2
Ethics

Lynn Gillam
Clare Delany

Key Points

- Good ethical practice involves using a clear ethical decision-making framework: identifying possible courses of action, identifying the ethical pros and cons of each (including the benefits and burdens of each option to the child); and comparing options to find the one that offers best overall fit to ethical principles.
- In paediatrics, three key ethical principles are:
  a. Promoting the well being and interests of the child
  b. Appropriate respect for the developing autonomy of the child
  c. Respect for parents' role and moral authority to make decisions for their child
- Considering a child's interests encompasses physical and psychosocial aspects of a child's life, paying attention to the subjective aspects - how life feels to the child.
- It is helpful to recognise standard types of ethically challenging situations in paediatrics: parents refusing medically indicated treatment; parents requesting a medically inappropriate or non-beneficial procedure; a younger child resisting treatment; and an adolescent (possible mature minor) refusing treatment.
- When parents' wishes differ from medical advice, the concept of the Zone of Parental Discretion (ZPD) can help in making a judgement about whether there is sufficient risk of harm to the child that intervention is ethically required.

Introduction

Good ethical practice is one of the cornerstones of good clinical practice. Good ethical practice involves:
- Considering ethically sound approaches to everyday situations, AND
- Using a clear ethical decision-making framework in complex, contested and challenging situations.

Ethical decision-making is guided by principles. Ethical principles reflect the fundamental values that are of ultimate importance in child and adolescent health care. Principles are not rules, which can be applied to all clinical practice according to an algorithm; they are general, need to be interpreted within context and may be in conflict with each other. Ethics is therefore a matter of professional and personal judgement.

Good ethical practice is not always obvious. While some practices are clearly unethical, and others are clearly ethically required, there is also room for reasonable, well-informed, and well-intentioned people to have different views. This chapter aims to give guidance on how to think through ethical aspects of paediatric and adolescent practice. A good ethical decision is one that is reached by a sound, considered process.

What is distinctive about Paediatric ethics?

Several aspects of the paediatric context make it inherently complex in ethical terms.

Paediatric Handbook, Tenth Edition. Edited by Kate Harding, Daniel S. Mason and Daryl Efron.
© 2021 John Wiley & Sons Ltd. Published 2021 by John Wiley & Sons Ltd.

Decision-making

Because the patient is a child, decisions are almost always being made not by the child (patient) but by the parents (or others with decisional authority) in conjunction with clinicians. The ethical weight of parents' wishes and decisions is explained further below (Key ethical principles II. Respect parents as decision-makers and care-givers for their child).

Best interests

The principle of ensuring treatment is in the best interests of a child is also more complex. What counts as best for a child can be viewed differently by parents and the clinicians involved in a child's care. The child, unlike an adult, does not count as the moral authority of their own best interests. In fact it is a defining feature of childhood that children need guidance and protection from adults, because they do not yet have the capacity to clearly identify their own interests, and to see which course of action will best promote these interests.

It is important to note that a child's interests and well-being are strongly intertwined with their parents and family, who in many ways enable the child to have a good life. But they are not *the same as* the interests of their family member's interests.

Ethics and law

Ethics and law do not have the same functions, though both guide practice. Law sets the boundaries — it delineates what is legally permissible or not. Within the category of 'legally permissible' there is still space for clinicians to make decisions about what is ethically appropriate. Law also provides processes for dealing with disagreements with parents about medical treatment or care of the child, for example child protection cases and/or court proceedings to seek a ruling about whether a child should have some form of treatment.

Key ethical principles
I. Promote the well-being and best interests of the child

The key ethical goal in child and adolescent health is to promote the well-being of the child. The phrase 'act in the child's best interests' is often used to reflect this principle. However, this is not as obvious and clear-cut as it might sound. Well-being is an overall term which encompasses physical and psychosocial aspects of a child's life. It is about how life feels to the child as well as their physiological condition.

Questions to ask yourself and colleagues when thinking about whether an intervention would promote a child's well-being:

1. What is life like for this child now? (How does this child *feel?*)
2. What would the child's life be like after the proposed intervention?
3. What would the child's life be like if the intervention wasn't done?
4. Does the difference between numbers 2 and 3 suggest that doing the intervention would promote the child's well-being overall?

Options Benefit Burdens Analysis (OBBA)

To clarify further, think in terms of **benefits** and **burdens** to the child of the proposed intervention. Benefits and burdens include physical, psychological, emotional, and social impacts on the child's life. Remember to also factor in the **probability** that the intended benefits will actually happen, as well as the probability of any expected burdens or known risks, and to also consider the **long-term** as well as **short-term** effects.

The child's best interests

'Interests' is an ethical term which provides another way of thinking about well-being. A child has *multiple* interests, which can *vary independently* from each other. An assessment of 'best interest' involves identifying and evaluating the effect a decision or practice has on all of these interests, and coming to an overall summation. There may not be one obvious 'correct' answer.

Questions to ask when considering what is in the child's best interests:

• What impact would the possible treatment options have on each of the child's interests?
• Might a treatment option make the child better off in relation to some interests, but worse off in relation to others?

- Is the short-term effect different from the long-term effect for any of these interests?
- Is there one treatment option that would produce an outcome that would count as being in the child's best interests overall? Or would different options equally promote the child's interests in different ways?

II. Respect parents as decision-makers and care-givers for their child

Parents have default decision-making authority for their child in both ethics and law. Giving parents information with appropriate explanation about their child's medical condition and management options is a basic ethical requirement. Parents' informed consent should be sought before undertaking any intervention. When there are multiple acceptable options for management (rather than a clear standard of care) it is particularly important to help parents think through the differences between the options, and the pros and cons of each option. This demonstrates respect for parents as decision-makers, and allows them to participate effectively in shared decision-making.

Concern about parents' decisions for their child

When concerned about the decision parents are making for their child ask:
- Are the parents adequately informed? What do they believe/think/understand?
- Have they been given a clear recommendation with the reasons explained?
- What do they think is important for their child?
- Are parents aware of what their child knows and wants? And have they taken this into account?
- What are the other factors which might be influencing their thinking?

The aim is to encourage and assist parents in making a decision that will best promote their child's well-being, and to also be open to the parents' ways of thinking about the situation.

When to go against parents' wishes

Parents' authority in decision-making for their child is not absolute. Parents are acting as proxy decision-makers for their child, and the acceptable scope of their decision-making is limited by considerations of the child's interests and well-being.

The *Zone of Parental Discretion* is an ethical tool (see Figure 2.1) which provides a way of understanding and making decisions about the ethical limits of parental decision-making for children. The Zone of Parental Discretion refers to an ethically and legally protected space in which parents can make decisions for their child, even if those decisions are not optimal in clinicians' eyes. The limit to the zone comes when parents' decisions would cause significant avoidable harm, or put the child at high risk of avoidable harm. When this occurs, the parents' decision should not be acted upon. A decision to go against parents' wishes should be discussed wherever possible with senior colleagues. Advice may be needed about whether there are any legal or procedural steps that need to be taken before acting.

III. Respect the child as a person with developing autonomy
Including the child in the conversation

A child is a person with their own experience of the world, their own desires and wishes, hopes and goals, worries and fear – and their own drive to understand and have some control over what happens to them. It is ethically important to acknowledge the child as a person, and to include them, in an age-appropriate way, in their health care. This means talking directly to them, not just to their parents, giving them the opportunity to ask questions, offering them choices where appropriate, seeking their agreement (technically, their 'assent', as distinction from 'consent') to treatment in an age-appropriate manner.

A child's wishes have some ethical weight, and should be taken into account in decision-making. However, they are not determinative. There is no absolute ethical obligation to act in accord with a child's wishes, just because that is what the child wants. The child's well-being and the parents' wishes are the two primary ethical considerations.

Adolescents and decision-making

While a younger child should clearly not be regarded as the authoritative decision-maker, what about older adolescents? When do they become sufficiently competent (as a 'mature minor') to make their own decisions?

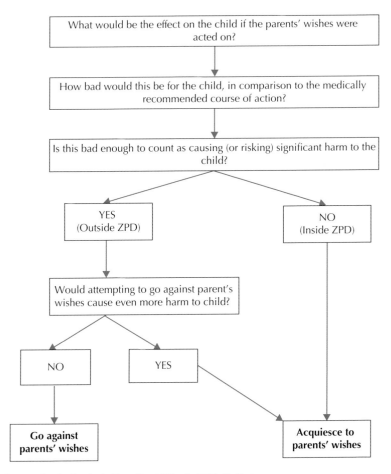

Figure 2.1 Flowchart for using the 'Zone of Parental Discretion' (ZPD) ethical tool.

In ethical terms, competence means having the cognitive and evaluative capacities to be able to identify one's own interests and values, understand information about medical treatment options, and make a decision that accords with those interests and values. Competence is assessed in relation to a particular decision; it is not a global assessment.

Clinical Pearl: Gillick competence
'Gillick-competence' is a legal term, derived from a case in the UK in which the House of Lords ruled that in certain circumstances, children under 16 years of age could consent to medical treatment (specifically to the prescription of contraceptives) without involvement of their parents, and that parents could not veto the treatment. This requires the child to have 'sufficient understanding and intelligence to understand fully what is proposed'.

When does an adolescent become competent?

There are no hard and fast rules about the age at which an adolescent becomes a 'mature minor'. Each situation must be assessed on its own merits, in relation to the particular decision that is being made. The higher the decision related consequences, and/or the more complex the information, the higher the level of understanding that is required for competence. Factors including the patient's level of emotional and psychological development, and their willingness and capacity to engage in the decision-making process should be considered in addition to their age when determining their ability to make independent or semi-independent decisions. Not every 16–18-year-old is equally ready to make decisions, and some 12–14-year-olds may be mature enough to have a fully informed and considered opinion that should be given significant weight.

Clinical Pearl: Assessing adolescent decision making capacity

- Engage the young person in a discussion about their wishes and the decision they are making in a non-judgemental way, seeking to understand their reasons and reasoning.
- Use this to form an assessment of their capacity to understand the relevant information and relate it to their own situation.
- Do this without their parents present, so that you have the best chance of hearing the authentic voice of the young person.
- In situations where the decision related consequences are high, seek a formal assessment from an adolescent psychiatrist.

When does an adolescent's competence really matter?

In most cases, it is not vital to establish whether a patient is competent or not. The adolescent's competence matters ethically if:

- The adolescent does not want to have their parents involved in their treatment (eg they present without their parents).
- The adolescent does not want information about their medical condition or other significant issues shared with their parents.
- The adolescent's view about treatment is different from their parents.
- The adolescent is refusing medically recommended treatment and is at risk of harm without it.

Making ethical decisions

The need to make an ethical decision can be obvious, especially when there is frank disagreement or people are openly expressing concern about what the right thing to do is. On other occasions it can be more subtle, such as a feeling of discomfort or unease with a particular decision. These feelings serve as an indicator that there might be an ethical problem that needs to be addressed. Remember, however, that a gut feeling that something is wrong does not automatically make it wrong. The next step is to ask the question 'what is the ethically appropriate thing to do here?' and work through an ethical decision-making process to answer it (Table 2.1).

Making decisions at end of life

All of the standard ethical principles and decision-making processes apply to end of life decision-making. Due to the context, certain issues and questions come to the forefront, and need particular attention. These include:

- **Withdrawing treatment vs not-initiating treatment.** Ethically speaking, there is no in- principle difference between withdrawing life-sustaining treatment (eg ventilatory support), and not starting it. Both are equally ethically justifiable, based on considerations of benefits and burdens to child relative to other management options.
- **Benefit and harm at end of life.** The standard ethical position in Western medicine is that prolonging life does not necessarily bring benefit – it depends on the quality of the life that is prolonged (how it feels to the child). Attempts to prolong life may cause harm to the child. Some families may hold a very different view. These situations require very careful handling, and great sensitivity. Seek advice from the Palliative Care and Clinical Ethics teams (as available).

Table 2.1 A process for ethical decision-making.

Step in process	Comments / Considerations
1. Identify the options	Questions to ask: • What are the options or pathways forward from here? • What would each one look like for *this* child?

2. Ethically evaluate each option
Using the basic ethical principles
	• What are the implications of this pathway for the child's interests?
	   ○ How does it relate to the parents' goals and values?
	   ○ How does it relate to the child's concerns and wishes?
	
	Use key concepts (Zone of Parental Discretion, interests, benefits and burdens) to help decide which option is ethically best.
	These tools provide a guide to weighing up competing ethical principles.

3. Decide which option best satisfies the relevant ethical principles overall	Bearing in mind that there will probably be no ethically 'perfect' option.

• **Prolonging the child's life for the sake of the parents.** This may be ethically justified, particularly for a short time, to give parents the best chance of healthy grieving (see chapter 34 Palliative Care). However, if this involves distress, suffering, or discomfort for the child it becomes ethically problematic.

Common ethical challenges in child and adolescent health

This typology of common ethical challenges is drawn from the cases referred to the Clinical Ethics Service at RCH, and situations discussed in departmental clinical ethics sessions. Each of these challenges involves some level of conflict, disagreement or uncertainty involving parents, clinicians and sometimes the child patient.

Parental refusal of a medically indicated procedure

Example: Parents of a 10-year-old girl with cerebral palsy, severe intellectual disability, and gross under-nutrition refuse nasogastric or gastrostomy feeding to improve her nutritional status.

Step 1 – Encourage parents to re-think and agree to procedure:
• Talk with parents in non-confrontational way to understand their reasons for refusal.
• Provide any information that parents seem not to have, and explain as clearly as possible:
  a. How the procedure will help the child.
  b. What is involved in doing the procedure, including how discomfort, anxiety, etc will be managed; and
  c. What the child will experience if the procedures is not done.
• Offer some compromise options if available and not medically detrimental – eg a trial of oral intake first.
Step 2 – If parents still don't agree: use Zone of Parental Discretion concept to decide whether intervening in some way to get procedure to happen is ethically justified.
The key questions to ask for the Zone of Parental discretion are:
• What will be the effect on the child if the parents' decision against the procedure is accepted?
• How detrimental would this be for the child, in comparison to having the medically recommended procedure?
• Does this difference equate to 'sub-optimal but not harmful' to the child, or is it bad enough to count as causing (risk of) significant harm to the child?
  ○ If counts as 'sub-optimal but not harmful', go along with parents' refusal, keep them engaged, and keep quietly working towards achieving best possible outcomes for the child over time.
  ○ If counts as risk of significant harm, go against parents' wishes (unless that would have an even worse effect on the child) to undertake the procedure.
Step 3 – *If child is at risk of significant harm:*
• Start with firm but respectful direction to parents.
• Involve senior clinicians to get support for this decision.

- Referral for a clinical ethics consult may be useful, if the timeframe allows.
- Notification to child protection and/or court orders for procedure may be required.

Parental request for medically inappropriate or non-beneficial procedures

Clinicians have no ethical or legal obligation to provide a treatment or undertake a procedure which they believe will not benefit a child, or would do more harm than good, even if parents strongly insist on it. The primary ethical responsibility is toward the child; to not cause burden or risk to the child for no, or disproportionally minimal, benefit. Responsible stewardship of health care resources and public health is also a consideration. On the other hand, in the interests of the child's long-term well-being it is important to maintain a good therapeutic relationship with the parents and maintain their engagement in the child's health care.

Such situations need to be handled with care. There may be unusual situations where doing something to a child just because their parents want it would be ethically justified – but only if the child would not suffer harm, and there were compelling reasons to do something non-beneficial. In general, doing procedures to address parental anxiety is risky, as it is likely to set up or re-inforce a pattern in which parents' anxiety leads to more and more procedures, with increasing risks and burdens to the child.

Example: Parents of a 4-year-old girl, who has been sick with a number of viral illnesses since starting daycare request IV insertion for antibiotics for her illness. Examination shows evidence of another viral infection, and no evidence of bacterial infection.

Step 1 – Talk with parents in a non-confrontational way to understand their reasons for wanting this procedure.
- For example what are they worried about? Is there anything unusual about their child's current situation? Have they had past bad experiences?
- Respond to parents: if you still think the procedure would be non-beneficial or inappropriate, offer reassurance as appropriate, provide any information that parents seem not to have, and explain as clearly as possible (a) why the procedure they want will not help the child, and (b) what downsides (burdens, risks) it will have for their child.

Step 2 – If parents continue to insist on the procedure:
- Respectfully but firmly explain that you will *not* do the procedure.
- Emphasise the care that you *will* provide.
- Advise parents about what to expect next in relation to their child's health, what changes would indicate they should seek further assistance.

Younger child resisting treatment

Example: 10-year-old boy referred by his GP with 2 weeks of fevers, abdominal pain, weight loss, and bloody diarrhoea (mother has Crohns disease). Requires investigations including blood tests, stool samples, imaging, and admission to hospital. He agrees to come into hospital, but adamant that he won't have any tests.

Step 1 – Listen to the child and take them seriously. Try to understand their concerns and reasons.
Step 2 – Address their concerns as far as possible. The goal is that the child's resistance dissipates, and they are able to co-operate with the procedure. All of the following are ethically appropriate responses:
- Explain at child's level of understanding how the procedure will help them, and what will be done to make it as comfortable as possible for them.
- Involve parents in offering reassurance and support.
- Offering to modify the way in which the procedure is done, or who does it, or where are all ethically appropriate, provided that procedure can still achieve its therapeutic goal. *Giving the child choice even over very small matters respects them as a person.*
- Involve nursing and allied health staff who have expertise in helping children cope with procedures, if at all possible.
- Delay, if not medically necessary to do the procedure right now and you think this will help the child.

Step 3 – If the child continues to resist, and will be harmed or suffer detriment to their health without the procedure, holding or restraining may have to be considered.
- It is important to recognise that holding or restraining is an ethically significant matter, which should be done only after an ethical decision-making process, not as a matter of course.
- Involve nursing and allied health staff who have expertise in helping children cope with procedures, if at all possible.
- Use the least restrictive/intrusive method.
- Seek parental consent.
- Offer parents the option to be involved or not.
- Use restraint as a last resort.

Adolescent (possible mature minor) refuses medically recommended treatment

Example 1 – 15-year-old girl with laceration to forearm from bicycle accident refuses suturing.
Example 2 – 16-year-old boy refuses amputation for osteosarcoma.

An older child or adolescent who is opposed to a form of treatment may be competent to make such a decision, but this is not certain, and is not guaranteed by their age alone. See Figure 2.2. Remember that the requirements for competence increase as the consequences associated with the decision increase (see key ethical principles *III. Respect the child as a person with developing autonomy*). It is ethically appropriate to encourage an adolescent to involve their parents in these situations, however this should not take the place of speaking directly with the adolescent about their concerns, or be done solely to pressure the adolescent into agreeing.

It may in the end be ethically necessary to restrain an adolescent to administer life-saving treatment as a last resort. It is important to be aware that no Australian court has supported a young person's refusal of medically

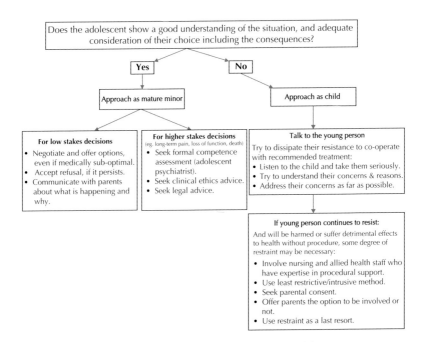

Figure 2.2 Flowchart for decision-making when adolescent is refusing medically recommended treatment.

recommended treatment when there is risk to life, even where the court has found the adolescent to have good understanding of the situation and the consequences of their refusal.

Ethics and conflict

Different opinions about the value and effectiveness of treatment options for a child can result in interpersonal conflict between clinical teams and between clinicians and parents. This can be particularly challenging in relation to withdrawing life-sustaining treatment, or not offering escalation of treatment at the end of life.

When conflict arises, this is always ethically important – it really matters how the conflict is handled. The basic ethical principle in conflict situations is **respect**: *respect for the thoughts and feelings of the other/s involved, recognition of their right to a voice*. Respect for others does not require agreeing with them or doing what they want – but it does require hearing and taking seriously their perspective and concerns.

Not all conflict can be fully resolved, and not everyone can get everything they want. In the end, *the key ethical principle is promoting the well-being of the child, rather than minimising conflict*. However, minimising or addressing conflict is often a necessary part of achieving this.

USEFUL RESOURCES
- *When doctors and parents disagree. Paediatrics, Ethics and the Zone of Parental Discretion (Book).* McDougall, R, Delany, C & Gillam, L 2016 (Eds.). New South Wales: Federation Press.
- *Essential Ethics podcasts RCH* https://www.rch.org.au/podcasts/essential-ethics/; informative podcasts about relevant paediatric ethics.
- The Royal Childrens Hospital childrens bioethics centre website https://www.rch.org.au/bioethics/about_us/About_the_Childrens_Bioethics_Centre/.
- *Clinical ethics in pediatrics: a case-based textbook (Book).* Diekema, Douglas S., Mark R. Mercurio, and Mary B. Adam, eds. Cambridge University Press, 2011.
- 'What Really Is in A Child's Best Interest? Toward A More Precise Picture Of The Interests Of Children' Malek, J (2009), *Journal of Clinical Ethics:* 175–182.
- Caring Decisions: A handbook for parents when making end of life decisions https://www.rch.org.au/uploadedFiles/Main/Content/caringdecisions/130890%20Caring%20Decisions%20book_v1.pdf.

CHAPTER 3

Resuscitation and medical emergencies

Michael Clifford
Tali Gadish
Joanne Grindlay

Key Points

- Regular training, education and simulation in paediatric resuscitation is essential to maintain skills and support best practice.
- Avoidance of the need for CPR by prompt recognition and management of the deteriorating patient prior to cardiopulmonary arrest is best practice.
- In the event of cardiopulmonary arrest, defibrillator pads should be attached as soon as possible and cardiac compressions commenced to 1/3 the depth of the chest. Though less common than in adults, defibrillation should occur immediately if a shockable rhythm is identified.
- Family members must be supported should they choose to remain present during cardiopulmonary arrest and resuscitation.
- Age-appropriate VICTOR charts are used across the state of Victoria to trace observations of paediatric inpatients. If your patient's vital signs are outside the acceptable age-appropriate value, you should follow your hospital's escalation pathway.

Cardiorespiratory arrest

- Cardiorespiratory arrest may occur in a wide variety of conditions that cause hypoxaemia or hypotension, or both.
- In hospital, respiratory arrest alone is more common than cardiorespiratory arrest.
- The initial cardiac rhythm during early resuscitation is most frequently severe bradycardia or asystole.
- Ventricular fibrillation (VF) may occur more frequently with congenital heart conditions or secondary to poisoning with cardioactive drugs.

Recognition and management of deterioration

- Most in-hospital cardiorespiratory arrests are preceded by a period of symptoms and signs suggesting physiologic compensation (e.g. tachypnoea and tachycardia).
- Decompensation with bradycardia and/or respiratory arrest is followed by loss of cardiac output unless prompt resuscitation occurs.
- Considerable focus is now placed on recognising and responding to deterioration *before* decompensation occurs.
- Mechanisms to systemise the recognition and response to clinical deterioration (e.g. VICTOR charts & mandatory escalation of care in response to specified parameters) have resulted in reduced rates of preventable cardiac arrest and are recommended by the International Liason Committee on Resuscitation.
- See https://www.victor.org.au/victor-charts/ for specific information regarding, and examples of, VICTOR charts.

Paediatric Handbook, Tenth Edition. Edited by Kate Harding, Daniel S. Mason and Daryl Efron.
© 2021 John Wiley & Sons Ltd. Published 2021 by John Wiley & Sons Ltd.

Diagnosis and initial management

- Cardiorespiratory arrest should be suspected when the patient becomes unresponsive or unconscious, is not moving or breathing normally or appears pale or cyanosed.
- Call for help immediately.
- Assess airway and respiration by observing movement of the chest, listening and feeling for expired breath while positioning the head and neck to open and maintain the airway. *Movement of the chest without expiration indicates a blocked airway.*
- Unlike adult arrests, airway opening and provision of ventilation is the first priority.
- DO NOT delay resuscitation while feeling for a pulse in the unconscious apnoeic patient.
- Cardiopulmonary resuscitation (CPR) must commence with basic techniques and be continued using advanced techniques (Figure 3.1).
- Start compressions in the presence of severe bradycardia before the pulseless state or if other signs of circulation (adequate ventilation, movement, consciousness) are absent.

Airway maintenance and ventilation

- If airway obstruction is present, quickly inspect the pharynx; clear secretions/vomitus by brief suction under direct vision using a Yankauer sucker.
- Maintain the airway with backward head tilt, chin lift or forward jaw thrust (Photo 3.1).
- *If adequate spontaneous ventilation does not resume:*
  - Ventilate the lungs mechanically for 2 initial breaths with a self-inflating resuscitator (e.g. Laerdal, Ambu, Air-viva) with added oxygen 8–10 L/min, T-piece or a mouth-to-mask technique.
- Select the appropriately sized resuscitator bag
  - Infant up to 2 years – 500 ml bag
  - Child/adult > 2 years – 2 litre bag
- Select an appropriately sized mask.
- Obtain an airtight seal.
- An *oropharyngeal airway* will facilitate maintenance of the airway and bag and mask ventilation.

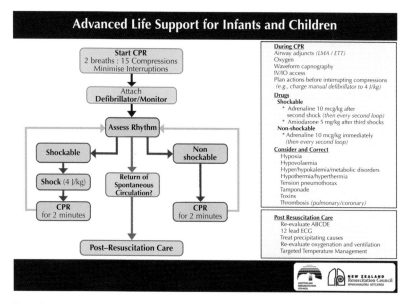

Figure 3.1 Management of cardiorespiratory arrest. *Source*: Australian and New Zealand Committee on Resuscitation. Reproduced with permission from guidelines at https://resus.org.au/guidelines/flowcharts.

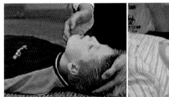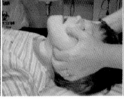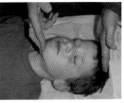

Photo 3.1 Airway opening manoeuvres. From left to right: head tilt, chin lift, jaw thrust. *Source*: Royal Children's Hospital Clinical Practice Guidelines - Resuscitation. Reproduced with permission of the Royal Children's Hospital.

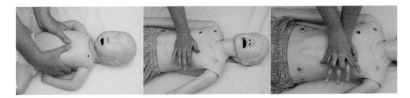

Photo 3.2 External cardiac compression techniques. From left to right: Two thumb technique (newborn / infant), Heel of one hand technique (small child), Two handed technique (larger child). *Source*: Royal Children's Hospital Clinical Practice Guidelines – Resuscitation. Reproduced with permission of the Royal Children's Hospital.

- Whatever technique is used, ensure that ventilation expands the chest adequately.
- Intubate the trachea via the mouth with appropriate endotracheal tube (ETT) size and depth (see below), if there is inadequate ventilation or once adequate help arrives.
- If intubation unsuccessful, continue ventilation via an appropriate rescue method, e.g. laryngeal mask airway (LMA) or ongoing bag and mask ventilation.
- Avoid hypoxaemia by prolonged unsuccessful attempts; *maintenance of ventilation is more important than method of ventilation.*

Endotracheal tube size and position
- Micro-cuffed tube size (internal diameter) = (age/4) + 3.5 mm (for patients > 1 year of age).
- Uncuffed tube size (internal diameter) = (age/4) + 4 mm (for patients > 1 year of age).
- Depth of insertion is approximately (age/2) + 12 cm from the lower lip.
- *For neonatal patients see chapter 27 Neonatal medicine.*
- Secure the tube with cotton tape around the neck or affix it firmly to the face with adhesive tape to avoid endobronchial intubation or accidental extubation.
- Confirm ETT placement by detecting end-tidal CO_2 & visualising on CXR as soon as is practicable.

External cardiac compression
Start external cardiac compressions (ECC) over the lower sternum if:
- There are no signs of life OR
- A pulse is not palpable within 10 seconds OR
- A pulse is less than
  - 60 beats/min (for infants)
  - 40 beats/min (for older children) OR
- Other signs of circulation (adequate ventilation, movement, consciousness) are absent.

Place the patient on a firm surface and depress the lower sternum one-third the depth of the chest whilst avoiding pressure over the ribs and abdominal viscera (Photo 3.2).
- Newborn or an infant (<1 year) – two-thumb technique in which the hands encircle the chest
- Small child (1–8 years) – the heel of one hand
- Larger child (>8 years) and adult – the two-handed technique

Table 3.1 Compression–ventilation ratios for cardiopulmonary resuscitation.

	Give two initial breaths, then	
	One rescuer (expired air resuscitation) Compression:Breaths	Two rescuers (bag–mask ventilation) Compression:Breaths
Newborn infants	3:1	3:1
Infants, Children	30:2	15:2
Adults	30:2	30:2

Source: The Australian Resuscitation Council. Adapted with permission from guidelines at www.resus.org.au/policy/guidelines.

Compression–ventilation rates and ratios
- The rates and ratios recommended for health-care rescuers by the Australian Resuscitation Council (https:// resus.org.au/) are shown (Table 3.1).
- Outside of the neonatal age range use a ratio of 30:2 if a sole rescuer or 15:2 when two rescuers are present.
- When using bag-to-mask ventilation or mouth-to-mask ventilation, the rescuer giving compressions should count aloud to allow the rescuer giving ventilation to deliver effective breaths during pauses between compressions (aim for minimal interruption in compressions).
- If the patient is intubated, DO NOT interrupt compressions.
- The *rate* of compressions should be 100–120/min.
- Aim for an end-tidal CO_2 of >15 mmHg.

Clinical Pearl: Cardiopulmonary resuscitation
Do not interrupt compressions apart from for ventilation if not intubated (as above), or for defibrillation if indicated.

Correct reversible causes
- During cardiopulmonary resuscitation, correct reversible causes
  - Hypoxaemia
  - Hypovolaemia
  - Hypo/hyperthermia
  - Hypo/hyperkalaemia
  - Tamponade
  - Tension pneumothorax
  - Toxins/poisons/drugs
  - Thrombosis

Management of cardiac dysrhythmias
If an automated external defibrillator (AED) is used, follow its instructions.
If not:
- Determine the cardiac rhythm with defibrillator paddles or pads or chest leads, ensuring they are in the correct position.
- Give a single 4 J/kg DC shock if ventricular fibrillation (VF) or pulseless ventricular tachycardia (VT) is present (Figure 3.1).
- Continue CPR for 2 minutes before checking rhythm
- Obtain Intraosseus (IO) access unless IV is available or is obtained in <30 sec
- Give **adrenaline** (epinephrine) if any other pulseless rhythm is present. The dose is:
  - IV and IO: 10 mcg/kg (0.01 mL/kg of 1:1000 solution) or 0.1ml/kg of 1:10000 solution
  - ETT: 100 mcg/kg (0.1 mL/kg of 1:1000 solution)
Other drugs (Table 3.2) include:

Table 3.2 Table of drugs, fluid volume, endotracheal tubes and direct current shock for paediatric resuscitation.

Age	0	2 months	5 months	1 year	2 years	3 years	4 years	5 years	6 years	7 years	8 years	9 years	10 years	11 years	12 years	13 years	14 years
Bodyweight (kg)[a]	3.5	5	7	10	12	14	16	18	20	22	25	28	32	36	40	46	50
Height (cm)[a]	50	58	65	75	85	94	102	109	115	121	127	132	138	144	151	157	162
Adrenaline (epinephrine) 1:1000 (mL)																	
10 mcg/kg	0.035	0.05	0.07	0.10	0.12	0.14	0.16	0.18	0.2	0.22	0.25	0.28	0.32	0.36	0.4	0.46	0.5
100 mcg/kg	0.35	0.5	0.7	1	1.2	1.4	1.6	1.8	2	2.2	2.5	2.8	3.2	3.6	4	4.6	5
Adrenaline (epinephrine) 1:10,000 (mL)																	
10 mcg/kg	0.35	0.5	0.7	1	1.2	1.4	1.6	1.8	2	2.2	2.5	2.8	3.2	3.6	4	4.6	5
100 mcg/kg	3.5	5.0	7.0	10	12	14	16	18	20	22	25	28	32	36	40	46	50
Lidocaine (lignocaine) 1% (mL)																	
1 mg/kg	0.3	0.5	0.7	1.0	1.2	1.4	1.6	1.8	2.0	2.2	2.5	2.8	3.2	3.6	4.0	4.6	5.0
Sodium bicarbonate 8.4% (mL)																	
1 mmol/kg	3.5	5	7	10	12	14	16	18	20	22	25	28	32	36	40	46	50
Fluid volume (mL)																	
10ml/kg	35	50	70	100	120	140	160	180	200	220	250	280	320	360	400	460	500
20 mL/kg	70	100	140	200	240	280	320	360	400	440	500	560	640	720	800	920	1000
Endotracheal tube																	
Uncuffed Size (mm) [Age/4 + 4]	3	3.5	3.5	4	4.5	4.5	5	5	5.5	5.5	6	6	6.5	6.5	7	7	7.5
Cuffed Size (mm) [Age/4 + 3.5]	2.5	3.0	3.0	3.5	4.0	4.0	4.5	4.5	5.0	5.0	5.5	5.5	6.0	6.0	6.5	6.5	7.0
Oral length (cm) [Age/2 + 12]	9.5	11	11.5	12	13	13.5	14	14.5	15	15.5	16	16.5	17	17.5	18	18.5	19
Direct current shock (J) unsynchronised																	
VF, VT 4 J/kg	10	20	30	50	50	50	70	70	70	100	100	100	150	150	150	200	200
Direct current shock (J) synchronised																	
SVT 1 J/kg	3	5	7	10	10	10	20	30	20	20	30	30	30	30	50	50	50

Modified from: Oakley P, Phillips B, Molyneaux E, and Mackway-Jones K. (1993) Paediatric resuscitation. Updated standard reference chart. *British Medical Journal* 1993;306(6892):1613. (Oakley 1993. Reproduced with permission by BMJ.)
[a] 50th percentiles.

Amiodarone
- The only antidysrhythmic shown to be of benefit for VT/VF.
- Dose: 5mg/kg bolus after 3rd shock. Can cause hypotension.

Calcium
- *Only used in dysrhythmia if caused by hypocalcaemia, hyperkalaemia, or calcium channel blocker toxicity.*
- Potentially harmful for asystole, ventricular fibrillation, or electromechanical dissociation.
- IV dose: 10% calcium chloride (0.2 mL/kg) or 10% calcium gluconate (0.7 mL/kg).
- Do not administer calcium via ETT and do not mix it with bicarbonate.
- Consider in trauma with blood products administration > 20 ml/kg.

Adenosine
- Preferred drug treatment for supraventricular tachycardia (SVT – see chapter 15 Cardiology).

Atropine
- For persistent asystole / bradycardia.
- Dose: 20mcg/kg (min 100mcg, max 600mcg).

Lidocaine (lignocaine)
- Second line in VT/VF, where amiodarone not available.
- amiodarone is preferred agent, never give lidocaine (lignocaine) after amiodarone.
- Dose (1mg/kg) (0.1ml/kg of 1%).

Magnesium Sulphate
- For hypomagnesaemia or polymorphic VT (torsade de pointes).
- Dose: 50% solution: 0.05–0.1ml/kg (0.1–0.2mmol/kg) (max 2 g)
  Infuse over 5 mins.

Clinical Pearl: Cardiac dysrhythmias
Sodium bicarbonate, calcium, and doses of adrenaline> 10mcg/kg/dose **have no place in *routine* resuscitation.**

Extracorporeal life support (ECLS)
- Centres with the capacity to provide paediatric cardiopulmonary bypass should consider the role of extracorporeal life support in cardiorespiratory arrest.
- ECLS for refractory cardiac arrest (ECPR) has been associated with increased survival. This is usually reserved for in-hospital arrests (IHA).
- For out of hospital arrests (OHA), a decision whether or not to proceed with ECPR is the responsibility of the ICU consultant who assesses the patient on arrival.
- Considerations determining suitability include:
  1. Immediate bystander CPR
  2. Shockable rhythm on first monitoring (VF or VT)
  3. Effective CPR during transport ($_{ET}CO_2$ >15)
  4. Duration of arrest (arrest to PICU arrival time) <90 minutes
  5. pH >7.0 on arrival in PICU
  6. Pupils reactive or small (NOT fixed and dilated) *or* patient spontaneously moving

Post-resuscitation care
- Ensure adequate ventilation and normocarbia.
- Provide adequate sedation.
- Confirm optimal positioning of the ETT with a supine CXR.
- Maintain adequate blood pressure and perfusion with infusion of fluids and inotropic support as needed.
- Monitor for further arrhythmias.
- Do not actively rewarm; if the child remains unconscious after resuscitation, mild hypothermia has an acceptable safety profile. There is currently no consensus to use therapeutic hypothermia (32–34°C) but after ROSC strict control of temperature must be obtained to avoid hyperthermia (>37.5°C) and severe hypothermia (< 32°C).
- Ensure normoglycaemia.

Parental presence

- Parents or caregivers witnessing their child's resuscitation believe their presence to be beneficial to their child.
- Their presence may allow them the opportunity to say goodbye and be beneficial for their own adjustment and grieving.
- When parents are present, a member of the resuscitation team should be allocated to them to explain the process and ensure they do not interfere with or distract the resuscitation.
- When appropriate, physical contact should be allowed; and wherever possible the parents should be allowed to be with their child during their final moments before death.

Acute upper airway obstruction

- The most common cause is laryngotracheobronchitis (croup).
- Other causes include epiglottitis (see chapter 38 Respiratory medicine), an inhaled foreign body, allergic oedema, and trauma.
- Stridor is the hallmark symptom
  - If accompanied by a barking cough suggests croup
  - If accompanied by dysphagia/drooling suggests epiglottitis
- Severe obstruction stimulates forceful diaphragmatic contraction that results in a retraction of the rib cage, tracheal tug, and abdominal protrusion on inspiration.
- Cyanosis, decreased saturations or irregular respiratory efforts are terminal signs.

Management

- Allow the child to settle quietly in the position the child feels most comfortable.
- Observe closely with minimal interference.
- Treat specific cause (e.g. croup – see chapter 38 Respiratory medicine; anaphylaxis – see below; airway foreign body – see chapter 38 Respiratory medicine).
- Call **PICU** if worsening or severe obstruction occurs.
- Oxygen may be given while awaiting definitive treatment. This can be falsely reassuring (a child with quite severe obstruction may look pink in oxygen).
- Intravenous access should be deferred – upsetting the child can cause increasing obstruction.

Clinical Pearl: Imaging in acute upper airway obstruction

Lateral cervical soft tissue X-rays do not assist in the management of acute upper airway obstruction. In severe airway obstruction, x-rays cause undue delays in definitive treatment and may be dangerous (as positioning may precipitate respiratory arrest).

Anaphylaxis

The life-threatening clinical manifestations of anaphylaxis (see also Chapter 13, Allergy) are:

- Hypotension (due to vasodilatation & increased capillary permeability)
- Bronchospasm
- Upper airways obstruction (due to laryngeal or pharyngeal oedema)

Immediate treatment

See Figure 3.2.

- Vasopressor and bronchodilator therapy:
  - **Adrenaline (epinephrine) 10 mcg/kg IM** (0.01 mg/kg) i.e. 0.01 mL/kg of 1:1000 solution
  - **Adrenaline (epinephrine) 10 mcg/kg IV** (0.01 mg/kg) i.e. 0.1 mL/kg of 1:10,000 solution by slow IV injection over 10 minutes.
  - A continuous **adrenaline (epinephrine) infusion** (0.1–1.0 mcg/kg/min) may be required if manifestations are prolonged.
  - Note: Do not use subcutaneous adrenaline as absorption is less reliable.
- Oxygen by mask

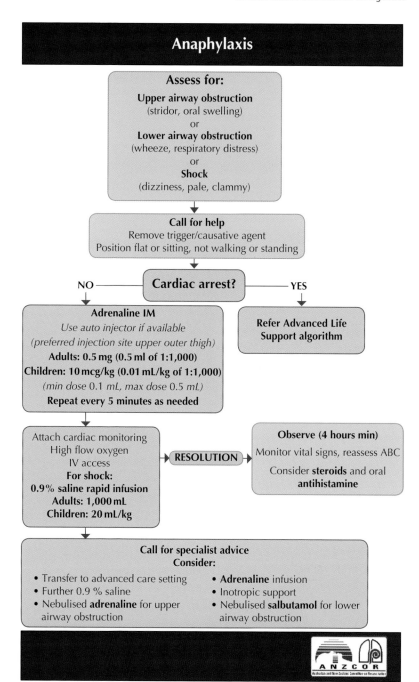

Figure 3.2 Management of anaphylaxis. *Source*: Australian and New Zealand Committee on Resuscitation. Reproduced with permission from guidelines at https://resus.org.au/guidelines/flowcharts.

- IV volume expander:
  - 0.9% saline at 20 mL/kg.
  - Give repeat boluses of 10–20 mL/kg until the blood pressure is restored.
- Bronchodilator therapy with salbutamol:
  - Continuous nebulised (0.5%) or IV 5 mcg/kg/min for 1 hour, then 1 mcg/kg/min thereafter.
- Secondary therapy with aminophylline may be helpful for prolonged bronchospasm.
- Nebulised adrenaline (epinephrine): mild to moderate oedema may respond to inhalation of:
  - Nebulised 1% adrenaline (epinephrine) (1 mL per dose diluted to 4 mL) or 5 mL of nebulised 1:1000 solution.
- **Escalation to endotracheal intubation may be required if persistent upper airway obstruction.**

Ongoing care

- Anaphylaxis can be biphasic, and the patient may deteriorate again over the next few hours, particularly when more than 1 dose of adrenaline in required.
- All children with anaphylaxis should be observed for at least 4 hours in a supervised setting with facilities to manage deterioration.
- Admission for a minimum 12 hour period of observation is recommended if, further treatment is required within 4 hours of last adrenaline administration (biphasic reaction), there is a history of biphasic reaction, there is poorly controlled asthma, or child lives in an isolated location with risk of delayed presentation to emergency services.
- All patients should be provided with a Medi-alert bracelet, an anaphylaxis plan and self-injectable adrenaline, and referred to an allergist for consideration of allergy testing.
- Hospitalised patients with a history of anaphylaxis should have an order/prescription for adrenaline 0.1 ml/kg (10 mcg/kg) IM documented prn.
- Refractory anaphylaxis has been shown to respond to both noradrenaline (norepinephrine) and vasopressin (argipressin) infusions.
- If drug-mediated anaphylaxis is suspected, a mast cell tryptase (serum tube) should be taken ideally between 1 and 4 hours after the reaction (earlier if hymenoptera (bee) sting suspected).

Septicaemic shock

- Hypotension is due to vasodilatation, (early) leakage of fluid from capillary beds and depression of myocardial contractility.
- Collect blood for culture, but do not delay administration of **antibiotics** if a blood sample cannot be collected.
  - Unknown pathogen: give flucloxacillin 50 mg/kg (max 2 g) IV 4 hourly and cefotaxime 50 mg/kg (max 2 g) IV 6 hourly.
  - Meningococcaemia: give cefotaxime 50 mg/kg (max 2 g) IV 6 hourly (benzylpenicillin 60 mg/kg (max 3 g) IV/IM 4 hourly if cefotaxime not available)
  - For specific circumstances / pathogens please consult local antimicrobial guidelines.
- Treat shock with **0.9% saline solution**, 20 mL/kg initially (further boluses of 10–20 mL/kg, up to 40ml/kg, may be needed).
- Give **oxygen** and monitor blood gases.
- Mechanical ventilation may be required.
- Commence **inotropic agent infusion early**; central vein administration is preferable however inotropes may be given peripherally as a dilute solution, e.g.:
  - Adrenaline (epinephrine) 0.01–0.1 mcg/kg/min; strength 0.15 mg/kg in 500 ml
  - Dobutamine 5–20 mcg/kg/min; strength 15 mg/kg in 500 mL; rate 10–40 mL/h
  - Noradrenaline (norepinephrine) 0.01–0.1 mcg/kg/min; strength 0.15 mcg/kg in 500 ml (third line)
- When central access obtained, change to central adrenaline (epinephrine) and noradrenaline (norepinephrine) concentrations (0.15 mg/kg in 50 mL 5% hep/dex at 1–10 mL/h = 0.05–0.5 mcg/kg/min).
- Defer lumbar puncture (if indicated) until the child has been stabilised.

Clinical Controversy: Resuscitation fluid volume

The optimal volume of fluid recommended for resuscitation is unknown. Large volume resuscitation (with the exception of anaphylaxis) is increasingly questioned and should be avoided unless there is evidence of fluid loss e.g. trauma. No isotonic fluid has been shown to be superior to others.

Drowning

- Results in a global hypoxic–ischaemic injury often associated with lung damage from aspiration of water and gastric contents.
- The differences between freshwater and saltwater drowning are not usually clinically important.
- Poor prognostic signs include
  o Immersion time >10 minutes
  o Rectal temperature <30°C
  o Absence of any initial resuscitative efforts
  o Arrival in hospital with CPR requirement or in coma
  o Initial serum pH <7.0

Management

- Adequate oxygenation and ventilation are of paramount importance.
- Mechanical ventilation is required for severe lung involvement, circulatory arrest or loss of consciousness (lung hypoxic–ischaemic injury is compounded by pulmonary oedema and/or aspiration of water or gastric contents).
- Decompress the stomach, which is usually distended with air and water.
- Support the circulation as per *Septicaemic shock* section above:
- Commence **inotropic agent infusion early**; central vein administration is preferable however inotropes may be given peripherally as a dilute solution, e.g.:
  o Adrenaline (epinephrine) 0.01–0.1 mcg/kg/min; strength 0.15 mg/kg in 500 ml
  o Dobutamine 5–20 mcg/kg/min; strength 15 mg/kg in 500 mL; rate 10–40 mL/h
  o Noradrenaline (norepinephrine) 0.01–0.1 mcg/kg/min; strength 0.15 mcg/kg in 500 ml (third line)
- When central access obtained, change to central adrenaline (epinephrine) and noradrenaline (norepinephrine) concentrations (0.15 mg/kg in 50 mL 5% hep/dex at 1–10 mL/h = 0.05–0.5 mcg/kg/min).
- If signs of cerebral oedema are present (i.e. a depressed conscious state), administer mannitol 0.25–0.5 g/kg IV once.
- Correct electrolyte disturbances (hypokalaemia in particular is common).
- Administer benzylpenicillin 60 mg/kg (max 3 g) IV 6 hourly if ventilation is required (to prevent the complication of pneumococcal pneumonia).
- If CPR is required, prevent hyperthermia and induce controlled hypothermia (33–34°C) for 72 hours for cerebral protection.
- Place a cervical collar if a diving injury is suspected. Early MRI will be required.

USEFUL RESOURCES
- Australian Resuscitation Council website https://resus.org.au/; has a wide variety of relevant resuscitation treatment algorithms and guidelines.
- Royal Children's Hospital Clinical Practice Guidelines https://www.rch.org.au/clinicalguide/; wide variety of guidelines including Resuscitation, Airway obstruction, Anaphylaxis, SEPSIS- assessment and management.
- Australasian society of clinical immunology and allergy (ASCIA) website https://allergy.org.au/; has Anaphylaxis information and action plans.
- Australian drug names due to change (April 2020) https://www.tga.gov.au/updating-medicine-ingredient-names-list-affected-ingredients; comprehensive list of updated medication names.

CHAPTER 4

Poisoning and envenomation

James Tibballs
Noel Cranswick

Key Points

- The majority of paediatric poisonings are of low severity, and mortality is unusual. Supportive care is usually sufficient in most cases, however local or national guidelines should always be consulted for management.
In Australia, 24-hour Poisons Information Centre advice is available through their hotline (13 11 26).
- Paracetamol poisoning is by far the most common childhood poisoning in the developed world, and should always be suspected in intentional ingestions.
- Life-threatening envenomation is caused by snakebite, Funnel-web and Red-back spider bites, by Box jellyfish and Irukandji jellyfish stings.
- Prompt provision of antivenom therapy (where available) and of life-support are required to prevent death and minimize morbidity.
- Specific antivenoms are available against Brown snakes, Tiger snakes, Black snakes, Taipans, Death adders and the Beaked sea snake. A polyvalent preparation contains all the above-named antivenoms except the beaked sea snake.

Poisoning

Poisoning during childhood occurs mainly among 1–3 year olds and most often is an ingestion of a substance that was improperly stored in the home. Other circumstances of poisoning are iatrogenic (particularly in infants) and the deliberate self-administration of substances by older children. Self-harm should always be considered, even in young children (see chapter 14 Behaviour and mental health).

Although poisoning in childhood is frequently minor in severity and mortality is low, serious illness may be caused by prescription and over-the-counter drugs as well as non-pharmaceutical products, including complementary medications (see chapter 8 Prescribing and therapeutics). Recovery is expected in the majority of cases if vital functions are preserved and the complications of poisoning and its management are avoided.

Clinical Pearl: Poisoning clinical presentation

Poisoning should always be considered in any child presenting with symptoms that cannot otherwise be explained, such as altered conscious state, fitting, unusual behaviour, hypoventilation, hypotension, and tachy- or bradycardia.

Prevention

- Action should be taken to prevent recurrence.
- Parents should be encouraged to store all medicines in childproof cabinets and toxic substances in places inaccessible to young children.

Paediatric Handbook, Tenth Edition. Edited by Kate Harding, Daniel S. Mason and Daryl Efron.
© 2021 John Wiley & Sons Ltd. Published 2021 by John Wiley & Sons Ltd.

- Urgent psychosocial help should be organised for children who have poisoned themselves intentionally.
- Steps should be taken to ensure that iatrogenic poisoning is not repeated.

General management
In Australia, call Poisons Information on **13 11 26** – a 24-hour nationwide service.

The principles of management for all poisonings are:
- Resuscitate the patient and remove the poison if indicated.
- Administer an antidote if one exists (Table 4.1).

A decision to remove the poison from the body should be dependent on the severity of the poisoning and the likelihood of success in removing the poison without further endangering the patient. Most poisonings in childhood are minor and observation alone or non-invasive treatment is indicated.

The severity of poisoning may be assessed by the:
- Established and expected effects
- Quantity of the poison(s)
- Preparation of the poison
- Interval since exposure

If removal from the body is required, this usually involves gastrointestinal decontamination but occasionally other methods (e.g. dialysis, exchange transfusion, charcoal haemoperfusion, plasmapheresis or haemofiltration) are utilised.

Gastrointestinal decontamination
If the conscious state is depressed, all methods of gastrointestinal decontamination carry a substantial risk of aspiration pneumonitis, even if the patient is intubated. *In the majority of childhood poisonings, activated charcoal administration is not required.* Gastric lavage and whole bowel irrigation having limited roles and there is no role for induced emesis in the hospital setting.

Activated charcoal
Activated charcoal is more efficacious than induced emesis or gastric lavage and is currently regarded as a 'universal antidote'. It adsorbs most poisons but not metals, corrosives or pesticides. Like other techniques, however, it is contraindicated if the patient is not fully conscious or has an ileus. If aspirated, charcoal may cause fatal bronchiolitis obliterans. Constipation is relatively common. The addition of a laxative does decrease transit time through the gut but does not improve efficacy in preventing drug absorption. It may also upset fluid and electrolyte balance. Repeated doses of activated charcoal can enhance elimination of slow-release preparations.

Whole bowel irrigation
Whole bowel irrigation should be limited to specialist involvement in children and may be useful in delayed presentations, the management of poisoning by slow-release drug preparations, and for substances not adsorbed by activated charcoal (e.g. iron).

Not recommended:
Gastric lavage
Gastric lavage has almost no application in the management of the poisoned child. It should only be employed under the direct advice of a toxicologist.

Induced vomiting
Syrup of ipecacuanha is not recommended for hospital use. It does not reliably empty the stomach and is specifically contraindicated where conscious state is impaired or potentially impaired due to the risk of aspiration pneumonitis. It is also contraindicated when the ingested substance is corrosive, a hydrocarbon or petrochemical.

Poisoning with unknown or multiple agents
- Suspect poisoning on presentation with convulsions, depression of the conscious state, hypoventilation, hypotension or an illness that is not otherwise readily explained.
- A urinary drug screen may be useful for diagnosis (but should not delay acute management).
- In all intentional poisonings, suspect the coadministration of paracetamol.

Table 4.1 Antidotes to poisons.

Poison	Antidotes and doses	Comments
Amphetamines	Esmolol 0.5 mg/kg IV over 1 minute, then 25–200 mcg/kg/min IV.	Treatment for tachyarrhythmia.
	Labetalol 0.15–0.3 mg/kg IV or phentolamine 0.05–0.1 mg/kg IV every 10 minutes.	Treatment for hypertension.
Benzodiazepines	Flumazenil 5 mcg/kg IV repeated at 1 minute, then 2–10 mcg/kg/h by IV infusion.	Specific antagonist at receptor. Titrate to effect. Caution: may precipitate convulsions or arrhythmia in multi-drug ingestion, especially with tricyclics.
Beta-blocker	Glucagon 50–150 mcg/kg IV, then 0.20–2.0 mcg/kg/min IV infusion. Isoprenaline 0.05–2 mcg/kg/min IV. Beware of b_2 hypotension. Noradrenaline 0.05–0.5 mcg/kg/min IV.	Stimulates non-catecholamine cAMP production. Preferred antidote.
Calcium blocker	Calcium chloride 20 mg (0.2 mL of 10%) per kg IV.	
Carbon monoxide	Oxygen 100%.	Hyperbaric oxygen may be required.
Cyanide	Hydroxycobalamin (Vit B_{12}) 70 mg/kg IV plus sodium thiosulfate 25% IV 1.65 mL/kg (max 50 mL) at 3–5 mL/min. Sodium nitrite 3% IV (0.33 mL/kg over 4 minutes) then sodium thiosulfate as above.	Chelates. Give 50 mL 50% glucose after each dose. Nitrites form methaemoglobin–cyanide complex (beware excess methaemoglobinaemia – restrict to <20%). Thiosulfate forms non-toxic thiocyanate from methaemoglobin–cyanide.
Digoxin	Digoxin Fab. Dose: acute ingestion 1 vial/2.5 tablet (0.25 mg); in steady state vials = serum digoxin (ng/mL) × BW (kg)/100.	
Ergotamine	Sodium nitroprusside infusion 0.5–5 mcg/kg/min. Heparin 100 units/kg IV, then 10–30 units/kg IV per hour according to clotting.	Treats vasoconstriction. Monitor BP. Treatment of coagulopathy.
Lead	If symptomatic or blood lead >2.9 μmol/L, dimercaprol (BAL) 75 mg/m^2 IM 4-hourly 6 doses, then calcium disodium edetate (EDTA) 1500 mg/m^2 IV over 5 days. If asymptomatic and blood lead 2.18–2.9 μmol/L, infuse calcium disodium edetate 1000 mg/m^2 per day for 5 days.	
Heparin	Protamine 1 mg/100 units heparin IV.	Heparin half-life 1–2 hours.
Iron	Desferrioxamine 15 mg/kg/h 12–24 hours if serum iron >90 μmol/L or >63 μmol/L and symptomatic.	Beware of anaphylaxis.
Methanol, Ethyleneglycol, Glycol ethers	Ethanol; infuse loading dose 10 mL/kg 10% diluted in glucose 5% IV and then 0.15 mL/kg/h to maintain blood concentration at 0.1% (100 mg/dL).	

Table 4.1 (Continued)

Poison	Antidotes and doses	Comments
Methaemoglobin, e.g. secondary to drug treatment	Methylene blue 1–2 mg/kg IV over several minutes.	
Opiates	Naloxone 0.01–0.1 mg/kg IV, then 0.01 mg/kg/h as needed.	
Organophosphates & carbamates	Atropine 20–50 mcg/kg IV every 15 minutes until secretions dry. Pralidoxime 25 mg/kg IV over 15–30 minutes, then 10–20 mg/kg/h for 18 hours or more. Not for carbamates.	Restores cholinesterase.
Paracetamol	N-acetylcysteine. IV: 150 mg/kg over 60 minutes, then 10 mg/kg/h for 20–72 hours. Oral: 140 mg/kg, then 17 doses of 70 mg/kg 4 hourly (total 1330 mg/kg over 68 hours).	Give for >72 hours if still encephalopathic.
Tricyclic antidepressants	Sodium bicarbonate IV 1 mmol/kg to maintain blood pH >7.45.	

Note: Recommended dosages may change – check dosage with local poisons information centre.
Antidotes should be administered in consultation with a toxicologist and/or PICU team at a tertiary centre where possible.

- Contact the Poisons Information hotline for advice (13 11 26).
- Specific constellations of symptoms may suggest a toxidrome (see table) and this may assist in identifying a possible poison and appropriate treatment.

Clinical Pearl: Poisoning & drug concentration
Determine blood concentration in suspected poisoning if there is any possibility of ingestion of paracetamol, iron, salicylate, theophylline, methanol, digoxin or lithium. Blood concentration may influence clinical management in such cases.

Individual poisons
Thousands of poisons exist. The most common serious poisons in young children presenting to the Royal Children's Hospital have been paracetamol, rodenticides, eucalyptus oil, benzodiazepines, tricyclic antidepressants and theophylline. Only the most common serious poisonings or poisonings peculiar to children are considered here briefly. Some have antidotes (Table 4.1), and details of the effects of specific poisons and suggested management should be obtained from a Poisons Information Centre and from appropriate, up-to-date references.

Consider the possibility of intentional drug ingestion. These children are often at 'high risk' for multiple psychological and social reasons.

Paracetamol (acetaminophen)
Paracetamol is the most common pharmaceutical poisoning.
- The liver metabolises it to a toxic product, N-acetyl-p-benzoquinone imine (NAPQI), which causes hepatic necrosis unless neutralised by the hepatic antioxidant, glutathione.
- Multi-organ failure and death may occur after 3–4 days if the ingested quantity exceeds 150–200 mg/kg or with smaller amounts if there is prior hepatic dysfunction or co-ingestion of alcohol or anticonvulsants.
- Most ingestions of paracetamol are initially asymptomatic but early symptoms can include anorexia, nausea and vomiting.

Specific management (Figure 4.1):
- N-acetylcysteine (NAC) is an effective antidote if given before hepatic necrosis occurs.

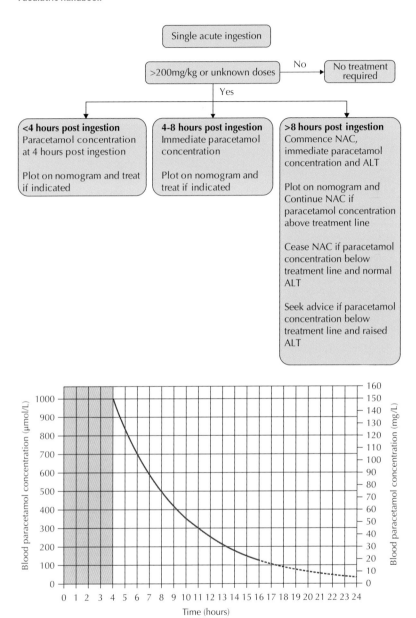

Figure **4.1** Paracetamol overdose treatment algorithm & normogram *Source*: Royal Children's Hospital Clinical Practice Guidelines – Paracetamol poisoning. Reproduced with permission of the Royal Children's Hospital.

- Adverse reactions (e.g. rash, bronchospasm and hypotension) occur more frequently when administered IV.
  - If reactions occur, cease NAC temporarily, administer promethazine and recommence the NAC infusion at a reduced rate.
- Since the outcome is related to serum concentration of paracetamol measured 4–16 hours after ingestion, a decision to administer NAC after a single overdose may be made according to time-related plasma concentrations (see nomogram).
- Local guidelines should be consulted for the dosing of NAC as recommendations change regularly.
- If the ingested dose is extremely large (>30g) or if initial paracetamol concentration is greater than double the nomogram value, gastrointestinal decontamination and specialist referral is required as liver failure can occur despite early administration of NAC.
- These recommendations do not apply to multiple smaller ingestions (see https://www.rch.org.au/clinicalguide/guideline_index/Paracetamol_poisoning/)

Iron

Small quantities (<20 mg/kg) of elemental iron may be toxic. This is usually ingested as iron tablets/capsules, mixtures or multivitamin preparations.

Toxic effects include:

- Immediate: nausea, vomiting, abdominal pain and possible gastric erosion.
- At 6–24 hours: hypotension, hypovolaemia and metabolic acidosis.
- At 12–24 hours: multi-organ failure – gastrointestinal (ileus, gastric erosion), CNS, cardiovascular, hepatic and renal.
- At 4–6 weeks: pyloric stenosis.

Specific management:

- Check serum iron concentration (mcg/dL × 0.1791 = µmol/L), *note*: absorption may be slow.
- Abdominal radiograph may reveal the quantity ingested.
- Consider whole bowel irrigation (not if ileus, obstruction or erosion is present).
  - Activated charcoal is ineffective
- Infusion of desferrioxamine no faster than 15 mg/kg/h for 12–24 hours is indicated if:
  - Patient clinically hypotensive or has depressed consciousness;
  - >60 mg/kg elemental iron has been ingested;
  - Iron concentration is >90 µmol/L; or
  - Iron concentration is >63 µmol/L and patient is symptomatic

Tricyclic antidepressants

Toxic life threatening effects include:

- CNS depression: coma, convulsions
- Non-cardiogenic pulmonary oedema
- Cardiac depression: hypocontractility, hypotension and sudden dysrhythmias (conduction blocks and ventricular ectopy, including tachycardia/fibrillation)
- Sudden death (cardiac arrest) may occur

Specific management:

- ECG monitoring: assess heart rate, QRS duration and QT interval.
- Alkalisation of blood to pH 7.45–7.50 with sodium bicarbonate infusion or hyperventilation, or both.
- Anticonvulsant therapy with diazepam 0.1–0.4 mg/kg (max 10–20 mg) if seizures.
- Antidysrhythmia therapy: give phenytoin slowly (over 30 minutes). Beware of hypotension.
- Treatment of hypotension with an alpha-agonist (noradrenaline 0.01–1 mcg/kg/min). Avoid beta-agonists and drugs with mixed alpha and beta actions.
- Treatment of ventricular tachycardia/fibrillation with DC shock, amiodarone (5 mg/kg IV) and a beta-blocker.
- Treatment of *torsade de pointes* with DC shock, magnesium sulfate (0.1–0.2 mmol/kg IV).

Salicylates

Toxicity is expected if >150 mg/kg is ingested.

Toxic Effects include:

- Coma, hyperpyrexia and respiratory alkalosis followed by metabolic acidosis

- Cardiac depression, pulmonary oedema and hypotension
- Hepatic encephalopathy (Reye syndrome) with chronic use

Specific management:
- Serum salicylate concentration, blood glucose, serum potassium and blood pH.
- Correction of dehydration.
- Correction of acidosis, maintenance of urine pH >7.5 (with sodium bicarbonate) and correction of hypokalaemia.
- Haemodialysis/haemoperfusion if the serum concentration is >25 mmol/L (mcg/mL × 0.0724 = µmol/L).

Eucalyptus and essential oils
Essential oils can be extremely toxic and may cause death even after small volume ingestions.
Toxic effects include:
- Initial: coughing, choking
- Rapid onset (30 minutes, occasionally delayed): CNS depression (convulsions and meiosis are rare).
- Vomiting and subsequent aspiration pneumonitis

Specific management:
- Exclude pneumonitis (perform chest radiograph and measure oxygenation).

Amphetamines and derivatives (e.g. methamphetamine ['Ice'] and 3,4-methylenedioxy methamphetamine ['Ecstasy'])
Toxic effects include:
- CNS stimulation
- Convulsions
- Hyperthermia (with secondary coagulopathy and rhabdomyolysis)
- Hypertension
- Cardiovascular collapse
- Adult respiratory distress syndrome

Treatment is largely supportive and may include sedatives (benzodiazepine), anticonvulsants, beta- and alpha-blockade, dantrolene, mechanical ventilation, inotropic and renal support.

Petroleum distillates
Inhaling the fumes of petrol, kerosene, lighter fluid, lamp oils, solvents and mineral spirits is often referred to as 'chroming' or 'sniffing'. There are significant social and cognitive effects of long-term abuse and these children are at high risk because of multiple psychosocial reasons.
Toxic effects include:
- CNS obtundation
- Convulsions
- Vomiting
- Hepatorenal toxicity

Specific management:
- Exclusion of pneumonitis (perform chest radiograph and measure oxygenation).

Button or disc batteries
- Battery ingestion may not be suspected on history and should be considered in young children with otherwise unexplained gastrointestinal symptoms.
- Ingestion may cause electrolysis, corrosion, the release of toxins or pressure effects.
- Impaction in the oesophagus is an emergency – it may cause perforation or an oesophagotracheal fistula and must be removed endoscopically as soon as possible.
- Surgical follow-up is essential.

Caustic substances
- Automatic machine dishwashing detergents, caustic soda, drain cleaners are strong alkalis and cause burns to the gastrointestinal tract when ingested.
- Significant oesophageal damage may occur in absence of proximal injury.
- Arrange surgical oesophagoscopy and follow-up.

Envenomation
Snakebite
This section applies to bites by Australian snakes of the family *Elapidae* in all States. Snakebites by species in other countries cause different effects and are not outlined in this handbook. Refer to local publications.

In young children, a history of snakebite is often uncertain. Without antivenom or in delayed treatment, envenomation (Table 4.2) culminates in respiratory and cardiovascular failure within several hours, but may be accelerated in a small child or after multiple bites.

Clinical Pearl: Snakebites

Although not all snakes are venomous and snakebite is not always accompanied by envenomation, **every snakebite should be regarded as potentially lethal**.

Of the many species of snakes in Australia, the principal dangerous species are from the genera of
- Brown snakes (*Pseudonaja* spp)
- Tiger snakes (*Notechis* spp)
- Taipans (*Oxyuranus* spp)
- Death adders (*Acanthophis* spp)
- Black snakes (*Pseudechis* spp)
- Copperheads (*Austrelaps* spp)
- Several marine genera

Symptoms and signs of envenomation
The bite site may be identifiable by fang or scratch marks surrounded by bruising or oedema. However, a bite site may be undetectable and the bite occasionally unnoticed by a victim. Clinical manifestations of envenomation include:
- Headache, nausea, vomiting and abdominal pain that may occur within an hour of envenomation.
- Early neurotoxic signs; ptosis, diplopia, blurred vision, facial muscle weakness, dysphonia and dysphagia.
- Advanced neurotoxic signs include weakness of limb, trunk and respiratory muscles.
- Spontaneous haemorrhage may occur from mucous membranes, occasionally into solid organs and from needle puncture sites.
- Hypotension secondary to haemorrhage and respiratory failure.
- Renal failure may occur, secondary to hypotension, haemolysis and rhabdomyolysis, particularly if treatment with antivenom is delayed or of the wrong type.
- Rapid cardiovascular collapse and cardiac arrest may occur which is probably due to pulmonary hypertension associated with thrombotic obstruction of the pulmonary vasculature.

Suspected envenomation
If there is a suspicious history of snakebite but the patient is asymptomatic, close observation should be maintained for approximately 12 hours.

Table 4.2 Common snake bite toxins & clinical manifestation of envenomation.

Venom toxin(s)	Clinical effects	Snake
Neurotoxins	Neuromuscular paralysis; secondary respiratory failure	All
Procoagulants	Consumption of clotting factors; secondary thrombocytopenia, coagulopathy, hemorrhage	Brown snake Tiger snake Taipan
Rhabdomyolysins	Rhabdomyolysis; skeletal muscle destruction & secondary complications	Tiger snake Black snake Taipan

- Test blood coagulation, as it is both a sensitive and reliable indicator of envenomation by major species (except death adders which do not cause serious coagulopathy).
  - Procoagulopathy is caused by Brown and Tiger snakes and by Taipans.
  - Anticoagulation is caused by Black snakes.
- Apply a pressure-immobilisation first-aid bandage (Figure 4.2). It can be removed after ensuring that antivenom is available.
- Perform a venom-detection test (see below). A positive test of a swab from the bite site or of a biological sample (urine or blood) indicates which antivenom to administer, if clinically indicated.

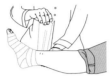

Apply a broad pressure bandage over the bite site as soon as possible. Do not remove clothing, as the movement in doing so will promote the entry of venom into the blood stream. Keep the bitten limb still.

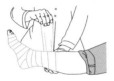

The bandage should be as tight as you would apply to a sprained ankle.

Note: Bandage upwards from the toes or fingers of the bitten limb to help immobilisation. Even though a little venom may be squeezed upwards, the bandage will be far more comfortable than if applied from above downwards; and may be left in place longer.

Extend the bandages as far up the limb as possible.

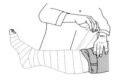

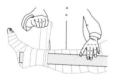

Apply a splint to the leg to immobilise joints on either side of the bite.

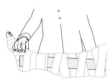

Bind it firmly to as much of the leg as possible. Bring transport to the patients.

Hospital staff:
Please note that first aid measures may usually be removed after availability of antivenom is confirmed. Do not leave on for hours.

Bites on the hand or forearm
1. Bind to elbow with bandages.
2. Use splint to elbow.
3. Use sling.

Figure 4.2 Application of a pressure-immobilisation first-aid bandage.

Definite envenomation

A number of measures may be required, depending on the severity of envenomation (Figure 4.3):

- Resuscitation with mechanical ventilation, oxygen therapy and fluid volume restoration where indicated.
- Application of a pressure-immobilisation first-aid bandage if not already in place. An elasticised bandage is preferred. Do not remove an existing first-aid bandage until antivenom has been administered. Cut a hole in the existing bandage to obtain a bite site swab if needed and then reinforce.
- Perform a venom test of urine (preferred) and blood and of a swab from the bite site.
- Administer antivenom IV (see below).
- Administer coagulation factors (fresh frozen plasma) after antivenom if haemorrhage present. Occasionally blood transfusion is needed.

Antivenom therapy

Specific antivenoms are available against Brown snakes, Tiger snakes, Black snakes, Taipans, Death adders and the Beaked sea snake. A polyvalent preparation contains all the above-named antivenoms except the beaked sea snake. All are given IV.

- Antivenom is required for clinical envenomation or for significant asymptomatic coagulopathy that may result in serious (e.g. intracranial) haemorrhage. A mild coagulopathy *may* resolve spontaneously but requires repeat testing until resolution.
- A course of prednisolone 1 mg/kg orally, daily for 2–5 days may prevent serum sickness, which may occur after polyvalent antivenom or after multiple doses of monovalent antivenom.
- Selection of antivenom should be based on the result of a venom-detection test or on reliable identification of the snake, as there is little cross-reactivity between antivenoms. Do not rely upon the victim's or witness' identification of the snake unless they are an expert.
- If antivenom therapy is required urgently without snake identification, administer antivenom according to location.
  - In Victoria, give both Brown and Tiger snake antivenom.
  - In Tasmania, give Tiger snake antivenom.
  - Outside of these states give polyvalent antivenom.
- Dilute with crystalloid and infuse IV over 30 minutes (faster in life-threatening envenomation).
- The dose of antivenom cannot be predetermined because the amount of venom injected and the patient's susceptibility to it are unknown. Initially administer 2 vials of the appropriate antivenom and then titrate additional doses against the clinical and coagulation status.
- However, be aware that:
  i. Established organ damage cannot be reversed by antivenom and that recovery is time-dependent on supportive treatment.
  ii. Improvement in coagulopathy will lag behind antivenom because endogenous hepatic production of new coagulation factors requires at least 6 hours.
  iii. Additional vials of antivenom may be required in moderate and severe envenomation, but minor envenomation may be treated satisfactorily with one vial.
- Administer antivenom before giving blood or coagulation factors to forestall their consumption.

Clinical Pearl: Antivenom adverse reactions & prophylactic premedication
Acute allergic reactions, including anaphylaxis, occur in approximately 20% of antivenom administrations. Monovalent antivenom is preferred to polyvalent preparations because there is a lower incidence of such reactions. *Always premedicate the patient prior to their first dose of antivenom with SC adrenaline 0.005–0.01 mg/kg to a maximum of 0.25 mg (0.25 mL of 1,1000).* Adrenaline is the only effective preventative treatment for antivenom adverse reactions.

Venom detection kit

The venom detection kit (VDK) is a useful but not totally reliable bedside or laboratory three-step enzyme immunoassay, able to detect venom in urine, blood or from a swab of the bite site in very low concentration.

- It takes about 25 minutes to perform and is highly operator dependent.
- If positive, it indicates which antivenom to administer (if clinically indicated), but not necessarily the species of snake.

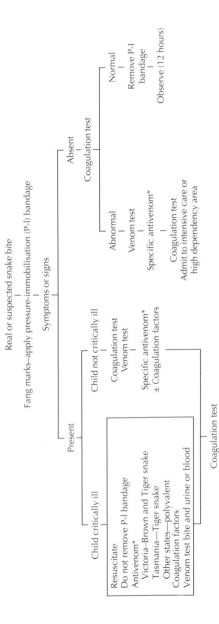

Real or suspected snake bite
|
Fang marks–apply pressure-immobilisation (P-I) bandage
|
Symptoms or signs

Present — Absent

Present:

Child critically ill | Child not critically ill

Child critically ill:
Resuscitate
Do not remove P-I bandage
Antivenom*
  Victoria–Brown and Tiger snake
  Tasmania—Tiger snake
  Other states—polyvalent
Coagulation factors
Venom test bite and urine or blood

Coagulation test

Child not critically ill:
Coagulation test
Venom test
|
Specific antivenom*
± Coagulation factors

Absent:

Coagulation test

Abnormal — Normal

Abnormal:
Venom test
|
Specific antivenom*
|
Coagulation test
Admit to intensive care or
high dependency area

Normal:
Remove P-I
bandage
|
Observe (12 hours)

Titrate specific antivenom* and coagulation factors against clinical state and coagulation
Admit to intensive care or high dependency area

Dangers and mistakes in management:
- Fang marks may not be visible
- Premature removal of P -I bandage may allow sudden systemic envenomation
- Erroneous identification may cause wrong antivenom (premedicate with adrenaline*)
  to be administered. If in doubt give polyvalent
- Delayed onset of paralysis may be missed
- Insufficient antivenom (premedicate with adrenaline*)
- Antivenom without premedication
- Antivenom without clinical or laboratory evidence of envenomation

* Premedicate with adrenaline 0.005–0.01 mg/kg s.c.; i.e. 0.05–0.1 mL/kg of 1:10,000 or 0.005–0.01 mL/kg of 1:1000 adrenaline.

Figure 4.3 Management of snakebite. *Source:* Sutherland SK, Tibballs J. "Australian Animal Toxins" 2nd edition, 2001. Oxford University Press. Reproduced with permission from the authors.

Spider Bites

Numerous species of spiders cause painful bites with only a mild local inflammatory reaction, although the reaction may sometimes be severe. *The bites of only a few species are life-threatening.*

Red-back spider

The venom of this spider (*Latrodectus hasselti*) contains a neurotoxin that causes release of neurotransmitters. Although potentially lethal, the syndrome of envenomation (latrodectism) develops slowly over many hours, and very few deaths have been recorded since an antivenom has been available.

Symptoms and signs include:

- Severe persistent local pain often worsened with movement and referred elsewhere.
- Local erythema, oedema, pruritus, sweating and regional lymphadenopathy.
- Systemic effects; may include distal limb and abdominal pain, hypertension, sweating, vomiting, fever and headache.
- Myalgia, muscle spasms, arthralgia, paraesthesia and weakness may last many weeks.

Management principles:

- Do not use a pressure-immobilisation bandage. The symptom onset is slow and application of a bandage may exacerbate pain.
- Severe local and systemic effects, or prolonged mild effects warrant administration of antivenom IM (occasionally IV). Sometimes several vials are needed. Antivenom has been effective even when administered months after envenomation.
- Although the rate of adverse reactions is low (<0.5%), premedication with promethazine may be used. In all cases, adrenaline should be at hand to treat anaphylaxis (see chapter 3 Resuscitation and Medical emergencies).

Funnel-web spiders

Several large aggressive species of Funnel-web spiders (*Atrax* and *Hadronyche* spp) and Mouse spiders (*Missulena* spp) can threaten life with protein toxins that release neurotransmitters and catecholamines. Several dangerous species exist in NSW and Queensland. In some other states (including Victoria), Funnel-web species exist but are not known to be dangerous. Envenomation does not always accompany a bite.

- Envenomation is indicated by (in approximate sequence):
  - Local muscle fasciculation, piloerection, vomiting, abdominal pain, profuse sweating, salivation and lacrimation;
  - Hypertension tachyarrhythmias and vasoconstriction;
  - The syndrome culminates in coma respiratory failure and terminal hypotension

Management includes:

- Application of pressure-immobilisation bandage.
- Administration of Funnel-web spider antivenom IV.
- Provision of mechanical ventilation, airway protection, atropine and cardiovascular therapy as required.

Jellyfish Stings

Numerous jellyfish stings may cause pain, including that of the Blue-bottle (*Physalia* spp) which may be relieved by immersion in hot water. Only the stings of the Box and 'Irukandji' jellyfish are life-threatening.

Box jellyfish

The Australian Box jellyfish (*Chironex fleckeri*) and related species are the world's most venomous animals. The Box jellyfish has a cuboid body (bell), approximately 30 cm in diameter, numerous trailing tentacles, and inhabits shallow northern Australian coastal waters.

- Stings are most common from October to May, but have been recorded throughout the year.
- Contact with the tentacles leads to the discharge of millions of nematocysts that fire barbs through the epidermis and blood vessels, releasing venom that contain neurotoxins, myotoxins, haemolysins and dermatonecrotic toxins. Severity of envenomation is related to the length of tentacles contacting the skin.
- Prevention is most important; envenomation is prevented by light clothing, unguarded waters must not be entered when these jellyfish are inshore, and beach warning signs should not be ignored.
- Symptoms and signs include severe pain, and possible cardiorespiratory arrest due to direct cardiotoxicity and apnoea due to the neurotoxin effects.

Management:
- Remove the victim from the water to prevent drowning.
- Cardiopulmonary resuscitation as required; immediately on the beach, en route to hospital and extracorporeal life support if indicated.
- Dowse adherent tentacles with vinegar/acetic acid to inactivate undischarged nematocysts (supplies of vinegar are stocked at popular beaches).
- Analgesia: parenteral for extensive stings, cold packs for minor stings.
- Antivenom IV (3 vials for life-threatening signs, 1–2 vials for analgesia or to prevent skin scarring).

'Irukandji' jellyfish

Numerous small jellyfish can cause 'Irukandji' syndrome, typified by the sting of *Carukia barnesi*. This tropical jellyfish has a bell measuring 2 × 2.5 cm and four tentacles – one from each corner, a few trailing up to 75 cm. It is almost transparent and very difficult to see in water. Although the sting is only moderately painful, it may be followed within an hour by:
- Nausea, vomiting, profuse sweating, agitation and muscle cramps.
- Vasoconstriction and severe systemic and pulmonary hypertension (due to catecholamine release). This may cause acute heart failure (Takotsubo cardiomyopathy) and require mechanical ventilation and cardiovascular support.

USEFUL RESOURCES
- Toxinology: http://www.toxinology.com/fusebox.cfm?staticaction=generic_static_files/site_directory.html; clinical toxinology resource from the Women's & Children's Hospital, Adelaide, Australia.
- Australian Venom Research Unit www.avru.org; information, research and resources.
- Images and ecological data on Victorian Snakes www.museumvictoria.com.au/bioinformatics/snake.
- RCH clinical practice guideline for initial management of poisoning https://www.rch.org.au/clinicalguide/guideline_index/Poisoning_-_Acute_Guidelines_For_Initial_Management/; including links to information on poisoning with specific substances.

CHAPTER 5

Procedures

Peter Archer
Leah Hickey
Ruth Armstrong

Key Points

- Procedures can be pain and anxiety free with good planning, parental involvement and procedural pain management and sedation. It is easier to perform any procedure with a calm child and family.
- Ideally, procedures should be carried out in a designated procedure room, with equipment ready before the child enters the room.
- Procedural pain management includes both non-pharmacological techniques such as distraction, presence of a parent, and pharmacological techniques with analgesia and sedation as required. Agents that provide sedation may not provide pain relief.
- Hand hygiene, and aseptic technique are critical to preventing procedure related infection. Universal precautions should be taken during any procedure. Gloves and protective eyewear should be worn and a hard plastic container should be within easy reach for the disposal of sharps.

Venepuncture

Suggested analgesia

- Topical local anaesthetic, for example amethocaine or EMLA (lignocaine (lidocaine), prilocaine), can be used for any age except preterm neonates.
- Sucrose in infants <3 months (max 2 mL, 0.5 mL in infants <1500 g).
- Consider nitrous oxide.
- Consider sedation, for example midazolam oral 0.5 mg/kg (max 15 mg) intranasal/buccal 0.3 mg/kg (max 10 mg).

Equipment

Needle (straight or butterfly), syringe, alcohol wipe, tourniquet, cotton ball, Band-Aid/tape, blood collection tubes.

Sites

- Cubital fossa
- Dorsum of the hand
- Others, as dictated by availability or necessity

Procedure

- In adolescents and older children, blood can be collected with a needle and syringe, as in adults. In infants and small children, a 23 gauge butterfly needle offers more stability.
- Wash the site with an alcohol preparation and allow to dry. Using a tourniquet around the limb, insert the needle into a vein and aspirate gently; once enough blood is collected, release tourniquet and apply local pressure with a cotton ball on the puncture site.
- Some visible veins are too small to be used to take blood. A palpable vein is more likely to be successful than a visible but non-palpable vein.

Paediatric Handbook, Tenth Edition. Edited by Kate Harding, Daniel S. Mason and Daryl Efron.
© 2021 John Wiley & Sons Ltd. Published 2021 by John Wiley & Sons Ltd.

- With small children, an assistant can hold the limb still and provide a tourniquet at the same time.
- An alternative technique is to insert a 21 or 23 gauge needle into a vein and allow the blood to drip out directly into collection tubes. Several millilitres can be collected this way.

Clinical Pearl: Capillary blood sampling
Skin-prick capillary blood sampling is frequently used to minimise the trauma of venipuncture and can be used for a number of point-of-care tests, as well as low volume paediatric biochemistry and haematology samples.

Blood culture collection
- Strict asepsis is required.
- Use alcoholic chlorhexidine or 70% alcohol-based preparations for skin preparation and wait at least 1 minute before taking blood. Do not touch the venepuncture site after skin preparation.
- Most paediatric blood culture bottles require 1–4 mL of blood; take as close to 4 mL as possible for optimal sensitivity.
- Consider anaerobic blood cultures (as well as aerobic) in neonates where there has been prolonged rupture of membranes or maternal chorioamnionitis, poor dentition, severe mucositis, sinusitis, abdominal sepsis, perianal infections, bite wounds or in immunosuppressed children.
- In children with central venous access devices take paired peripheral and central line cultures.
- There is no need to change needles between venepuncture and injecting the blood culture bottles. Inject blood culture bottles first (before dividing blood into other specimen tubes).

Intravenous cannula insertion
See the RCH Peripheral IV access CPG available at www.rch.org.au/clinicalguide/guideline_index/Intravenous_access_Peripheral/

Suggested analgesia
- As for venepuncture above.
- Consider injectable local anaesthetic in older children, for example lignocaine (lidocaine) 1%, applied intra-dermally with a 30G needle.

Equipment
Dressing pack, antiseptic solution, IV cannula, blood collection tubes and syringe if needed, 0.9% saline flush, three-way tap/connection tubing (primed with 0.9% saline), tourniquet, splint, tapes, bandage.
For ultrasound guided insertion, a sterile probe cover and sterile gel is required. A long IV cannula may also be required.

Sites
- Dorsum of the non-dominant hand is preferred, the vein between 4th and 5th metacarpals is most frequently used.
- Alternative sites include the anatomical snuffbox, volar aspect of the forearm, dorsum of the foot, great saphenous vein or cubital fossa.
- The site usually requires splinting and this should be taken into consideration (e.g. foot in a mobile child is less desirable).
- If available ultrasound should be considered when cannulation is predicted to be difficult, or prolonged treatment is anticipated. The cephalic vein in the forearm is the best site.
- Scalp veins should only be used when there are no other possibilities.

Procedure
- Apply tourniquet and look carefully for the best site. Ensure the child is warm, fed if possible and there is adequate light. Consider vein tap and use of gravity to improve vein size.
- Application of a cold trans-illumination light directly to the skin in a darkened room can be helpful in neonates and infants.

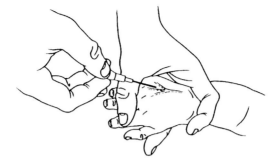

Figure 5.1 Intravenous cannula insertion.

- Decontaminate skin with alcohol 70% chorhexidine 2% and leave to dry for at least 30 seconds. Use a no touch technique.
- If using the back of the hand in infants, grasp the wrist between the index and middle fingers with the thumb over the child's fingers, flexing the wrist. This achieves both immobilisation and tourniquet (Figure 5.1). Use an assistant to immobilize the joint above.
- Insert the cannula just distal to and along the line of the vein at an angle of 10–15°. When a large vein is entered, a 'flash' of blood will enter the hub of the needle.
- Advance the cannula a further 1–2 mm along the line of the vein, then remove the needle while advancing the cannula along the vein. If the cannula is in the vein, blood will flow back out along the cannula.
- Safety IV cannulae have a clip or mechanism which covers the needle tip when the needle is retracted fully from the cannula. It may be necessary to insert the cannula (with needle in situ) slightly further into the vein initially, as the safety mechanism often produces a backward movement as it retracts and may dislodge the cannula.
  - When trying to cannulate a small vein, there may not be a flashback of blood. Insert the cannula and when it is likely to be in the vein, partially remove the needle and watch for blood moving slowly back along the cannula. Advance the cannula along the vein gently. With safety cannulae it is not possible to remove the needle and reinsert.
- Take required blood samples at this stage. In neonates and young infants, blood may be collected by allowing it to drip directly into collection tubes or with a syringe/blunt needle.
- Connect a primed three-way tap/connector and tape the cannula. Place tape over the cannula, then a clear plastic dressing and further tape over the top.
- Secure the plastic hub with sterile tape and a plastic transparent dressing. Ensure that the skin just proximal to the hub always remains visible to allow assessment for inflammation and extravasation.
- Apply padding (cotton wool) under the hub to prevent pressure injury.
- Flush the cannula with 0.9% saline to confirm IV placement. Connect the IV tubing and splint the arm to an appropriately sized board. Wrap the entire length of the board in a bandage.

Clinical Pearl: Intravenous access
- In young children, preparation and planning are important for successful cannulation. This may involve the use of topical analgesia, distraction techniques, the parent to hold / re-assure the child, and the use of assistants to stabilize the limb being cannulated.
- Judicious use of the IV route is encouraged when there are other ways to give fluids, medication and achieve blood sampling.
- Multiple attempts at IV cannulation are traumatic for children and families. It is important if access is predicted to be difficult that more experienced help should be sought.
- Where vascular access is needed immediately, intraosseous access should be obtained.

Intraosseous needle insertion

Indications
For emergency vascular access when efforts to cannulate a vein are unsuccessful.

Suggested analgesia
Performed in emergency situations. Injectable local anaesthetic (lignocaine (lidocaine) 1%) if the child is conscious.

Equipment
Intraosseous needle (if not available, a short large-bore lumbar puncture needle or bone marrow aspiration needle are alternatives), syringe with 0.9% saline flush, three-way tap/connection tubing (primed with 0.9% saline), alcohol wipe, syringe, blood collection tubes.

Alternately, The EZ-IO drill is a powered drill alternative that enables rapid and less painful insertion of the EZ-IO needles, IO needles pink 15 mm (3–39 kg), blue 25 mm (>40 kg), yellow 45 mm (excess tissue), EZ connect tubing, EZ stabilizer dressing.

Sites
Preferred sites of insertion are:
- Proximal tibia (depending on size, 1–3 cm inferomedial to tibial tuberosity)
- Distal femur (approximately 3 cm above the condyles on anterolateral surface) (Figure 5.2)
- Proximal humerus
- Avoid fractured bones and limbs with proximal fractures

Procedure
- Prepare the insertion site.
- Insert the needle at 90° to the skin (Figure 5.2). Apply downward pressure with a rotary motion to advance the needle. When the needle passes through the bony cortex into the marrow cavity, resistance suddenly decreases. The needle should stand without support (except in a very young infant).

EZ-IO insertion
- Attach the EZ-IO needle to the driver and ensure it is securely seated.
- Remove the safety cap.
- Position the driver at the insertion site.
- Push the needle set tip through the skin until the tip rests against the bone ensuring 5 mm of the catheter is visible.

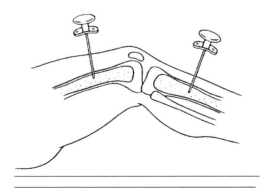

Figure 5.2 Intraosseous needle insertion sites.

- Squeeze the driver's trigger with steady downward pressure to penetrate the bone cortex.
- A sudden give will be felt when the medullary space is entered.
- Stabilise the hub, place stabiliser.
- Remove the stylet and attach primed connector.

Clinical Pearl: IO
- An IO may be first line access if child is in extremists.
- Fluids will need to be pushed e.g. with 50 ml syringe.
- If the head of humerus is used, secure the arm in AD-duction / internal rotation (i.e. on the chest) to prevent damage to the cannula.
- Lignocaine 0.5 mg/kg may reduce the pain of infusion.

Umbilical arterial and venous catheterisation

Normally there are two arteries and one vein which spirals through the umbilical cord. These vessels can be used to provide direct central access in the unwell neonate and may be used up to 10 days old. The umbilical vein can be used in an emergency to provide volume and resuscitation drugs.

Emergency Insertion of UVC
- This is not a sterile procedure. An X-ray is not required before use.
- Short term umbilical venous access is acceptable as a route for resuscitation drugs and fluids.
- Use a 5Fr feeding tube if an umbilical venous catheter is not immediately available.
- Insert the tip 3–5 cm beyond the muco-cutaneous junction (this will be low lying).
- Secure and use immediately.

Umbilical artery catheter (UAC)
Indications
- Acid-base and oxygen monitoring
- Blood sampling for other investigations
- Continuous invasive arterial blood pressure monitoring

Precautions/contraindications
- Peritonitis
- Omphalitis
- Abdominal wall defects (gastroschisis, exomphalos)
- Evidence of local arterial compromise in lower limbs or buttocks area
- Necrotising enterocolitis

Equipment
- Instrument pack: 1 scalpel blade handle, 2 probes: fine and medium, 4 mosquito artery forceps: 2 curved, 2 straight, 2 pair dissecting forceps: toothed, non-toothed, 2 iris forceps
- Sterile field: Surgical mask, Sterile gown and gloves, Sterile plastic drape (transparent is better for visualisation), 2% aqueous chlorhexidine solution as skin prep. (dilute 1:1 with sterile water if infant <750 g).
- Catheter: 1 umbilical artery catheter, 3.5 Fr <1200 g baby, 5 Fr =1200 g baby.
- Other equipment: 1 pair vein scissors, 1 pair suture scissors, 1 needle holder, 2 bowls, cotton wool swabs, gauze swabs, tape measure, 1 scalpel blade no. 11, 1 packet 3/0 black silk suture with a cutting edge needle, 1 cm wide leukoplast for taping of catheter (non sterile, 3-way tap and syringe, 1 x 5 mL syringe and 18G needle, 1 x 10 mL ampoule 0.9% saline, 1 mL ampoule heparin 1000 units/mL (labelled).

Procedure
- **Prepare the Infant:** Place on open heated cot, monitor the infant throughout (oximetry and cardiorespiratory), use appropriate measures to relieve distress which may include oral sucrose, containing the infant by holding, ensuring all four limbs are gently restrained throughout the procedure, avoiding clamping or suturing the skin.

- **Identification of the umbilical artery:** Small, round and white, thick walled, lumen often pinpoint due to muscle constriction, stands proud (protrudes) from the cut surface.
- **Strict sterile technique throughout the procedure**
- **Prepare the catheters:** Calculate UAC insertion length (cm)
  [weight (kg) x 3] + 9cm + umbilical stump length (cm)
  or
  Distance from umbilicus to shoulder tip (cm) + umbilical stump length (cm)
  ○ Attach to the 3-way tap
  ○ Prime the line with **heparinised** saline
  ○ Leave the syringe attached to the 3-way tap throughout the procedure
  ○ The 3-way tap should be closed at the remaining port
  ○ All catheters and their 3-way tap connections must be filled with fluid prior to insertion to prevent air embolism from flushing the catheters in situ prior to aspiration of blood.
- **Prepare the umbilicus**
  ○ Cleanse the umbilical stump and surrounding 3–4 cm of abdomen with the chlorhexidine-based solution
  ○ Wait two minutes to allow to dry
  ○ Drape around the umbilical stump with sterile towels and/or the plastic drape with a fenestration (approx. 3 cm diameter)
  ○ Tie a short piece of umbilical tape around the base of the cord to maintain haemostasis – not too tight to prevent passage of the catheter(s)
  ○ Grasp the cord clamp with the straight forceps and pass the forceps to an assistant. Whilst the assistant applies gentle upward traction, slice the cord horizontally with the straight blade scalpel, 1–1.5 cm from the skin margin – avoid a tangential slice
  ○ Blot the cut surface and identify the umbilical vessels
  ○ Immobilize the cord by grasping the Wharton jelly at the cord edges with two artery forceps at 3 and 9 o'clock, taking care not to include the vessels
- **Catheterisation:** Gently dilate, then probe the orifice of an artery prior to inserting the catheter:
  ○ Initially insert one tip of the iris forceps, then both tips, allowing them to spring apart.
  ○ The tips should be gradually advanced to the curve of the forceps.
  ○ Then insert the straight probe using its weight to further dilate the artery prior to cannulation.
  ○ Gently introduce the primed catheter into the artery, advancing steadily with gentle pressure. Take care not to force.
  ○ Obstruction may be encountered at the anterior abdominal wall or bladder. This is usually overcome by 30–60 seconds of gentle, steady pressure.
  ○ Advance the catheter the desired length.
  ○ Make sure that blood can be freely aspirated and check for 'pulsation' of blood/saline in the catheter.
- **Securing the UAC:** Secure catheter with 3/0 black silk suture by placing a purse string suture at the base of the umbilical cord through the Wharton jelly:
  ○ Commence the suture close to the catheter. Take care not to pierce the catheter
  ○ Take several small 'bites' around the base of the cord and tighten. Do not include skin.
  ○ Knot the purse string securely at the base of the catheter
  ○ Tie the secured suture around the catheter tightly
  ○ Strap with goal post strapping
- Label the UAC and UVC clearly
- Connect the catheter to the infusion fluid (heparinised saline) but do not run until tip position has been confirmed.
  ○ The correct final position of the UAC tip is above the level of T10 in the descending aorta, away from the origin of mesenteric and renal arteries (avoids occlusion).
  ○ Obtain a chest/abdominal X-ray *prior* to use.
  ○ **On X-ray:** Aims caudally prior to ascending via the left or right internal iliac artery into the descending aorta.
- Check for arterial waveform on arterial transducer after it is connected and calibrated

---

Clinical Pearl: Difficulties with UAC insertion
- If unsuccessful, seek advice from a more experienced clinician.
- The most common error inserting a UAC arises after cannulating the layer between the vascular intima and the muscle (usually occurs if dilatation has been inadequate).
- Correcting tip position
  - Too high (in brachiocephalic arteries): pull back by an appropriate amount and repeat X-ray.
  - Too low (at the origin of mesenteric and renal arteries or within pelvic arteries): insert a new catheter to avoid contamination (may use the other artery).

Umbilical vein catheter (UVC)
Indications
- Preferred venous access route in infants weighing <800 g
- Rapid intravenous access during resuscitation (see below)
- Need for exchange transfusion (tertiary neonatal setting only)

Precautions/contraindications
- Peritonitis
- Omphalitis
- Abdominal wall defects (gastroschisis, exomphalos)
- Portal venous hypertension
- Relative caution in necrotising enterocolitis

Equipment
- **Instrument pack:** 1 scalpel blade handle, 2 probes: fine and medium, 4 mosquito artery forceps: 2 curved, 2 straight, 2 pair dissecting forceps: toothed, non-toothed, 2 iris forceps, 1 pair vein scissors, 1 pair suture scissors, 1 needle holder, 2 bowls, cotton wool swabs, gauze swabs, tape measure
- **Sterile field:** Surgical mask, Sterile gown and gloves, Sterile plastic drape (transparent is better for visualisation), 2 per cent aqueous chlorhexidine solution as skin prep. (dilute 1:1 with sterile water if infant <750 g)
- **Catheter:** single lumen catheter can be inserted for short-term use, 3.5 Fr <1500 g, 5.0 Fr >1500 g, 8.0 Fr >3500 g. In an emergency (or if umbilical lines are unavailable) use a feeding tube (size 5)
- **Other Equipment:** 1 scalpel blade no. 11, 1 packet 3/0 black silk suture with a cutting edge needle, 1 cm wide leukoplast for taping of catheter (non sterile), 3-way taps and syringes with NaCl 0.9% flush for each lumen

Procedure
- **Prepare the Infant:** Place on open heated cot, monitor the infant throughout (oximetry and cardiorespiratory), use appropriate measures to relieve distress which may include oral sucrose, containing the infant by holding, ensuring all four limbs are gently restrained throughout the procedure, avoiding clamping or suturing the skin.
- **Identification of the umbilical vein:** Large, thin walled, patulous/gaping lumen, 12 o'clock position at base of umbilical stump.
- **Strict sterile technique throughout the procedure**
- **Prepare the catheters:** Calculate UVC insertion length (cm): Distance between umbilicus to xiphisternum (cm) + umbilical stump length (cm).
  - Attach all lumens to a 3-way tap
  - Prime all lumens via their 3-way tap with 0.9% saline
  - Leave the syringes attached to the 3-way taps throughout the procedure
  - The 3-way taps should be closed to the atmosphere
  - Note: Air embolism is a particular risk in UVC insertion where negative pressure from deep inspiration by the infant, may draw air into the catheter.
  - All catheters and their 3-way tap connections must be filled with fluid prior to insertion to prevent air embolism from flushing the catheters in situ prior to aspiration of blood.

- **Prepare the umbilicus**
  - Cleanse the umbilical stump and surrounding 3–4 cm of abdomen with the chlorhexidine based solution.
  - Wait two minutes to allow to dry.
  - Drape around the umbilical stump with sterile towels and/or the plastic drape with a fenestration (approx. 3 cm diameter).
  - Tie a short piece of umbilical tape around the base of the cord to maintain haemostasis – not too tight to prevent passage of the catheter(s).
  - Grasp the cord clamp with the straight forceps and pass the forceps to an assistant. Whilst the assistant applies gentle upward traction, slice the cord horizontally with the straight blade scalpel, 1–1.5 cm from the skin margin – avoid a tangential slice.
  - Blot the cut surface and identify the umbilical vessels.
  - Immobilize the cord by grasping the Wharton jelly at the cord edges with two artery forceps at 3 and 9 o'clock, taking care not to include the vessels.
- **Catheterisation** Gently and repeatedly dilate the vein (this may not be necessary if the lumen is gaping):
  - Insert the tips of the iris forceps into the lumen of the vein.
  - Allow the forceps tips to spring apart.
  - Remove any visible clot where possible to prevent dislodgement into the circulation.
  - Gently introduce the primed catheter into the vein, advancing cautiously in a cephalad direction. Take care not to force a false passage.
  - Resistance at the level of entry into the body may be overcome by gentle, steady pressure or by pulling the cord gently caudally in the midline.
  - Advance the catheter the desired length.
  - Make sure that blood can be freely aspirated, collect specimens at this stage, then flush the catheter gently.
- **Securing the UVC:** Secure catheter with 3/0 black silk suture by placing a purse string suture at the base of the umbilical cord through the Wharton jelly:
  - Commence the suture close to the catheter. Take care not to pierce the catheter
  - Take several small 'bites' around the base of the cord and tighten. Do not include skin.
  - Knot the purse string securely at the base of the catheter
  - Tie the secured suture around the catheter tightly
  - Strap with goal post strapping
- Label the UAC and UVC clearly
- Connect the catheter to the infusion fluid (maintenance fluid / intravenous nutrition / IV medications) but do not run until tip position has been confirmed.
  - A UVC may sit 'high' or 'low'. The ideal position of the UVC tip is at T8–9 just above the right diaphragm and not within the right atrium. Placement of the catheter tip in the portal circulation is not acceptable
  - Obtain a chest/abdominal X-ray *prior* to use unless using a 'short' UVC in an emergency.
  - **On X-ray:** Aims cephalad via the ductus venosus into the inferior vena cava.

Clinical Pearl: Difficulties with UVC insertion
- If unsuccessful, seek advice from a more experienced clinician
- The most common error inserting a UVC is the creation of a false passage within the Wharton jelly
- Correcting tip position
  - Too high (inside right atrium): pull back by an appropriate amount and repeat X-ray
  - Too low (below the diaphragm, within the hepatic contour): insert a new catheter to avoid contamination **or** partly withdraw the catheter to the safe 'short' position (inserted 3 to 5 cm + stump length, where it will be below the liver.

Post procedure care for umbilical catheters
- Maintain infant supine or in lateral position for 24 hours post procedure to observe for haemorrhage from umbilical stump.

- For UAC: Observe for complications: Note blanching or bruising of limbs, toes or buttocks prior to, during and following the procedure, and at any time that catheter is in situ. If one limb is involved; warm opposite limb to induce reflex vasodilation of affected limb.
  - If these measures fail, the catheter may be withdrawn 0.5–1 cm and observe, remove catheter if blanching persists >30 minutes.
- For UVC: Check infusion solution is correct and prepared to the stage where it can immediately run into the catheter. Start infusion once correct placement is confirmed.

Complications
- Infection, prophylactic antibiotics not required.
- Bleeding
  - UAC: vascular perforation of the umbilical arteries, haematoma formation and retrograde arterial bleeding.
  - UVC: disconnection of tubing.
- Vascular
  - UAC: arterial occlusion/thrombosis (Femoral artery: limb ischaemia, gangrene, Renal artery: hypertension, haematuria, renal failure, Mesenteric artery: gut ischaemia, necrotising enterocolitis); Embolism (blood clot or air in the infusion system); Vasospasm (Femoral artery).
  - UVC: thrombosis, embolism.
- Perforation, never cut the rounded end of any indwelling catheter.
- UVC malpositioning, effects include cardiac arrhythmias, hepatic necrosis, portal hypertension.

Removal of umbilical catheters
Removal is performed by medical staff or experienced nursing staff
- Turn infusion pump off and clamp infusion line
- Clean the stump with an alcohol swab
- Remove sutures with a sterile stitch cutter
- Keep the infant in supine position during removal of the catheter and for the immediate 4 hours after removal
- Leave the abdomen visible for inspection, not covering the umbilicus with a nappy or dressing, so that inadvertent bleeding from the umbilicus does not go unnoticed
- Send the tips for culture only if infection is suspected
- Withdraw UAC to within 3–4 cm of skin.
  - Tape the catheter to skin
  - Wait for pulsation in catheter to stop (usually 10–20 minutes)
  - Remove rest of catheter
  - If bleeding occurs, press firmly just below the umbilicus
- Withdraw UVC gradually in a single action
  - If bleeding occurs, press firmly just above the umbilicus

Accessing central venous catheters
Types
- Catheter devices, for example Hickman or Broviac catheters, are central venous access devices that are tunneled subcutaneously before they enter a central vein. They may be either single or double lumen. The external part of the line has a clamp and a connector which is accessed.
- Infusaports are central venous access devices that have a small chamber attached to the intravenous cannula. This chamber is placed completely under the skin, so no part is exposed. The chamber can be accessed through the skin.

Suggested analgesia
- Topical local anaesthetic, for example amethocaine or EMLA (lignocaine (lidocaine), prilocaine), for Infusaport access.
- Consider sedation and nitrous oxide in children >2 years.
- A procedural pain management plan should be developed for all children with a central venous access device.

Equipment

Sterile gloves, dressing pack, alcohol-based chlorhexidine, Huber point needle (90° bend) for Infusaport, short three-way tap or minimum volume extension tubing, giving set, sterile adhesive strips, syringe with sterile 0.9% saline flush, additional syringes/blood collection tubes, gauze, two occlusive clear plastic dressings.

Procedure

Generic (Hickman, Broviac, Infusaport)

- Strict asepsis is required.
- Central venous access devices are flushed with heparin-containing solutions when not in use.
- For short-term disconnection use 50 units heparin per 5 mL 0.9% saline.
- For long-term disconnection (e.g. on discharge) use 1000 units heparin per 1 mL 0.9% saline ×1 mL diluted to 10 mL with 0.9% saline (i.e. 100 units heparin/1 mL final concentration).
- For both types of flush use 4–5 mL volume. Stop backflow immediately by clamping catheter devices and in Infusaports by turning tap to off (short-term flush) or removing needle (long-term flush).
- Catheter devices require weekly flushing; Infusaports require monthly flushing.
- Catheter devices require dressing changes weekly. The exit site is washed with antiseptic solution (applied radially from centre outwards) and the tubing is also washed. The solution is allowed to dry, then two clear adhesive dressings are used to 'sandwich' the tubing. The distal tubing is then taped to the child's chest wall and the remainder safety-pinned to clothing to avoid pulling on the line. In younger children tape the clamp and tap to avoid little fingers exploring.

Infusaport specific

- Wash the site with antiseptic preparation and allow it to dry.
- Attach Huber point needle to minimum volume extension tubing connected to a three-way tap and prime the line with 0.9% saline.
- Insert Huber point needle into the centre of the port chamber. Aspirate 5 mL of blood back through three-way tap (may be used for blood cultures), then take other bloods using a second syringe as required. Ensure tap is turned to 45° to avoid backflow when connecting/disconnecting syringes. Flush line with 5 mL 0.9% saline.
- Make a pillow of gauze under the Huber point needle and secure with sterile adhesive strips; then apply airtight adhesive clear plastic dressing.
- Remove the stylet and attach a syringe; aspirate to confirm that the needle is in the bone marrow (this is not always possible). Flush the needle with saline to confirm correct placement and connect IV tubing. Often fluids will not flow by gravity into the marrow – a three-way tap and syringe or pressure infusion may be needed.
- Watch the infusion site for fluid extravasation, or the calf becoming tense. A pair of artery forceps clamped around the base then taped along the limb (with appropriate padding underneath) can provide stability. The needle should be removed once IV access has been obtained.
- Any fluid or drug that can be given IV can be administered through the intraosseous route.

Suprapubic aspiration

See the RCH Suprapubic aspirate CPG available at www.rch.org.au.clinicalguide.guideline_index.Suprapubic_aspirate.

Indications

Sterile urine collection for suspected urinary tract infection (UTI) as part of septic workup. This is most successfully performed by confirming urine in the bladder with a bedside ultrasound.

Note: Not recommended in age >24 months (unless the bladder is palpable or percussible).

Suggested analgesia

Topical local anaesthetic. Sucrose if <3 months of age

Equipment

- Alcohol wipe, 23 gauge needle and 2 or 5 mL syringe, cotton ball, adhesive tape, sterile urine collection pot.
- Bladder ultrasound increases the success of the procedure.

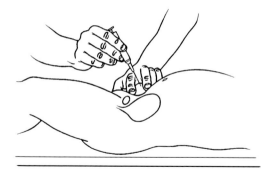

Figure 5.3 Suprapubic aspiration.

Site
Midline in the skin crease above the symphysis pubis

Procedure
- If multiple procedures are planned, aim to perform the Suprapubic aspiration (SPA) first as the child may void whilst having a venepuncture or lumbar puncture.
- Give fluids and wait at least 30 minutes after the last void, or if bladder appears empty on ultrasound.
- Use ultrasound if possible; attempt SPA only if >20 mL urine present, or bladder size is visualised to be >3cm in the transverse axis.
- Position the child with legs either straight or bent in the frog-leg position. Have a sterile bottle handy for a midstream clean catch in case the child voids.
- Prepare the skin with an alcohol wipe. Insert a 23 gauge needle attached to a 2 or 5 mL syringe perpendicular to the abdominal wall (Figure 5.3). Pass almost to the depth of the needle and then aspirate while withdrawing. If urine is not obtained, do not remove the needle completely. Change the angle of the needle and insert it again, first angling superiorly and then inferiorly.
- In the event of obtaining no urine, either: (1) perform urethral catheterisation; or (2) wait 30 minutes, giving the child a drink during this time. Repeat the SPA. It is a good idea to put a urine bag on to determine if the child has voided before proceeding with a further SPA.

Clinical Pearl: Suprapubic aspiration
- Never undo the nappy until you have an open urine jar and someone ready to catch urine.
- The anterior bladder wall may collapse completely against the posterior bladder wall during slow needle insertion, in this event urine may only be aspirated during withdrawal of the needle.

Urethral catheterisation
Indications
- Suspected UTI where midstream specimen is not possible
- Acute urinary retention

Suggested analgesia
- Local anaesthetic topical gel (e.g. lignocaine (lidocaine) 2% gel) – takes 10 minutes for full effect
- Consider nitrous oxide. Sucrose if <3 months of age

Equipment
- Sterile drapes and gloves, water-based antiseptic solution, catheter, catheter bag, sterile urine collection pot, and bowl/kidney dish (to hold urine) tapes to secure and syringe with sterile water for balloon (if indwelling catheter).

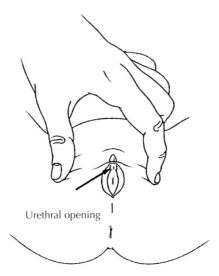

Figure 5.4 Urethral orifice in girls.

- For diagnostic catheterisation, use a 5 FG feeding tube (depending on age). For indwelling catheters, use a silastic catheter with an inflatable balloon. Appropriate sizes are: 0–6 months 6 FG, 2 years 8 FG, 5 years 10 FG, 6–12 years 12 FG; this may vary with the size of the child. Lubricants or xylocaine gel syringe will aid insertion.

Procedure
- The child lies with legs apart in the frog-leg position. Prepare and drape the area, apply local anaesthetic gel and wait.
- Using a sterile technique, locate the urethral orifice. In girls, see Figure 5.4. In boys the foreskin need not be retracted for successful catheterisation. Gently advance the catheter posteriorly until urine is obtained.
- For indwelling catheters: inflate balloon only when urine has been obtained, attach catheter to collection device and tape catheter securely to leg.

Clinical Pearl: Catheterisation
- In girls, urethral visualisation is assisted by gentle cleaning with a downward motion from pubis to introitus.
- In boys, avoid urethral injury by not forcing a catheter against resistance, when the sphincter is first reached await relaxation before passing, ask the child to take a deep breath and try to pass urine. Consider a second tube of lubricant before trying reinsertion.

Lumbar puncture
See the RCH Lumbar Puncture CPG available at www.rch.org.au/clinicalguide/guideline_ index/Lumbar Puncture Guideline/

Indications
- A febrile, sick infant or child with no focus of infection
- Fever with meningism
- Prolonged seizure with fever

Contraindications

- Coma, i.e. reduced conscious state and absent or non-purposeful responses to painful stimuli. Elicit by squeezing the earlobe hard for up to 1 minute. Children should localise response and seek a parent. If in doubt, do not proceed with lumbar puncture.
- Focal neurological signs
- Focal seizures, recent seizures (within 30 minutes) or prolonged seizures (>30 minutes)
- Signs of raised intracranial pressure (ICP): altered pupil responses, decerebrate or decorticate posturing, papilloedema (unreliable and late sign in meningitis)
- Cardiovascular compromise/shock
- Respiratory compromise
- Thrombocytopenia/coagulopathy
- Local superficial infection
- Strong suspicion of meningococcal infection (typical purpuric rash in ill child)

Note:
- Drowsiness, irritability, vomiting and isolated tonic–clonic, myoclonic, absence or atonic seizures are not in themselves contraindications.
- A bulging fontanelle in the absence of other signs of raised ICP is not a contraindication.

Suggested analgesia
Topical local anaesthetic plus:
- Sucrose in infants <3 months of age.
- Injectable local anaesthetic (lignocaine (lidocaine) 1%).
- Consider nitrous oxide.
- Consider sedatives (e.g. nitrous oxide, midazolam) with appropriate monitoring, although this may complicate assessment of conscious state.

Equipment
- Sterile drapes, gown, mask and gloves, antiseptic solution, sterile dressing pack, specimen collection tubes, cotton ball, band-aid/adhesive dressing.
- A lumbar puncture needle with introducing stylet should be used. A 22 or 25G needle is usually appropriate.
  The correct needle length is:
  o 20 mm for preterm infants
  o 30 mm for <2 years old
  o 40 mm for 2–5 year olds
  o 50 mm for 5–12 year olds
  o 60 mm for older children
  o Longer needles may be required in large adolescents

Insertion site
- The iliac crests are at the level of L3–L4. Use this space or the space below (Figure 5.5).
- At birth the conus medullaris finishes near L3, but in adults it finishes at L1–L2.

Procedure
- Using a strict aseptic technique, cleanse the skin and drape the child.
- Positioning of the child is crucial, and an assistant is needed. Restrain the child in the lateral position on the edge of a flat surface. A line drawn between the iliac crests should be perpendicular to the table surface. Maximally flex the spine without compromising the airway. In small babies, flex from the shoulders only; neck flexion can cause airway obstruction. Alternatively, the child can be held in the sitting position with the trunk flexed.
- Anaesthetise the area (with injectable lignocaine 1%) until the proximity of the dura (i.e. about two-thirds the length of the appropriate lumbar puncture needle).
- Grasp the spinal needle with the bevel facing upwards. With the needle perpendicular to the back, insert it through the skin between the spinous processes slowly, aiming towards the umbilicus (i.e. slightly cephalad).

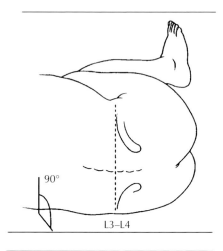

Figure 5.5 Position for lumbar puncture.

Continue advancing the needle until there is decreased resistance (having traversed ligamentum flavum), or the needle has been inserted half its length. Remove the stylet and advance the needle about 1 mm.
- Wait at least 30 seconds for CSF to appear in the hub. Rotation of the needle 90–180° may allow CSF to flow. Advance 1 mm at a time if no CSF has appeared. If no CSF is obtained when bone is contacted or the needle is fully inserted, withdraw the needle very slowly until CSF flows, or the needle is almost removed. Reinsert the stylet, recheck the child's position and needle orientation, and repeat the procedure.
- Collect 0.5–1 mL of CSF (10–20 drops) in each of two tubes, for microbiological and biochemical analysis. Remove the lumbar puncture needle swiftly. Press on the puncture site with a cotton ball for about 30 seconds. Cover with a light dressing.

Clinical Pearl: Lumbar puncture
- Movement is common in infants and young children. Insert the needle through skin in the marked midline interspinous position and wait until this settles.
- Maintain an awareness of midline with a finger of non dominant hand either side of spinous processes at L3–L4.
- Keep needle midline and aim for umbilicus (slightly cephalad).
- Ultrasound may be a useful adjunct assisting in guiding angle and depth of needle insertion (measurement of skin to dura distance).
- In infants and neonates, a sitting position over a towel roll may facilitate identification of the midline, and successful lumbar puncture.

Needle thoracocentesis
Indication
For emergency evacuation of tension pneumothorax, providing temporary relief until definitive intercostal catheter (chest drain) placement. It is an emergency procedure only.

Contraindication
An infant with vital signs stable enough to allow intercostal catheter placement.

Preparation
- Monitor spontaneously breathing infants to determine ongoing need for intubation and ventilation.
- Consider appropriate pain relief which should not delay treatment but may include:
  - Oral sucrose
  - Infiltration of the insertion site with 1 per cent lignocaine 0.5–1 mL before preparing and draping the field (to allow greater time for the anaesthetic to take effect)
  - Intravenous infusion of morphine

Equipment
- Sterile gloves
- 70 per cent isopropyl alcohol swab
- 10 mL syringe
- 3-way stopcock
- Butterfly needle
  - 25G for <32 w or <1500 g
  - 23G for >32 w or >1500 g

Procedure
- Maintain asepsis.
- Connect male end of the 3-way stopcock to the female end of the butterfly needle. Connect syringe to the 3-way stopcock.
- Position infant supine, prepare skin with alcohol wipe.
- Insert needle into the pleural space (directly over the top of the rib in the second or third intercostal space in the midclavicular line) aspirating whilst advancing. Stop when air is aspirated into the syringe.
- Expel air through the three-way stopcock.
- Minimise movement in the needle to avoid lacerating the lung or puncturing blood vessels.

Post procedure care
- Insertion of an intercostal catheter is required for ongoing management.
- It may be necessary to seek help with this procedure – consultation and assistance will be available through PIPER or the receiving NICU.

Nasogastric tube insertion
Indications
- Oral rehydration
- Administration of medication (e.g. charcoal, bowel washout solutions)
- Decompression of stomach (e.g. bowel obstruction, abdominal trauma)

Suggested analgesia
Topical anaesthetic spray (e.g. co-phenylcaine) and lubrication with lignocaine (lidocaine) containing lubricant. Sucrose in infant <3 months.

Equipment
- Nasogastric tube, tape or adhesive dressing, litmus paper
- Select the correct tube size (size may vary depending on the use of the nasogastric) 8 FG for newborns, 10–12 FG for 1–2 year olds, 14–16 FG for adolescents.

Procedure
- Measure the correct length of insertion by placing the distal end of the tube at the nostril and running it to the ear and to the xiphisternum. Add a few centimetres. Mark the tube with permanent marker at this point so the position can be checked.
- If the tube is too pliable, stiffen it by immersing in cold water or freezing briefly.
- Grasp the tube 5–6 cm from the distal end and insert it posteriorly. Advance it slowly along the floor of the nasal passage (Figure 5.6). Firm pressure is needed to pass the posterior nasal opening.
- If the child is cooperative, once the tube is in the nasopharynx/oropharynx, ask the child to flex their neck and swallow.

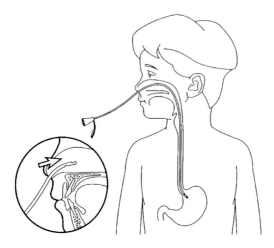

Figure 5.6 Nasogastric tube insertion.

- If the child coughs and gags, their voice becomes hoarse or the tube emerges from the mouth, pull the tube back into the nasopharynx and start again.
- Once the tube has been passed to the measured length, there are two methods for checking the position: (1) by aspirating fluid and testing for an acid pH; (2) with radiograph if necessary.
- Secure the tube to the side of the face using adhesive tape.

Clinical Pearl: Nasogastric tube insertion
- Secure the tube so it is flat against the face with a protective layer dressing e.g. Comfeel against the skin.
- Use measures as required to prevent removal of the nasogastric by small fingers.
- Do not use tube until happy it is correctly positioned.
- Do not use syringe of air to confirm position.

Gastrostomy tube replacement

See the RCH Gastrotomy acute replacement of displaced tubes CPG available at www.rch.org.au/clinicalguide/ guideline_index/Gastrostomy_Acute_replacement_of_displaced_tubes/

Indications
- Burst balloon/malfunctioning parts
- Displacement/extrusion of tube

Suggested analgesia
Nitrous oxide or sedation (e.g. midazolam)

Equipment
Gastrostomy tube, syringe and sterile water, lubricant. When a replacement gastrostomy tube is not available, a sterile indwelling urinary catheter can be used as a temporary measure to keep the stoma patent.

Procedure
- Slide the skin flange on the new tube to the 8–10 cm mark. Close off the feeding ports and apply a small amount of lubricant to the tube.
- If the old tube is still *in situ*, attach an empty syringe to the side port and deflate the balloon by removing the water. Note: There is usually less than the expected 4 or 15 mL of water left in the balloon.
- Gently pull on the tube and rotate it slowly until it is removed.

- Place the tip of the new tube at the opening of the stoma. Hold the distal end of the tube and slowly put pressure on the tube to push it into the hole.
- The new tube should insert easily. Insert it to 6–8 cm.
- Inflate the new tube to either 4 or 15 mL (i.e. not to full capacity) with water. Slowly pull back on the tube until resistance is felt.
- Slide the skin flange down until there is a snug fit, but not too tight. This is usually at the 2–4 cm mark.
- In the case of a MIC key, the correct tube for that child should be inserted to its full depth before inflating the balloon.
- Gastrostomy buttons or Malecot catheters need introducers and should only be replaced by experienced staff.

Note: If there is any difficulty inserting the tube, a radiographic study (i.e. contrast through the tube) should be performed to check correct positioning.

> **Clinical Pearl: Gastrostomy tube replacement**
> PEG tubes /catheters should be placed without delay to avoid stomal closure. If unable to insert the replacement, a smaller size catheter will often pass and maintains the stomal opening.

Wound (laceration) management

See the RCH Lacerations CPG available at ww.rch.org.au.clinicalguide.guideline_index. Lacerations.

Assessment

Lacerations are common in childhood. Most are superficial and tend to occur on the face, scalp and extremities. When assessing a wound consider:

- Is the wound contaminated or could it contain a foreign body (e.g. glass)?
- Are there likely to be other associated injuries?
- Is there injury to deeper structures?
- Is blood supply impaired or is this an area of end-arteriolar supply? Do **not** use local anaesthetic with adrenaline on such wounds.

Cleaning wounds

- Superficial wounds can be cleansed with normal saline or aqueous chlorhexidine.
- Adequate analgesia is required for complete examination, cleaning and repair of all but the most superficial wounds.
- Radiograph (particularly for glass and metal objects) or ultrasound is indicated if there is a possibility of a foreign body.

Suggested analgesia

Topical local anaesthetic

- Laceraine (amethocaine 0.5%, lignocaine 4% (lidocaine) adrenaline0.1%/). Dose = 0.1 mL/kg bodyweight.
- Apply on a piece of sterile gauze or cotton wool placed **inside** the wound and held in place with an adhesive clear plastic dressing.
- Leave for 20–30 minutes. An area of blanching (~1 cm wide) will appear around the wound. Anaesthesia lasts about 1 hour.
- Test the adequacy of anaesthesia by washing and squeezing the wound: if pain free, suturing will usually be painless.
- The sensations of pulling and light touch are preserved. This should be explained to the child and parent.

Injectable local anaesthetic (lignocaine (lidocaine) 1%)

Injectable lignocaine (lidocaine) 1% (max 0.4 mL/kg (4 mg/kg)) can be used to supplement topical local anaesthetic if adequate anaesthesia has not been achieved.

There are several ways to decrease the pain from injecting local anaesthetic:

- Use topical anaesthesia first.
- Use 27 or 30G needles.
- Inject slowly.
- Place the needle into the wound through the lacerated surface, not through intact skin.

- Pass the needle through an anaesthetised area into an unanaesthetised area.
- Use 1% lignocaine (lidocaine) rather than 2% at body temperature.
- Buffer lignocaine (lidocaine) with sodium bicarbonate (10,1 dilution).

Sedation
- Nitrous oxide or sedation (e.g. midazolam).
- Ketamine may be used in children >12 months by staff experienced in its use.

Regional blocks
- Regional blocks provide excellent analgesia. See page 57.

Wound closure
Tissue-adhesive glues
- Tissue glue (e.g. Dermabond) is an alternative to suturing in wounds that are small (<3 cm), straight, easily approximated and under no tension. It must not be used on mucosal surfaces.
- Topical anaesthesia will reduce bleeding from the wound and the discomfort of gluing.
- Clean the wound with normal saline or aqueous chlorhexidine and let dry. Hold the edges firmly together and apply a small amount of glue (~0.05 mL) to the line of the laceration. 3 thin layers applied to wound gives maximal strength. Do not allow glue to enter the wound itself.
- Hold the wound edges together for 30 seconds. Steristrips should be applied to prevent the child picking the glue off.
- The wound should be kept dry for 2 days. It then can be washed. The scab will come off in 1–2 weeks.

Suturing
- Rapidly absorbable sutures (e.g. fast catgut, Vicryl rapid) are appropriate for use on areas where the cosmetic advantages of non-absorbable sutures are not required (e.g. scalp and hand). Using absorbable sutures avoids the stress and potential pain of suture removal.
- Non-absorbable sutures (e.g. nylon and polypropylene) are used in areas where cosmetic appearance is important.
- Deep sutures (absorbable) should be used to close deep tissues; this reduces cavitation and dead space, which increase the risk of infection.
- The size of suture and timing of suture removal depends on the area affected.
  - Scalp: 4/0–5/0, 5–7 days.
  - Face: 5/0–6/0, 5–7 days.
  - Arm/hand: 4/0–5/0, 7–10 days.
  - Trunk/legs: 4/0–5/0, 10–14 days.
  Note: Areas of stress (e.g. over joints) need longer.
- Splint any sutured wound that is under tension (e.g. across joints or on the hand), for at least 1 week. This decreases pain and promotes healing.

Special circumstances
- **Lips:** Accurate approximation of vermilion border and skin is essential.
  - May need general anaesthesia and plastic surgical repair in small or uncooperative children.
  - Sutures: mucosa/muscle 4/0 gut, skin 6/0 nylon or fast gut in the young child. Remove sutures in 5 days.
  - Lacerations of the inner lip rarely need intervention, but degloving to the gum margin requires specialist referral.
- **Palate:** Rarely requires suturing unless laceration is wide, extends through posterior free margin or is actively bleeding.
  - Beware retropharyngeal injury (needs specialist opinion).
- **Tongue:** Small lacerations do not require suturing.
  - Plastic surgical opinion is required if the laceration is large, bleeding actively, extends through the free edge or is of full thickness.
- **Fingertips:** Areas of skin loss up to 1 cm^2 are treated with dressings and heal with good return of sensation. Greater areas require specialist referral.
  - Involvement of the nail bed requires plastic surgical consultation.

- **Scalp:** For small lacerations suitable for tissue-adhesive glue use hair from each side of the laceration to approximate the wound; twist hair together, pull across the wound and glue over the hair.
- **Other:** Lacerations involving cartilage (e.g. nose, ear) require specialist opinion.

Tetanus prophylaxis
See the RCH Management of Tetanus prone wounds CPG available at www.rch.org.au/clinicalguide/guideline_index/Management_of_tetanusprone_wounds/

Antibiotics
Antibiotics are not indicated for simple lacerations. They are usually given for bites and wounds with extensive tissue damage, but are of secondary importance to the initial decontamination of the wound (Appendix: Antimicrobial guidelines).

Femoral nerve block
Indications
Pain relief for femoral fractures (in addition to other techniques including splinting the fractured leg).

Equipment
Monitoring, ultrasound machine (high frequency linear probe), Sterile probe cover, Sterile gloves, dressing pack, antiseptic solution, Nerve block needle for injection and extension tubing 23G needle, and syringes, local anaesthetic solution, adhesive tape.

Procedure
- It may be appropriate to use nitrous oxide or sedation when giving a femoral nerve block.
- This is best performed using ultrasound localisation of the nerve and guided injection ideally with an assistant.
- Prepare ultrasound position opposite side, with gel onto probe, and cover.
- After skin preparation, use in-plane technique with marker pointing to ASIS. Observe landmarks. infiltrate lateral to the artery with lignocaine (lidocaine) 1%.
- Introduce needle through anaesthetized skin and advance slowly ensuring tip of needle is always visible.
- Aspirate to ensure that the needle is not in a blood vessel. When lateral to nerve and between layers of fascia iliaca infiltrate small amount.
- Continue to infiltrate anaesthetic Ropivocaine 0.5ml/kg of 0.75% or Bupivicaine 0.4ml/kg of 0.5%, gradually aiming to encircle the nerve.

Bier's block
Indications
Children over 5 years with forearm fractures requiring manipulation.

Equipment
Dressing pack, antiseptic solution, two IV cannulae (and associated equipment), lignocaine (lidocaine) 1%, monitored tourniquet system, equipment for plaster application.

Procedure
- Give adequate pain relief. Consider also intranasal fentanyl (1.5 mcg/kg, half in each nostril) for long bone fractures.
- Two trained staff must be present and full resuscitation equipment available. Radiology should be notified for timely post reduction images.
- Insert an IV cannula into a distal vein on each hand.
- Elevate the affected arm above the level of the heart while compressing the brachial artery for 1 minute.
- Inflate the tourniquet cuff to 75 mmHg above the child's systolic blood pressure. This reading should be maintained throughout the procedure.
- Infuse lignocaine (lidocaine) 0.5% 3 mg/kg (0.6 mL/kg, max 40 mL). Full anaesthesia takes 5–10 minutes.
- Release tourniquet cuff **at least** 20 minutes after lignocaine (lidocaine) infusion, after procedure is complete and position confirmed radiologically.

Digital/proximal nerve block

Indication

Anaesthesia of finger for minor surgical procedures (e.g. suturing, drainage of paronychia).

Equipment

Dressing pack, antiseptic solution, 25 gauge needle and syringe, local anaesthetic, for example lignocaine (lidocaine) 1%.

Procedure

Digital nerve block

- With the palm facing down, insert a 25 gauge needle at the base of the finger on either medial/lateral side at a 45° angle to the vertical (Figure 5.7).
- Inject when needle hits periosteum.
- Rotate needle to vertical and inject along the side of the finger to at least three-fourth of the depth of the finger.
- Remove needle and repeat on the other side.

Proximal nerve block

- Insert a 25 gauge needle between the fingers at the interdigital fold in line with the web space (Figure 5.7).
- Insert until needle tip is level with the head of the metacarpal bone.
- Inject 1–2 mL at this level.
- Repeat on the other side, or for index/fifth finger; inject half ring wheal around the outer side of the finger.

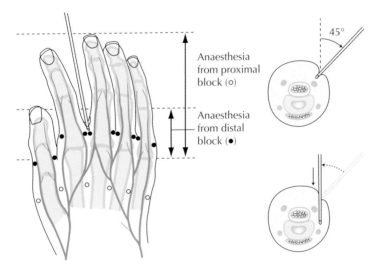

Figure 5.7 Digital nerve block.

USEFUL RESOURCES
- The RCH Clinical practice guidelines www.rch.org.au/clinicalguide for procedural CPGs
- Neonatal eHandbook www.bettersaftercare.vic.gov.au/resources/clinical-guidance/maternity-and-newborn for neonatal procedure guidelines.
- Comfort kids www.rch.org.au/comfortkids/for_health_professionals/ and the RCH Communicating procedures to families CPG www.rch.org.au.clinicalguide. guideline_index.Communicating_procedures_to_families. For some simple ways of communicating procedures to parents and children.

CHAPTER 6

Pain management

George Chalkiadis
Greta Palmer
Ian McKenzie

Key Points

- Unrelieved or inadequately treated pain may have acute and longer term negative physiological and psychological consequences.
- Advise parents on when and how to appropriately wean analgesia.
- Psychological distress contributes to the pain experience. For procedural pain, the use of non-pharmacological strategies may build the child's resilience and capacity to cope during future episodes of pain. Careful planning before the procedure reduces the likelihood of a poor outcome.
- Early pain specialist (where available) and allied health referral is appropriate for children with persistent pain that is significantly impairing their physical, social, sleep and school functioning.
- For chronic non-cancer pain, opioid analgesics are rarely indicated.

Assessment of acute pain

Pain scores are the fifth vital sign on patients' observation charts. Pain assessment includes a combination of the following:

History

- Includes: site, onset, duration, quality, radiation, triggers and relievers, impact on functioning (including sleep disturbance & other activities), treatments tried and their effectiveness.
- In children who can communicate, ask the child directly about their pain using appropriate tools
- In neonates, pre-verbal children and cognitively impaired children, parents and regular caregivers are often best equipped to reliably interpret the child's pain.

Examination

- Behavioural observation (e.g. vocalisation, facial grimacing, posturing, movement).
- Physiological parameters (e.g. heart rate, respiratory rate, blood pressure) and physical signs (e.g. muscle spasm).
- Function: for example, the ability to move (e.g. sitting up after laparotomy) and the tolerance of touch to the painful area usually signify adequate analgesia, whilst inadequate analgesia may result in a withdrawn child lying still and reluctant to move.

Clinical Pearl: Postoperative pain

Postoperatively always enquire where the pain is located. Pain remote to the site of surgery may indicate postoperative complications such as compartment syndrome or urinary retention

Paediatric Handbook, Tenth Edition. Edited by Kate Harding, Daniel S. Mason and Daryl Efron.
© 2021 John Wiley & Sons Ltd. Published 2021 by John Wiley & Sons Ltd.

Use of pain-rating scales

- Observe the trends in an individual's pain score or function (e.g. ability to turn in bed comfortably, ability to walk to the toilet) rather than the 'raw' pain score.
- Verbal children:
  - FACES scales for children >4 years, e.g. Wong–Baker FACES Pain Rating Scale (Figure 6.1) or Faces Pain Scale – Revised.
  - Visual analogue scale (e.g. 100 mm ruler).
  - Verbal numerical rating scale (e.g. 'out of 10.......').
- Non-verbal children including neonates and cognitively impaired are particularly vulnerable to inaccurate assessments of pain (see Chapter 28, Neurodevelopment and disability; section on Irritability in children with profound intellectual and physical disability):
  - FLACC: Face, Legs, Activity, Cry and Consolability (Figure 6.2).
  - PATS (for neonates): Pain Assessment Tool Score.

Wong Baker Faces Pain Scale

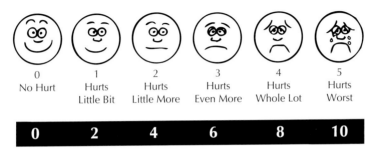

0	1	2	3	4	5
No Hurt	Hurts Little Bit	Hurts Little More	Hurts Even More	Hurts Whole Lot	Hurts Worst

| 0 | 2 | 4 | 6 | 8 | 10 |

Figure 6.1 Wong–Baker FACES Pain Rating Scale. *Source*: Hockenberry MJ, Wilson D, Winkelstein ML: Wong's Essentials of Pediatric Nursing, ed. 7, *St. Louis*, 2005, p. 1259. © Mosby. Reproduced with permission from authors.

FLACC scale

Behavioral Observation Pain Rating Scale

Categories	Scoring		
	0	**1**	**2**
Face	No particular expression or smile; disinterested	Occasional grimace or frown, withdrawn	Frequent to constant frown, clenched jaw, quivering chin
Legs	No position or relaxed	Uneasy, restless, tense	Kicking, or legs drawn up
Activity	Lying quietly, normal position, moves easily	Squirming, shifting back and forth, tense	Arched, rigid, or jerking
Cry	No crying (awake or asleep)	Moans or whimpers, occasional complaint	Crying, steadily, screams or sobs, frequent complaints
Consolability	Content, relaxed	Reassured by occasional touching, hugging, or talking to. Distractable	Difficult to console or comfort
Each of the five categories (F) Face; (L) Legs; (A) Activity; (C) Cry; (C) Consolability is scored from 0–2, which results in a total score between 0 and 10.			

Figure 6.2 FLACC pain rating scale. *Source*: The FLACC: A behavioural scale for scoring postoperative pain in young children. Merkel S, Voepel-Lewis T, Shayevitz JR, et al. *Paediatric nursing* 1997; 23:293–797. © Elsevier. Reproduced with the permission from authors.

Analgesics for acute pain

- Multimodal analgesia (MMA) refers to using more than one analgesic drug class and/or method of controlling pain to obtain additive beneficial effects, reduce side effects, or both.
- MMA use is ideal for acute pain management including pain due to surgery, trauma or cancer, as it allows analgesia to be optimised and directed according to the multiple sources of pain (somatic, visceral and/or neuropathic).
- Analgesic options include:
  - Paracetamol
  - NSAIDs (non-selective or COX-2 inhibitors)
  - Opioids (e.g. morphine, oxycodone or fentanyl)
  - Tramadol
  - Tapentadol
  - Clonidine
  - Ketamine
  - Muscle relaxants (e.g. buscopan for smooth and diazepam for skeletal muscle spasm)
  - Antineuropathic agents (such as gabapentin, pregabalin or amitriptyline)
- Drugs can be administered by various routes.
- Specialised infusions (e.g. local anaesthetics via perineural, epidural or wound catheters or ketamine and opioid intravenously) can be via continuous infusion and/or intermittent bolus.
- Use an analgesic ladder approach to managing acute pain (Table 6.1). Progress up or down the steps varies according to the:
  - Intensity of pain experienced.
  - Anticipated duration.
  - Expected recovery period.

Each step up employs all the analgesics listed in the steps below. Once pain is controlled, wean back to the previous step. This varies with the speed of resolution of the painful condition and the number of breakthrough or rescue agents that are required in the higher category. If pain is poorly responsive to these measures, get consultant assistance. Table 6.2 outlines common pain medications, preparations and dosing.

Table 6.1 Analgesic ladder approach.

Degree of pain and setting	Analgesic 'steps'
Severe pain	
Inpatient	Add specialised infusion, e.g. ketamine, epidural, perineural or wound catheter local anaesthetic infusion Add IV opioid by infusion (nurse or patient controlled) Use adjuncts for neuropathic pain e.g. gabapentin or pregabalin, amitriptyline if sleep is impaired
Outpatient or Emergency presentation	Add IV or IN opioid by bolus or regular oral opioid (consider controlled release when pain is constant and of long duration) Consider IV tramadol, NSAID, paracetamol if NBM Consider nerve block e.g. femoral where appropriate Address sleep impairment and anxiety if present
Moderate pain	Add one (or combination) of: strong opioid e.g. oral morphine or oxycodone 'atypical opioids': tramadol or tapentadol Address environmental/psychosocial contributors
Mild pain	Begin with paracetamol and/or NSAIDs

Table 6.2 Analgesic medications, preparations and dosage information.

Analgesic	Dose per kg (maximum)	Route(s)	Indications	Side effects	Special notes/ Contraindications
Paracetamol	**Short-term oral total daily maximum:** 90 mg/kg/day for 48 h **Chronic or unsupervised community setting oral maximum:** 60 mg/kg/day *Oral:* 15 mg/kg (max 1g) per dose 4 hourly prn or 30 mg/kg as initial dose *Rectal:* 20–40 mg/kg (max 1g) one-off dose, rounded to appropriate suppository dose *IV:* 15 mg/kg (max 1gm) 6 hourly	Oral: syrup/tablet Oral preferred to rectal; absorption more reliable & earlier peak concentration (oral 30–60 m vs rectal 2-3 h) I.V. (onset 15m)	Mild to moderate pain Has antipyretic effects **but** physical measures better	Hepatotoxicity Otherwise well tolerated	Check strengths of different syrup (suspensions) Hepatotoxicity reported in children. Use with caution in severe liver disease, jaundice, malnutrition, glutathione depletion, dehydration and long-term ingestion Significant opioid sparing effects
Opioid					
Oxycodone	0.1–0.2 mg/kg (usual max 5-10mg) 4 hourly *Oral* *IV*	Oral tablet and oral liquid solution (onset 30–60 min) Also available in IV form (see below) and slow release (SR) form alone as OxyContin® and mixed with SR naloxone as Targin®	Strong opioid for moderate to severe pain	Nausea, Vomiting Constipation Urinary retention Sedation, Dysphoria/Euphoria Dreams, hallucinations Ventilatory impairment Less itch than morphine	Cost is only slightly greater than morphine and no metabolism issues Avoids morphine stigma
IV Oxycodone IV Morphine	Titrate as 10-20mcg/kg boluses or for severe pain 50-100mcg/kg (max 10mg)	IV – both as 10mg/mL ampoules	Strong opioid	As above	
Morphine	0.25–0.5 mg/kg (usual max 15-30mg)4 hourly	Oral (onset 40–60 min) Also available in controlled release (CR) form	Strong opioid	As above	Stigma Metabolite accumulation issues

Drug	Dose/Route	Indication	Adverse effects	Comments
Tramadol	1–2 mg/kg (usual max 50–100mg) 6 hourly	Oral; 50 mg capsules, IR (onset ~30–60 min) Can suspend contents in water and disperse in syringe for smaller children Also available in: SR tablet I.v. form (onset same as i.v. morphine)	2 mechanisms of action via noradrenaline/serotonin reuptake inhibition; opioid effects via metabolite M1 (requires CYP2D6 for conversion) For moderate to severe pain	Nausea and vomiting, dizziness, sedation Not constipating; less itch and respiratory depression than opioids	Off-licence use in <12 y but has been studied in all age groups: requires anaesthetist-only prescription or Drug Usage Committee approval at RCH Use with caution if active seizures
Fentanyl	1.5 mcg/kg (half into each nostril) [RCH guideline max. 75mcg] (50mcg boluses titrated 5 minutely in adult sized children to a maximum of 200mcg by the Victorian ambulance service]	Intranasal (initial studies have used a specially designed Mucosal atomisation device (MAD) which is cushioned and well accepted by children – alternative is 1mL tuberculin syringe drop technique)	Short-term analgesia for moderate to severe pain (including procedural pain)		Due to slower absorption from the nasal mucosa – lower peak of plasma level to explain the reduced rate of ventilatory impairment vs IV administration 100mcg/2mL now used (to avoid confusion with more concentrated formulation)

Non-selective NSAIDS

Drug	Dose/Route	Indication	Adverse effects	Comments
Ibuprofen	5–10 mg/kg tds–qid (usual max on product information can be exceeded with medical supervision to 600-800mg]	Oral: Syrup 100 mg/5 mL 200 mg tablets (including enteric coated] or capsules	For mild to moderate pain Particularly for muscular, bony or visceral pain	Gastrointestinal Renal Platelet inhibition **avoid in severe bleeding	Caution in low volume status, poor urine output, bleeding and asthma Avoid in severe asthma with nasal disease (because of NSAID/aspirin-exacerbated respiratory disease (ERD)) Can be used in mild asthma Generally NSAIDs are avoided in infants <6 months in Australia and <12 months in USA
Diclofenac	1 – 2 mg/kg bd–tds [usual max. 50-75 mg]	Oral and rectal 25 and 50 mg tablet			

(continued)

Table 6.2 (*Continued*)

Analgesic	Dose per kg (maximum)	Route(s)	Indications	Side effects	Special notes/ Contraindications
Piroxicam	0.2–0.4 mg/kg (max. 10–20 mg) daily	Oral tablet			
Meloxicam	0.1–0.25 mg/kg [max. 15mg] daily	Oral tablet			
Naprosyn	5–7.5 mg/kg (max. 500 mg) twice daily	Oral tablet IR and SR			
Indomethacin	0.5–1.0 mg/kg per dose (adult 25–50 mg) 8 hourly (max. 6 hourly)	Oral tablet			
Ketorolac	0.2 mg/kg i.v. (**not** i.m.) [max. 10 mg]	I.V. available for anaesthetists to use at RCH			Off-licence use <16 years
COX-2 inhibitor					
Celecoxib	1.5–3 mg/kg bd [max. 200mg]	Oral capsule Oral suspension 10mg/mL made up by pharmacy		No platelet inhibition	COX-2s are OK in NSAID-ERD Off-licence use <18 years Used in RCH post-tonsillectomy analgesic pathway
Local anaesthetics					
Lignocaine (lidocaine) 1–2% (1 mL of 1% = 10 mg)	Max. doses: Lignocaine (lidocaine) with adrenaline: 7 mg/kg Without adrenaline: 3 mg/kg	Injectable	Wound infiltration Nerve blocks/infusion	Neurological Cardiac	
Bupivacaine 0.25–0.5%	Max. dose: 2–2.5 mg/kg e.g. <0.5 mL/kg of 0.5% or <1 mL/kg of 0.25%				**Do not** inject local anaesthetic **premixed with adrenaline** into 'end organs' such as fingers, toes, penis, nose or ears due to the risk of ischaemia

Drug	Dose	Preparation	Indication	Side effects	Notes
Levobupivacaine 0.25–0.5%	Max. dose: 2–2.5 mg/kg e.g. <0.5mL/kg of 0.5% or <1 mL/kg of 0.25%				
Ropivacaine 0.2-1.0%	3 mg/kg				Some vasoconstrictive effect
Adjuvants					
Gabapentin	5-10 mg/kg [max 600 mg] tds	Capsule 100, 300, 400, 800 mg	Neuropathic pain, anxiety, dystonia	Dizziness, sedation, impaired concentration, nausea	
Pregabalin	2.5-5mg/kg [300 mg] bd	Tablets 25, 75, 150 and 300mg	Neuropathic pain, anxiety, dystonia	Dizziness, sedation, impaired concentration, nausea	
Amitriptyline	0.25-2mg/kg [max 100mg]	Tablet 10 and 25mg	Neuropathic pain, impaired sleep initiation, anti-anxiety and depression at higher dose level	Dizziness, postural hypotension sedation, hangover effect, nausea	
Clonidine	0.05-2mcg/kg [usual max. 150mcg]	Oral tablet 100 and 150mcg and suspension 10mcg/mL made by RCH pharmacy IV 150mcg /mL	Neuropathic pain, analgesia (deepening of regional or peripheral blockade), anxiety, dystonia, analgesia (antihypertension)	Dizziness, bradycardia/ hypotension sedation	
Melatonin	0.05-0.1mg/kg [max. 6-10mg] nightly	IR and SR tablet, Suspension available at RCH Retail pharmacy 3 or 6 mg/mL	Used to assist sleep initiation adjust sleep wake cycle eg in as in and outpatient		IR used for sleep initiation issues SR used for sleep maintenance early morning waking issues

---

Clinical Pearl: Discharging on opioid analgesia

Take special care when discharging patients with opioid analgesics. Prescribe an amount and quantity appropriate for the cause of pain or type of surgery. Parents must be instructed on the safe storage and disposal of unused medication and the potential for drug diversion and inadvertent ingestion.

Suggested management for specific cases of severe pain
Femoral fracture
- Single shot local anaesthetic femoral nerve block or ideally insertion of femoral nerve catheter with ultrasound guidance to facilitate repeat administration.
- Anticipate need for stronger (opioid) analgesia when the nerve block wears off.
- Immobilise in back slab or traction.
- Give other analgesics (e.g. paracetamol regularly).
- Avoid NSAIDs preoperatively to reduce bleeding risk.
- Diazepam as needed for muscle spasm.

Bowel obstruction requiring laparotomy
- The patient will be nil orally and will require parenteral analgesia for severe pain.
- It is important that analgesia be commenced even if the child is to be transferred to a larger centre.
- The following are suggested options:
  - Regular intravenous paracetamol **and**
    - Opioid intravenous infusion via nurse-controlled or patient-controlled analgesia (PCA).
    - Ketamine intravenous infusion can be added if above measures are inadequate.
    - Postoperatively, epidural analgesia may also be used.

Metastatic cancer with bony metastases and large intra-abdominal mass
- May benefit from regular dosing with a long acting slow-release opioid such as MSContin (morphine) or Targin, (oxycodone and naloxone combination) or fentanyl patch (applied every 3 days).
- Manage breakthrough pain with immediate release morphine, oxycodone, fentanyl lozenges, sublingual tablets or intranasal spray.
- If analgesia inadequate, consider intravenous or subcutaneous opioid infusion and/or ketamine infusion
- Consider intrathecal local anaesthetic and opioid analgesia if analgesia is still sub-optimal.

Procedural pain management
Procedural pain management (see also Chapter 5, Procedures) is better approached as aiming to minimize distress related to clinical procedures. This is because fear and anxiety can contribute as much to distress as the experience of pain. Any distressing clinical event (even when there is no pain) can sensitise a child to future events creating anticipatory anxiety and worsen the distress associated with the next procedure. This includes amplifying the actual pain experience if the procedure is painful. Therefore, the aim is to minimize distress associated with any clinical procedure, even if painless.
- For procedures that can be associated with a painful stimulus, the quality of the child's experience can be optimized by appropriate planning to minimize associated anxiety as well as the pain stimulus.
- The number of procedures required for a child's care should be kept to the minimum required. For example, ensuring all blood tests are ordered for a single sampling time or multiple procedures are coordinated if formal sedation or anaesthesia are required can minimize the procedural burden for the child and family.
- Children with conditions that require multiple interventions over time are at significant risk of developing heightened anxiety about procedures. The program to minimise distress related to procedures should start from the first procedure.
- Diagnosing anxiety about procedures in children with chronic illnesses is obvious and can be highly motivating for staff to ensure these patients receive appropriate care.

- However, a child who has a single significant distressing experience can still have long term trauma that impacts medical care for the rest of their life, and underlines the importance of minimising distress for all clinical interventions.
- Minimising procedural distress can be considered in the three phases of before, during and after a procedure.

Before the procedure

Consider:

- The patient: age, previous experiences, emotional and physical condition.
- The procedure: is it needed and how urgently; is all required equipment and material available.
- The proceduralist: availability of appropriately skilled staff.
- Who will be the child's support person (commonly a parent) and what will be their role and have they been prepared for that role?

General principles – preparation is the key

- Prepare yourself and other staff involved.
- Ensure parents and the child are appropriately informed about the procedure. The younger the child, the closer to the procedure it is appropriate to give information. Older children may benefit from discussion prior to this time.
- The language of explanation should not only be appropriate to allow understanding for the parent as well as developmentally appropriately for the child, but should instill confidence in the process, purpose and benefits of having the procedure and use positive framing of the planned intervention.
  - Avoid medical jargon; explain what is going to happen and in what order.
  - Calico dolls (or similar) can be very useful to assist explanations, especially in an age appropriate way.
  - If a Child Life Specialist is available, they also may contribute at all phases of a procedure.
- Obtain consent from the parents (verbal or written as required).
- Set up your equipment before the child enters the procedure room.
- Encourage parents to play an active role during the procedure by involving them in distraction/engagement techniques and comfort strategies. Avoid asking them to restrain their child.
- Thoughtfully arrange the 'choreography' of who will be where during the procedure accounting for "positioning for comfort" (see https://www.rch.org.au/comfortkids/), how the parent is physically engaged with the child and where the 'line of sight' of the child will be in relation to the procedure.
- Children may be assisted to develop their own personal procedure routine, comfort or distraction / engagement strategies
- An explanatory video may be helpful in preparing the child and their parent for the procedure.
- If considering procedural sedation, ensure adequate staffing and resources are available.
- Plan what "non-pharmacological" techniques will be used. In general, behavioural techniques are always applicable.
- Attention focus / Engagement / Distraction techniques may have concepts and possibilities introduced prior to the procedure: selection of a book, screen interaction, favourite things that can then be familiar and expected at the time of the procedure.
- For children with special needs, such as those with autism spectrum disorder, more extensive preparation such as with 'story boards' can be very effective. Using quiet low stimulus spaces in both a pre-procedure waiting area and the treatment area may be beneficial.
- Plan what, if any, pharmacological techniques will be used.
- Implement pharmacological strategies that need initiation prior to the procedure in a timely manner: such as:
  - Topical local anaesthetics for skin puncture (e.g. AnGel or EMLA)
  - Laceraine for wounds
  - Anxiolytics (e.g. midazolam)

- ○ Analgesics (e.g. paracetamol, ibuprofen, oxycodone or fentanyl)
- ○ Sedatives (e.g. chloral hydrate) if indicated
- ○ Clonidine, dexmedetomidine and ketamine can all have a role in appropriate settings and have complex multiple actions contributing to sedation, anxiolysis and analgesia.
- *Please note: the use of combinations of agents significantly increases the risks of excess sedation and associated complications and should only be used in suitable settings with appropriately trained staff.*

During the procedure
General principles
The developmental stage, previous experience and potentially the effects of pharmacological agents can all influence how the child should be communicated with during the procedure. Having a clear lead person who will speak to and engage the child is important. *This is the 'one voice' principle.*

- Giving the child some feeling of control may be very helpful especially in older children.
  - ○ If choice is provided, care must be taken to make sure the choices are limited to things that are available and acceptable for the procedure (e.g. choice of hand for i.v., sitting up or lying down).
- Many children will feel more anxious if they have to lie down for a procedure so this transition should be planned or managing the procedure with the child in the sitting position arranged.
- Prompt the child to use the previously planned coping methods.
- Monitor effectiveness of pain / distress minimization techniques during a procedure and if the child is not coping well, consider changing the strategies being used or aborting the procedure if clinically appropriate.

Comfort techniques
- Position for comfort (i.e. infants on parents' lap with physical/eye contact with parent).
- Have parents comfort child with gentle massage/touch or holding hands.
- Calm breathing.
- Swaddling for infants (<6 months).

Attention focus/Distraction/Engagement techniques
- Choosing and playing an interactive I-pad game, music CD or watching a favourite movie.
- Playing with developmentally appropriate toys.
- Counting objects in the room or looking at posters on the wall or ceiling.
- Reading interactive storybooks.
- Visual imagery (e.g. ask the child to imagine a place where they would like to be and to tell you about it).

Pharmacological techniques (see Table 6.3)

After the procedure
- Encourage the parent to remain with their child.
- Continue monitoring until appropriate recovery to baseline has occurred.
- Provide ongoing analgesia as needed.
- Document techniques used to minimize pain and distress and their perceived efficacy.
- Depending on the procedure, the child may need the opportunity to debrief.
  - ○ For example, staff & parents should focus on the helpful things the child did during the procedure.
  - ○ Staff may also like to suggest alternative techniques for any further procedures that may be planned.
  - ○ Providing positive feedback in a calm post procedure setting can positively influence the approach to future procedures.

Table 6.3 Pharmacological techniques for procedural sedation.

Pharmacological technique	Notes	Considerations
Oral Sucrose	*For Infants:* 2 mL of 33% sucrose	Give 0.25 mL 2 min before start of procedure onto infant's tongue Offer dummy/pacifier if indicated Give remainder slowly during the procedure.
Anaesthetic agents		
Topical EMLA, AnGel for skin; Cophenylcaine for mucosa	EMLA (prilocaine 2.5% & lignocaine (lidocaine) 2.5%) AnGel (amethocaine 1%) Faster onset than EMLA Lignocaine+phenyephine topical to mucosa (Cophenylcaine)	Apply LA cream 60–90 min before needling procedures (to ensure skin analgesia a few mm deep). Creams remain effective for up to 4 h after application. EMLA causes vasoconstriction to area AnGel causes erythema & itch
Local anaesthetic infiltration	Lignocaine (lidocaine) Ropivacaine Bupivacaine Levobupivacaine	Skin & subcutaneous tissues can be effectively infiltrated with LA solutions. Lignocaine (lidocaine) stings as it is injected (1% lignocaine stings less than 2%). Stinging may be reduced by adding 1 mL of 8.4% sodium bicarbonate to 9 mL of lignocaine (lidocaine) solution.
Regional	Peripheral nerve block or I.V. regional anaesthesia (e.g. Bier's block) suitable for specific procedures	
Analgesics Anxiolytics Sedatives		Require environment with adequate monitoring, resuscitation equipment & appropriate staffing. Monitoring involves a minimum of in line of sight clinical observation & pulse oximetry if patient sedated. Patient monitoring continues until return to baseline conditions. Relative contraindications agents include conditions which reduce cardiorespiratory reserve or have depressed mental state.

(continued)

Table 6.3 (Continued)

Pharmacological technique	Notes	Considerations
Inhaled Nitrous Oxide	Rapid onset and offset. Efficacy for analgesia & sedation can commence at low concentrations, unconsciousness (unusual) can occur at higher concentrations (such as 70%).	Useful inhalational analgesic agent. Potent short-term analgesia and sedation for painful procedures e.g. vascular access, wound dressings & removal of catheters. Can combine with LA. Person administering should have adequate training including airway management skills. SE include sedation, nausea and vomiting. Careful titration is required if combined with other agents. Contraindications include conditions where closed gas filled space might expand. e.g. pneumothorax, & avoid excess sedation in obtunded patients
Intranasal Fentanyl	Mucosal atomizer device (MAD300). Initial dose of 1.5 mcg/kg & if required follow up doses of 0.75–1.5 mcg/kg.	
Oral Midazolam	Oral midazolam 0.5 mg/kg (usual max. 15 mg). Administer 15–30 m before treatment.	Intranasal delivery stings & usually avoided. Amnestic effect should be considered if giving instructions to patient (may not be remembered). Agitation associated with midazolam is unusual, self limiting & reversed with flumazenil. Useful for anxiolysis & can facilitate cooperation. Not analgesic; analgesia (including local analgesia where appropriate) is required if the procedure is painful.
Clonidine	Slow onset (45–60m) & slow offset (hours). Can be given orally (2–5 mcg/kg) or IV.	Complex sedative analgesic & anxiolytic effects mediated by central alpha 2 adrenergic agonist action. Can also cause hypotension & bradycardia + initial hypertension if given rapidly IV.

Chronic or persistent pain management

Acute and chronic pain are distinct entities that require vastly different diagnostic and management skills (Table 6.4).

- Chronic pain is classified as primary, or secondary to an underlying disease (cancer-related, neuropathic, visceral, posttraumatic and postsurgical, headache and orofacial and musculoskeletal).
- Whilst its definition by the International Association for the Study of Pain (IASP) requires it to be present for at least 3 months, some persistent pain problems are evident earlier and should be suspected when pain after traumatic injury or surgery persists longer than expected.

Assessment

General principles

- Interdisciplinary assessment and treatment is ideal (multimodal treatment provided by a multidisciplinary team collaborating in assessment and treatment using a shared biopsychosocial model and goals).
- Assess the physical and psychosocial contributors to, and sequelae of the chronic pain presentation.
- Outcomes are best when the child or adolescent, their family and therapists share the same treatment goals.
- Functional impairment often includes school absenteeism, poor sleep, social withdrawal and reduction in sport participation.
- Treatment goals are usually to do with functional restoration, not elimination of pain.
- When an interdisciplinary approach is not used, ensure good communication between involved healthcare providers.

History

- Is the pain:
  - Nociceptive (arising from peripheral or visceral nociceptors)?
  - Neuropathic (arising at any point from the primary afferent neurone to higher centres in the brain)?
  - Primary (occurs in the absence of any identifiable noxious stimulus or injurious process)?
    - Chronic primary pain refers to pain that has persisted for more than 3 months and is associated with significant emotional distress and/or functional disability, and the pain is not better accounted for by another condition.

Table 6.4 Comparison of the qualities and clinical course of acute versus chronic or persistent pain.

Acute pain	Chronic or persistent pain
Tangible & understandable by the patient, family, friends & treating doctor	Often nothing to 'see' & minimal evidence of tissue damage
Usually brief, evoked by a recognised noxious stimulus and associated with an adaptive biological significance (e.g. protection of injured part to encourage healing)	Present for prolonged duration
Usually improves rapidly & associated with functional improvement & pain score reduction on a daily basis	May be evoked by minor trauma
Usually related to the nature and extent of tissue damage	Generally improves slowly over time with an undulating course
Responds to pharmacological intervention	Improvement and deterioration may be linked to life stresses
	Not necessarily related directly to the nature and extent of tissue damage
	Does not always respond to pharmacological intervention
	Often associated with secondary gains (e.g. school, sport or chore avoidance)

- Consider:
  - Fixed factors: age, cognitive level, previous pain experience, witnessed examples of how other family members react to pain, domestic situation.
  - Situational factors; social and academic functioning at schools, bullying, pain triggers, pain-reducing strategies including medications tried.
  - Suffering; fear, anxiety, anger, frustration, depression.
  - Pain behaviour (overt distress, moaning, splinting, complaining of pain). Pain behaviour is exacerbated when:
    Pain is central to communication (e.g. to receive a diagnosis or treatment, or for secondary gain).
    - There is an absence of reinforcement for non-pain communication.
    - The child is fearful of increased pain with moving (fear avoidance).
    - The meaning of pain is fear-inducing.
    - The child and their parents hold unhelpful beliefs and inadvertently maintain suffering, disabiity and dependency
    - The parents or child obtain significant secondary gain from the child's maintained pain
- Assess for:
  - Unhelpful belief systems of child and/or family (e.g. if pain were cured, the other problems would not exist).
  - Unrealistic expectations (e.g. it is others' responsibility to fix the problem).
  - Functional impact (e.g. inability to play sport, socialise with peers, attend school). Impaired sleep often occurs.

Clinical Pearl: Chronic pain & emotional distress
When pain is out of proportion to what one would expect from the inciting event, enquire about emotionally upsetting events that might have occurred around the onset of that pain.

Examine the painful site:
- What is causing the pain?
- Are there signs of complex regional pain syndrome? (see section below).
- Is there secondary deconditioning? Muscle wasting, joint stiffening, and tendon shortening can occur rapidly, especially when fear of touch or movement exists.

Management
- The goals are to manage pain, restore function and reduce pain behaviour.
- It is desirable to identify the cause of pain, treat and eliminate it; however, this is not always possible. Therefore, management aims to achieve a more active and fulfilling lifestyle, less constrained by pain with improved coping.
- Coordinating outpatient appointments facilitates achieving these goals, minimising school absenteeism and time off work for parents.
- **A multidisciplinary pain team** ideally includes a pain medicine specialist, physiotherapist, psychologist, occupational therapist and child and adolescent psychiatrist. The team should have access to surgeons (orthopaedic, neuro-, urologic, general and gynaecological), a paediatrician, paediatric rheumatologist, neurologist, gastroenterologist and a rehabilitation specialist.
  Refer when:
  - Pain is more intense or persists longer than anticipated (e.g. after an injury).
  - Character of pain is different to that expected.
  - Pain responds poorly to medication.
  - Loss of function results in secondary deconditioning (e.g. muscle wasting).
  - Pain interferes with sleep, socialising with peers, school attendance and leisure activities.
  - Pain behaviour manifests.
  - Complex regional pain syndrome (CRPS) is present.
  - Pain is neuropathic.

Non-pharmacological techniques in chronic pain management

- Pain education:
  - Help the patient and their family understand pain and how stress, anxiety and anger may contribute to pain. Identifying stressors (often school, friendship or family related) and managing the feelings that arise more effectively may reduce or eliminate pain.
  - Where appropriate, explain that pain does not always mean damage, and that pain is not a hindrance to return to function.
  - Provide further information and pain resources (see additional resources at end of chapter).
- Acceptance and commitment therapy (ACT), cognitive behavioural therapy (CBT) or their combination employ acceptance, values-based and mindfulness strategies, promote psychological flexibility and address the (often unhelpful) thoughts that maintain pain and disability e.g. catastrophisation.
  - Thought stopping or challenging techniques.
  - Behaviour modification techniques: based on modifying the consequences of the child's pain experience and pain behaviour by rewarding positive behaviour.
- Pain coping strategies include
  - Relaxation techniques: muscle relaxation via body awareness techniques, meditation, self-hypnosis or biofeedback.
  - Distraction techniques: art, play or music therapy.
- Physiotherapy reconditioning programs:
  - Involve gradual return to function.
  - Utilise: muscle stretches, postural exercises, reconditioning programs and stress loading (e.g. 'scrub and carry' techniques for the upper limbs, weight bearing for lower limbs).
  - Ultrasound treatment.
  - Heat/cold treatment.
  - Transcutaneous electrical nerve stimulation (TENS): activates large, myelinated primary afferent fibres (A fibres) that act through inhibitory circuits within the dorsal horn to reduce nociceptive transmission through small unmyelinated fibres (C fibres). TENS is more likely to be effective if pain responds to heat or cold.
- Pacing activity with reasonable and achievable goals.
- Management of setbacks.
- Sleep management.
- Family therapy:
  - Family dynamics may contribute to and maintain pain.
  - Pain affects the rest of the family (e.g. lack of attention for well siblings, family holidays or activities).
- Parental counselling:
  - Parents may inadvertently encourage illness behavior and disability, and ignore non-pain activities.
  - Addresses parental feelings of helplessness and loss of control.
  - Equips parents with strategies to manage pain behaviour.
- Assertiveness training
- School liaison:
  - Address bullying.
  - Modifications to allow return to school despite disability.
  - Equip teachers with strategies to deal with pain behaviour.
  - Graded return-to-school programs with involvement and education of teachers.
- Vocational counselling.
- Hydrotherapy.
- Acupuncture.

Pharmacological techniques in chronic pain management

- Paracetamol: limit dosing for long-term administration to 60 mg/kg per day.
- Steroids
  - Triamcinolone used for joint injections, trigger point injections, tendon sheaths and neuralgias.
  - Dexamethasone administered by iontophoresis for soft tissue injuries.
  - Epidural steroid administration for localised nerve root irritation (radiculopathy) due to disc herniation.

- NSAIDS
  - Topical gels (diclofenac, piroxicam, ibuprofen).
  - Oral preparations (described in Table 6.2).
- Anti-neuropathic medications:
  Tricyclic antidepressants (TCAs)/newer serotonin or serotonin and noradrenaline reuptake inhibitors may improve pain even if depression is not present by suppressing pathological neural discharges. Provide effective analgesia, usually within days, once appropriate dose reached.
  Indications include:
  - Severe unremitting pain, especially if neuropathic.
  - Complex regional pain syndrome (CRPS).
  - Associated depression and anxiety.
  - Poor sleep.
- Amitriptyline is the most commonly used TCA:
  - Start at 0.2 mg/kg per day increasing over 2 weeks to 2 mg/kg per day (up to max of 75mg).
  - Administer as a single dose before bed to take advantage of sedative properties.
  - Increase dosage until the desired treatment goal is achieved or side effects become unacceptable, e.g. dry mouth, morning somnolence.
- Fluoxetine (SSRI) or Duloxetine (SNRI) may be indicated when anxiety is assessed to be a significant contributor,
- Anticonvulsants (e.g. A2d ligands Gabapentin or Pregabalin, Carbamazepine) indicated for neuropathic pain and CRPS.
  - Dosage should be in the therapeutic anticonvulsant range, although there is no evidence of any relationship between analgesic effect and the plasma level.
  - Some recommend increasing the dosage to the point of side effects or analgesia.
  - Side-effects include clouded mentation.
- Opioids
  - Only partially modulate central and peripiheral sensitization to pain stimuli
  - Indicated in cancer pain and nociceptive pain.
  - Usually ineffective in controlling neuropathic pain or pain secondary to CRPS.
  - Avoid if possible in children and adolescents with chronic pain – there may be temptation to escalate the dose to further improve analgesia if partially effective or tolerance is evident, to continue long term prescription with risk of physiological and psychological dependence.
- Other pharmacological measures include:
  - Ketamine and clonidine
  - Muscle relaxants e.g. diazepam or baclofen may be indicated where muscle rigidity or spasm is present.
  - Interventional techniques rarely indicated in paediatric patients.
  - Sympathetic and peripheral nerve blocks can diagnose and/or treat some pain problems
  - Lignocaine patches may be useful for superficial persistent pain.

Complex regional pain syndrome (CRPS), types I and II

This condition is of unknown aetiology and is relatively common in children and adolescents. The diagnosis is clinical, and treatment is easier when the condition is recognised early.

- **Type I** (formerly known as reflex sympathetic dystrophy; RSD) often occurs after a noxious stimulus to the affected limb (e.g. minor trauma or surgery). Symptoms are disproportionate to the inciting event. It is most commonly present in a lower limb in children and adolescents.
- **Type II** was formerly referred to as causalgia. It differs from type I because it occurs after peripheral nerve injury.

Clinical manifestations

The affected area, usually a limb, manifests autonomic, sensory and motor symptoms consisting of:

- Pain:
  - Regional non-dermatomal distribution.
  - Hyperaesthesia (diffuse pain exacerbated by touch).
  - Allodynia (pain elicited by a stimulus that is not usually painful).

- Temperature change (affected limb often colder).
- Changes in skin blood flow – often red/purple colour change
- Abnormal sweating
- Oedema.
- Loss of function/reduced range of motion
- Motor dysfunction – weakness, tremor, dystonia
- Abnormal hair growth, skin and/or nail atrophy

Investigations
Investigations maybe performed to exclude underlying injury but are not required to make the diagnosis.
- Acute phase markers – normal.
- Bone scan often abnormal – increased or decreased uptake.
- Plain radiograph – osteopenia in protracted cases.
- MRI – diffuse marrow infiltration or oedema sometimes present.

Management
- Management requires early identification, skillful physical therapy, avoidance of immobilisation and multidisciplinary pain team input.
- Consider psychiatric or psychological assessment, pharmacological and interventional techniques.

Neuropathic pain
- Typified by continuous burning with an intermittent electric shock, stabbing or shooting-type discomfort.
- May be paroxysmal or spontaneous.
- Pain in an area of sensory loss.
- Pain in the absence of ongoing tissue damage.
- Associated with dysaesthesia (unpleasant, abnormal sensation, e.g. ants crawling on skin), allodynia and hyperalgesia (increased pain in response to noxious stimuli).
- Increased sympathetic activity may be present.
- Causes include CRPS type II, tumour, spinal cord injury, nerve damage (e.g. neuropraxia or avulsion, neuroma).
- Usually poor response to simple (paracetamol and NSAID) and opioid medications.
- Consider the use of anti-neuropathic medications and early referral to a pain specialist and/or multidisciplinary pain management team if prolonged or refractory.

Pain in children and adolescents with disabilities
Pain assessment in individuals with cerebral palsy, cognitive impairment and/or communication difficulties can prove challenging. No simple pain assessment tool exists for this cohort of patients. General considerations include:
- Caregivers are best placed to distinguish pain from 'normal' behaviour for the individual.
- Pain may manifest as crying, screaming, frequent waking, grimacing, arching, muscle spasm or self-injurious behaviour, however some individuals with cerebral palsy or intellectual disability may exhibit these behaviours without experiencing pain.
- Differential diagnosis includes seizures, muscle spasm, anxiety, depression and anger.
- A thorough search for the cause of pain will guide treatment options.
- Causes include the common causes of pain in all children.
- Additionally, children with disabilities may also develop hip joint subluxation or dislocation, constipation, renal and salivary gland calculi, gastro-oesophageal reflux and urinary tract infection.
- See also Chapter 28, Neurodevelopment and disability; section on Irritability in children with profound intellectual and physical disability.

Sleep disturbance:
- Occurs frequently and has implications for the functioning of the whole family.
- Most young children settle with re-positioning.
- Tricyclic antidepressants, via their analgesic and sedative effects (e.g. amitriptyline nocte) and melatonin, may be useful in initiating sleep faster and reducing the frequency of waking (amitriptyline nocte).

USEFUL RESOURCES

- RCH Acute Pain Management Service clinical practice guidelines: www.rch.org.au/anaes/pain_management/Acute_Pain_Management_CPMS/
- RCH procedural pain management clinical practice guideline: https://www.rch.org.au/rchcpg/hospital_clinical_guideline_index/Procedural_pain_management/
- RCH analgesia & sedation clinical practice guidelines (including links to Nitrous oxide & Ketamine guidelines): https://www.rch.org.au/clinicalguide/guideline_index/Analgesia_and_sedation/
- RCH parent information sheets: www.rch.org.au/kidsinfo/fact_sheets/Reduce_childrens_discomfort_during_tests_and_procedures/
- RCH children / patient resources: www.rch.org.au/comfortkids/for_kids
- Canadian centre for Pediatric Pain Research, containing useful downloadable pamphlets and protocols: *www.pediatric-pain.ca*
- Chronic pain resource; understanding pain and what's to be done about it in 10 minutes; https://www.youtube.com/watch?v=KfYC6zfrV80
- Low cost Mindfulness Apps to aid in self regulation of pain include: www.smilingmind.com.au/smiling-mind-app; www.headspace.com/headspace-meditation-app; www.calm.com/

CHAPTER 7

Fluids and electrolytes

Sarah McNab
Trevor Duke

Key Points

- The hierarchy of fluids for a sick child (depending on availability, disease state and tolerance) are: breast milk; other enteral formula by mouth or nasogastric tube; enteral clear fluid such as oral rehydration solution; then intravenous fluid.
- When prescribing maintenance intravenous fluid, an isotonic fluid should be used.
- The hydration state of a child can be estimated by clinical signs. Where available, a change in weight from a pre-illness state can be very helpful in estimating the degree of dehydration.
- Hospitalised children, particularly those with increased losses or receiving nasogastric or intravenous fluid, should be frequently assessed for hydration – both dehydration and overhydration.

Fluids

Sick children should be given enteral fluids/feeds where possible. If oral fluids are not tolerated, consider giving fluids/feeds via a nasogastric (NG) or nasojejunal (NJ) tube. Clear intravenous (IV) fluids provide no nutrition.

Oral rehydration and feeds

- Dehydration without shock can generally be managed with oral rehydration fluid and solid or semi-solid feeds, unless there is a contraindication (e.g. imminent surgery).
- Even where vomiting is present, frequent administration of small volumes of fluid are often sufficient; in gastroenteritis, ondansetron may be given to facilitate this.
- If diarrhoea is present, fluid with high sugar content (e.g. undiluted juice or soft drink) should not be given and fortification of formula feeds should cease during the acute illness.

Latest Evidence: Optimal rehydration fluids

In mild gastroenteritis, administering preferred fluids may be more beneficial than using standard electrolyte replacement fluids. Fluid with a high sugar content (e.g. juice or soft drink) should be diluted.

Nasogastric feeds

Nasogastric (NG) fluids may be given where oral feeds have been unsuccessful.

- NG fluids are less likely to be associated with electrolyte imbalances compared with intravenous (IV) fluids, but an NG tube tends to be poorly tolerated in older children.
  - Rapid NG rehydration using oral rehydration solution at 25 mL/kg/h may be given over 4 hours for most children with gastroenteritis and moderate dehydration.
  - NG rehydration should be slower in infants <6 months old, children with comorbidities, complications such as hypernatraemia and those with significant abdominal pain.

Paediatric Handbook, Tenth Edition. Edited by Kate Harding, Daniel S. Mason and Daryl Efron.
© 2021 John Wiley & Sons Ltd. Published 2021 by John Wiley & Sons Ltd.

- If a child has an existing nasojejunal (NJ) tube, this can also be used for rehydration. NJ tubes are sometimes used for medium- to long-term feeding children at high risk of aspirating or with delayed gastric emptying; *they are not usually placed for acute rehydration.*

Intravenous fluid (outside neonatal period)

Intravenous fluids are used where enteral fluids are not tolerated or contraindicated, or in severe dehydration.

- They are more likely to be associated with electrolyte imbalances and other adverse effects.
- Children receiving intravenous fluid should be clinically assessed and have electrolytes checked regularly (see Principles of safe fluid management below).

Hypovolaemic shock

- Children with shock caused by hypovolaemia should be given parenteral fluid immediately: **administer 20 mL/kg of an isotonic fluid such as 0.9% sodium chloride (NaCl), Plasmalyte148 or Hartmann's solution, then reassess the cardiovascular and hydration state.**
- Fluid can be given IV or via an intraosseous needle.
- NG fluid rehydration is not effective in shock.
- Any child with shock who requires more than 40 mL/kg in fluid boluses should be urgently reviewed to consider the need for vasopressor or inotropic support (it is important to consider the adverse effects of additional fluid boluses on lung function).

Replacement and maintenance therapy

Four basic aspects are considered:
- Existing fluid deficit
- Continuing losses
- Maintenance requirements
- Principles of safe fluid management

Existing fluid deficit/dehydration

The fluid deficit is most reliably estimated from the loss of body weight if a recent pre-illness weight is available. Any loss of weight is equal to the fluid deficit (e.g. if 600g have been lost, there is a fluid deficit of 600 mL, which represents 6% dehydration in a 10 kg child).

Clinical signs may be used to determine approximate fluid deficit; these signs are an approximate guide:

- **Mild dehydration (<4%)**
  ○ Thirst, but usually no clinical signs
- **Moderate dehydration (4–6%)**
  ○ Delayed capillary refill time
  ○ Increased respiratory rate
  ○ Mildly decreased tissue turgor
  ○ Dry mucous membranes
  ○ Absent tears
  ○ Sunken fontanelle
  ○ Tachycardia
- **Severe dehydration (≥7%)**
  ○ Sunken eyes
  ○ Very delayed capillary refill >3 seconds, mottled skin
  ○ Tachycardia, low pulse volume
  ○ Hypotension or narrowed pulse pressure
  ○ Central nervous system signs of shock (irritable, lethargic or reduced conscious level)
  ○ Deep, acidotic breathing
  ○ Decreased tissue turgor
  ○ Oliguria

Clinical Pearl: Hypotension in the dehydrated child

In children, hypotension is a late sign and should warrant escalation of care. Normal blood pressure does not exclude severe dehydration or shock.

- The child's weight as well as the estimated degree of dehydration can be used to calculate an approximate fluid deficit (e.g. a 10 kg child who is 7% dehydrated has lost 700 mL of fluid).
- In general, intravenous fluids to replace the existing deficit are given over the first 24 hours using an isotonic fluid with a similar sodium concentration to plasma.
- For hypernatraemic or hyponatraemic dehydration, they should be given over at least 48–72 hours (see hypernatraemia and hyponatraemia below).

Continuing losses
- Fluid balance charts should accurately record – volumes of vomitus, gastric aspirates, drainage from fistulae/stoma, diarrhoea, urine output and other fluid losses to guide fluid replacement.
- In practice, it can be difficult to accurately measure all losses; *body weight should be measured regularly (at least daily)*, as this is an important marker of ongoing losses and hydration status.

Maintenance requirements
Maintenance fluid requirement is the daily water requirement for well children to excrete an iso-osmotic urine (Table 7.1 & 7.2). This is relatively high (per kg of bodyweight) in infancy and gradually decreases throughout childhood. indicate the maintenance volumes required in well children. This volume differs in disease states.
- Many acutely ill children have high levels of **antidiuretic hormone (ADH)**, resulting in reduced free water excretion. This particularly occurs in children after surgery and those with brain or lung disease (meningitis, encephalitis, bronchiolitis, pneumonia), although many other hospitalised children have high ADH levels.
- As urinary output is reduced, the total fluid required to maintain normal intravascular volume is reduced.
- If these children receive maintenance IV fluid at standard rates, fluid overload and hyponatraemia may occur.

Clinical Pearl: Fluids in children with risk of inappropriately high ADH

In children at particular risk of inappropriately high ADH, a total fluid intake (TFI) of about 60% of the usual maintenance volumes should be the starting point for IV administered fluid.

- In contrast, some sick children will have increased fluid requirements (e.g. those with high fever, capillary leak, third-spacing of fluid into the abdomen or those with continuing losses). These children may need more than the standard maintenance fluid rate to maintain normal hydration.

Table 7.1 Daily maintenance intravenous fluid requirements.

Bodyweight	Requirements
3–10 kg	100 mL/kg per day
10–20 kg	1000 mL + (50 mL/kg per day for each kg over 10 kg)
20 kg and over	1500 mL + (20 mL/kg per day for each kg over 20 kg)

Table 7.2 Hourly maintenance intravenous fluid requirements.

Bodyweight	Requirements
3–10 kg	4 mL/kg/h
10–20 kg	40 mL + (2 mL/kg/h for each kg over 10 kg)
20 kg and over	60 mL + (1 mL/kg/h for each kg over 20 kg)

Table 7.3 Commonly used intravenous solutions.

	Na+ mmol/L	Cl– mmol/L	K+ mmol/L	Lactate mmol/L	Ca2+ mmol/L	Glucose g/L
0.9% NaCl (isotonic)	154	154	–	–	–	–
0.9% NaCl with 5% glucose and 20 mmol/L of potassium chloride (isotonic)	154	174	20			50
0.45% NaCl with 5% glucose (hypotonic)	77	77	–	–	–	50
Plasmalyte148 solution (isotonic)	130	110	5	30	2	–
Plasmalyte148 solution with 5% glucose (isotonic)	130	110	5	30	2	50
Hartmann's solution (similar in ionic composition to Ringer's lactate) (isotonic)	131	111	5	–	2	29

- Prescribing fluid volumes can be complex; some ill children have clinical features that imply a need for increased *and* decreased fluids. These children need regular assessments, including weight, to ensure adequate hydration is achieved.
- In general, maintenance fluids should be isotonic, containing a similar sodium concentration as plasma (Table 7.3). A glucose concentration of 5% is generally recommended.
- 0.45% NaCl (or 1/2 saline) contains 77 mmol/L of sodium, and 0.18% NaCl (or 1/5 saline) contains only 30 mmol/L of sodium. These are hypotonic fluids and are **not** appropriate for maintenance hydration.

Clinical Pearl: 0.9% NaCl
0.9% NaCl contains a higher chloride concentration than plasma. This can lead to hyperchloraemic acidosis – particularly if large volumes are given or if additional potassium chloride is added. If this occurs, consider using a balanced fluid, such as Plasma-Lyte148 or Hartmann solution instead.

Principles of safe fluid management
Calculate the total fluid intake (TFI)
Calculate the TFI once a day in both mL/h and in mL/kg/day. The prescribed TFI should take into account: deficit replacement + maintenance + estimation of continuing losses.
   Remember to factor in the following:
- IV fluid for drug lines
- Blood products
- Enteral feeds
- Any other fluid intake

The balance of enteral and parenteral fluid should be adjusted around this prescribed TFI.

Regular monitoring
The key to good fluid management is regular clinical monitoring. Signs of dehydration should be corrected, but signs of overhydration, such as rapid weight gain and eyelid oedema, avoided.
- Children receiving IV fluids must be weighed at least every day.
- Children receiving deficit replacement fluid should be weighed at least every 6 hours.

- In a child on maintenance fluid an increase in weight of 5% or more over 24 hours is likely to indicate fluid overload. Manage by stopping or slowing IV fluids, measure serum sodium and consult senior medical staff. A decrease in weight of 5% or more is likely to indicate dehydration.
- Assess for oedema every day. Check for eyelid and lower limb swelling. If either is present, stop or slow IV fluids and consult senior medical staff.
- Check serum electrolytes and glucose at least daily. Senior medical staff should be consulted if:
  - Serum sodium is ≤130 mmol/L or has fallen by >5 mmol/L (even within normal limits).
  - Serum sodium is ≥150 mmol/L or has risen by >5 mmol/L (even within normal limits).

Acid–base problems

- The maintenance of pH within narrow limits is a result of two mechanisms.
  - Buffer systems: the bicarbonate system is quantitatively the most important in plasma (70% of total).
  - Excretory mechanisms: via the kidneys and lungs.
- Acidosis (low pH) and alkalosis (high pH) may be respiratory or metabolic in origin (Table 7.4).

The four primary disorders are:

1. **Metabolic acidosis.**
   This is due to:
   - Increased production of acid (e.g. ketoacids and lactic acid);
   - Failure of the kidney to excrete acid or conserve base; and
   - Excess loss of buffer base (e.g. gastroenteritis or intestinal fistula).
2. **Metabolic alkalosis.**
   This is due to:
   - Excess loss of acid (e.g. pyloric stenosis);
   - Excess intake of buffer (e.g. bicarbonate infusion); and
   - Conditions where hydrogen ions are lost in the urine (e.g. renal tubular syndromes, diuretic therapy) or from vomiting (e.g. pyloric stenosis).
3. **Respiratory acidosis**
   - Hypercapnia is the result of alveolar hypoventilation from any cause (e.g. central, neuromuscular or pulmonary disease).
4. **Respiratory alkalosis.**
   - This is caused by hyperventilation.
   - Blood gas abnormalities are often mixed, with a metabolic and a respiratory component.
   - Usually one is the primary disorder and the other occurs secondary and tends to correct the change in pH.
   - However, sometimes primary metabolic and respiratory disturbances occur together; for example in severe acute respiratory distress syndrome (ARDS), acidosis may be caused by both carbon dioxide retention resulting in respiratory acidosis and hypoxia or sepsis leading to lactic acid accumulation and subsequent metabolic acidosis (Table 7.5).

Table 7.4 Changes in arterial capillary blood (before compensation).

	pH (mmol/L)	Pco_2 (mmHg)	Base excess (mmol/L)	Actual bicarbonate (mmol/L)
Normal range	7.36–7.44	36–44	−5 to +3	18–25
Metabolic acidosis	Decrease	Normal	Decrease	Decrease
Metabolic alkalosis	Increase	Normal	Increase	Increase
Respiratory acidosis	Decrease	Increase	Normal	Normal
Respiratory alkalosis	Increase	Decrease	Normal	Normal

Table 7.5 Change in indicators of acid–base status seen in combined disorders.

	pH (mmol/L)	P_{CO_2} (mmHg)	Base excess (mmol/L)	Actual bicarbonate (mmol/L)
Normal range	7.36–7.44	36–44	–5 to +3	18–25
Primary metabolic acidosis + compensatory respiratory alkalosis (e.g. gastroenteritis, diabetic ketosis)	Decrease or normal	Decrease	Decrease	Decrease
Primary metabolic alkalosis + compensatory respiratory acidosis (e.g. pyloric stenosis)	Increase or normal	Increase	Increase	Increase
Combined primary respiratory and metabolic acidosis (e.g. respiratory distress syndrome)	Decrease	Increase	Decrease	Normal or low

Hyperkalaemia

Potassium may be elevated as an artefact where haemolysis is present. This is more common on a capillary specimen or where venepuncture has been difficult. If hyperkalaemia is an unexpected finding, consider repeating the sample using venepuncture.

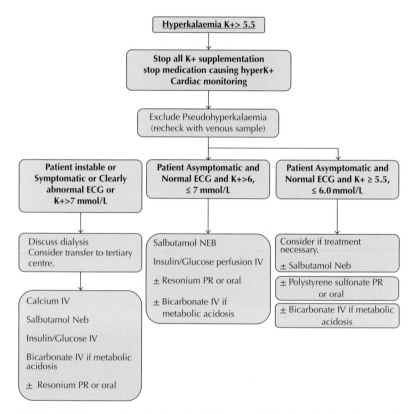

Figure 7.1 Hyperkalaemia support algorithm. *Source*: Royal Children's Hospital Clinical Practice Gudelines – Hyperkalaemia. Reproduced with permission of the Royal Children's Hospital.

- The management of hyperkalaemia depends on the underlying cause (Figure 7.1). Causes include:
  - Decreased excretion (e.g. renal failure, mineralocorticoid deficiency)
  - Transcellular shift (e.g. acidosis)
  - Increased production (e.g. trauma, rhabdomyolysis)
  - Exogenous source (e.g. ingestion, iatrogenic)
  - Medication (e.g. potassium sparing diuretic)
- A 12-lead ECG should be obtained. Indications of a conduction disturbance include
  - Peaked T wave (early)
  - Prolonged PR, flattening of P wave, widening of QRS (increased risk of arrhythmia)
  - Absence of P wave, sine wave (fusion of QRS and T wave)
  - Ventricular arrhythmia, asystole

Clinical Pearl: hyperkalemia & arrhythmia
A normal ECG does not eliminate the risk of subsequent arrhythmia in hyperkalaemia.

If cardiac arrhythmias or severe hyperkalaemia are present, rapid but temporary benefit may be achieved by giving (while arranging dialysis).
- Salbutamol nebulizer.
- Short-acting (regular) insulin 0.1 unit/kg given with 10 ml/kg of IV 10% dextrose.
- IV sodium bicarbonate 2 mmol/kg.
- IV calcium gluconate 10% 0.5 mL/kg, given slowly Rectal or NG sodium polystyrene sulfonate (Resonium) 1 g/kg may also be given to reduce total body potassium, but has a longer onset of action.

Hypokalaemia
Metabolic alkalosis may cause hypokalaemia, but this resolves if alkalosis is treated. Severe hypokalaemia causes long QT interval, often with prominent U waves. Management is usually sufficient with supplementation of oral potassium or by adding potassium to IV maintenance fluid.
- Potassium should rarely be given faster than 0.2 mmol/kg/h and never faster than 0.4 mmol/kg/h. ECG monitoring should be considered with potassium replacement at those rates, and infusions of concentrated solutions should be controlled with the use of a pump.
- Concentrated potassium infusions can cause chemical burns if extravasation occurs. Concentrations of potassium >40 mmol/L should be used with extreme caution and generally only through a central line. Infusions of potassium at concentrations of ≥60 mmol/L should only be given in the intensive care unit.
- In hyperkalaemia and hypokalaemia the causes should always be identified and treated.

Hypernatraemia
Hypernatraemia is most frequently due to a water deficit (e.g. increased losses or reduced intake). In rare cases it is due to an increase in total body sodium (e.g. ingestion of large quantities of sodium, incorrect preparation of formula).
- If the patient is shocked, provide volume resuscitation with an isotonic fluid as required in 20 mL/kg boluses (see Hypovolaemic shock above).
- After the correction of shock, the aim is to lower the serum sodium slowly at a rate of no faster than 12 mmol/L in 24 hours (0.5 mmol/L/h). This should be even slower if the hypernatraemia is chronic.

Clinical Pearl: Sodium correction in hypernatremia
Serum sodium levels should be corrected slowly; if sodium is corrected too rapidly, cerebral oedema, seizures and permanent brain injury may occur. Monitor and manage for concurrent hyperglycaemia and other electrolyte abnormalities.

Moderate hypernatraemic dehydration, [Na⁺] 150–169 mmol/L
After initial resuscitation, replace the deficit plus maintenance **over 48 hours**.
- Use nasogastric oral rehydration solution (Gastrolyte) where possible, but remember that Gastrolyte has a lower sodium concentration than plasma (60 mmol/L). Electrolytes will need to be monitored.

- If requiring IV rehydration use **an isotonic fluid with glucose**. Add maintenance KCl if required once urine output is established.
  - Initial daily volume (mL) = Daily maintenance fluids (mL) + (remaining fluid deficit (mL)/2)
  - Initial hourly rate (mL/h) = Daily volume (mL)/24(h)
- Check UEC and glucose every hour – if serum sodium is falling faster than 0.5 mmol/h, slow down rate of infusion by 20%. Recheck the serum sodium in 1 hour.
- If after 6 hours of rehydration therapy the sodium is decreasing at a steady rate then check the U&Es and glucose 4 hourly.
- If there are persistent neurological signs, consider urgent cerebral imaging.

Severe hypernatraemic dehydration, [Na⁺] >169

- Consult with intensive care team (as available).
- After initial resuscitation, replace deficit and maintenance with **an isotonic fluid with glucose over 72– 96 hours**.
  - Initial daily volume (mL) = Daily maintenance fluids (mL) + (remaining fluid deficit (mL)/3)
  - Initial hourly rate (mL/h) = Daily volume (mL)/24 (h)

Hyponatraemia

- Hyponatraemia may be caused by excessive water intake or salt loss.
- Hyponatraemia is frequently iatrogenic, caused by the administration of hypotonic intravenous fluid (fluid containing less sodium than plasma). This is worsened when ADH levels are elevated, leading to reduced excretion of water.

Hyponatraemia with seizures or decreased conscious state

- Resuscitation should occur, including the use of anticonvulsants, where indicated.
- The sodium level should be increased using 4 mL/kg of 3% NaCl intravenously. If central access is readily available, this should be used.
- Ongoing seizures with persistent hyponatraemia will require further 3% NaCl.

Hyponatraemia without symptoms

- A low serum sodium should be corrected slowly, especially if the abnormality is long-standing. It should never be increased faster than 0.5 mmol/L/h and usually an increase of 0.25 mmol/L/h or less is more appropriate.

Clinical Pearl: Sodium correction in Hyponatermia

Serum sodium levels should be corrected slowly; *if sodium is corrected too rapidly in hyponatraemia, cerebral (especially pontine) demyelination and permanent brain injury may occur.*

- Management of asymptomatic hyponatraemia depends on the hydration status and severity of sodium imbalance.
  - If the child has a *normal or increased volume state*, restrict fluids to slowly remove excess water.
  - If the child is *moderately dehydrated with a serum sodium of 130–135 mmol/L*, aim to rehydrate orally or via a nasogastric tube. Note that the sodium concentration of gastrolyte is low (60 mmol/L) – **rapid nasogastric rehydration is not appropriate where hyponatraemia is present**. If it is not possible to give enteral fluid, use isotonic fluid with glucose.
  - Where there is *severe dehydration with a serum sodium of <130 mmol/L*, isotonic fluid should be administered.
- Electrolytes should be monitored regularly (at least every 4 hours) until stable.

The newborn/neonate

- Babies (<4 weeks of age) are different from older children because they have
  - Proportionately more body water in all compartments.
  - Greater insensible water losses.

- ○ Higher metabolic requirements.
- ○ Reduced renal capacity to compensate for biochemical abnormalities.
- ○ Less integrated and responsive endocrine controls.
- Any baby needing IV therapy should be in a level 2 or level 3 nursery.
- For fluid & electrolyte requirements & management in neonatal patients see chapter 27 Neonatal medicine.

USEFUL RESOURCES
- Royal Children's hospital clinical practice guidelines; succinct and practical guidelines on multiple topics including:
  - ○ https://www.rch.org.au/clinicalguide/guideline_index/Gastroenteritis/
  - ○ https://www.rch.org.au/clinicalguide/guideline_index/Dehydration/
  - ○ https://www.rch.org.au/clinicalguide/guideline_index/Intravenous_fluids/
  - ○ https://www.rch.org.au/clinicalguide/guideline_index/Hypokalaemia/
  - ○ https://www.rch.org.au/clinicalguide/guideline_index/Hyperkalaemia/
  - ○ https://www.rch.org.au/clinicalguide/guideline_index/Hyponatraemia/
  - ○ https://www.rch.org.au/clinicalguide/guideline_index/Hypernatraemia/
  - ○ https://www.bettersafercare.vic.gov.au/resources/clinical-guidance/maternity-and-newborn

CHAPTER 8

Prescribing and therapeutics

Noel Cranswick
Antun Bogovic
David Metz

Key Points
- Dosing in children depends upon both age and size (as well as kidney and liver function).
- Care should be taken in dose calculation and based upon current weight (unless in an emergency).
- All suspected adverse drug reactions should be reported – for the benefit of the individual and the community.
- Pharmacogenomic testing has an expanding role in identifying individuals at risk of specific serious adverse drug reactions and guiding therapies.
- Knowledge of the medicines with high potential for harm (e.g. with the acronym APINCHS), and resources to check for drug interactions, can help to minimize iatrogenic adverse outcomes.

Knowledge of how children and infants differ physiologically and pharmacologically from adults, and how their bodies handle and respond to medicines and approved drugs, is essential to the practice of paediatrics. Most registered medicines do not have licensed (official medication body) indications or dosing for children, and we rely on specialist paediatric information sources to provide guidance.

Unlicensed and off-label drug use
These are commonplace in paediatric practice as a result of inadequate paediatric data.
- *Unlicensed drug* use is the use of
  - a drug that has not been approved by the Therapeutic Goods Administration (TGA), **or**
  - an untested formulation of an approved drug, **or**
  - a non-pharmacopoeial substance as a medicine.
- *Off-label prescribing* is the use of a drug in a manner other than that recommended in the manufacturer's product information.

Dosing in children
The major determinants of dose size and frequency in children are body size and organ function (kidneys and liver). Dosage regimens thus need to account for:
- Age (due to immaturity of renal and hepatic drug clearance in infancy)
- Body size (with dose scaled to appropriate size metric, see Dose calculation)
- Renal or hepatic disease

Paediatric Handbook, Tenth Edition. Edited by Kate Harding, Daniel S. Mason and Daryl Efron.
© 2021 John Wiley & Sons Ltd. Published 2021 by John Wiley & Sons Ltd.

Table 8.1 Guidelines for best prescribing practice.

DO check the dose:
- Use a calculator for dosing by weight/BSA
- Ensure it does not exceed the maximum adult dose

DO check for allergies and contraindications

DO write legibly

DO write UNITS (not IU) after insulin doses – and other medications where the dose is expressed as 'units'

DO include generic drug name. Generic names should always be used – avoid trade names if possible. Dose, frequency, route and date of start, finish or review should also be provided.

DO only use recognised abbreviations for prescription instructions

Do refer to accepted RCH and paediatric prescribing and dosing formulary, including local clinical practice guidelines.

DO write a leading zero before a decimal point, for example 0.6 mg not .6 mg

DO NOT write a trailing zero after a whole number, for example 8 mg not 8.0 mg

DO NOT abbreviate drug names, for example AZT could be azathioprine or azithromycin

Source: Courtesy of the Pharmacy Department, The Royal Children's Hospital, Melbourne.

Dose calculation

- Most medicines in children are dosed by weight. Of note, the per-kilogram total daily dose (e.g. mg of medicine per kg of child weight) may differ by age strata, e.g. a higher per-kilogram total daily dose in pre-school age than older children. Infants also require a separate dose size +/- frequency, due to immaturity of clearance mechanisms.
- Alternatively, some medications such as cytotoxic drugs are dosed by body surface area.
- Always attempt to obtain an accurate weight before calculating the appropriate initial dose. Height is required for dosing by BSA.
- In an emergency, a child's weight (in kg) can be estimated by the formula (age + 4) × 2 for children aged from 1 to 8 years. Standardised centile charts for weight and height may be utilised for BSA calculations.
- Remember to confirm an accurate weight +/- height at the first available opportunity.
- Consider using ideal body weight in obese children (BMI >95th% for age and sex).
- See general guidelines in Table 8.1.

Drug errors

The Australian Commission on Safety and Quality in Healthcare has defined the acronym APINCHS (from the original APINCH), to identify groups of medicines associated with high potential for medication-related harm, wherein extra care should be taken when prescribing:

- **A**ntimicrobials: aminoglycosides, vancomycin, amphotericin
- **P**otassium and other electrolytes (including K, Mg, Ca, 50% dextrose, hypertonic sodium chloride)
- **I**nsulins
- **N**arcotics and other sedatives
- **C**hemotherapeutics
- **H**eparin and other anticoagulants
- **S**ystems (as a reminder to use medication safety systems such as independent double checks, safe administration of liquid medications, standardised order sets and medication charts etc.)

Children are at increased risk of drug errors due to the need for dose calculation and changing dose with age.

- Errors in the prescription of IV fluids are also more frequent in children and may have more severe outcomes. Administration rate of IV fluids (including parenteral nutrition) must take into account concurrent administration of oral and enteral fluids.

- A safety check that is frequently effective in adults, to reassess the dose if more than one ampoule of the drug is required, does not provide as much assurance with paediatrics. A small child can be severely overdosed on administration of less than a single ampoule.

When prescribing for children, the following factors should be taken into consideration:
- Children's doses vary widely and so there is no standard dose (as there is with adults).
- Clarify if drug doses are given in mg/kg per day in divided doses (or mg/kg per dose given x times per day). When prescribing, always write as **mg/kg per dose given x times per day.**
- Calculations are required for most childhood dosing and errors may occur during this step.
- Some paediatric preparations may cause confusion in those unfamiliar with their use, for example IV versus enteral paracetamol, or Painstop Night-Time (which contains three active agents) vs other paracetamol containing products.
- The small doses used in children may cause measuring and administration errors.
- Misplacing or misreading of decimal points can lead to error.

Therapeutic drug monitoring
Relatively few drugs need therapeutic drug monitoring (TDM).
- TDM can be useful for
  - Antibiotics e.g. gentamicin, vancomycin.
  - Anticonvulsants, e.g. phenytoin, phenobarbitone.
  - Immunosuppressants e.g. tacrolimus, cyclosporin, mycophenolic acid, methotrexate.
  - Drug overdose e.g. paracetamol, iron.
- Routine testing is not beneficial for
  - Carbamazepine
  - Valproate
- Most benefit will be derived from reference to specific monitoring programs and guidelines e.g. www.rch.org.au/clinicalguide/guideline_index/Vancomycin/, or through liaison with specialist services.
- Timing of samples for monitoring will vary depending upon the actual drug but accurate recording of the drug dose, administration time and sample time is essential.

Nonlinear kinetics
Most drugs involved in TDM have *linear* kinetics within the range of doses used, whereby concentration increases proportionally with dose. For drugs with *nonlinear* kinetics e.g. phenytoin being the most commonly encountered example, small dose increments can lead to large increases in drug concentrations, leading to adverse effects. Particular care is required at the upper end of the dosing range.

Latest Evidence: Model-informed precision dosing
For certain high-risk drugs or scenarios, drug safety and effectiveness can be further enhanced by adjusting dose based on estimation of an individual's pharmacokinetics, rather than single drug concentrations in isolation. Clinical benefit of 'model-informed precision dosing' has been shown in prospective trials for the immunosuppressant mycophenolic acid and the antimicrobial vancomycin, with supportive data for various other immunosuppressants, cytotoxic agents and antimicrobials.

Pharmacogenomics
Certain individuals are at increased risk of toxicities or inefficacy to a drug due to polymorphisms in genes that produce drug metabolizing enzymes, drug transporters or drug receptors. These include:
- HLA-B*5701 and abacavir/flucloxacillin
- HLA-B*5801 and allopurinol (important in Han-Chinese, Thai, Korean populations)
- HLA-B*1502 and carbamazepine/oxcarbazine (important in Asian populations)
- Thiopurine methyltransferase (TPMT) and azathioprine/mercaptopurines
- CYP2D6 and codeine inefficacy/toxicity
The Pharmacogenomics Knowledge Base (www.pharmgkb.org) provides guidance on indications for and use of pharmacogenomic testing.

Adverse drug reactions (ADRs)

ADRs are common but under-recognised in children.

- All suspected and proven ADRs should be reported, even if seemingly trivial. For types see Table 8.2.
- Reporting ADRs benefits the individual (through facilitation of further assessment where appropriate, or documentation of need for avoidance) and the community (through ongoing pharmacovigilance assessment of the safety profile of drugs).
- The relevant points to document on history are:
  - The illness the medication was prescribed for, as it may be causing confusion with symptoms or contributing to the ADR (e.g. intercurrent viral infections may also cause urticaria).
  - The name of the medication and preparation.
  - Whether this was the first exposure to the medication.
  - The time of onset of the reaction, and lag in time from the last dose given.
  - How many doses were given before a reaction occurred?
  - The symptoms of the reaction and its total duration.
  - Any other reactions or allergies the child may have OR a family history of reaction/allergy?
- Suspected allergic reactions should be assessed and followed up (e.g. by a drug allergy clinic). This allows for confirmatory testing, testing for cross-reactivity and, in some instances, 'de-labeling' (see Antibiotics and skin reactions)
- When an avoidable ADR is identified, children should be given a permanent record (e.g. card or medical alert bracelet) as appropriate.

There may be variation in the ADRs experienced in different age group (e.g. neonates, children, adolescents). Some specific examples include:

- Jaundice (hyperbilirubinemia) in neonates or very young children taking sulfur-containing drugs, such as cotrimoxazole.
- Biliary sludging with neonates/very young children receiving ceftriaxone.
- Grey baby syndrome associated with chloramphenicol – although this drug is now rarely prescribed.
- Valproic acid hepatotoxicity in early childhood.
- Reye syndrome in children receiving moderate to high doses of aspirin.
- Cefaclor and serum-sickness like reaction.
- Prednisolone and reduced height velocity.

Antibiotics and skin reactions

One of the most common ADR presentations in children is a non-specific skin rash following the commencement of an antibiotic. These children should be followed up with confirmatory tests (e.g. intradermal or controlled oral re-challenge in a specialist facility). The majority of children who are tested are found not to be allergic to or intolerant of the antibiotic.

Table 8.2 Types of ADRs.

Type A	Type B
Predictable from the known pharmacology of the drug. Dose dependent.	Uncommon. Generally unpredictable. Not clearly dose dependent.
Examples: • opiate sedation • tachycardia with β_2-agonists	Include: • Immunoallergic (Gell & Coombs Type 1-4) • Pseudo-allergic • Metabolic intolerances • 'Idiosyncratic' reactions
	Type B reactions can be severe/life-threatening, requiring immediate cessation and ongoing avoidance of the drug (+/- structurally related molecules).
	Important examples include anaphylaxis, and the 'severe cutaneous adverse reactions': • Stevens–Johnson syndrome / Toxic Epidermal necrosis (most commonly associated with anticonvulsants) • **D**rug **R**eaction (or Rash) with **E**osinophilia and **S**ystemic **S**ymptoms (DRESS syndrome)

Drug interactions

Drug interactions are always possible when using more than one medicine, however, only a few drug combinations result in clinically significant sequelae.

- Be aware that drug interactions are more common when:
  - More drugs are prescribed, where possible, aim for monotherapy.
  - Children are sick, especially with multiple organ pathologies.
- Drugs with a narrow therapeutic window are more likely to result in more significant interactions.
- Certain drugs used together can have additive risk, e.g. multiple nephrotoxins increasing the risk of acute kidney injury (NSAIDs, gentamicin, vancomycin, ACE inhibitors), particularly in the setting of dehydration/sepsis.
- Drug interactions do not just occur between drugs that are recognized as traditional pharmaceutical products. They can occur between drugs and:
  - Feeds e.g. azoles and fatty foods, calcineurin inhibitors and grapefruit juice.
  - Supplements e.g. complementary therapies, see below.
  - Fluids and other agents e.g. IV administration of ceftriaxone to neonates receiving fluids containing calcium can cause widespread precipitation, with severe and possibly fatal consequences.
- Interactions listed in reference books can be difficult to interpret. Likelihood and consequences may best be assessed through discussion with specialist pharmacologists or medicines information pharmacists.
- Drug interaction 'checkers' are available in certain electronic formularies, e.g. 'Lexicomp' and 'Medscape'.

Complementary medicines

Specific history of these should be sought, as:

- Complementary medicines and many herbal products are available 'over the counter' or through alternative medicine practitioners.
- Families often do not offer this information, either as they feel uncomfortable in admitting the use such products or they do not consider something 'natural' could cause harm.
- Such products can be involved in ADRs and interactions.

Examples of potential drug interactions with Complementary medicines

- **St John's wort:** anticoagulants, antidepressants, digoxin, MAO inhibitors, dextromethorphan, decreases effects of cyclosporin and antiviral drugs, and prolongs effect of general anaesthetics.
- **Ginseng:** anticoagulants, stimulants, antihypertensives, antidepressants, phenelzine, digoxin, potentiates effects of corticosteroids and oestrogens.
- **Ginger:** anticoagulants, antihypertensives, cardiac drugs, hypoglycaemic drugs and enhances effects of barbiturates.

USEFUL RESOURCES
- Frank Shann's drug doses www.drugdoses.net.
- Australian Prescriber Journal www.australianprescriber.com/ an independent journal with articles relevant to both paediatric and adult prescribing.
- AMH children's dosing companion https://childrens.amh.net.au/ Australian Children's Dosing Guide cover commonly used medicines.
- Prescribing medicines in pregnancy database www.tga.gov.au/hp/medicines-pregnancy.htm
- BNF for Children www.bnf.org/bnf/org 450055.htm.
- Micromedex www.micromedex.com/ a US-based comprehensive database of drug monographs (subscription required).
- The Australian Commission on Safety and Quality in Healthcare www.safetyandquality.gov.au/our-work/medication-safety/.

CHAPTER 9

Immunisation

Daryl Cheng
Nigel Crawford

Key Points
- Timely vaccination is paramount in the prevention and reduction in severity of vaccine preventable diseases (VPD).
- Consumer and health professional resources are helpful for both education, information, and immunisation planning.
- For up-to-date immunisation information, consult the MVEC guidelines or the Australian Immunisation Handbook.
- Report any suspected AEFI via state-based vaccine safety surveillance systems e.g. Victoria- SAEFVIC.
- To help address immunisation queries, stay up to date with the routine immunisation schedule and your local VPD epidemiology.

Since they were first discovered in 1796, immunisations have been a success story of modern public health. They prevent clinical manifestations or substantially reduce severity of a growing number of diseases. In Australia, vaccinations are now captured for all-of-life via the Australian Immunisation Register (AIR). Immunisations are also detailed in the state-based childhood health book and whilst vaccination is not compulsory in Australia, immunisation status must be detailed at childcare and school entry. In recent times, "No Jab No Pay" and "No Jab No Play" policies have been introduced by federal and state governments respectively, with the aim to improve vaccination rates and reduce the spread of vaccine preventable disease.

Modern vaccines are both safe and effective. As a disease becomes less common through a successful immunisation programme, the occurrence and perception of side effects assume greater relative importance. Health care providers may need to explain the risks of the diseases themselves and inform parents clearly that disease complications far outweigh the potential vaccine side effects. With adequate and informed discussion and explanation, parents feel more comfortable about immunising their children.

Health professionals have a responsibility to ascertain the immunisation status of children in their care and to offer due or overdue vaccinations. Every health care visit is an opportunity to do this. The AIR can be used to check vaccination status for all ages (see Useful resources), and electronic health records also enable consumer access to this information. The Australian Commonwealth Government website has extensive information including the latest Australian Immunisation Schedule, parent fact sheets and The Australian Immunisation Handbook as a regularly updated online resource (see Useful resources). The Melbourne Vaccine Education Centre (MVEC) also has local up-to-date resources, including an Immunisation Schedule App (see Useful resources).

Current Australian standard vaccination schedule
Current vaccines, their abbreviations and available forms with trade names are indicated in Table 9.1. The Australian schedule, at 1 April 2019, is shown in Table 9.2. The schedule differs slightly in different states, depending on the vaccine(s) purchased and schedules applicable to specific states are updated regularly and available in The Australian Immunisation Handbook or via state health departments.

Paediatric Handbook, Tenth Edition. Edited by Kate Harding, Daniel S. Mason and Daryl Efron.
© 2021 John Wiley & Sons Ltd. Published 2021 by John Wiley & Sons Ltd.

Table 9.1 Current immunisation schedule vaccines, their abbreviations and available forms with trade names.

Disease	Vaccine	Available products
Diphtheria, tetanus, pertussis, hepatitis B, Haemophilus influenzae type B, polio	DTPa-hepB-Hib-IPV	Infanrix-hexa
Diphtheria, tetanus, pertussis, polio	DTPa-IPV, dTpa-IPV	Infanrix-IPV, Quadracel
Diphtheria, tetanus, pertussis	DTPa, dTpa	Infanrix, Boostrix, Adacel
Diphtheria, tetanus	dT	ADT Vaccine
Haemophilus influenzae type B	Hib (PRP-T)	Act-Hib
Haemophilus influenzae type B – meningococcal C	Hib (PRP-T)-meningococcal C conjugate vaccine	Menitorix
Hepatitis B	HepB	Engerix-B, H-B VaxII
Human papillomavirus	HPV 9-valent vaccine	Gardasil 9
Influenza	Quadrivalent influenza vaccine[a]	Fluquadri Junior, Fluarix-tetra, FluQuadri, Afluria Quad, Influvac Tetra
Measles, mumps, rubella	MMR	MMR II, Priorix
Measles, mumps, rubella, varicella	MMR–VZV	ProQuad, Priorix-Tetra
Meningococcal B disease	MenB	Bexsero, Trumemba
Meningococcal disease A, C, W, Y	4-valent Meningococcal conjugate vaccine	Nimenrix, Menveo, Menactra
Pneumococcal	Pneumococcal	Prevenar 13, Pneumovax 23
Poliomyelitis	IPV	IPOL
Rotavirus	Rotavirus vaccine	Rotarix, RotaTeq
Varicella	VZV	Varilrix, Varivax

[a] For appropriate influenza vaccines for specific age ranges, please refer to Table 9.3.

Table 9.2 Australian immunisation schedule (from 1 April 2019).

Age	Vaccines		
Birth	HepB		
2 months (can be administered from 6 weeks of age)	DTPa-hepB-IPV-Hib	Rotavirus	13vPneumococcal
4 months	DTPa-hepB-IPV-Hib	Rotavirus	13vPneumococcal
6 months[a]	DTPa-hepB-IPV-Hib		
12 months	Men ACWY	MMR	13v Pneumococcal
18 months	DTPa	MMR–Varicella[b]	Hib
4 years	DTPa-IPV		
School year 7	dTap	HPV[c] 2doses	
School Year 10	Men ACWY[d]		

[a] Influenza vaccine can be given to all infants ≥6 months. Children in special risk groups are highly recommended to have an annual influenza vaccine.
[b] Varicella vaccine is funded for infants aged 18 months, administered as combined MMR-V vaccine. This is the second dose of MMR, separated by minimum of 4 weeks.
[c] HPV9 vaccine is funded for males and females aged 12–13 years. Two doses spaced 0, 6 months.
[d] This booster dose commenced from April 2019.

Contraindications to vaccination

There are few complete contraindications. Anaphylaxis to a vaccine or one of its constituents is considered a contraindication and requires allergy specialist assessment. Immunosuppression is generally a contraindication to live vaccines such as BCG, varicella and measles, mumps, rubella (MMR) vaccines, see Immunisation guidelines for various special groups, below, for further information. Consultation with an immunisation specialist is required if there is uncertainty regarding vaccine contraindications.

Vaccine administration

- Cold chain: never use a vaccine if there is any doubt about its safe cold chain storage. Vaccines should be kept in a refrigerator reserved for vaccine/medicine storage at 2–8 °C and never frozen.
- Prevent immunisation errors: always check about a vaccine dose, route of administration and potential side effects before prescribing. If in doubt check, with a pharmacist or immunisation service.
- Post-vaccine observation: Recipients of any vaccine should remain in the vicinity of medical care for approximately 15 minutes. Although anaphylaxis is very rare, it can occur with any vaccine and should be treated with adrenaline urgently; see Chapter 3, Resuscitation and medical emergencies.

Common misconceptions for missing vaccinations

Children may be under-immunised for their age when health professionals miss opportunities to vaccinate, when parents forget appointments or when parents actively oppose vaccination (only 1–2%). Some common misconceptions about vaccination include:
- Natural infection is the best way to achieve immunity.
- Vaccination weakens the immune system or is too much for the immune system to handle.
- Herd immunity is sufficient for protection.
- 'Homeopathic immunisation' is safer and more effective.

Vaccine Confidence

For reasons above, it is essential to address parental concern, to emphasise the well-established risks associated with not vaccinating their child and to provide reassurance about vaccine safety.

There has been some controversy over the introduction of the "No Jab No Pay" and "No Jab No Play" policies. Whilst there has been some criticism of these policies as blunt instruments, there have been signs of their impact on maintaining Australia's childhood immunisation rates as one of the highest in the developed world. As clinicians, it is important to help children and their families understand the legislation and their impacts on the individual situation, but particularly in the context of the risk: benefit evaluation of vaccination.

Other families may be vaccine hesitant, and it is important for clinicians to maintain a balanced and positive approach to what can be an emotional subject. There are a growing number of resources that address vaccine confidence and the effects of vaccines and diseases. These include Vaccine Confidence Project and the Sharing Knowledge About Immunisation (SKAI) initiatives.

Catch-up doses

When infants and children have missed scheduled vaccine doses, a 'catch-up' schedule should be recommended. Sometimes, a catch-up schedule is relatively simple to plan; for example, the 2- and 4-month vaccines can be given 1 month apart, hence a late 2-month vaccine given at 3 months can be followed by the routine 4-month vaccines just 1 month later. Comprehensive catch-up dose information along with an overdue vaccine catchup-calculator is available from the MVEC website.

Adverse events following immunisation (AEFI)

All vaccines are medications and all medications have side effects. For each individual vaccine there are a known list of fairly common, relatively minor symptoms and a small but important, list of significant major side effects.
- The vast majority of adverse events experienced after the scheduled vaccinations are minor (e.g. fever, local redness, swelling or tenderness) and do not contraindicate further doses of the vaccine.
- Parents who have questions regarding potential adverse events should discuss these with their vaccine provider.

Surveillance of adverse events following vaccinations in the community

When symptoms occur in the hours or days after a vaccination, they may be directly due to the vaccine or totally unrelated and coincidental in nature.

- AEFI should never be dismissed and often require individual assessment to provide accurate advice for the family about the actual adverse event and about options for further doses of the same vaccine.
- Maintaining confidence in immunisations following an adverse event is very important.
- Notifying significant or unexpected adverse events is also important to assist with safety monitoring of vaccines used in Australia, via the Adverse Events Following Immunisation – Clinical Assessment Network (AEFI-CAN/SAEFVIC).

Vaccines in the Australian schedule

Pertussis vaccines

Although the pertussis vaccine is highly effective, it does not provide lifelong immunity against disease. There is limited clinical protection against pertussis following a single vaccine dose.

- In childhood, the inactivated acellular combination vaccine is highly effective once the three-dose primary course is completed.
- A childhood pertussis booster is recommended at 4 years of age and again in adolescents, as part of the secondary school immunisation program.
- Adults can contract pertussis 5–10 years after their most recent pertussis vaccine and spread it to infants, causing serious illness.
- The vaccine can be considered for parents, close household contacts and childcare workers who are in contact with infants <6 months of age.
- In particular, pertussis in pregnancy is also now recommended for all mothers between 20 and 32 weeks of pregnancy. This has been shown to protect infants by passive antibody passage and reduced maternal exposure.

Hepatitis B vaccine

Neonatal and infant schedule

This inactivated vaccine is recommended to be given within seven days of birth. Infants born to mothers who are positive for hepatitis B surface antigen should receive passive protection with 100 IU hepatitis B immunoglobulin (0.5 mL) preferably within 12 hours of birth. Their active hepatitis B vaccination should be commenced at the same time. Three further doses of hepatitis B vaccine are required for all infants (Table 9.2).

Preterm infants

Preterm babies do not mount as strong an antibody response to hepatitis B-containing vaccines, so those born at <32 weeks gestation or <2000 g should have a 'booster' given at 12 months of age (Table 9.1).

Pneumococcal vaccines

S. pneumoniae is an important cause of bacterial infections in children. Invasive pneumococcal disease (IPD) includes meningitis, septicaemia and pneumonia. S. pneumonia is also a cause of otitis media. A 7-valent killed conjugate pneumococcal vaccine (PCV7) was licensed for use in Australia in December 2000 and replaced by an extended 13-valent (PCV13) vaccine in 2011. It is highly effective against IPD caused by the 13 vaccine serotypes. The vaccine is safe and effective in children, with the primary doses administered in early infancy due to the high morbidity and mortality in children <2 years of age.

Schedule

Conjugate pneumococcal vaccine (PCV13) is given routinely at 2 and 4 months of age and the third booster at 1 year of age. This change in schedule, moving the third dose from 6 months to 12 months of age occurred in 2018, and will provide protection (immune memory) later into childhood.

- Children with special risk medical conditions (e.g. asplenia, preterm <28 weeks, cystic fibrosis, cardiac disease, nephrotic syndrome, haematological malignancies) are at higher risk of IPD.
- These children are also recommended to have a 23-valent-polysaccharide pneumococcal vaccine at 4–5 years of age and an additional PCV13 at 6 months of age.
- The recommendations for indigenous children living in other areas of Australia vary; refer to The Australian Immunisation Handbook for details.

Meningococcal vaccines

There are at least 13 meningococcal serogroups. Group B is currently the most common in Australia. A vaccine against MenB is licensed in Australia (Bexsero® GSK), but is not currently part of the National Immunisation Program schedule. A second Men B vaccine (Trumemba) is only licensed for children ≥10 years of age and the dose requirements by age are detailed on the MVEC website.

Conjugate 4-valent meningococcal ACWY vaccine

Meningococcal serogroup C was the main cause of disease in the late 1990s to early 2000s and has dramatically decreased following the protein-conjugated group C vaccine introduction in 2003. In 2015 there was an emergence of serogroup W nationally. In addition, serogroup Y disease was also emerging, so an adolescent conjugate ACWY vaccine was introduced by all states and territories to ensure broader coverage. In 2018, this MenACWY vaccine (Nimenrix) was included on the NIP at 12 months of age and at 14–16 years of age in 2019. (Table 9.2). These vaccines are safe and effective at preventing group ACWY meningococcal disease at all ages. The killed conjugate vaccine does provide long-term immunity, with boosters recommended at 5 years for at risk SRG.

A single MenACWY vaccine is given routinely to all 1-year olds. Whilst meningococcal ACWY disease is rare under the age of 1 year, families can choose to purchase the vaccine for infants from 6 weeks of age. Infant doses under 12 months of age still require the booster dose at 1 year of age to provide lasting immunity. Newly arrived refugees should receive a catch-up meningococcal ACWY vaccine. See Chapter 35, Refugee health, for further details on this group of children.

MMR vaccine

Two doses of live-attenuated MMR vaccine are given to improve serum immune response and long-term protection. The two doses were previously given at 12 months and 4 years, since July 2013 it has been given at 12 months and 18 months of age. The 18-month dose includes varicella (chickenpox), as MMR-V.

- If children are travelling overseas to a measles endemic country, we recommend an early additional dose from >6-months of age. These children will still require the routine doses at 12 and 18 months.
- The MMR vaccine is safe for children with egg allergy or anaphylaxis, as the vaccine is produced in chicken fibroblast cell cultures, not eggs.
- There is no link between MMR vaccination an autistic spectrum disorder. Families with further concerns about this topic should discuss them with a specialist.

Co-administration with other vaccines

The MMR vaccine can be given on the same day as the varicella vaccine, at a separate site. If MMR is not given on the same day as the separate varicella vaccine, they should be spaced at least 4 weeks apart. MMR-V is recommended to be the second dose of MMR vaccine, administered at 18 months of age.

Post-exposure prophylaxis

The MMR vaccine can be administered to susceptible contacts >9 months of age within 72 hours of exposure to measles as post-exposure prophylaxis. NHIG can be given within 7 days of contact as an alternative for those with contraindications to MMR such as immunosuppression.

Previous proven measles, mumps or rubella

Children require protection from all components of MMR. Monovalent measles vaccine is not available in Australia. As vaccination of children who have been previously infected with any of the three components of this vaccine is not dangerous, MMR should be given to all children.

Varicella vaccine

Chickenpox disease used to be considered a childhood rite of passage, however, many children are hospitalised, and a few die each year in Australia from chickenpox. The most common complication is secondary bacterial infection of varicella skin lesions, but more severe sequelae include pneumonitis and encephalitis.

How many varicella doses? One or two?

Varicella vaccine is a live attenuated vaccine, highly effective against severe varicella disease. When a single dose is used the chance of mild breakthrough cases is about 7% in the next 10 years. The USA introduced a two-dose schedule in 2006 to reduce the rate of breakthrough varicella from 7% to 2%. Australia currently only funds a single dose, but a second dose can be considered and bought privately (a minimum of 4 weeks between doses).

Who should be given varicella vaccine?

- According to the 2019 schedule, a single varicella vaccine at 18 months of age is recommended for all immunocompetent children who do not have a definite history of varicella. Families can purchase this dose earlier if required. The vaccine is not required if they have had confirmed chickenpox infection, although it is safe to give if uncertain.
- Individuals ≥14 years of age without a definite history of chickenpox and those with serologically proven non-immunity, are recommended two doses, at least 4 weeks apart.
- Varicella vaccine should be spaced at least 4 weeks apart from the MMR, if it is not given on the same day.
- It is highly recommended for non-immune health care workers and family members who are in contact with immunosuppressed subjects.
- Health care workers with a negative or uncertain history of varicella should have serology checked and vaccinated if negative. Checking serology after vaccination is not routinely needed.
- Non-immune women immediately postpartum or women planning a pregnancy should be given two doses of varicella vaccine ≥4 weeks apart and should not become pregnant for 1 month after a varicella vaccine dose.

Note: Approximately 40% of adults who do not think they have had chickenpox are found to be immune on serology and do not need vaccination. However, there is no known harm giving the vaccine to immune subjects.

Varicella vaccine rash

Rash and/or fever can occur in 2–5% of vaccines during a period of 5 days to 3 weeks after the vaccine. This can occur over the injection site or be generalised, and the appearance is either maculopapular or vesicular. Although rare, varicella vaccine virus can be spread from vesicular rash lesions. If children develop a rash they should avoid contact with immunocompromised persons for the duration of the rash. If a health care worker develops a vesicular rash following the vaccine, they should be reassigned to duties that do not require patient contact or placed on sick leave for the duration of the rash (not for 4–6 weeks as the product information states) usually <1 week. Florid vesicular rash after the vaccine is highly suspicious of wild-type varicella.

Post-exposure prophylaxis

Varicella vaccine is effective in preventing varicella in those already exposed if used within 3–5 days, with earlier administration preferable. It is not 100% effective but, as with pre-exposure vaccination, if breakthrough varicella occurs it is usually milder. Post-exposure varicella vaccine can be considered in children >9 months of age, with a second dose still recommended at the routine 18 months of age.

Oral rotavirus vaccine

Rotavirus is the leading cause of severe childhood gastroenteritis in children <5 years. There are at least four main serotypes. Infection with any two of the natural strains provides broad protection to most children.

Schedule

The vaccine currently on the National Immunisation Program (NIP) is: Rotarix, two doses, given at the routine 2- and 4-month immunisations. The rotavirus vaccines have been associated with a very small increased risk of intussusception (two additional cases of intussusception among every 100,000 infants vaccinated, or 14 additional cases per year in infants in Australia). Therefore, Rotarix is recommended for use in children within the specified age range: first dose is recommended by 14 weeks and second dose by 24 weeks. The vaccine is not licensed or funded for use beyond these age limits and hence infants late for the routine immunisation doses may miss out on a rotavirus vaccine dose. Knowledge of this should encourage parents and immunisation providers to have the 2- and 4-month immunisations on time. Preterm and hospitalised infants can have the oral rotavirus vaccine.

Contraindications

There are some groups of infants for whom this live attenuated vaccine is contraindicated:

- Infants with severe combined immunodeficiency (SCID).
- Previous history of intussusception or a congenital abnormality that may predispose to intussusception.
- Anaphylaxis following a previous dose of either rotavirus vaccine.

Human papillomavirus vaccine

Human papillomavirus (HPV) is responsible for most cervical carcinoma in females, as well as anogenital warts in both sexes. There are multiple types with approximately 70% cervical carcinoma caused by types 16 and 18. HPV types 6 and 11 are responsible for 90% of genital warts. Two killed vaccines are licensed in Australia, derived from inactive virus-like particles. Gardasil9 contains types 6, 11, 16, 18, 31, 33, 45, 52, 58 and Cervarix contains types 16 and 18.

Schedule

The funded Australian HPV vaccine program is with the 9-valent HPV vaccine (Gardasil) and since 2013, has been recommended for both sexes. The female HPV program commenced in 2007 and has already had an impact on cervical cancer screening programs and the incidence of anogenital warts. The vaccine is administered as part of the secondary school program or at the local doctor at age 12–13 years. The HPV vaccination is most effective when it is given before exposure to HPV. Even if young people have already begun to have sexual contact, the HPV vaccine will provide excellent protection against types an individual may not have been exposed to. The two doses are administered 6 months apart. There is no need to recommence the schedule if there is a delay between doses. Special risk immunocompromised groups are recommended to have a 3-dose course at 0, 2 and 6 months.

Influenza vaccine

Schedule

All children and adolescents, >6 months of age, can have the annual influenza vaccine. It is funded for all children aged between 6 months and 5 years of age, and children of all ages with medical special risk conditions that predispose them to an increased risk of influenza-related complications. This includes children with chronic illnesses requiring regular medical follow-up, such as chronic suppurative lung disease (e.g. cystic fibrosis), congenital cardiac disease and those receiving immunosuppressive treatments (e.g. childhood cancer). Health care workers and family members of those at increased risk of severe influenza disease are highly recommended to be vaccinated to reduce risk of transmission to at-risk individuals.

Vaccine dose

The dose requirements vary by age and are detailed in Tables 9.3 and 9.4. In children 9 years and under, two doses are recommended in the first year that an annual influenza vaccine is received.

Clinical Pearl: Influenza vaccine

- The majority of influenza vaccines are inactivated and currently contain four strains (two Type A and two Type B influenza). This is updated annually based on virulence patterns worldwide.
- Influenza vaccine can be administered concurrently with most childhood vaccinations.
- Influenza vaccination is carried out during a season where it is common to have regular intercurrent illness. Symptoms post vaccine may be due to the killed vaccine dose or may be due to a coincidental intercurrent illness.

Table 9.3 Influenza vaccine brand and dosing guidelines for children aged <5 years.

Age group	Brand and dose		
	FluQuadri Junior®	Fluarix-tetra®	FluQuadri®
<6-months	Too young to receive vaccine [N/A]		
≥6-months to <3-years*,˟	0.25 mL	0.5 mL	N/A
3-years to <5-years*,˟	N/A	0.5 mL	0.5 mL

* 2 doses, minimum of 4 weeks apart should be given to children in this age group in the first year of receiving the influenza vaccine.
˟ For all children < 9-years, a single dose is recommended in subsequent years.
N/A not registered for use in this age group.
Source: Melbourne Vaccine Education Centre (MVEC) 2019. https://mvec.mcri.edu.au/immunisation-references/influenza-vaccine-recommendations/. Reproduced with permission of MVEC.

Table 9.4 Influenza vaccine brand and dosing guidelines for 5-years to ≤64-years.

Age group	Brand and dose			
	Fluarix-tetra®	FluQuadri®	Afluria Quad®	Influvac tetra®
5-years to <9-years*,¥	0.5 mL	0.5 mL	0.5 mL	N/A
9-years to <18-years	0.5 mL	0.5 mL	0.5 mL	N/A
18-years to ≤64-years	0.5 mL	0.5 mL	0.5 mL	0.5 mL

* 2 doses, minimum of 4 weeks apart should be given to children in this age group in the first year of receiving the influenza vaccine.
¥ For all children <9-years, a single dose is recommended in subsequent years.
N/A not registered for use in this age group.
Source: Melbourne Vaccine Education Centre (MVEC) 2019. https://mvec.mcri.edu.au/immunisation-references/influenza-vaccine-recommendations/. Reproduced with permission of MVEC.

Immunisation guidelines for various special groups
Additional vaccine requirements for consideration
- Some preterm infants require additional hepatitis B and pneumococcal vaccines. For infants born
  - <28 weeks gestation: Pneumococcal conjugate vaccine and hepatitis B vaccine at 12 months, pneumococcal polysaccharide vaccine at 4 years.
  - <32 weeks gestation and/or <2000 g birth weight: Hepatitis B vaccine at 12 months of age.
- Aboriginal and Torres Strait Islander (ATSI) children require additional influenza, meningococcal and pneumococcal vaccines.

Vaccines in the setting of immunosuppression
Live vaccines (e.g. varicella vaccine, MMR, BCG) are generally not recommended for immunosuppressed individuals.
- Children who have recently received high-dose oral steroids (prednisolone 2 mg/kg per day for >1 week, or 1 mg/kg per day for >1 month):
  - Delay live vaccine administration until at least 1 month after treatment has stopped.
  - The use of inhaled steroids is not a contraindication to vaccination with either live or inactivated vaccines.
- Children who have recently received immunoglobulin products:
  - Varicella vaccine should be delayed for 5 months in children who have received zoster immunoglobulin.
  - Delay MMR and varicella for 9–11 months if immunoglobulin has recently been given to avoid potential reduced effectiveness of the vaccine(s).
- Children who have received bone marrow transplants:
  - Require booster doses or complete revaccination, depending on their serological and clinical status, as per guidelines in the Australian Immunisation Handbook.
- Children who receive cancer chemotherapy:
  - Require booster doses 6 months after completion of treatment
  - Inactivated vaccines (such as pertussis), modified toxins (such as diphtheria and tetanus vaccines) and subunit vaccines (such as Hib and hepatitis B vaccines) can be safely given to children receiving immunosuppressive treatments, but may produce a diminished serum immune response and additional doses are recommended.
  - Influenza vaccine is an important safe vaccine for children with immunosuppression, even though it may not work optimally because of the reduced immune function.
- Children on disease modifying agents (e.g. monoclonal antibody treatment).
- Functional or anatomical asplenia:
  - Immunisation status should be reviewed every five years
  - All children post-splenectomy should receive pneumococcal and meningococcal vaccinations in addition to the vaccinations of the standard schedule, as well as annual influenza vaccine.

○ In cases of elective splenectomy, the vaccinations should ideally be given at least 2 weeks before the operation.
○ A detailed immunisation protocol for children (and adults) with asplenia is available from the MVEC website.
• The MMR vaccine can be given to some children with HIV but the safety of this should be assessed in each case in discussion with their treating physician.

For further details of immunisation in immunosuppressed special risk children refer to The Australian Immunisation Handbook.

Household contacts of children with immune deficiency

Siblings and close contacts of immunosuppressed children are recommended to ensure vaccination status is up to date for MMR, varicella and pertussis (whooping cough).
• Annual influenza vaccines are also recommended for household contacts.
• Immunisation will ensure that they have less chance of infecting their immunosuppressed siblings.

Vaccination of newly arrived immigrants to Australia

Catch-up schedules for newly arrived immigrants can be complex, see Chapter 35, Refugee health, and the RCH Immigrant Health resources available at https://www.rch.org.au/immigranthealth/clinical/Clinical_resources/.

USEFUL RESOURCES
• Australian Immunisation Register (AIR) – available within Australia on 1800 653 809
• Australian Immunisation Handbook https://immunisationhandbook.health.gov.au/ Provides a comprehensive up-to-date online resource for the Australian context
• The Melbourne Vaccine Education Centre (MVEC) https://mvec.mcri.edu.au/ MVEC is a resource developed by MCRI and provides up-to-date immunisation information for healthcare professionals, parents and the public
• AEFI-CAN SAEFVIC https://www.aefican.org.au/ Vaccines safety and AEFI surveillance system in Victoria
• National Centre for Immunisation Research and Surveillance of Vaccine Preventable Diseases www.ncirs.usyd.edu.au NCIRS VPD website includes fact sheets related to specific vaccines, vaccine-preventable diseases and vaccine safety
• RCH Immunisation Service www.rch.org.au/immunisation/ RCH immunisation services resources
• Victorian immunisation schedule app www.rch.org.au/rch/apps/vicvax/Victorian_immunisation_schedule_app/
• Victorian Department Health Immunisation Section http://w ww.health.vic.gov.au/immunisation
• Sharing knowledge about immunisation http://www.talkingaboutimmunisation.org.au/ a vaccine confidence initiative

CHAPTER 10

Nutrition

Liz Rogers
Evelyn Volders
Victoria Evans
Zoe McCallum
Julie E. Bines

Key Points
- Breast feeding is almost always the best method for feeding infants. Solids can be introduced around 6 months of age, including high allergen foods.
- Malnutrition is common in hospitalised children and screening should occur on hospital admission and weekly whilst an inpatient.
- Enteral tube feeding can provide full or supplementary nutrition support for short or longterm treatment.
- Children requiring enteral tube feeding or parenteral nutrition should undergo a full nutritional assessment.
- Parenteral nutrition is a complex intervention that requires oversight from a multidisciplinary nutrition team and should be limited to children with a non-functioning gastrointestinal tract or contraindications to enteral tube feeding.

General Nutrition
Breastfeeding
Breastfeeding is almost always the best method of feeding infants and all efforts should be made to promote, encourage and maintain breastfeeding. The World Health Organisation recommends exclusive breastfeeding for the first six months of life, and thereafter continued breastfeeding with appropriate introduction of solids. Breast milk:
- Provides passive immunity to protect infants from infection until the immune system is fully functional.
- Provides complete nutrition for an infant to 6 months of age, with the type and level of protein, carbohydrate and fat ideal for the optimal growth and development of the infant.
- Is readily available, environmentally and economically friendly and assists in the establishment of a healthy microbiome in infants.

Breastfeeding decreases rates of respiratory, gastrointestinal infections and necrotizing enterocolitis. It has also been shown to impact on rates of asthma, obesity, some cancers and neurodevelopmental outcomes. For hospitalised neonates and infants, the provision of breast milk should be encouraged, and mothers supported to maintain supply.

Breast milk production is reliant on effective removal of milk from the breast.
- The frequency, intensity and duration of suckling will impact on supply.
- Most women will produce around 800ml of milk per day when exclusively breastfeeding.
- Normal patterns of breastfeeding are very variable: Many infants will feed eight to ten times in a 24-hour period, with irregular gaps between feeds or clusters of feeds.

Paediatric Handbook, Tenth Edition. Edited by Kate Harding, Daniel S. Mason and Daryl Efron.
© 2021 John Wiley & Sons Ltd. Published 2021 by John Wiley & Sons Ltd.

- The effectiveness of breastfeeding can be assessed by the observation of positioning (of mother and baby, i.e. chest to chest, chin to breast), attachment, sucking and swallowing rhythms as well monitoring the baby's growth.
- A thriving breastfed infant will be growing with frequent wet nappies and bright yellow, soft stools.
- Expressing breast milk is not as effective in removing milk as the infant suckling and is not an accurate indicator of milk supply.
- Test weighing (infant weight pre and post breastfeed) is sometimes used to assess milk production but can be perceived by mothers as a measure of "lactation performance" and contribute to maternal stress. If further evaluation is required, 24-hour weighing is likely to be a better indicator of intake.

Growth in breastfed infants
Growth patterns differ between breastfed and formula fed infants. Average weights of breastfed babies are similar to or higher than formula-fed babies until 4–6 months, then slows. Length and head circumference remain similar (See Chapter 11, Growth).

The WHO growth charts (0–2 yrs), are based on optimal growth in fully breastfed infants.
- If poor growth occurs in a breastfed infant, then an assessment by a lactation consultant is advised. Interventions can include optimising positioning and attachment, increasing frequency of feeds or expressing to increase milk supply, and breast compression during feeds.
- If supplementation is required the first choice is mothers own breast milk, then donated milk, then formula. A top up (30 to 40 ml) after 3–4 breast feeds per day may be adequate to increase energy intake (by ~25%) and meet the dual goals of increasing weight gain and continuing breastfeeding.

Vitamin D
Exclusively breastfed infants of Vitamin D deficient mothers should be supplemented with 400IU D3 daily for at least the first 12 months of life.

Formula feeding
If breast milk is not available, a commercially prepared formula is required. Most standard infant formulas are based on cow's milk, modified to lower the protein, calcium and electrolytes to levels better suited to infants and contain added amino acids, lactose, vitamins and minerals, to meet the needs of the growing infant. The 2012 NHMRC Infant Feeding Guidelines state that for formula fed babies, it is preferable to use a formula with a lower protein content due to a link between higher protein intake in young children and later obesity.

There is a wide range of infant formula options available.
- 'From-birth' (Stage 1) formula should be selected for infants from 0 to 12 months.
- For infants >6 months, follow-on formulas (Stage 2) may be used but they are not necessary. Follow-on formulas tend to contain more protein, electrolytes and minerals and have a higher renal solute load.
- Toddler formulas (Stage 3 and 4) are extensively marketed for infants older than one year. They are not nutritionally complete, contain sugar and may displace solid intake and encourage reliance on fortified milk drinks rather than encouraging a varied diet.
- Whole cow milk or soy milks are not suitable as a main drink until 1 year of age but they may be used on cereal and in cooking from 6 months.
- Plant based milks including rice, oat, and almond milks are low in energy, protein, fat and calcium (unless fortified) and are not an appropriate substitute for full cream dairy or soy milk in children younger than 2 years.
- Some formulas have been supplemented with 'functional food micronutrients' to mimic breast milk constituents, such as pre- and probiotics and long-chain polyunsaturated fatty acids.

There are a number of special formulas for specific medical indications.
- These include soy, AR (anti-reflux), low-lactose and hypoallergenic or partially hydrolysed formulas.
- These should not be encouraged unless there is evidence that they are required.
- Partially hydrolysed formulas are not recommended for the prevention of food allergy.

A key component of the history in the formula-fed infant with feeding problems is a review of formula preparation technique.
- When changing between formulas, ensure that the correct scoop and dilution is used as these can vary significantly between brands.

Introduction of solids

The introduction of solids allows the increase in intake of some nutrients (i.e. iron) and provides stimulus for the development of gross motor, fine motor and oro-motor skills.

- Solid food should be introduced at around 6 months, in parallel with continued breastfeeding.
- Initial solids include iron-fortified baby cereal, smooth vegetables or fruits, and iron rich foods such as meats.
- Texture should be increased so that by 8–9 months the infant is offered lumps, varying textures and finger foods. Commercial foods are a finer texture and can be sweet, which may discourage the infant from eating family foods.
- The amount of solid food is typically only 1–2 teaspoons per serve initially, gradually increasing over the second 6 months to become nutritionally significant.
- To avoid choking small, hard pieces of food such as whole nuts, whole grapes and pieces of carrot should not be offered. All children should be seated and supervised when eating.

Introduction of high allergen foods

- NHMRC and ASCIA guidelines recommends this from 6 months, even in high risk families.
- Includes nuts (as nut butters), fish, eggs, dairy and wheat.
- Introduction should not be delayed beyond the first year of life as there is little evidence this will reduce food allergies.

By 12 months

- Most family foods can be offered.
- Increasing the intake of solids should result in a reduction of milk intake to 400–500 mL per day.
- Higher intakes of cow's milk can limit the intake of other foods and is associated with iron deficiency.
  - Iron deficiency with associated anaemia is the most common nutrient deficiency in Australian children.
  - It is associated with the early introduction of cow's milk, high intake of cow's milk in the second year and low intake of iron-rich foods.

Toddler Eating

Early childhood is a critical time for the development of food preferences and eating patterns. Many toddlers go through a period of food refusal which is developmentally normal as the growth rate slows and choosing and refusing food is an expression of independence. Some toddlers also develop a fear of new things, including food.

An assessment of the toddler who refuses food (who seems otherwise healthy) includes the following steps:

- Clarify the dietary history, exploring intake, volume, pattern, mealtime routine, and reactions to food refusal. Many children are given milk, juice or foods (e.g. yoghurt, banana) if they do not eat their meals and may 'hold out' for these options. Check that drinks are not suppressing appetite for food. Water or plain milk are the only drinks most children require.
- Plot weight, height and head circumference to assess the child's growth. Use the growth chart to demonstrate that growth rate slows in the second year with a subsequent drop in appetite.

The approach to child feeding is based on the concept of the 'Division of Responsibility' whereby it is the parents' job to choose and prepare food, to offer regular meals and snacks, make meal-times pleasant and to respect the child's hunger and satiety cues. Respect their 'right to refuse'. The child can decide if they will eat and how much.

- Self-feeding is encouraged. Aim for a range of foods, to increase learning about taste and texture.
- Many children go through fads of liking particular food. Continued offering of less preferred foods, while including some healthy food choices that they like, increases familiarisation. It is suggested that up to 15 exposures to new foods can be needed to learn to 'like' new foods.
- Parents eating with their children allows role modeling of healthy eating.
- Multivitamins are generally not required and contain minimal amounts of key nutrients such as calcium and iron.
- Many parents are surprised at how little children of this age need (Table 10.1). However, because total needs are small there is limited place for extra high-fat and high-sugar foods.

Cues for further intervention include extreme picky eating where a child has long-standing food group restrictions, changes in growth rates and bizarre food and eating habits.

Table 10.1 Guide to the quantities suitable for children 1–3 years of age.

Food Group	Number of serves/day	One serve equals
Dairy	1–1.5 serves	250 mL of milk, 200 g of yoghurt or 35 g of cheese
Grains	4 serves	one slice of bread, half cup of pasta or two cereal wheat biscuits
Vegetable	2–3 serves	approx. half a cup
Fruit	½–1 serve	approx. one cup
Meat and alternatives	1 serve	65 g of lean meat, fish or chicken, 1 cup of beans or 2 eggs

---

Clinical Pearl: Raising a healthy eater
- Eat together so parents can role model enjoyment of healthy foods
- Repeated exposure to new foods leads to acceptance and enjoyment
- Remember the division of responsibility to allow children to learn and respond to hunger and satiety – 'parent provides, child decides'
- Do not use food as a reward or punishment. It only increases its power!

Nutritional Screening

As malnutrition is common in hospitalised children, weekly nutritional screening should be undertaken, to prevent children developing malnutrition during their hospitalisation. There are a number of paediatric screening tools available. The PNST (Paediatric Nutrition Screening Tool) is a quick, simple, validated tool that involves four simple nutrition screening questions that can be undertaken as part of the nursing admission for children (see Useful resources). At risk children should be referred to a dietitian for a full nutritional assessment.

Nutritional Assessment

See Table 10.2.

Clinical Pearl: Measuring micronutrients
Many micronutrients are acute phase reactants; therefore serum levels cannot be reliably interpreted during infection or inflammation. C-reactive protein level taken concurrently can assist with interpretation of these results.

Establishing a nutrition treatment plan

Calculating nutritional requirements

Energy

Estimated energy requirements for the sick infant or child can be calculated by using either:
- the requirements of a normal well infant/child of the same sex and age (NRVs).
- an estimate of basal requirements (BMR) with additional stress and activity factors.

Energy requirements are increased in the following conditions:
- Malnutrition
- Very low birthweight (VLBW, <1500g) infants
- Respiratory disorders (Chronic lung disease, Cystic fibrosis)
- Cardiac defects
- Chronic infection
- Diseases causing malabsorption (liver, intestinal failure, allergic enteropathy)
- Trauma or Burns
- Malignancy

Energy requirements are decreased below those recommended for healthy children, in critically ill children who are ventilated and/or hypothermic.

Table 10.2 Nutritional assessment of sick children.

Assessment	Features
Current medical problem and past medical history	Type and duration of illness Degree of metabolic stress Treatment (medications or surgery, or both) Developmental, social and family history History of recent weight loss
Nutritional intake/feeding history	24–hour diet recall Supplemental enteral feeds or oral supplements
Physical examination	General assessment: wasting, oedema, lethargy and muscular strength Specific micronutrient deficiencies: pallor, bruising, skin, hair, neurological and ophthalmological complications
Anthropometry	Weight, length, head circumference – serial measurements plotted. Correct for age for preterm infants Mid-arm circumference, skinfold thickness provides additional information on fat and muscle stores
Fluid requirements	Document current intravenous and enteral fluid intake, fluid restrictions and losses
Laboratory data	**Assessment of gastrointestinal status absorptive status:** stool microscopy, pH and reducing sugars **Protein status:** albumin, total protein, pre-albumin, urea, 24-hour urinary nitrogen **Fluid, electrolyte and acid–base status:** serum electrolytes and acid–base, urinalysis **Iron status:** serum ferritin and full blood examination **Mineral status:** calcium, magnesium, phosphorus, alkaline phosphatase, bone age and bone density **Vitamin status:** vitamins A, C, B_{12}, D, E/lipid ratio, folate, and INR **Trace elements:** zinc, selenium, copper **Lipid status:** serum cholesterol, HDL cholesterol and triglycerides **Glucose tolerance:** serum glucose, HbA1c Note: Blood test are often performed when children are acutely unwell. This can result in falsely high levels of ferritin and copper and falsely low levels of zinc, vitamin A, C, D and selenium

Protein

Increased protein intake is recommended in:
- Protein-losing states e.g. enteropathy and nephrotic syndrome
- Chronic malnutrition
- Trauma or Burns
- HIV
- Dialysis and Haemofiltration (~2–2.5 g/kg per day)

Reduced protein intake is recommended in:
- Hepatic encephalopathy
- Severe renal dysfunction (not dialysed)

Fat

- Infants/children have higher fat needs than adults.
- Fat is a concentrated source of energy and essential for transport of fat-soluble vitamins and hormones, and brain development in infancy.
- Fat restricted diets are **not** suitable for infants and young children.

Micronutrients

Special consideration is needed when estimating the micronutrient requirements of sick children (Table 10.3).

Table 10.3 Diseases that increase micronutrient requirements.

Disease	Increased requirement
Burns	Vitamins C, B complex, folate, zinc
HIV/AIDS	Zinc, selenium, iron
Renal failure: dialysis	Vitamins C, B complex, folate (reduce or omit copper, chromium, molybdenum)
Haemofiltration	Vitamins C, B complex, trace elements
Protein–energy malnutrition	Zinc, selenium, iron
Refeeding syndrome	Phosphate, magnesium, potassium, thiamine
Short bowel syndrome, chronic malabsorption states	Vitamins A, B_{12}, D, E, K, zinc, magnesium, selenium
Liver disease	Vitamins A, D, E, K, zinc, iron (reduce or omit manganese, copper)
High fistula output, chronic diarrhoea	Zinc, magnesium, selenium, folate, Vitamins B complex, B_{12}
Pancreatic insufficiency	Vitamins A, D, E, K
Inflammatory bowel disease	Folate, Vitamin B_{12}, zinc, iron

Feeding the sick infant or child

Infants and children with acute or chronic disease often require additional nutrition support. This can include energy dense foods, supplemental feeds, enteral tube feeding or PN.

Appropriate feeds for sick infants

Breast-milk feeding should be the primary aim for all sick babies. When babies are too ill or too premature to suckle at the breast, most mothers can establish lactation by expression. EBM can be fed via a tube until the baby is well enough to be placed on the breast. In this way breast-milk feeding can be achieved in extremely premature babies and in babies with serious illness.

- The only situations where breast-milk feeding is not possible are:
  - When an informed mother chooses not to express
  - Some inborn errors of metabolism, which require specific formulas
  - Complex malabsorption syndromes
- Breast-milk fortifiers
  - Available in hospital to add to EBM to increase its protein, energy and nutrient content.
  - Generally reserved for preterm infants who have increased nutritional requirements but can be used for term infants who are fluid restricted.
  - EBM can also be fortified with a standard infant formula which can then be used upon discharge if still required.

When formula feeding is required, fortification of formulas is most commonly achieved by adding additional formula powder (Table 10.4).

- This increases the energy/protein ratio and provides additional nutrients, which can be beneficial in fluid restricted infants and those with high catch-up growth requirements. However, may reduce total intake if taken orally and needs to be monitored especially if receiving a 420kj/100ml feed.
- Formulas containing 420kj/100mls have a higher renal solute load and osmolality, and their use needs to be monitored carefully.
- It is possible to fortify some specialised formulas, but care should be taken particularly in infants with renal or liver impairment.
- Infants and young children who develop gastroenteritis should have fortification withheld until vomiting and diarrhoea resolve, in order to avoid hypernatraemic dehydration.
- Due to potential risks associated with fortification of infant formula this should only be done under the supervision of a paediatric dietitian or paediatrician.

Table 10.4 Increasing concentration of infant formula.

Standard Concentration ~280kj/100mls	1.25 x Concentration ~350 kj/100mls	1.5 x Concentration ~420 kj/100mls
1 scoop* + 60 mL water	1 scoop + 50 mL water	1 scoop + 40 mL water
1 scoop + 50 mL water	1 scoop + 40 mL water	1 scoop + 35 mL water
1 scoop + 30 mL water	1 scoop + 25 mL water	1 scoop + 20 mL water

*Always use the scoop provided from the formula tin.

Preterm infants
Preterm infants are at greatest risk of rapid nutritional depletion due to their limited muscle and nutrient stores.
- Very Low Birth Weight (<1500 g) babies require higher levels of phosphorous, folate, iron, sodium and vitamins A, C, D, E and K.
- Breast milk plays an important role in the prevention of necrotizing colitis (NEC) in this cohort and should be encouraged and supported.

Born <1500 g or delay in starting feeds
- Commence PN on Day 1 of life and progress to full PN by Day 4–5.
- Introduce enteral feeds slowly (20–30 mL/kg/d per 24 hrs) and wean PN as appropriate.
- At 120 mL/kg/d – transition to fortified EBM or preterm formula.
- Aim for 180–200 mL/kg/d fortified EBM or preterm formula.
- Monitor growth. Correct for gestation on centile charts.
- Cease fortified EBM or preterm formula when fully breastfed, reach term or upon discharge.
- If formula fed can use post discharge formula formulated for preterm infants.
- Commence iron supplementation four weeks post birth for all babies on EBM or term formula. Other vitamins as per unit protocol.

Born <32 weeks or <1800 g
- Commence EBM or term formula on D 1 of life at 60 mL/kg/d.
- Increase by 20–30 mL/kg/d.
- At 120 mL/kg/d, transition to fortified EBM or preterm formula.
- Aim for 180–200 mL/kg/d fortified EBM or preterm formula.
- Monitor growth. Correct for gestation on centile charts.
- Cease fortified EBM or preterm formula when fully breastfed, reach term or upon discharge.
- If formula fed can use post discharge formula formulated for preterm infants.
- Commence iron supplementation four weeks post birth for all babies on EBM or term formula. Other vitamins as per unit protocol.

Born >32 weeks or >1800 g
- Commence EBM or standard infant formula on Day 1.
- Formula volumes
  - D 1 60–90 mL/kg/d
  - D2 90–120 mL/kg/d
  - D3 120–150 mL/kg/d
  - Up to 180 mL/kg/d
- Monitor growth. Correct for gestation on centile charts.
- Fortify feeds if necessary.
- Gradually transition to oral feeds.

Feeds for older infants/children
Young children often maintain oral intake when they are ill. However, those with chronic disease generally require additional nutrition to maintain growth such as:
- High energy eating strategies, to help boost food intake density including energy dense food, the addition of infant formula or milk powder to dairy products, cream/yoghurt to fruits and additional fats to all meals.

- Paediatric supplements
  - Complete supplements, for example Pediasure, Kids Essentials or Sustagen drinks, which can be used in addition to food to increase energy, protein and nutrient intake.
  - High energy milkshakes can be used with added milk powder.
- Energy supplements: Glucose polymers (Polyjoule) or fat emulsions (Calogen/Liquigen) or combined fat and carbohydrate (Duocal) can be added to normal foods and fluids. Skim milk powder or infant formula can be added to foods/fluids.
- Enteral Tube Feeding
  - Overnight feeding or top-up feeds post meals.
  - In cases where there is an unsafe swallow, complete nutritional requirements are provided via tube feeds.

Note: Any supplement taken can displace food intake and regular re-assessment is necessary.

Specific diet related disease

Infants and children with chronic diseases such as cystic fibrosis, complex cardiac anomalies, liver or renal impairment, complex allergy, malignancy, intestinal failure or inborn errors of metabolism often require additional nutritional support and disease specific formulas. They should be managed by a multidisciplinary team including a dietitian with expertise in that nutrition field.

Enteral tube feeding

Enteral tube feeding is the provision of nutrients to the gut through a feeding tube.
Advantages over parenteral nutrition include:
- Lower risk of serious infection (central line infection)
- Lower risk of metabolic abnormalities
- Nutrients provided to the gastrointestinal tract enhance intestinal growth and function
- Inexpensive, safer and easier to administer

If enteral tube feeding is considered (Figure 10.1), a nutritional assessment should be completed by a paediatric dietitian to establish an appropriate nutrition plan comprising of recommending the optimal feed (Table 10.5), volume of feed, method of feeding (continuous versus bolus) and the length of time the feeding may be required.
- The most commonly used route for enteral tube feeding is nasogastric, the main benefit being ease of insertion.
- When long-term feeding is required, a gastrostomy tube may be indicated.

Blended diets (vitamised solid foods) delivered via a tube are becoming increasingly popular. Parents may choose to use a blended diet to provide whole foods and to incorporate tube feeding into the pattern of routine family meals.
In some children, blended diets:
- Decrease symptoms of tube feeding intolerance.
- Can lead to inadequate calorie intake due to dilution of both the energy and nutrient content with fluid that is required to achieve a suitable consistency for tube feeding.
  - Children are particularly vulnerable due to their increased nutrition and hydration requirements and small gastric capacity.
- Have been associated with tube blockage and microbial contamination, particularly if there has been inadequate cooking, or prolonged storing and hanging time of feeds.

Once the feeding plan has been fully implemented, regular assessment of the child's nutrient requirements is needed to ensure that nutritional support has been adequate, and to indicate when enteral feeding can be reduced or ceased. This should include assessment of serum micronutrients including Vitamins A, E, D, B12, folate, iron (ferritin) and zinc 12 monthly.

Common problems with enteral tube feeding

- **Gastrointestinal disturbance:** This is the most common problem (diarrhoea, cramping, nausea, vomiting, constipation) and can be managed by reviewing formula selection and medications administered. High gastric residues can be managed by reducing the rate of feeds, feeding smaller volumes, reassessing the concentration of feed and gastrointestinal function. In children with slow gastric emptying, a trial of jejunal tube feeding may be considered. Fibre containing formula and adequate fluid volumes can assist with constipation. Additional laxatives may be necessary especially in children with a neurological diagnosis.

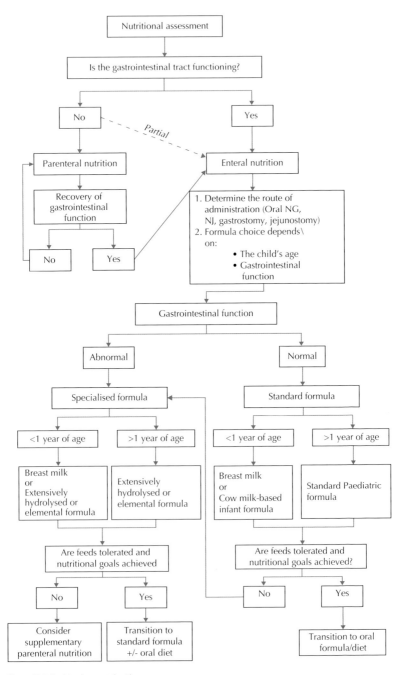

Figure 10.1 Nutritional support algorithm.

Table 10.5 Standard feeds for different ages.

Age	Normal gut function	Impaired gut function
0–12 months	Expressed breast milk (EBM), standard infant formula or follow on formula (>6 months) ± • Additional formula • Energy supplement e.g. Polyjoule or Calogen	EBM All formula below can be fortified if necessary: Lactose free formulas, soy formulas, CHO free formulas
	High energy infant formula e.g. Infantrini (420 kJ/100 mL)	Extensively hydrolysed formula e.g. Peptijunior, Alfare
		Elemental formula e.g. Neocate, Elecare, Alfamino, Novalac Allergy (Rice based)
1–6 years (8–20 kg)	Standard paediatric formulas:e.g. Nutrini, Pediasure, Resource for kids 420 kJ/100 mL (1 kcal/mL)	Concentrated hydrolysed infant formula e.g. Peptijunior, Alfare
	Higher energy feeds: e.g. Nutrini Energy, Pediasure Plus 630 kJ/100 mL (1.5kcal/mL)	Hydrolysed Paediatric formula e.g. Peptamen Junior, Nutrini Peptisorb 420 kj/100ml
	+ Fibre	Elemental paediatric formula e.g. Neocate Junior, Elecare 1+, Alfamino Junior 420 kj/100ml
>6 years (>20 kg)	Paediatric feed may still be appropriate. Standard adult formula: e.g. Nutrison Standard, Osmolite, Ensure and Resource 420 kJ/100 mL (1 kcal/mL)	Hydrolysed Paediatric formula e.g. Peptamen Junior, Nutrini Peptisorb Elemental Paediatric formula (at 420 kj/100m concentation)
	High Energy Adult Formula: e.g. Nutrison Energy, Ensure Plus, Fortisip, Resource Plus 630 kJ/100 mL (1.5 kcal/mL) e.g. Nutrison Concentrated, NovaSource 2.0, TwoCal HN 840 kJ/100 mL (2 kcal/mL)	Adult Elemental Formula e.g Vivonex TEN, Peptamen OS
	+ Fibre	

• **Food aversion:** Non-nutritive sucking (dummies) and mouth contact (bottle or breast) can help infants to establish feeding. Introduction of solids at age appropriate times and taking small amounts of appropriate food/fluid orally will help establish or maintain eating and feeding skills. Assessment by a speech pathologist may be required.

Clinical Pearl: Enteral tube feeding
Oversight by a multidisciplinary team has been shown to minimize the risk of prolonged tube dependency and balance the requirements for growth and development with the quality and quantity of nutritional intake, irrespective of the route of delivery (oral, tube or parenteral nutrition).

From enteral to oral feeding
Once the child is able and willing to eat by mouth, enteral feeds can be reduced in proportion to oral intake.
• Often, weaning from a tube occurs quite rapidly but for some children, this can be prolonged.
• Younger children (< 3years) have been found to be more readily weaned from enteral tube feeds than older children.
• Prior to attempting tube weaning, children should have stable growth and normal nutritional status.
• They should be able to sit at a table and accept a bite of food.
• Transition from continuous feeds to overnight feeds may help establish oral intake while ensuring the child is not nutritionally compromised.

- Early teaching of skills that promote chewing and oral intake and exposure to tasks requiring oral motor skill acquisition is critical.
- Assessment of the parent-child interaction to develop an approach that will meet the child's nutritional requirements within the family lifestyle is also important.

Children who have been dependent on enteral tube feeding and have failed routine approaches to weaning require a multidisciplinary team approach. In the outpatient or inpatient setting, this approach uses a combination of behavioural techniques and nutrition modifications for successful tube weaning. Most protocols focus on changing the child's perceptions and interactions with food through play while reducing tube feedings to encourage hunger. Structured meals, social modeling and positive reinforcement are sited as being crucial for success.

Parenteral Nutrition

Parenteral Nutrition (PN) is a sterile intravenous solution of protein, glucose, electrolytes, vitamins, trace elements and water administered along with a fat emulsion solution. If the child has a functioning gastrointestinal system, they should be fed enterally.

PN prescribing, administration and monitoring is a potential source of medical and nursing error and requires specialist education, oversight and review by multidisciplinary nutrition support teams comprising dietitians, nurses, doctors and pharmacists.

General Indications for PN

- When enteral nutrition is not possible
  Day 1 for a preterm neonate less than 2.5 kg.
  >2 days in a term neonate
  >3 days in infants
  >5 days in an older child
- Weight loss of >10% with a poorly functioning gastrointestinal tract
  AND
  Anticipated need for PN support for (minimum) of 5 days

The following are recommended prior to PN commencement

1. Determine appropriate venous access (a central venous access device is required for any solution with a dextrose content greater than 10% due to risk of extravasation and potential significant tissue injury).
2. Child's weight.
3. Nutritional assessment by a dietitian, including estimated energy and protein requirements.
4. Baseline blood samples: UEC CMP LFTs, Triglyceride levels and VBG.
5. Fluid available for PN: taking into consideration any fluid restriction, other IV infusions and oral/enteral intake.
   Note: replacement of losses (i.e. nasogastric losses) is in addition to PN and IV medications.
6. Identify if the child is at risk of refeeding syndrome (see below). Ensure any electrolyte derangements are corrected prior to the commencement of PN and then monitor electrolytes and acid base status closely whilst grading up PN.
   Note: In cases of severe refeeding syndrome it may take several days to meet nutritional requirements.
7. Consider the PN solution required; aiming to meet approximately 50% of nutritional requirements on Day 1, grading up to approximately 75%–100% by Days 2–3.
8. Commence lipid (SMOF) on day 1 at 0.5–1g/kg/d and grade up as appropriate.
9. The following investigations should be performed daily until full PN provision is reached and results remain stable: UEC, CMP, LFTs, VBG and triglyceride levels.

Children receiving PN for more than 1 month require additional nutritional monitoring

- Monthly: Iron Studies, Vitamin B12, Red Cell Folate, Vitamins A, D and E, Zinc and Copper, if a child has been NBM for one month Free and Total Carnitine should be considered as carnitine is not standard in PN solutions
- 6-monthly: selenium and manganese
- Annually: Vitamin C, Chromium and Aluminium
- CRP with all bloods

Refeeding syndrome

After a period of prolonged starvation, aggressive nutritional support may precipitate a cascade of potentially fatal metabolic complications. These include:

- Hypokalaemia, hypophosphataemia, hypomagnesaemia
- Glucose intolerance
- Cardiac failure
- Seizures
- Myocardial infarction/arrhythmias

Children at particular risk are those with:

- Anorexia nervosa
- Classical marasmus or kwashiorkor
- No nutrition for 7–10 days in adolescents (much less in infants and children)
- Acute weight loss of ≥10–20% of usual body weight and possible metabolic stress, or weight loss of >20% of usual body weight
- Morbid obesity with massive weight loss (i.e. postoperative)

Management

- Identify risk and chronicity.
- Identify and treat metabolic stress if present (e.g. infection).
- Establish baseline status: weight, height, head circumference, fluid status, electrolytes, urea, creatinine, calcium, phosphate and magnesium, liver function and albumin, blood sugar, lipid status and acid base balance prior to commencing nutritional rehabilitation.
- Assess micronutrient and trace element status at baseline.
- Establish modest nutritional goals initially (e.g. basal requirements until stability is assured), then aim to provide for catch-up growth. During the first week of nutritional support, weight gain may not be seen or, if present, may reflect fluid gain rather than muscle or fat gain. Children at high risk of refeeding syndrome should be started on less than 50% of their estimated energy requirements.
- Monitor closely over the first week until a nutritional plan is established with pulse rate, fluid balance, weight, energy intake, glucose, electrolytes, urea, creatinine, calcium, phosphate and magnesium levels.
- Administer vitamin and mineral supplements. Children who are severely malnourished may require supplementation with thiamine, folate, vitamin A, and a multivitamin, and consideration of prophylactic antibiotics.
- Iron supplementation should be avoided in the initial management of refeeding.

USEFUL RESOURCES

Breastfeeding

- Australian Breastfeeding Association https://www.breastfeeding.asn.au/ resources for families and health professionals
- RCH Breastfeeding clinical guideline www.rch.org.au/rchcpg/hospital_clinical_guideline_index/Breastfeeding_support_and_promotion/
- Lactmed https://toxnet.nlm.nih.gov/newtoxnet/lactmed.htm a website database for information on drugs in breastfeeding

General Nutrition

- Paediatric Nutrition Screening tool www.childrens.health.qld.gov.au/wp-content/uploads/PDF/pnst-form.pdf
- RCH nutrition department resources www.rch.org.au/nutrition/resources/
- WHO guidelines for severe malnutrition www.who.int/elena/titles/full_recommendations/sam_management/en/
- RCH refeeding guideline www.rch.org.au/uploadedFiles/Main/Content/gastro/Refeeding%20syndrome%20guideline.pdf
- RCH Clinical Nutrition www.rch.org.au/gastro/clinical_nutrition/

Nutrition related professional bodies:

- ESPGHAN www.espghan.org/
- AUSPEN www.auspen.org.au/
- ASPEN www.nutritioncare.org/

CHAPTER 11
Growth

Jane Standish
Zoe McCallum
Daniella Tassoni
Peter Simm

Key Points
- Serial measurements plotted on appropriate growth chart are needed to optimally assess growth.
- Stature should always be assessed in the context of the midparental height/genetic height potential.
- In childhood BMI is plotted on age and gender specific charts to ascertain weight status. Waist circumference is an easy marker of central adiposity.
- Obesity is a chronic disease and requires consideration of the social determinants of health. Children and young people with physical or intellectual disability are at increased risk of obesity.
- Short stature is most commonly due to familial short stature, maturational delay or a combination of both.

Slow weight gain
Slow weight gain may also be referred to as 'poor weight gain', 'poor growth' or 'faltering growth'. Slow weight gain has historically been called 'failure to thrive (FTT)', however this term may be misleading and is potentially distressing to parents/families. There is no consensus definition, but slow weight gain describes a child whose current weight, or rate of weight gain is significantly below that expected.
- Consider further assessment when a child has dropped ≥2 major percentile lines over time on an appropriate growth chart.
- Most commonly, linear growth and head circumference are initially preserved.
- In severe or prolonged situations of insufficient nutrition, linear growth and head circumference may also be affected, along with broader systemic consequences of severe malnutrition.

Slow weight gain can result from a wide variety of medical and psychosocial issues, often in combination, culminating in 'insufficient usable nutrition'. A good history, assessment of family growth patterns and examination of the child is often adequate to exclude significant pathology, and guide investigation and intervention. Short stature is discussed separately on page 120. See Chapter 10, Nutrition for nutritional assessment.

Is this weight normal or is it slow weight gain?
When assessing children's growth, it is important to recognize that being in the lower/lowest percentiles does not necessarily indicate a problem. Serial measurements of all growth parameters over time give the best assessment of a child's growth. Weight and height are distributed in the population, and growth standards are developed from population based studies. By definition, children who are growing along a percentile line (including the 3rd percentile line) have normal growth. Children who have a discrepancy between their height and weight percentiles may still have normal growth if both parameters are tracking, although they will be lean, and may have a body mass index (BMI) that is low. Normally growing children appear healthy, with good muscle bulk, adequate subcutaneous fat, and normal activity and development. It is important to plot parental height to estimate

Paediatric Handbook, Tenth Edition. Edited by Kate Harding, Daniel S. Mason and Daryl Efron.
© 2021 John Wiley & Sons Ltd. Published 2021 by John Wiley & Sons Ltd.

Table 11.1 Causes of slow weight gain.

	Examples
Inadequate caloric intake/retention	Inadequate nutrition (breastmilk, formula and/or food volume) Breast feeding difficulties Restricted diet e.g. low fat, vegan, sensory Structural causes of poor feeding e.g. cleft palate Persistent vomiting Anorexia of chronic disease Error in infant formula dilution Early (before 4 months) or delayed introduction of solids
Psychosocial factors	Parental depression, anxiety or other mood disorders Substance abuse of one or both parents Attachment difficulties Disability or chronic illness of one or both parents Coercive feeding (including feeding child whilst asleep) Difficulties at mealtimes Food insecurity Behavioural disorders Poor social support Poor carer understanding Exposure to traumatic incident/family violence Neglect of this infant or siblings Current or past Child Protection involvement
Inadequate absorption	Coeliac disease Chronic liver disease Pancreatic insufficiency e.g. Cystic fibrosis Chronic diarrhoea Cow milk protein allergy
Excessive caloric utilization	Urinary tract infection Chronic illness Chronic Respiratory disease e.g. Cystic Fibrosis Congenital heart disease Diabetes Mellitus Hyperthyroidism
Other Medical Causes	Genetic syndromes Inborn Errors of Metabolism

expected height potential (mid parental height page 121). In Australia, it is recommended that WHO growth standards are used in the first 2 years of life, and CDC growth charts for children over 2 years. Condition specific growth charts (e.g. Down syndrome, Turner syndrome) should be used where appropriate. See Useful resources.

Birthweight percentile does not predict future weight. In the first months of life, many infants will equilibrate to their 'true' growth channels and cross percentile lines. After the first months, crossing percentile lines does usually represent slow weight gain.

Slow weight gain can be approached through the framework of considering potential underlying causes (Table 11.1), which guides targeted investigation and management strategies. It is important to understand age of onset of weight concerns and surrounding events. There are frequently multiple contributing factors or conditions, and there can be significant overlap between 'organic' and 'non-organic' causes.

Clinical Pearl: Assessing slow weight gain
- Remember to correct for prematurity (<37 weeks) until 24 months of age
- Birth weight is not necessarily representative of genetic growth potential

---

History

History is focused on intake, output and identifying other potential contributing factors including psychosocial stressors and symptoms of specific underlying medical conditions.

- **Intake**: breast/bottle feeding history, number and volume/duration of feeds per day, impression of breast milk supply, formula dilution, age solids commenced, age when three meals and two snacks per day achieved, composition and quantity of meals (including quantifying 24 hr milk intake in toddlers).
- **Output**: vomiting (frequency, volume, blood/bile), stool (frequency, consistency, mucus/blood), urine losses, other losses (e.g. stoma if present). Any identified triggers to increased output (e.g. specific food)
- **Food behaviour**: acceptance of food (or parents feeling need to coerce/distract), mealtime set-up, duration, behaviour/attitudes (child and parent/caregiver).
- **Pregnancy/birth**
- **Past history:** chronic and current illness, recurrent infections
- **Family growth:** pattern of weight gain and growth in other family members
- **Family medical/mental health issues and social situation:** medical issues, mental health issues, household situation, food access, engagement with community services e.g. maternal-child health nurse (MCHN).

Examination

- **General:** does the child appear well and proportionate, or sick, scrawny, irritable or lethargic.
- **Pattern of growth:** plot serial measures of weight, height and head circumference, clarify family and health situation at times where growth trajectory changed, e.g. solids introduction.
- **Expected growth:** plot mid-parental height.
- **Assess** muscle bulk and subcutaneous fat stores, consider anthropometry. Assess for micronutrient deficiency including skin, hair, gums, eyes, nails. For full nutritional assessment details, see Chapter 10, Nutrition.
- **Physical examination** for signs of underlying systemic diagnosis.
- **Observe** developmental status of child, interaction between child and parent/caregiver, and observe feed if practical to do so.

Investigations

Investigations may not be necessary and should be guided by a thorough clinical assessment. If there is significant clinical concern and the cause of slow weight gain is not readily apparent after history and examination, investigation may include:

- **Blood:** FBE*, ESR* UEC, LFT, ferritin (include full iron studies if presence of systemic inflammation suspected, otherwise ferritin gives best measure of iron stores), calcium, phosphate, thyroid function, blood glucose, coeliac serology (if on solid feeds containing gluten)
- **Urine:** urinalysis, microscopy and culture*, electrolytes
- **Stool:** Microscopy, fat (globules/fatty acid crystals)

*First line investigations

Other investigations to consider

- Specific investigations for underlying cause as guided by history, examination, and initial investigation results may include immune function testing, cystic fibrosis investigations, or genetic testing. These will likely be performed in consultation with specialist services.
- A dietitian review will help clarify intake and provide information on estimated energy requirements and whether the child is meeting these requirements.

Management

The underlying cause will determine the management. Follow up plan should be clear and individualised. Weekly weight monitoring at most is usually sufficient to monitor growth. More frequent weights can increase anxiety and cloud the growth trajectory in the setting of normal fluctuations in weight. A community based multidisciplinary approach may appropriately include GP, MCHN, dietitian and paediatrician.

Admission to hospital should be considered in some circumstances:

- Severe under nutrition, significant illness, significant dehydration
- Failed outpatient management
- Concern re potential child abuse or neglect
- Significant mental health concern in a parent.

Admission may facilitate further assessment of feeding technique, parent–child interaction and allow the involvement of a multidisciplinary team.

Obesity

One-in-four (25%) Australian 2–17 year olds are overweight or obese, with one-in-three predicted to be overweight or obese by 2025. In addition to the rate of obesity increasing over recent decades, the degree or severity of obesity for individuals has increased. Subsequently, the incidence of weight-related comorbidity has also likely to increase.

Paediatric obesity arises from a complex interplay between genetic and environmental factors. Whilst the theory of increasing energy expenditure and restricting energy intake should result in decrease in Body Mass Index (BMI) the actual sustained practice of this is clearly very difficult in reality. Like other chronic diseases, obesity is strongly influenced by the social determinants of health, with socioeconomic adversity, education, family disharmony and intergenerational trauma being risk factors for obesity. Neurodevelopmental disability (including both ID and physical disability) is also a risk factor for obesity. Table 11.2 outlines some of the causes or contributors to childhood obesity.

Children with exogenous (non-medical) obesity are usually of normal intellect, have normal development, and are either of normal or relatively tall stature. Endocrine or genetic causes of obesity in childhood are rare. Endocrine causes are usually associated with growth failure. Syndromal causes are often recognised by the presence of a significant developmental/intellectual disability and less frequently by dysmorphic features.

Clinical Pearl: Clues to syndromal or endocrine causes of obesity
- Height <50th centile (or less than genetic potential)
- Dysmorphic features
- Developmental/intellectual disabilities
- Cushingoid features (including abdominal striae)
- Hypogonadism

Table 11.2 Causes of obesity in children and adolescents.

Causes of Obesity in Children and Adolescents
Societal
• Poverty • Parental mental illness • Abuse
Environmental
• Excess energy intake (nutrition) • Decreased activity levels (physical activity, screen time, sleep)
Hormone problems
• Hypothyroidism • Cushing's Syndrome, Congenital Adrenal Hyperplasia • Other hormonal problems
Medications
• Behaviour-related medications (such as psychotropics) • Anticonvulsants • Steroids
Genetics/Genetic syndromes
• Overweight/ obese parents • Perinatal programming • Prader Willi syndrome • Other genetic syndromes (e.g. MC4R deficiency)

Childhood obesity is likely to lead to adult obesity, with an increased long-term risk of mortality and morbidity. Parent obesity appears to be one of the strongest risk factors for persistence of obesity in children; this underpins the need for family-based change for successful weight. Overweight/obese children who enter adulthood at a healthy weight have a significantly reduced risk of obesity-related complications in adult life, thus timely intervention for early-onset obesity can improve health outcomes significantly for an individual.

Complications

Previously only diagnosed in older adults with longstanding obesity, obesity-related complications are now being diagnosed in school-aged children (Table 11.3). Health consequences of obesity increase with increasing age- and sex-adjusted BMI, the degree of co-morbidities in obese children and adolescents is not clearly associated with the severity of obesity and as such should be considered for investigation where a strong family history is present.

Assessment

A simple, clinically useful definition that reflects excess body weight is the BMI. However, it does not reflect body composition and thus people with significant muscle mass may have a high BMI. This is usually clinically apparent.

$$BMI\,(kg/m^2) = weight\,(kg)/height^2\,(m^2)$$

In children and adolescents, BMI changes with normal growth; BMI is high in the first two years of life and this drops to a nadir, before gradually increasing to normal adult levels (see Useful resources). The rise after the nadir is termed the **adiposity rebound** and usually occurs around the age of 6 years. The timing of the adiposity

Table 11.3 Complications of obesity in childhood and adolescents.

Category	Complication
Psychosocial	Body dissatisfaction Low self-esteem Depression Bullying/teasing School avoidance
Cardiovascular	Dyslipidaemia Hypertension Metabolic syndrome
Endocrine	Glucose intolerance Insulin resistance Type 2 diabetes Accelerated linear growth and bone age Earlier onset of puberty Polycystic ovary syndrome and menstrual abnormalities Thyroid dysfunction
Respiratory	Obstructive sleep apnoea (OSA) ± possible links to asthma
Gastrointestinal	Non-alcoholic fatty liver disease (NAFLD)
Orthopaedic	Blount disease Slipped capital femoral epiphysis
Renal	Obesity-related glomerulopathy
Dermatological	Intertrigo Furunculosis Acanthosis nigricans (marker of insulin resistance)
Neurological	Idiopathic intracranial hypertension

Table 11.4 Definition of childhood and adolescent overweight and obesity.

Growth Category	CDC BMI Growth Chart – age and gender specific
Overweight	85–95th percentile
Obese	Above the 95th percentile

rebound may be important for later risk of obesity. Bioimpedance can assist interpret BMI by providing body composition and waist circumference is a helpful maker of central adiposity. See Table 11.4 for BMI based definition of overweight and obese growth categories. Figure 11.1 describes the approach to assessment and management of obesity.

History

A detailed personal, family, developmental and past (including perinatal) history, complemented by a thorough dietary history, activity history and physical examination is sufficient. Consider the following:

- Early life history including pregnancy complications, birthweight, and development incl. features suggestive of an underlying cause, e.g. poor postnatal feeding and hypotonia during infancy (Prader–Willi syndrome)
- Medical and medication history
- Family history
  - Obesity (+/- weight loss surgery) and obesity related complications
  - Ethnicity. Children from certain ethnic backgrounds (e.g. Indigenous Australians, Pacific Islanders, Asians and Indians) have a higher tendency for central weight gain and display greater levels of co-morbidity for a given level of obesity.
- Age of onset of obesity
- Complications history, including risk factors for co-morbidities, e.g. symptoms of OSA.

Examination

- Plot height, weight and BMI on percentile charts.
- Document pubertal and developmental status.
- Assess body build and distribution of adiposity.
- Measure waist circumference (at midpoint between lowest ribs and iliac crests, include any apron of abdominal fat).
- Measure blood pressure with an appropriate-sized cuff.
- Look for acanthosis nigricans (darker pigmentation on the neck and/or axilla).
- Look for clues to a syndromal/endocrine cause.
- Consider other associated problems, for example look for dental caries.

Investigations

For aetiology:
- For underlying cause, if clinically indicated, consider genetic tests (Chromosomal microarray, Prader Willi methylation) or endocrine causes (thyroid function, hormonal assays).
For complications:
- Hyperlipidaemia, full fasting lipid profile (cholesterol and triglyceride).
- Type 2 diabetes, puberty is associated with a significant reduction in insulin sensitivity in normal individuals and investigation for Type 2 diabetes may be needed in peri-pubertal children. Formal oral glucose tolerance testing is preferred in adolescents, although fasting glucose and insulin is often sufficient in younger children. HbA1C can be used as a substitute for formal oGTT in some circumstances.
- Hepatic steatosis, liver function tests.
- Vitamin D.
- Other investigations (e.g. sleep studies in significant OSA) should be performed as clinically indicated.
- Malnutrition in the form of micronutrient deficiency can be present in the overfed but undernourished. Young people with dietary restriction relating to sensory preferences or extreme fussy eating, e.g. ARFID, where complete food groups are avoided should be screened for micronutrient deficiency.

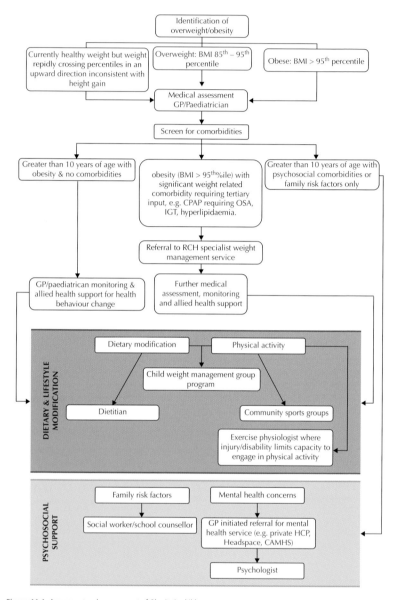

Figure 11.1 Assessment and management of Obesity in children.

Tip for consultations

• Use the appropriate growth charts as a reference for assessing a child's weight. This will reassure the child/parent that you are making a standardised assessment rather than giving your own opinion of their child's weight.

- Focus on:
    - Health, the aim of weight management is to diminish risk of morbidity and mortality with an emphasis on improving health and fitness.
    - Improving physical and social functioning rather than aesthetic ideals.
- Use an encouraging and empowering approach that is age appropriate. Avoid using negative language such as 'fat', 'chunky' or 'obese'. Use phrases like 'above his/her healthiest weight' or 'the healthiest weight for your child is…'.
- Explore the family's:
    - motivation for making healthy lifestyle changes.
    - barriers to being able to make changes – consider referrals to other healthcare professionals, e.g. social work or psychologist, to assist with overcoming these hurdles.
- Get the whole family involved in the conversation – what is good for one child is good for the entire family – same rules for everybody.
- Try not to label food/activities as 'good' and 'bad', uses words like 'healthy', 'healthier option/choice', 'sometimes/occasional food'.
- **No diets:** diets often encourage unhealthy and, at times, unsafe eating behaviours. When considering suggesting a dietary change you should consider whether the child/family will be able to incorporate this change into their regular meal pattern for the rest of their life. If you are unsure you can seek advice from a healthcare professional, e.g. dietitian.

Management
Nutrition
Dietitians are university-qualified specialists in the area of nutrition and its role in health and disease. Where possible, overweight and obese children and adolescents should be referred to a dietitian for weight management to ensure a thorough assessment and safe recommendations for weight management. Dietitians can be accessed through local community health centres or in private practice.

- Drinks
    - Water is the best drink! Sugar-sweetened drinks include soft drinks, fruit juices, flavoured mineral water, nutrient water, cordial, sports drinks and flavoured milks should be avoided.
    - Low-fat (2% fat) milk (<500 mL per day) is preferred for children >2 years of age.
- Snacks
    - Avoid pre-packaged snacks where possible.
    - Almost everything commercially marketed to be sold to children should not be given!
    - Encourage children to have at least one fruit AND one vegetable snack per day.
- Regular meals and snacks
    - Avoid skipping meals/snacks.
- Portions
    - Portion size is just as important as the type of food we eat. There is such a thing as 'too much of a good thing'. Portion sizes should be appropriate for your child's age. See Chapter 10, Nutrition.

Physical activity, sedentary behaviour and screen time
See Table 11.5.

Clinical Pearl: Physical activity
Any increase in activity is an improvement!
- Aim for 'lifestyle' exercise: using the stairs, walking to school, walking the dog.
- Involve the whole family.
- Use after-school time to get outdoors and be active.
- Can the family/children walk part or all of the way to/from school?

Sleep
Sleep should be assessed, and sleep hygiene optimised. See Chapter 40, Sleep medicine.

Table 11.5 National physical activity, sedentary behaviour, and sleep recommendations.

Age (years)	Physical Activity	Sedentary Behaviour	Screen time (per day)
<1	Being physically active several times in a variety of ways, particularly through interactive floor-based play; more is better. For those not yet mobile, this includes at least 30 minutes of tummy time spread throughout the day while awake	Not being restrained for more than 1 hour at a time (e.g., in a stroller or car seat)	Not recommended
1–2	At least 180 minutes spent in a variety of physical activities, of which at least 60 minutes is energetic play	Not being restrained for more than 1 hour at a time (e.g. in a stroller or car seat) or sitting for extended periods.	<2 years - Not recommended 2 years - <1 hour
3–5	At least 180 minutes spent in a variety of physical activities, of which at least 60 minutes is energetic play	Not being restrained for more than 1 hour at a time (e.g. in a stroller or car seat) or sitting for extended periods.	<1 hour
5–17	60 minutes of moderate to vigorous intensity activity per day	Avoid long periods of sitting where possible	<2 hours of recreational screen time

Mental Health
Optimal mental health is critically important for a young person being able to engage in sustainable and safe weight management. If a young person presents with low mood/depression, anxiety, poor body image or low self-esteem, they should be referred to appropriate counselling or psychology services. See Chapter 14, Behaviour and mental health.

Bariatric Surgery
In Australia and New Zealand bariatric surgery should only be considered where there is a persistence of the level of obesity despite supervised involvement in a formal multidisciplinary service for diet and lifestyle modification for at least six months. It should only be considered for severe obesity BMI >40 kg/m^2 or 35 kg/m^2 in the presence of severe complications. Bariatric surgery is not recommended for patients with an untreated or untreatable psychiatric or psychological disorder.

Health care team
Obesity without comorbidity or complications should be managed in primary care by a GP or paediatrician with supporting allied health as appropriate e.g. dietitian, psychologist, exercise physiologist, etc.
Referral to a specialist service should be considered for:
- A suspected pathological cause
- Presence of obesity related complications
- Specific medical therapies in obese adolescents, e.g. Metformin may be useful in reducing obesity-associated insulin resistance.

Short stature
When assessing stature, it is important to consider parental heights and the child's pubertal status. While stature is cross sectional, growth is a dynamic process and therefore multiple measures are required to determine growth velocity. This should be compared with age-matched peers as well as the child's pubertal status/bone age. A number of factors affect longitudinal growth. These include familial growth patterns, nutritional status, general health, presence of a normal skeleton, GH/IGF1 axis, adrenal function, thyroid status and the actions of sex steroids.

Assessment
Stature
Measure the child and, wherever possible, both biological parents.
- Height should always be measured with shoes off, with the child standing upright and fully extended against a vertical surface, with a calibrated, fixed measuring device.

- The head should be facing directly forward.
- Gentle pressure can be applied beneath the mastoid processes to ensure full neck extension.
- The child's height and the mid parental height (MPH) should be plotted on the appropriate centile chart. MPH is assessed using the following equation:

$$\text{For boys}: \frac{(\text{Mother's height} + 13\,\text{cm}) + (\text{Father's height in cm})}{2}$$
$$\text{For girls}: \frac{(\text{Father's height} - 13\,\text{cm}) + (\text{Mother's height in cm})}{2}$$

- A child's projected final height (extrapolated from their height centile and observed growth pattern) should fall within a range of MPH ± 7.5–8 cm (one standard deviation).
- Questions to consider:
  ○ Is the child short in relation to other children of the same age (i.e. below the third percentile).
  ○ Is the child unexpectedly short for the family?

Growth rate
- Serial measurements over time are required to fully assess stature and growth. Ideally measurements should be performed by the same clinician; however, previous height measurements, if available, are also useful to help assess the pattern over time.
- Calculate the height velocity and check this against a growth velocity (GV) chart. Growth velocity can only be reliably calculated from measurements taken over 6–12 months (with a minimum of 3–4 months between consecutive readings). In most children, GV tends to fluctuate and only a consistently low GV will lead to a falling-off in height percentile. Further investigation is required in a short child with a GV below the 25th percentile.
- Questions to consider:
  ○ Is the child growing slowly/crossing height centiles.
  ○ If the child's growth really is slow, what is the reason.
  ○ Is the child growing at the rate expected for pubertal status. A growth spurt should always accompany puberty.

Skeletal Proportions
Measure the skeletal proportions (arm span/height and upper/lower segment ratios):
- The lower segment should be greater than half the height beyond the age of 10 years.
- The arm span should be within a few centimetres of height at all ages.

Causes of short stature
Physiological
Constitutional delay of growth and puberty
- This is a common normal variant.
- Family history of delayed puberty is often present.
- Growth slows at about 2 years of age, producing a fall in the height percentile. Thereafter, growth usually follows a centile, but the prepubertal decline in growth is exaggerated and the onset of the pubertal growth spurt is later than average.
- Bone age is delayed; however, height for bone age is usually within the expected mid-parental range. The final height is likely to be in keeping with that of other family members.

Familial short stature
- Several adult family members are short.
- Skeletal proportions and GV are normal.
- Bone age is equivalent to the chronological age.
- Some children from short families also have constitutional delay in maturation.

Note: Parents who have suffered protein–calorie malnutrition as children may not have achieved their own genetic potential and may be on a lower percentile than their children.

Table 11.6 Organic causes of short stature.

	Examples	Clues to diagnosis
Intrauterine	Placental insufficiency, Russell–Silver syndrome	Birth weight <3rd centile for gestational age
Skeletal	Bone dysplasia (e.g. achondroplasia), Spinal irradiation	Skeletal disproportion (short limbs) - Low upper: lower segment ratio
Nutritional	Malabsorption (e.g. coeliac disease/short gut)	Poor weight gain ± abdominal distension
	Rickets	History of poor nutrition or limited sunlight/ dark skin
	Protein–calorie malnutrition (world's leading cause)	Low weight-for-height (if not chronic)
Chronic illness	Renal failure, inflammatory bowel disease, JCA, CF, inborn errors of metabolism, organic or amino acidurias	Anaemia, high ESR, findings specific to associated pathology
Iatrogenic	Corticosteroid treatment	Cushingoid features
Chromosomal/ other genetic	Turner, Down, Prader–Willi, Noonan, Cornelia de Lange, Rubinstein–Taybi syndromes (amongst many others)	Specific dysmorphic features
Endocrine	Hypothyroidism, growth hormone deficiency, Cushing syndrome/disease, pubertal delay/ arrest, pseudohypoparathyroidism, Albright hereditary osteodystrophy (AHO)	Height centile < weight centile, associated examination findings specific to diagnosis
Other	Psychosocial deprivation	Additional child protection concerns

Organic
Organic causes of short stature are classified in Table 11.6. Clues to the diagnosis may emerge from the history and the child's general appearance. Some serious medical conditions (e.g. chronic renal failure, coeliac disease, inflammatory bowel disease, craniopharyngioma) may present with slow growth as the only abnormal sign.

Clinical Pearl: Clinical features suggestive of an organic cause for short stature
- Dysmorphic features, e.g. Turner syndrome.
- Cutaneous changes, e.g. café au lait markings (Silver–Russell syndrome, neurofibromatosis).
- Hand and wrist changes, e.g. short fourth/fifth metacarpals, narrow deep-set nails (Turner syndrome), Madelung deformity of the wrist (SHOX gene abnormality).
- Fundal changes, e.g. optic atrophy.

Investigations
The bone age is often the first investigation performed, depending on features as discussed above. The younger a child is, the less predictive the bone age. If the GV is <25th percentile for bone age, or the height is out of keeping with genetic potential, or other concerns on history and examination, then further tests are indicated. The differential diagnosis will be based on history and examination findings in a given case, but the following can be considered:
- Thyroid function tests, TSH is the usual screening test, check free T4 (FT4) if central (pituitary) dysfunction is considered.
- Full blood count and erythrocyte sedimentation rate (ESR) (inflammatory bowel disease).
- Renal function and urine microscopy and culture.
- Liver function tests
- Serum calcium, phosphate and alkaline phosphatase.

- Coeliac antibodies.
- Karyotype (all short girls: lack of dysmorphism does not exclude Turner syndrome).
- Skeletal survey (if disproportionate).
- Baseline IGF-I level (needs to be interpreted in the context of bone age).

If above are all normal and concerns persist (for example, ongoing falling growth velocity), more definitive assessment of GH axis may be considered, even if the baseline IGF1 is normal. Stimulated growth hormone (GH) studies are a more definitive test. Growth hormone can be assessed in response to either:

- Exercise
- Pharmacological stimulation (e.g. glucagon stimulation used at RCH; other agents include clonidine, insulin, arginine). These should be performed at a centre with experience in carrying out the tests.

Clinical Pearl: GH deficiency

Basal GH is not a useful test as due to the pulsatile nature of GH release – a low random level does not define GH deficiency.

Management

Treatment of the underlying cause if found e.g. thyroxine replacement, gluten free diet, where applicable.

Growth hormone treatment

Recombinant human GH is government-controlled in Australia; it costs an average of $20 000–$30 000 per year per child. To qualify on the basis of stature, children must meet one of the following criteria:

- Growth hormone deficiency
- Turner syndrome or SHOX gene disorders
- Chronic renal disease
- Short and slow growth, defined as height below the 1st percentile and GV below the 25th percentile for bone age
- Prader Willi syndrome (further criteria exist for this indication)
- Additional criteria that must be met in all cases include:
- Bone age <13.5 years for girls, or <15.5 years for boys

Exclusion criteria include diabetes mellitus (unless proven biochemical GHD and excellent diabetes control), known risk of malignancy (e.g. Down or Bloom syndrome) or active malignancy (tumour activity needs to be stable for 12 months before commencement).

Children with GH deficiency would be expected to get to near their MPH with treatment, in the absence of any other comorbidities/early commencement of treatment. Predicted height gain with growth hormone treatment in "idiopathic short stature" is difficult to judge due to the highly heterogenous nature of this group, but most studies suggest a 3-7cm increase on final height expectation. In Australia, the starting dose of growth hormone is 4.5–7.5 mg/m2 per week divided into 6–7 doses. Children with Turner syndrome/SHOX haploinsufficiency/renal insufficiency can commence treatment at a higher dose (7.5–9.5 mg/m2 per week).

Psychological support should also be offered as short children can experience teasing or bullying and are often treated as younger than their chronological age.

Tall stature
Assessment

See Short stature assessment above for assessment of stature, growth rate and skeletal proportions.

Height must be considered in the context of mid-parental expectation and pubertal status. For example, if puberty is 2–3 years earlier than average, the child may appear to be very tall for chronological age but have a normal final height expectation for the family. Repeated height assessments are important in assessing tall stature, to determine growth velocity. Review of associated symptoms may help with differential diagnosis. Clinical assessment should also include:

- Assessment for dysmorphic features
- Intellectual development
- Pubertal staging

- Thyroid status
- Assessment of arachnodactyly
- Cardiovascular system
- Palate and joint mobility (Marfan syndrome)
- Eyes (Marfan syndrome/homocystinuria)
- Skin and visual fields (if pituitary adenoma suspected)

Causes
- Familial
- Precocious puberty
- Hyperthyroidism
- Syndromes: Marfan, Klinefelter, triple X, homocystinuria and Sotos.
- Pituitary gigantism (juvenile acromegaly).
- Lifestyle-related obesity is associated with increased stature in childhood, but normal adult final height (maturational advancement).

Investigations
Consider:
- Bone age
- Thyroid function
- Karyotype
- Urine metabolic screen/antithrombin III/coagulation/lipids (homocystinuria)
- Baseline IGFI, with 3 hours oral glucose tolerance test assessing for failure of suppression of GH/IGF1 if acromegaly is further suspected
  - MRI pituitary and further assessment of pituitary function are indicated if this test is consistent with GH excess

Management
- Management of any underlying disorder, for example precocious puberty.
- High-dose oestrogen was previously used in very tall girls, to hasten epiphyseal closure; however, long-term follow-up indicated a reduction in fertility in treated girls and so this treatment is now rarely used.

USEFUL RESOURCES
- Growth charts and calculators www.rch.org.au/gastro/about-us/Growth_charts_and_calculators/
- APEG https://apeg.org.au/clinical-resources-links/growth-growth-charts/ Growth and growth chart resources.
- National obesity guidelines www.nhmrc.gov.au/about-us/publications/clinical-practice-guidelines-management-overweight-and-obesity
- International Association for the Study of Obesity www.iaso.org
- RACP Guidelines on Bariatric Surgery in Adolescents www.racp.edu.au//docs/default-source/advocacy-library/recommendations-for-bariatric-surgery-in-adolescents.pdf?sfvrsn=f0a12f1a_10

CHAPTER 12

Adolescent medicine

Susan Sawyer
Michelle Telfer
Colette Reveley
Kathy Rowe
Adam Scheinberg

Key Points

- The burden of disease in adolescents differs greatly from infants and children.
- As many of the health outcomes and risks faced by adolescents are hidden, every consultation should go beyond the presenting complaint and involve a psychosocial assessment, as this can identify health outcomes and important risk and protective factors within the family, peer group, school, and community.
- Building an independent therapeutic relationship with the adolescent by seeing them on their own, while respectfully engaging parents, promotes engagement, psychosocial assessment, enhancement of health literacy and ultimately improves health outcomes.
- Regardless of the quality of family relationships, confidential health care is an integral aspect of quality care for adolescents.

Adolescence is a highly dynamic period of human development that brings major changes in health outcomes (e.g. mental health, overweight, and obesity), health risks (e.g. diet, physical activity, substance use) and the social determinants of health (e.g. education). Prioritising adolescent health is increasingly appreciated to yield a triple dividend through advancing health and well-being during adolescence, achieving healthier trajectories into adulthood, and laying the foundations of optimal health for the next generation. As such, adolescence is increasingly viewed as a developmental phase for acquiring the assets for later health and well-being, which requires both protection from harm and empowerment.

Definition of adolescence

Adolescence encompasses elements of biological growth (e.g. reproductive maturation, linear and bone growth, and brain maturation) leading to cognitive, social, and emotional development which underpins a series of social role transitions to adulthood. Earlier onset of puberty has accelerated the start of adolescence in nearly all populations, while delayed timing of role transitions, including completion of education, marriage, and parenthood, is shifting perceptions of when adolescence ends. Physical, cognitive, social, and emotional maturation during adolescence underpins the growing interest and relevance for young people around:

- Autonomy and independence from family
- Personal identity, self-esteem, and body image
- Peer relationships
- Sexuality
- Educational and vocational goal
- Financial independence

Paediatric Handbook, Tenth Edition. Edited by Kate Harding, Daniel S. Mason and Daryl Efron.
© 2021 John Wiley & Sons Ltd. Published 2021 by John Wiley & Sons Ltd.

A 'child' is defined as under 18 years old.

- Although certain adult legal privileges start at 18, many start at a younger age, and the adoption of adult roles and responsibilities generally occurs later.
- The WHO defines 'adolescents' as 10–19 years olds (i.e. under 20), but the years from 10–24 years are increasingly referred to as 'adolescence'.
- Terms such as 'youth', 'young people', and 'adolescents and young adults' are typically used interchangeably.

Adolescence and adolescent health care

The burden of disease in adolescents differs greatly from infants and children. Many causes of ill health in adolescents reflect unhealthy patterns of behaviour that are largely preventable, as well as mental disorders. Young people with chronic disease and disability can be especially disadvantaged.

Marginalised young people who are poorly connected to their families and schools have poorer health outcomes. High-risk vulnerable young people include those with:

- Significant health risk behaviours (e.g. regular drug use)
- Mental health problems (e.g. severe depression, psychosis, eating disorders)
- Families who are impoverished or chaotic
- Parents who have a severe mental illness or substance use issue

High-risk young people commonly experience a range of co-morbidities for which they uncommonly receive appropriate health care. Close consultation and liaison with case managers in the community is a priority and is generally more effective than referral to new services.

Understanding the elements of quality health care for adolescents, also known as 'adolescent friendly health care' is the key to providing the best care possible to young people. Clinicians should recognise the dynamic changes that occur across adolescence and reflect this in the care they provide. Key steps to achieving quality health care for adolescents (and their parents or carers) include:

- Actively engage young people in their health care.
- Assess psychosocial concerns even if not the presenting problem.
- Consult with adolescents alone for part of each consultation.
- Support families to understand healthy adolescent development.
- Promote self-management and adherence to treatment regimens, including medication.
- Support healthy engagement with peers and schools.
- Support the process of transition to adult health care.
- Liaise with health and community professionals involved in the young person's care.
- Ensure the physical environment is appropriate and welcoming for young people.

When young people require admission to hospital, they prefer to be nursed with other people their own age. Adolescent inpatient wards provide developmentally appropriate nursing, recreation and peer support. They also facilitate links to educational and mental health support.

Starting the consultation

The challenge of consulting with adolescents is to build an independent relationship with adolescents while respectfully engaging and supporting their parents.

- Greet the young person by name. When parents are present, greet the young person first, then introduce yourself to the parents.
- If parents are present, spend time with both the parents and the adolescent together to understand the presenting complaint, past history and parent concerns.
- Explain the issue of confidentiality at the beginning of the first contact with every adolescent (Table 12.1). It is important for parents to hear this as well.
- Spend some time alone with the young person as they must learn to increasingly function independently of their parents which includes health consultations.
- Allow adequate time.
- Listen and acknowledge the young person's viewpoint and opinions.

Table 12.1 Explaining confidentiality.

- Define the term at the start of the interview*.
- Consider all information from an adolescent as confidential until discussed or clarified.
- In most Australian States, confidentiality is a legal requirement over 16 years of age.
- Negotiation or compromise may be required for adolescents under 16 years.
- Exceptions to confidentiality are when the adolescent is at risk of significant harm, such as risk of suicide or if they are subject to physical or sexual abuse.
- Ensure that information to be kept confidential from parents is appropriately highlighted in the medical record.

* An example: 'In addition to spending time with you and your parents together, we also spend time with young people alone without their parents. This part of a consultation is confidential. That means that I cannot talk about anything we discuss today with your parents or anyone else, unless you and I have agreed to do so. However, there are some exceptions. I cannot maintain confidentiality if you are at risk of harm, such as threat of suicide, self-harm, or sexual abuse.'

- Always attempt to confidentially 'go beyond' the presenting complaint to identify wider psychosocial risks – as it is uncommon for these to be the presenting complaint.
- A clinician who listens respectfully and acknowledges a young person's point of view will have made an excellent start in establishing a therapeutic relationship.
- Young people benefit from reminders about confidentiality when sensitive information is discussed (Table 12.1).

Clinical Pearl: Tips for engaging adolescents and families
- Greet the young person by name. When family are present, greet the young person first, then introduce yourself to the family.
- Explain what confidential health care means for adolescents when parents are present to ensure consistent expectations around disclosure of patient information over time.
- Framing the benefits of consulting alone as a strategy that helps build adolescents' confidence and health literacy (that are both required to manage future independent health care as a young adult), is consistent with the family's goals of wanting to support their child's healthy development.

Psychosocial screening and developmental assessment
Consultations should go beyond the presenting complaint to identify broader psychosocial concerns e.g. bullying at school, school disengagement and academic failure, common mental disorders (e.g. anxiety, depressed mood), self-harm (including suicidal ideation), disordered eating, unsafe sex, family illness. One approach to taking a psychosocial history is to use the HEADSS framework (Table 12.2).
- Questions can be asked in any order, although the first three domains generally involve less sensitive questions than the last three.
- Taking a psychosocial history is a powerful way of engaging a young person and establishing rapport.
- It also provides an opportunity to assess developmental stage (maturity), identify the balance of health risk and protective factors, and identify opportunities for early intervention and health promotion.

Physical examination
- Reassure and explain the reason for the particular exam.
- Conduct a thorough physical examination whenever appropriate.
- Consider use of a chaperone.
- Ensure privacy from others and protect modesty as much as possible.
- Many young people are anxious about many aspects of normal development and benefit from reassurance.
- Provide feedback on the examination findings as much as possible (e.g. "I note you have some pimples on your forehead which is normal for your age").
- Monitor height, weight, and pubertal development. Plot growth on a growth chart and explain what this means in the context of normal growth patterns.

Table 12.2 Adolescent developmental screening: the 'HEADSS' psychosocial assessment.

Domains	Potential topics to discuss	Tips on contextualising and addressing these domains
Home	• Where they live, with whom • Housing security (tenure), recent moves • Physical environment and resources (e.g. electricity, transport, phone) • Social environment, key supports	Physical living arrangements and social and psychological supports available to young people at home are all key to understanding and addressing health conditions, especially chronic conditions (such as mental health). Living arrangements of young people can be quite complex – it is important not to make any assumptions.
Education/ employment	• Current education/employment • Educational attendance, performance, literacy and numeracy • Relationships with peers and superiors • Employment, finances, and financial security/supports • Future aspirations	Education and employment are important determinants of health and well-being. Health status is also a significant determinant of young people's capacity to engage in education and employment. In addressing this domain, it is important to appreciate how hard it can be for young people to be honest about bullying at school, or to acknowledge that they are not as academically successful as they or their families expected.
Eating/exercise	• Number and nature of meals • Body image; satisfaction, are others concerned? • Recent change in weight (increase/decrease) • Exercise patterns	Capitalize on the opportunity to address nutrition and exercise: both under- and over- nutrition are important determinants of individual and intergenerational health. Avoid using language like 'fat', 'chubby', or 'bony'– young people are sensitive about their weight and body image, irrespective of their body habitus.
Activities	• Activities and interests, including weekends/holidays • Family contact, shared activities, supports • Friend and peer networks • Social media use	Personal, peer, and family activities are all important determinants of health. Interests and hobbies may also provide a lever for change (e.g. ability to play sport may be an incentive to take asthma medication). Social media can be a platform for engagement with peers as well as creating risks (e.g. sexting, exposure to violence, pornography). It is often hard for adolescents with few friends to acknowledge this.
Drugs	• Peer and family substance use • Individual substance use, recent changes • Effects of substance use and regrets (e.g. injuries, loss of friends) • Injected substances (blood-borne virus risk) • Knowledge gaps	Family, peer, and personal drug use all impact on health outcomes and behaviours. Adolescence is a period of experimentation, and drug use is often modifiable. Before asking these questions, reaffirm confidentiality. Asking first about peer and family substance use helps normalize and contextualize this. Use this opportunity to provide education and advice around harm reduction.
Sexuality	• Sexual orientation • Gender identity • Romantic relationships, experience of sexual intercourse (including unwanted sex) • Concerns around sex (coercion, unplanned pregnancy, STI) • Knowledge/use of contraception and safe sex • Females: menstrual periods • Knowledge gaps	Sexual debut is common during adolescence. STIs and unplanned pregnancy disproportionately affect adolescents. Explain why you are asking these questions and use the opportunity to educate and promote sexual reproductive health and rights. Do not assume that young people are heterosexual or cis-gender. Be sensitive; sexual coercion is common and not all sexual experiences may be desired or pleasurable. When asking questions, remember that some young people have been sexually abused as younger children.

Table 12.2 (*Continued*)

Domains	Potential topics to discuss	Tips on contextualising and addressing these domains
Suicide and depression	• Sleep, appetite, energy, • Low mood and anxiety, including panic attacks (common mental disorder) • Self-harm/suicidal thoughts, attempts, plans	Poor mental health is a significant health issue but an uncommon reason for accessing health care. Additionally, mental health is an important determinant of many other health outcomes. In addressing this domain, be cognisant of the stigma of mental illness; a sensitive approach and reassurance of confidentiality (and its exceptions) are important. There is no evidence that asking about suicide or self-harm increases risk of these behaviours.
Safety	• Safety at home, school, and within the community • Reasons for not feeling safe (e.g. driving with someone affected by alcohol or drugs) • Carriage of weapons (e.g. knives) • Exposure to interpersonal violence within the home • Use of seatbelts, bicycle helmets, off-road motorbikes etc.	Injury is a leading contributor to the burden of disease experienced by young people globally. Health consultations provide an opportunity to identify key risk behaviours and can help the young person identify ways to improve their safety.
Strengths and spirituality	• Culture and identity • Strengths, both as identified by the individual, and strengths that others identify about them.	Culture and identity can be powerful protective factors. This domain also promotes a strengths-based approach and may help reassure young people of the skills and strengths they have and the active role they can play in improving their health. Importantly, culture and identity of young people can be different to that of their family or community.

Source: Modified from Azzopardi PS, Creati MB, Sawyer SM. Adolescent Health. In: Nelson B, ed. Essential Clinical Global Health Medicine. Wiley Blackwell Publishing. 2015. p. 168. (Nelson 2014). Reproduced with permission from Wiley & Sons Ltd.

Common issues when working with young people with chronic diseases and disabilities

Young people with chronic conditions are typically the most experienced consumers of the paediatric health system. Most young people greatly benefit from the support provided by parents around their health care. However, as young people mature, they should be supported to take on increasing responsibility for managing their health. Both clinicians and parents need to have appropriate expectations of what adolescents can (and can't) do, while supporting greater self-management over time.

Specific elements of self-management that young adults need to be able to take responsibility for, independent of their parents, include being able to:

- Name and explain their condition.
- Explain why each medication is necessary.
- Remember to take their medication.
- Arrange repeat prescriptions before medication runs out.
- Be able to consult with doctors (see the doctor alone, ask and answer questions, arrange and cancel appointments).
- Understand Medicare and health insurance.
- Develop a desire to be independent with health care.
- Prioritise their health over (some) other desires.

Adolescents with intellectual disability (and their families) should also be supported to develop greater self-management capacities around their healthcare and to have expectations that adolescence is also a time that they become more independent, with the extent being highly variable.

Conflict of priorities

At times there may be a conflict of priorities between the therapeutic goals of the clinician (focused on disease control and management) and the developmental goals that are frequently the main concern of young people. For example, a young person with persistent asthma who goes on a school camp may be too embarrassed to take their preventer medication while on camp, preferring instead to put up with the unknown consequences (and the unspoken wishful thinking that their asthma will be fine).

Practical tips include:

- Negotiate management approaches in ways that the young person is developmentally comfortable with.
- Provide the young person with a choice of acceptable management options.

Adherence

Promoting adherence with treatment regimens is a challenge for clinicians irrespective of the age of the patient. It can be especially difficult with adolescents with chronic disease, as they are generally less influenced by long-term health goals than adults. There may be conflict between the young person's (developmentally appropriate) pursuit of increasing autonomy and independence, and the clinician and parents' desire to improve their health. Don't assume adolescents are informed, even if their parents are.

Practical tips include:

- Provide a clear rationale for all treatments.
- Simplify the treatment regimen (e.g. choose daily dosing rather than tds dosing options when available).
- Use simple language and write down all instructions.
- Don't use threats.
- Help the adolescent develop routines about each treatment. Use technology, for example, phones can assist with reminders.
- Discuss the acceptability of treatment in relationship to peers and education.
- Work with both parents and young people. Parents may need to be more involved or encouraged to step back and be less overprotective.

Working across teams and across sectors

- Multidisciplinary team input can be very valuable for young people with complex health conditions.
- Excellent communication is required: different team members need to repeat the same key messages to the young person and family.
- It can be valuable to seek information from others who know the young person better, both within the health sector (e.g. mental health counsellor) and beyond (e.g. year level coordinator at school).
- Young people must provide their consent for doctors to contact school-based professionals.

Transition to adult health care

Transition is the purposeful and planned movement of adolescents with chronic diseases and disability from child-centred to adult-oriented health care systems. 'Transition' refers to the process of facilitating developmentally appropriate self-management and generally requires the acquisition of knowledge, attitudes, and skills over time. This skill set starts to develop well before 'transfer' to adult health care, the actual timing of the physical move, with the process of transition continuing well after transfer. From the time of diagnosis, anticipation of transfer to an adult setting is one way of ensuring that the physical move is truly part of a broader transition process.

Practical tips for successful transition

- Start seeing young people alone for at least part of the health consultation from about the age of 14 years. This helps remind parents that their children are growing up, can prompt young people 'stepping up' within health consultations and facilitate successful transition to adult health care.
- Use a checklist and resources to support success transition (See www.rch.org.au/transition/).
- Planning and coordinating transfer to adult health care is essential. Some young people may no longer need specialist health services. Others will transfer to adult specialist services in public hospitals or to private specialists, including psychiatrists. In all cases, GPs are the critical resource.

- When adult tertiary care is indicated, identify an adult specialist team that is both interested and capable of providing tertiary care. This is fundamental, but sometimes challenging.
- Documentation to support the transfer is important: a detailed health care summary should be compiled and clearly communicated to adult providers. It is important the adolescent and their GP also receive a summary of this information. Discuss with the adolescent whether there is some information that they would prefer was not communicated to the adult team. This may (or may not) be appropriate to withhold.

Management of specific health problems in adolescence
Fatigue

Fatigue is a common presenting complaint in adolescent medical consultations. It is often accompanied by other constitutional and neuropsychological symptoms (commonly sleep disturbance, headaches, abdominal pain, nausea, postural, and depressive symptoms).

Differential diagnoses include:

- Inadequate sleep (e.g. obstructive sleep apnoea, excessive nocturnal computer use)
- Mental Health Issues (e.g. depression, anxiety)
- Hypothyroidism
- Anaemia
- Malabsorption syndromes (e.g. coeliac disease)
- Chronic Illness (e.g. inflammatory bowel disease, connective tissue disease, renal disease)
- Chronic Fatigue Syndrome (CFS)

Chronic Fatigue Syndrome

Chronic Fatigue Syndrome is a condition of unknown aetiology, characterised by a new onset of fatigue persisting for at least three months and associated with constitutional symptoms (Table 12.3). Many young people have a preceding history of a suspected or confirmed viral illness or trigger event (e.g. injury/surgery). It is more common in adolescence but can occur in younger children and is three times more common in females.

Chronic Fatigue Syndrome is a clinical diagnosis and requires exclusion of other causes of fatigue (see above) together with the presence of CFS Diagnostic criteria (Table 12.3). Orthostatic intolerance (e.g. Postural Orthostatic Tachycardia Syndrome, see chapter 15, Cardiology) is common, often associated with hypermobility, and this should be assessed during the examination, using lying standing heart rate and blood pressure at baseline, 1 and 5 minutes with self-reported symptoms and a Beighton Score.

Recommended investigations in those without red flag symptoms or signs on examination are:

- FBE, Ferritin
- UEC, CMP, LFT, glucose
- ESR, ANA
- TFT, Vitamin D
- Coeliac serology
- Urinalysis
- It is not usually necessary to perform cranial imaging or extensive rheumatological screening.
- EBV/CMV serological testing does not alter management or effect diagnosis.
- Overseas travel or farm/country living may prompt additional screening including: Ross River Virus, Barmah Forest Virus, Murray Valley Virus, Q fever, and stool testing for parasites.
- Lyme disease has not been proven to exist in Australia so testing for this is not recommended in the absence of a travel history to an endemic area; serological testing for Lyme disease has low sensitivity and specificity and prior to any treatment being commenced consultation with an infectious disease specialist is recommended (especially given that there is evidence that functional outcome/recovery is not improved by treatment).

The management of CFS involves making the diagnosis (i.e. stopping ongoing investigations and specialist appointments) and educating the young person and the family regarding the prognosis (life altering but not life threatening, with most adolescents recovering good function over a few years). The average duration of CFS is 5 years, with a range of 1–16 years, with 68% reporting recovery by 10 years.

Table 12.3 CFS diagnostic criteria.

CFS Diagnostic criteria
1. Chronic fatigue that is persistent over 3 months and is not a result of ongoing exertion, not substantially alleviated by rest and results in reduction of the previous level of education/social/personal activity.

2. Concurrently:
• Post Exertional Malaise/Fatigue (occurs with physical/cognitive exertion and has delayed recovery)
• Unrefreshing sleep/sleep disturbance
• Pain, often widespread affecting either: myofascial/joint or head/chest/abdominal
• Two neurocognitive symptoms e.g. reduced memory, reduced concentration, word finding difficulties, reduced speed of thought, sensory or perceptual disturbances
• One of either
   ○ autonomic symptoms e.g. orthostatic intolerance, pallor, IBS symptoms urinary frequency, palpitations, exertional dyspnoea
   ○ neuroendocrine symptoms e.g. dysmenorrhea, loss of thermal stability, marked weight change
   ○ immune symptoms e.g. recurrent sore throats, tender lymph nodes, new food/medication sensitivities

It is important to address symptoms with lifestyle modifications and medications (where necessary) in order to promote function.

• Due to the multiple symptoms present it is best to focus on the one that the young person identifies as most troublesome. Commonly sleep initiation, phase-shift, or sleep disturbance need to be managed initially followed by any remaining symptoms, one at a time.
• Review and refinement of lifestyle measures should be undertaken prior to the introduction of medication.
• Medication can be useful for symptom control, but in order to minimize side effects, which are common in this patient group, it should be commenced slowly, at low doses and reviewed over time. Useful medications are listed with symptoms in Table 12.4. Careful enquiry regarding alternative medicine use is required as this is particularly common in this patient group and could be contributing to symptoms.

Table 12.4 Useful medication in CFS.

Useful Medications for symptoms in CFS	
Sleep disturbance **Initiation:** **Interrupted:**	Melatonin 2–10mg nocte Endep 5–10mg nocte Dothiepin 25mg nocte
Chronic daily headaches	Pizotifen 0.5–1.5mg nocte Periactin 4–12mg nocte Endep 5–50 mg nocte Topiramate 25mg nocte – 50mg bd Riboflavin 400mg daily Co-enzyme Q 100mg bd Magnesium 250mg daily
GI/IBS symptoms	Endep 5–10 mg nocte
Muscular pain	Endep 5–10 mg nocte Dothiepin 25 mg nocte
Orthostatic symptoms **(as add on if lifestyle measure unsuccessful)**	Propanolol 10–40mg bd Fludrocortisone/midodrine: under cardiology guidance
Concentration **(once sleep/headache and workload have been addressed)**	Methylphenidate 5–30mg prn (intermittently for assignments/exams)
Mood/anxiety	Fluoxetine 10–20mg daily Sertraline 50–150mg daily

- The adolescent and family should be encouraged and supported to develop a 'return to function' plan, incorporating school, social interaction, physical activity, and an enjoyable activity outside the home. The young person should be supported to plan how to spend their energy over the week to incorporate each of these activities.
- Feedback from young people has indicated the importance of: 'being believed', feeling supported, having an advocate for their educational needs, and regular follow up by a professional.
- Take a multidisciplinary approach with engagement of one or all of the following: the GP, school-based professionals (well-being or year coordinator, school counsellor, visiting teacher), clinical psychologist, occupational therapist, and an exercise physiologist/physiotherapist.
- Regular review to assess progress and manage troublesome symptoms should occur every 2 to 3 months with close attention being paid to the psychosocial aspects of the illness.
- Annual vaccination with the fluvax is recommended, together with annual monitoring of TFT, FBE, ferritin, ESR whilst symptoms persist.
- Letters to the school should be provided every 12 months outlining the diagnosis and asking for an Individual Learning Plan and Special Consideration. Useful educational considerations include modified timetables, additional time to complete projects, rest breaks during exams, use of computers or scribes, sitting exam in a separate room, access to food/drink/medication.
- During VCE students should be made aware of the Special Consideration Process, the possibility of extending over 3 or more years, and the SEAS process for tertiary education. Remaining engaged in education was identified as the best predictor of later functioning.

Somatic Symptom and Related Disorder

Adolescents presenting with somatic symptom and related disorder (SSRD) may have specific symptoms (e.g. localised pain) or non-specific symptoms (e.g. fatigue).

- Symptoms may be single or multiple and commonly occur in conjunction with known organic illness.
- Conversion disorder is commonly used when neurological symptoms are involved, while Somatic Symptom Disorder refers to other presentations.
- The individual's suffering is authentic, whether or not it can be medically explained.
- The impact on the adolescent and their family's daily life can be severe, with functional impairment impacting on school attendance, family functioning, educational, social, and emotional development.
- Clinically significant somatoform disorders are remarkably common; SSRDs account for 10–15% of primary care visits in children, and due to the variety of symptoms that can present, can be seen in every hospital department.

The diagnostic criteria for Somatic Symptom Disorder include:

- One or more somatic symptoms that are distressing or result in significant disruption of daily life.
- Excessive thoughts, feelings, or behaviours related to the somatic symptoms or associated health concerns with disproportionate concern about the seriousness of one's symptoms, persistent anxiety, or excessive time and energy devoted to them.
- Although any one symptom may not be continuously present, the state of being symptomatic is persistent and typically lasts more than 6 months.

Management involves reassurance and provision of psychological support whilst addressing possible underlying psychosocial contributing factors such as depression, anxiety and family stressors. Avoidance of excessive medical investigations and interventions is necessary and a functional approach to recovery, including use of multidisciplinary rehabilitation services, may be necessary. Parent understanding of the somatization process predicts recovery, hence the importance of working closely with parents.

Substance use and misuse

- Assess other psychosocial risks as adolescents who use substances are more likely to experience other health risks, including mental health concerns.
- Take a non-judgemental, 'harm minimisation' approach to preserve rapport. Over time, important health messages can be conveyed and reasons for using drugs explored.
- Motivational interviewing can be especially helpful in eliciting 'change talk'.
- Referral to specialist drug services is generally not helpful unless the young person wishes to reduce substance use.

Mental health

Adolescence is characterised by a marked increase in a wide range of emotional and mental health disorders. The presence or extent of these may not be appreciated by adolescents themselves or by their parents, hence the importance of opportunistic assessment using the HEADSS framework, with more detailed assessment and referral according to responses. See also Chapter 14, Behaviour and mental health.

Eating disorders

Eating disorders typically arise in early to mid-adolescence. Dieting is a common antecedent to a clinical presentation. More severe dieting behaviours are associated with a greater risk of developing an eating disorder, although the majority of those who go on to develop an eating disorder have more moderate levels of dieting. Abnormal eating behaviour and a preoccupation with weight or body shape that interferes with normal adolescent social or emotional functioning requires further assessment, especially when it is associated with significant weight loss (even if the adolescent is not underweight) and always if it results in amenorrhoea.

Anorexia nervosa

The diagnostic criteria of anorexia nervosa includes:
- Restriction of energy intake relative to requirements leading to a markedly low body weight.
- Intense fear of gaining weight or becoming fat or persistent behaviour that interferes with weight gain, even though at a significantly low weight.
- Disturbance in the way in which one's body weight or shape is experienced, undue influence of body weight or shape on self-evaluation, or persistent lack of recognition of the seriousness of the current low body weight.

Atypical anorexia nervosa describes those who have lost a large amount of weight (e.g. 5–20 kg in 6–12 months) and have all the diagnostic features of anorexia nervosa except they are not underweight. They are generally over their healthiest weight prior to weight loss, which is why they are not underweight. They are managed the same way.

Anorexia nervosa can be of either restricting type or binge-eating/purging type (self-induced vomiting or the misuse of laxatives, diuretics, or enemas in the last 3 months). Differential diagnoses include physical disorders (e.g. thyrotoxicosis, malabsorption) and other psychiatric disorders (e.g. major depression, obsessive compulsive disorder). Physical complications are potentially very severe, especially if the onset of the disorder occurs during the prepubertal or peripubertal stages where impaired growth and osteoporosis are of particular concern. Cardiac arrhythmias, substance abuse, self-harm and suicide contribute to a mortality rate that is greater than that of any other psychological disorder.

Management
- Confirm diagnosis by careful medical and mental health assessment (not electrolytes).
- Provide multidisciplinary outpatient care utilising family-based treatment which aims to empower the parents/carers to refeed the adolescent to a healthy body weight within the home environment. This is usually provided over 6 months.
- Brief hospital admission is required when evidence of physiological compromise (e.g. bradycardia or postural hypotension) signals lack of physical safety.
- Refeeding is the mainstay of acute admissions that aim to achieve physiological stability. The adolescent is supported to eat the meals provided to them; nasogastric feeding is required if the adolescent is unable to eat enough to appropriately gain weight.
- Refeeding syndrome is a potentially fatal acute complication that requires careful monitoring of electrolyte and cardiovascular status, especially within the first 72 hours following increased caloric intake.

Avoidant/Restrictive Food Intake Disorder (ARFID)

The diagnostic criteria of ARFID includes:

An eating or feeding disturbance (e.g. apparent lack of interest in eating or food; avoidance based on the sensory characteristics of food; concern about aversive consequences of eating such as vomiting or choking) with persistent failure to meet appropriate nutritional and/or energy needs associated with one or more of the following:
1. Significant weight loss (or failure to achieve expected weight gain or faltering growth in children).
2. Significant nutritional deficiency.
3. Dependence on enteral feeding or oral nutritional supplements.
4. Marked interference with psychosocial functioning.

The impact on physical health and psychosocial well-being can be of similar severity to that seen in anorexia nervosa and a similar approach to refeeding, including multidisciplinary outpatient care and intermittent hospital admissions, may be required. Common co-morbidities include anxiety disorders, obsessive-compulsive disorder and neurodevelopmental disorders such as autism spectrum disorder.

Bulimia nervosa

The diagnostic criteria of bulimia nervosa includes:

- Recurrent episodes of binge eating (consuming a large amount of food within a discrete period of time) with a sense of lack of control over eating during the episode. The young person may feel that they cannot stop eating or control what or how much one is eating.
- Recurrent inappropriate compensatory behaviour in order to prevent weight gain (e.g. self-induced vomiting, misuse of laxatives, diuretics, other medications, fasting or excessive exercise).
- The binge eating and inappropriate compensatory behaviours both occur, on average, at least once per week for 3 months.
- Self-evaluation is unduly influenced by body shape and weight.

Common co-morbidities and complications include depression, anxiety disorders and difficulties with impulse control in other areas (e.g. alcohol and substance use, self-harm behaviours). Potential complications include dental erosion, oesophagitis and severe electrolyte disturbance leading to cardiac arrhythmias.

Management

- Usually occurs on an outpatient basis.
- Focal psychotherapies such as cognitive-behavioural therapy are effective both in individual and group treatment settings.
- Antidepressant medication such as selective serotonin reuptake inhibitors (SSRIs) are indicated when severe depressive symptoms are present.

Binge Eating Disorder

The diagnostic criteria for binge eating disorder includes:

- Recurrent episodes of binge eating characterised by consumption of a large amount of food over a discrete period of time and a sense of lack of control during the episode.
- The binge eating episodes are associated with eating more rapidly than normal, eating until uncomfortably full, eating large amounts of food when not feeling hungry, eating alone due to embarrassment and feeling disgusted with oneself, depressed or very guilty after overeating.
- Marked distress regarding binge eating is present.
- The binge eating occurs, on average, at least once per week for 3 months and is not associated with recurrent use of inappropriate compensatory behaviour (e.g. purging).

While overeating is commonly seen within the general population, binge eating disorder is much less common, is far more severe and is associated with significant complications relating to the physical and psychological problems of obesity (see Chapter 11, Growth).

CHAPTER 13

Allergy

Joanne Smart
Dean Tey

Key Points

- Allergy is a reproducible immunological reaction to an ordinarily harmless substance called an allergen e.g. a food, pollen, house dust mite.
- Anaphylaxis is an acute life-threatening allergic reaction characterized by either respiratory, cardiovascular or severe, persistent gastrointestinal symptoms.
- Fatal anaphylaxis is strongly associated with delayed administration of intramuscular adrenaline and poorly controlled asthma or allergic rhinitis.
- Infant feeding guidelines in Australia recommend early introduction of allergenic foods in the first 12 months of life.
- Allergy testing (skin prick tests and serum specific IgE) is associated with false positive results, and should only be performed after careful clinical evaluation. Allergy testing should *not* be used as a screening tool as over-testing can lead to unnecessary allergen avoidance.

Definitions

- **Allergy** is an objective, reproducible reaction mediated via the body's immune system, initiated by exposure to a defined stimulus at a dose tolerated by normal persons.
- **Allergic diseases** affect up to 40% of children, and include food allergy, eczema, asthma, allergic rhinoconjunctivitis ('hay fever'), and insect sting & drug allergies.
- **Sensitisation** is defined by the production of IgE antibodies against an antigen, as detected via a skin prick test (SPT) or serum-specific IgE (sIgE).
- **Atopy** is the genetic tendency to develop sensitisation in response to ordinary exposure to allergens, which subsequently lead to the development of food allergy, eczema, asthma and allergic rhinoconjunctivitis.

Diagnostic methods
General principles

- 'Skin prick testing and serum specific IgE testing both detect evidence of IgE-sensitisation *in vivo*.
- Because SPT and sIgE are associated with possible false positive results, targeted testing of specific allergens is recommended only after a comprehensive clinical assessment.
- Screening with allergen panels or using food allergen mixes is **not** recommended as this leads to frequent false positive results, resulting in unnecessary allergen avoidance.
- A high SPT or sIgE result is associated with a strong likelihood of IgE-mediated allergy to that allergen, **but does not predict the severity** of allergic reactions or risk of anaphylaxis to that allergen.
- IgE mediated allergy is confirmed when there is a clinical history of recent immediate allergic reaction in association with a positive SPT or sIgE.

Paediatric Handbook, Tenth Edition. Edited by Kate Harding, Daniel S. Mason and Daryl Efron.
© 2021 John Wiley & Sons Ltd. Published 2021 by John Wiley & Sons Ltd.

- A positive SPT or sIgE in the absence of a clinical reaction raises the possibility of allergic disease, but may represent a false positive result.
- Where SPT or sIgE results are equivocal, an *in vivo* oral food challenge should be considered to assess if the child is allergic or tolerant.

Skin prick testing

- Highly sensitive, inexpensive, simple and rapid.
- Can be performed from early infancy (lower sensitivity <2y age).
- Uses single-, dual- or multi-point device to introduce allergen extract into the epidermis (usually back or forearm). Wheal diameter measured 15 minutes later. Histamine and saline used as positive and negative controls.
- False-negative results can occur after antihistamine use (within 4–5 days), or after recent anaphylaxis (within 6 weeks due to mast cell tachyphylaxis).
- False-positive results may occur with dermatographism.

Serum-specific IgE antibodies (sIgE)

- Useful in the primary care setting as initial investigation to confirm a suspected, **single** allergy. eg. confirmation of IgE-mediated food allergy to cow's milk, egg or peanut; or assessment for house dust mite, pet dander or pollen sensitisation in asthma or allergic rhinitis.
- Useful alternative to SPT if dermatographism, widespread skin disease, or if antihistamines cannot be discontinued.
- Compared to SPT, has reduced sensitivity, is more expensive and has slower turnaround time.

In-vivo challenges

- **Gold standard** for diagnosis of food allergy and antibiotic reactions.
- Performed if SPT or sIgE result equivocal, or to determine if previously diagnosed food allergy has resolved.
- Due to risk of anaphylaxis, should only be performed by experienced specialists in centres with facilities for resuscitation.
- Procedure involves administration of increasing quantities of an allergen until either a threshold dose is tolerated, or objective signs of an allergic reaction are observed.

Food Allergy Classification

- Food hypersensitivity is an objective, reproducible reaction initiated by exposure to a defined food (Figure 13.1). Food hypersensitivity reactions may be either mediated through the immune system (allergy) or not (intolerance e.g. lactose intolerance).
- Food allergies can be further classified as IgE-mediated, non-IgE-mediated, or mixed IgE-/non-IgE-mediated.

IgE mediated Food Allergy

- The prevalence of IgE mediated food allergies and infantile eczema has increased dramatically.
- HealthNuts, a population-based study in Melbourne in 2007, reported that more than 10% of 12-month-old infants have challenge-proven IgE-mediated food allergies (egg 9%, peanut 3%).
- Early onset, severe eczema in the first three months of life is strongly associated with an increased risk of IgE mediated food allergy.
- The majority (85%) of IgE-mediated cow's milk, egg, soy and wheat allergies resolve during childhood.
- The minority (10-20%) of IgE-mediated peanut, tree nuts, sesame, fish and shellfish allergies resolve by adulthood.

Clinical presentation

- Symptom onset within 30–60 minutes of food ingestion.
- Symptoms include lip swelling, urticaria, oral tingling, facial angioedema, vomiting and acute diarrhea.
- Duration of symptoms usually a few hours.
- Anaphylaxis is an acute severe allergic reaction involving the respiratory tract (throat tightness, stridor, hoarse voice, persistent coughing, wheezing, chest tightness) and/or the cardiovascular system (hypotension, collapse).
- Children with a food allergy usually have associated allergic disease, including eczema, asthma and allergic rhinitis

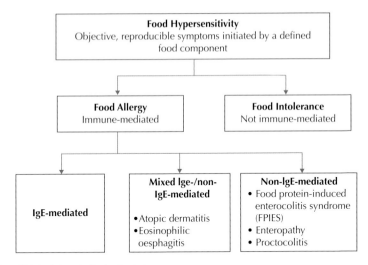

Figure 13.1 Food allergy classification flowchart.

Assessment & Diagnosis
- Take a comprehensive history of the reaction, including:
  - Age at time of reaction
  - Amount of food ingested
  - Form of food (raw, cooked or baked egg)
  - Time until onset of reaction
  - Presence of respiratory, cardiovascular or severe & persistent gastrointestinal symptoms to suggest anaphylaxis.
- History and severity of other food allergies, co-existing eczema, asthma and allergic rhinitis.
- Diagnosis relies on convincing clinical history of immediate allergic reaction **plus** demonstration of IgE antibodies by either positive SPT or sIgE antibodies.
- If the history is uncertain or diagnosis not supported by demonstration of sIgE, specialist referral is warranted where further evaluation by formal food challenge in hospital may be considered.

Management
- Strict elimination of the offending food allergen(s) from diet. Requires parental education and attention to reading ingredient labels.
- Written allergy or anaphylaxis action plan (available from *www.allergy.org.au*).
- The Australasian Society of Clinical Allergy and Immunology (ASCIA) guidelines recommend provision of an adrenaline autoinjector (Epipen®) when there has been a history of anaphylaxis. Prescription of an adrenaline autoinjector should also be considered in patients with limited access to emergency medical care, have co-morbid asthma, have a nut or insect sting allergy, or are in the adolescent age group.
- Dose for adrenaline autoinjector:
  - Child >20 kg: 300 mcg single dose.
  - Child 10–20 kg: 150 mcg single dose.
  - Child <10 kg: discuss with allergist immunologist
  (Note: this is different to current product information dosage guidelines, where the Epipen 300 mcg is recommended for children >30 kg).
- Long term follow-up involves:
  - Repeat SPT and/or sIgE to monitor for possible development of tolerance.
  - Regular education on allergic reaction management and checking adrenaline autoinjector technique.
  - Ensuring that co-existing allergic disease is optimally managed.

Prevention
ASCIA recommendations on infant feeding for food allergy prevention:
- Normal, healthy and balanced maternal diet rich in fibre, vegetables and fruit.
- Up to three serves of oily fish per week may reduce infantile eczema.
- If breastfeeding is not possible, use a standard cow's milk formula.
- Solids introduction
  - Introduction of solids around age 6 months, but not before 4 months, while continuing breastfeeding.
  - In the first year of life, all infants, including those at high risk of food allergy, should be given allergenic solid foods including dairy, wheat, egg and peanut butter.
- Hydrolysed formulas, either partially or extensively, are not recommended for the prevention of allergic disease.

Non-IgE mediated Food Allergy
- Non-IgE-mediated food allergies present in the first years of life, mainly with chronic manifestations of the gastrointestinal tract or atopic dermatitis.
- Prevalence in infancy is not known but may be as high as 10%.

Clinical presentation
- Delayed onset 24–48 hours after food ingestion (exception FPIES; see below).
- A **small** proportion of infantile eczema is triggered by non-IgE-mediated food allergy.
- Cow's milk, soy and wheat are the most common trigger foods for non-IgE-mediated reactions.
- Gastrointestinal symptoms include frequent regurgitation/vomiting, chronic diarrhoea, rectal bleeding, unsettled behaviour and abdominal pain.
- Feeding difficulties and food refusal are common in infants with non-IgE food allergy and may cause poor weight gain or failure to thrive.
- Natural history is generally good, with tolerance in majority by 12–24 months of age.

There are three main clinical syndromes of non-IgE-mediated gastrointestinal food allergy:

1. **Food-protein-induced proctocolitis**
   - Most common cause of rectal bleeding in early infancy.
   - Presents with mild rectal bleeding, increased mucus and low-grade diarrhea in first few months of life (breastfed & formula-fed infants).
   - Infant otherwise well and thriving.
2. **Food-protein-induced enterocolitis syndrome (FPIES)**
   - Acute, delayed-onset forceful, repeated vomiting associated with pallor and lethargy 2-4 hours after food allergen ingestion.
   - 20% of infants with FPIES develop severe dehydration and hypovolaemic shock.
   - Diarrhoea can persist for 24 hours & occasionally contains blood.
   - Reactions may be mistaken for gastroenteritis, sepsis or intestinal obstruction.
   - Typically occurs after first ingestion of formula (cow's milk, soy) or solid foods (egg, rice, oats, chicken).
   - Rarely occurs in exclusively breastfed infants.
3. **Food-protein-induced enteropathy**
   - Clinical picture similar to coeliac disease: irritability, persistent diarrhoea, vomiting (in two-thirds of cases) and poor weight gain/growth failure.
   - Signs of secondary lactose malabsorption, including abdominal bloating and perianal excoriation, may be present.
   - Usually formula-fed infants (cow's milk or soy), or after early introduction of intact cow's milk.

Assessment
- No specific *in vitro* test for non-IgE-mediated food allergy is available. SPT or sIgE is not indicated.
- Diagnosis requires demonstration of significant symptom resolution after food elimination (within 2–4 weeks), followed by relapse of objective symptoms with reintroduction of offending food.
- Some patients require additional investigations to exclude other diagnoses, such as such sigmoidoscopy and biopsy (atypical rectal bleeding) and HLADQ2/DQ8 testing, gastroscopy and biopsy (enteropathy).

Management of non IgE mediated cow's milk allergy (CMA)

- In infants with CMA, all cow's milk-based products should be eliminated;
  - In breastfed infants, a maternal dairy-free diet may be effective (see below).
  - In formula-fed infants, a soy-based or extensively hydrolysed rice-based formula can be used in infants from age 6 months, a calcium-fortified soy milk can be used from age 12 months.
  - In infants with soy allergy, an *extensively hydrolysed cow's milk formula* should be used.
- About 10% of infants will not tolerate an extensively hydrolysed formula (due to residual allergenicity) and require an elemental *amino acid based formula*.
  - Amino acid based formula is generally reserved for infants with complex or severe manifestations of food allergy, including enteropathy with failure to thrive, multiple (non-IgE-mediated) food allergy, or children with eosinophillic oesophagitis (EoE); and is prescribed under the PBS after discussion with an allergist immunologist or gastroenterologist.
- Maternal elimination diets
  - Food allergens can transfer from the maternal diet into breast milk and cause allergic reactions in the infant. The clinical relevance is determined via a maternal elimination then reintroduction diet over a 2–4 week period.
  - Maternal elimination of specific food proteins, usually milk and/or soy milk protein, may be effective in gastrointestinal food allergy e.g. food-protein-induced proctocolitis. It is rarely beneficial to avoid multiple food proteins.
  - The maternal elimination diet needs to be closely supervised by a dietitian, and maternal micronutrient/ vitamin supplementation is generally required (NB maternal RDI for calcium 1200 mg daily).

Clinical Pearl: Persistent chronic diarrhoea

In infants with persistent chronic diarrhoea and failure to thrive who are non-responsive to dietary changes, consider evaluation of other causes e.g. inflammatory bowel disease, severe combined immuno-deficiency disease (SCID) and other enteropathy.

Anaphylaxis

- Anaphylaxis is a serious, life-threatening, systemic allergic reaction which can result in death.
- In Australia, the majority of food-induced anaphylaxis admissions occur in children aged <5 years, whilst food-induced anaphylaxis fatalities predominantly occur in children aged >5 years.
- Fatal anaphylaxis in Australia is rare, with approximately 20 deaths occurring annually, primarily in adults.

Definition

- The Australasian Society of Clinical Immunology and Allergy (ASCIA) defines anaphylaxis as:
  a. An acute illness with typical skin features (urticarial rash or erythema/flushing, and/or angioedema), plus involvement of respiratory and/or cardiovascular and/or persistent *severe* gastrointestinal symptoms, **OR**
  b. Acute onset of hypotension or bronchospasm or upper airway obstruction where anaphylaxis is considered possible, even if typical skin features are not present.

Management

- See also Chapter 3 Resuscitation and Medical Emergencies.
- Adrenaline (epinephrine): the definitive management of anaphylaxis is the immediate administration of intramuscular adrenaline into the anterolateral aspect of the thigh. Fatal anaphylaxis is strongly associated with the delayed administration of adrenaline.
- Posture: patients should remain supine, or, if having difficulties breathing, remain in a sitting position (risk of unexpected cardiovascular collapse after change to standing position).
- Hospital admission: mitigate risk of secondary biphasic reaction several hours later. Most are mild cutaneous reactions, however biphasic anaphylaxis can occur. Patients with anaphylaxis should be observed for at least 4 hours in hospital, and at least 12 hours if history/concern for biphasic reaction.

- Long-term management:
  - ○ Allergen avoidance.
  - ○ Education on label reading & early recognition of symptoms.
  - ○ Provision of an adrenaline autoinjector ('Epipen') in at-risk patients.
  - ○ Implementation of a written anaphylaxis action plan.
  - ○ Ensuring optimal management of co-existing allergic disease, in particular asthma and allergic rhinitis.

Eosinophilic Oesophagitis
- See Chapter 21, Gastroenterology.

Atopic dermatitis (eczema)
- See also Chapter 18, Dermatology.
- Eczema is often the first allergic manifestation in infants and young children.
- Moderate-to-severe eczema in the first year of life is strongly associated with IgE-mediated food allergy.
- SPT & sIgE have a poor positive predictive value in determining offending foods that may be exacerbating eczema therefore are **not** recommended.
- The majority of children with eczema do not have an underlying food allergy driving their eczematous flares; dietary restriction is not generally recommended. Any elimination diets should be supervised by an allergist.

Allergic rhinitis and conjunctivitis
- Presents with paroxysmal sneezing, itching, congestion and rhinorrhea, caused by sensitisation to environmental allergens.
- Commonly unrecognised and may impact significantly on quality of life and school performance.
- Traditional classification into *perennial* (throughout the year), *seasonal* (for example, during summer and spring) or *triggered by a specific allergen* (e.g. cats or horses).
- Recent classification uses *persistent* (symptoms for >4 days a week **and** >4 weeks a year) or *intermittent* (symptoms <4 days a week or <4 weeks a year), and as *mild*, *moderate* or *severe*. Both classification systems may be used in combination.
- Diagnosis requires the demonstration of an allergic basis for symptoms.
- Other causes of rhinitis should be considered: non-allergic rhinitis with eosinophilia syndrome, infective rhinitis, vasomotor rhinitis, hormonal rhinitis or rhinitis medicamentosa (rhinitis induced by excessive use of topical decongestants).

Perennial allergic rhinitis
- Can occur at any age, however more common in preschool and primary school children.
- Sneezing & congestion prominent especially on waking in the morning
- Nasal obstruction & snoring at night can occur (associated risk of obstructive sleep apnoea)
- House dust mite is the most common allergen involved (and/or other pollens in older children).

Seasonal allergic rhinitis
- More frequent in teenagers and young adults.
- Seasonal sneezing, itching and rhinorrhoea.
- Nasal symptoms often associated with itchy, red and watery eyes.
- General pollination times/season: trees (early spring), grasses (late spring & summer), weeds (summer and autumn) with some overlap.
- Rye grass is the commonest provoking antigen in Australia.
- Examination: assess nasal mucosa and nasal airflow: pale, oedematous mucosa and swollen turbinates indicate ongoing rhinitis (may be normal outside pollen season).

Management
- Oral second-generation antihistamines (loratadine, desloratadine, cetirizine, levocetirizine) first-line for mild intermittent rhinitis; breakthrough whilst on nasal topical corticosteroid or prophylaxis prior to anticipated exposure. Terfenadine and astemizole should be avoided (risk cardiac arrhythmia).

Table 13.1 Nasal corticosteroids.

Nasal corticosteroid spray (generic)	Dose (mcg)	Age indicated for use in seasonal rhinitis	Age indicated for use in perennial rhinitis
Over the counter			
Rhinocort hayfever (budesonide)	32	≥12 year old	≥18 year old
Beconase allergy and hayfever 12 hours (beclomethasone)	50	≥12 year old	≥12 year old
Beconase allergy and hayfever 24 hours (fluticasone propionate)	50	≥12 year old	≥12 year old
Nasonex (mometasone)	50	≥3 year old	≥3 year old
Prescription-only			
Avamys (fluticasone dipropionate)	27.5	≥2 year old	≥2 year old
– Dymista (azelastine hydrochloride and fluticasone propionate)*	125/50	≥12 year old	≥12 year old
Rhinocort (budesonide)	64	≥6 year old	Adults
Omnaris (ciclesonide)	50	≥6 year old	≥12 year old

* Combination antihistamine and steroid spray.

- Topical corticosteroid nasal sprays (Table 13.1) first line for moderate–severe or persistent symptoms (both allergic and non-allergic rhinitis).
  Continuous use is safe and do not suppress the hypothalamic–pituitary–adrenal axis.
- Initial treatment 2–3 months (expect improvement from 3-4 wks); if seasonal rhinitis, commence 1 month prior to the relevant pollen season & continue through symptomatic period.
- **Allergen avoidance** measures may be of benefit to selected patients.
  - Dust mite reduction (wash bedding in hot water weekly, vacuum carpet dust and hard surfaces weekly, use allergen-impermeable bed covers).
  - Avoidance of grass pollens is challenging (close windows, shower post outdoors).
- **Immunotherapy:** systemic administration of house dust mite and/or grass pollen allergen extracts to achieve clinical tolerance (monthly s/c or daily p.o for 3y).
  Consider if refractory disease despite optimal pharmacotherapy.

Allergic conjunctivitis
Usually associated with allergic rhinitis (can occur in isolation)
- Red, watery, itchy eyes.

Management
- Eye toilette (normal saline) & cool compresses.
- Oral antihistamine +/- topical antihistamine eye drops (e.g. Patanol), and combination antihistamine/mast cell stabilisers eye drops (e.g. Zaditen)

Asthma
- Allergic factors may contribute to the symptoms of asthma, particularly if chronic asthma requiring ongoing corticosteroid therapy.
- The major allergens are indoor inhalational (house dust mite, cat and dog dander) pollens seasonal exacerbations) and moulds (arid climates).
- Untreated allergic rhinitis can also exacerbate asthma
- Food does not generally induce asthma symptoms in isolation.
- See Chapter 38, Respiratory medicine.

Urticaria and angio-oedema

- Urticarial rashes (hives) are papular, pruritic patches of erythema and oedema.
- Angioedema frequently accompanies urticaria and involves painful, rather than pruritic, swelling in areas of low tension (eg. eyelids, lips and scrotum).
- Hereditary angioedema should be considered in patients who present with isolated angioedema without urticaria (see Chapter 24, Immunology).
- Urticaria and angioedema are further classified as either acute (<6 weeks' duration) or chronic (>6 weeks' duration).

Acute urticaria and angioedema

- Acute urticarial reactions to foods generally subside within 24 hours.
- History should ascertain exposure to foods or drugs (especially antibiotics) that may have induced an immediate allergic reaction.
- Persistence or recurrence >24 hours is generally not due to food allergy. Usually no precipitating factor is identified, however some cases follow an intercurrent viral infection.

Chronic spontaneous urticaria and angioedema

- Can persist or occur intermittently for months or years.
- Rarely caused by specific allergic factors; therefore, investigation with SPT and sIgE not indicated.
- Consider physical urticaria (e.g. heat, cold, exercise, cholinergic), underlying connective tissue or autoimmune disorders.

Treatment

- Second-generation antihistamines are the mainstay of therapy, eg. cetirizine (Table 13.2). Can increase to 2–4× the usual daily dose if required.
- Refer to specialist for resistant cases, for consideration of additional therapy with an H_2 antihistamine (ranitidine), or combined H_1 and H_2 antihistamine (doxepin) and/or montelukast.

Hereditary angio-oedema

See Chapter 24, Immunology.

Antibiotic allergy and adverse drug reactions

- Self-reported antibiotic allergy is common, however, formal evaluation is important as the majority of patients can tolerate the medication.
- Penicillin reactions are the most commonly reported.
- Confirmed penicillin allergy confers 3% chance of reacting to first- and second-generation cephalosporins (third-generation cephalosporins usually tolerated).

History

- Reaction kind, severity, timing in relation to drug dose; prior and subsequent drug exposure; concurrent illness; and other concurrent new food or drug ingestion.
- Clarify for features of anaphylaxis (cardiovascular and/or respiratory involvement), mucocutaneous involvement (Stevens–Johnson syndrome) or signs of toxic epidermal necrolysis.

Investigation and management

- No reliable *in vitro* or *in vivo* tests for drug allergy are available.
- SPT and sIgE tests for drug allergy have low sensitivity and the majority of patients will require intradermal testing to the penicillin metabolites (major and minor determinants) and amoxicillin (for side chain reactions).
- In most cases, intradermal test results are negative or equivocal, and patients can undergo inpatient oral drug challenge to confirm or exclude allergy.
- If suspected multiple antibiotic allergies, a challenge to a single antibiotic is usually done (which is considered appropriate for future treatment).

Table 13.2 H₁ antihistamines.

Antihistamine	Common brand name	Doses
Loratadine	Claratyne (10 mg tablet, 1 mg/mL suspension)	1–2 years: 2.5 mg daily 3–6 years: 5 mg daily >6 years and adults: 30 mg daily
Desloratadine	Aerius (5 mg tablet, 0.5 mg/mL suspension)	6–11 months: 1 mg daily 1–5 years: 1.25 mg daily 6–11 years: 2.5 mg daily ≥12 years and adults: 5 mg daily
Fexofenadine	Telfast (30 mg, 60 mg, 120 mg, 180 mg tablets, 6 mg/mL suspension)	6–23 months: 15 mg b.i.d 2–11 years: 30 mg b.i.d ≥12 years: 120–180 mg daily
Cetirizine	Zyrtec (10 mg tablet, 1 mg/mL suspension, 10 mg/mL drops = 0.5 mg/drop)	2–12 years: • 8–14 kg: 2 mg b.i.d • 14–18 kg: 2.5 mg b.i.d • 18–22 kg: 3 mg b.i.d • 22–26 kg: 3.5 mg b.i.d • 26–30 kg: 4 mg b.i.d • >30 kg: 5 mg b.i.d Adults: 10 mg daily
Levocetirizine	Xyzal (5 mg tablet)	≥12 years and adults: 5 mg daily
First-generation antihistamines (sedating)		
Trimeprazine	Vallergan (1.5 mg/mL suspension) Vallergan Forte (6 mg/mL syrup) Vallergan tablets (10 mg)	Urticaria • ≥2 years: 2.5–5 mg t.d.s or q.i.d • Adults: 10 mg t.d.s or q.i.d (max 100 mg per day) Sedation (eczema) • 3–6 years: 15–60 mg per day • 7–12 years: 60–90 mg per day
Promethazine	Phenergan	Sedation (give 1–2 hours prior to procedure) • 2–12 years: 0.5–1 mg/kg • 12–18 years: 25–75 mg once daily Allergy • 2–12 years: 0.125 mg/kg/dose t.d.s and 0.5 mg/kg nocte • 12–18 years: 10–25 mg 2 or 3 times daily

Insect sting allergy
• Insect sting reactions in Australia commonly occur to honey bees, European wasps and jack jumper ants (Tasmania and regional Victoria).
• Majority transient local reactions; Minority large, localised or systemic allergic reactions.

Large localised reactions
• 5–15%
• Angioedema and erythema at the sting site, peak size at 24–48 hours, last ≥ 1 week.
• Risk of future systemic allergic reaction 10% (no further assessment needed).
• Management symptomatic; ice pack, simple analgesia, topical steroid, a second generation antihistamine and a single dose of oral steroid (if significant spreading angio-oedema).

Systemic allergic reactions
• <1% of children & 3% of adults.
• Rapid onset of gastrointestinal, respiratory and/or cardiovascular symptoms.
• Risk future systemic allergic reaction 40–70%.
• Investigations: sIgE, SPT and/or intradermal testing to confirm sensitisation to the suspected insect.

- Baseline mast cell tryptase to exclude mastocytosis, (risk of insect sting anaphylaxis).
- Management: Provision of adrenaline autoinjector & education
- Referral for venom immunotherapy (VIT) in all patients with insect sting anaphylaxis).

Latex allergy

- Two main agents: chemical additives causing dermatitis & natural proteins that induce immediate allergic reactions.
- Most reactions in hospital setting involve disposable gloves.
- Common community latex products include balloons, baby-bottle teats and dummies, elastic bands and condoms.

Irritant dermatitis

- Most common problem with latex glove use.
- Non-allergic skin rash: erythema, dryness, scaling and cracking.
- Caused by sweating and irritation from the glove or its powder.

Immediate allergy to latex

- IgE-mediated allergic reactions to latex proteins are serious and potentially life threatening.
- Secondary to direct contact or the inhalation of airborne powder particles containing latex proteins.
- Sensitisation may occur following direct exposure of mucosal surfaces to latex (e.g. catheterisation).
- SPTs and/or sIgE testing are useful in confirming suspected allergy.

Contact dermatitis

- Delayed hypersensitivity (Type IV) to chemical additives in latex.
- Reactions limited to site of contact (e.g. back of hands from glove exposure).
- Patients with irritant and contact dermatitis are at an increased risk of developing immediate hypersensitivity to latex and exposure to latex should be minimized.

Management

- Patients at high risk for latex sensitivity should be referred to a paediatric allergist/immunologist for further evaluation.
- Confirmed latex allergy (either immediate or delayed) should undertake strict latex avoidance including latex-free precautions during surgery.

USEFUL RESOURCES
- The Australian Society of Clinical Allergy and Immunology (ASCIA) website *www.allergy.org.au*; Contains excellent information for patients and health care professionals. Includes anaphylaxis action plans.

CHAPTER 14

Behaviour and mental health

Ric Haslam
Chidambaram Prakash
Christos Symeonides

Key Points

- Parent management training (psychoeducation, problem-solving, developing strategies, counselling) is an effective part of intervention for many childhood mental disorders.
- Children with behavioural or emotional symptoms may be 'symptom-bearers for wider family relationships or functional difficulties.
- Suicidal ideation is often unstable over time and key to the risk assessment is taking steps to establish and ensure follow-up.
- SSRIs are effective for treating anxiety and in some cases depression in children and adolescents, however, should be closely monitored during initiation for adverse effects.
- In prescribing psychotropic medications, it is important to specify target symptoms with the young person and family, to set expectations and monitor treatment response.

Introduction

Emotional, behavioural and mental health concerns in infants, children and adolescents are common presentations to medical services including GPs and paediatricians across all settings. Presentations can be non-specific and vary from healthy developmental challenges of emerging independence and personality, to symptoms of developmental (see Chapter 28, Neurodevelopment and disability) or mental health disorders as shown in Table 14.1. Common emotional, behavioural and mental health problems are listed in Table 14.2. Additional topics considered within this chapter include: psychosis, psychiatric emergencies and psychotropic medications.

Mental health

Mental health is defined as a state of emotional and social well-being in which individuals realise their own abilities, cope with the normal stresses of life, work productively and are able to make a contribution to their community. One in five people will experience mental health problems in their lifetime. The prevalence of mental health problems among children and adolescents in Australia (including subclinical symptoms) is approximately 14%. Most are managed in their community.

Childhood and adolescent mental health problems are predominantly managed by GPs, paediatricians, schools and community services. A relatively smaller number of children and adolescents with mental health problems of significant severity are treated by specialist mental health services/professionals. As medical practitioners are often well placed to identify mental health problems and facilitate management, it is important that they develop skills in mental health assessments.

The recognition and early diagnosis of child and adolescent mental health disorders is a clinical challenge. Presenting features may be different to those in an adult population. Many child and adolescent mental health problems continue into adulthood resulting in long lasting morbidity, hence the need for early diagnosis and referral for treatment.

Paediatric Handbook, Tenth Edition. Edited by Kate Harding, Daniel S. Mason and Daryl Efron.

Table 14.1 Mental state examination.

Observe the child's play and behaviour before, during and after the formal consultation. The young child communicates through play. Access to simple toys (e.g. a doll, a ball, or pencil and paper) allows the clinician to assess the child's level of self-organisation as well as their inner world of imagination and thought. Ask the child to draw a person or a house. Interview with the parents.

1. **General appearance and behaviour**
   - Observe the child's appearance, demeanour, gait, motor activity and relationship with examiner.
   - What is the child's apparent mood?
   - Do they seem sad, happy, fearful, perplexed, angry, agitated?

2. **Speech**
   - How does the child communicate?
   - Consider rate, volume (amount), tone, articulation and reaction time.

3. **Affect**
   - Observe the range, reactivity, communicability, and appropriateness to the context and congruence with the reported mood state.

4. **Thought**
   - Stream: Are there major interruptions to flow of thinking?
   - Content: What is the child thinking about?
   - Do they seem preoccupied by inner thoughts, obsessional ideas, delusions, fears or have suicidal ideation?

5. **Perception**
   - Are there hallucinations, illusions, imagery or disturbances in sensory modalities?

6. **Cognition**
   - Conscious state and orientation: Does the child know where they are, what time it is, who they are and who is around them?
   - Concentration: Is the child able to concentrate on developmentally appropriate tasks?
   - Memory: How well do they remember things of the recent and more distant past?
   - Do they understand questions posed to them and how well do they problem solve?

7. **Insight**
   - Does the child seem aware of their illness?

8. **Judgement**
   - Personal (as inferred from answers to questions about themselves), social (as inferred from social behaviour) and test situation (answers to specific questions).

Table 14.2 Common Emotional, Behavioural and Mental Health Problems by age group.

Infant	Infant Settling and Sleep Problems (see chapter 40 Sleep medicine), Infant Mental Health
Toddler	Behavioural Sleep Problems (see chapter 40 Sleep medicine), Tantrum Behaviours, Defiance (Independence), Food Issues
Preschool and Early Primary	Behavioural Sleep Problems (see chapter 40 Sleep medicine), Preschool and Early Primary Anxiety Disorders, Preschool Behaviour Disorders
Late Primary	School-aged Sleep Problems (see chapter 40 Sleep medicine), School-aged Anxiety Disorders, School-aged Behaviour Disorders
Adolescent	Adolescent Sleep Problems (see chapter 40 Sleep medicine), Depression, School-aged Anxiety Disorders, School-aged Behaviour Disorders
Other common problems	Grief and Loss, Mental Health associated with Chronic Illness, Psychosomatic Problems

Child mental health problems may have their origins in biological, attachment, developmental or family issues. Additionally, adolescent mental health problems may arise in the context of interpersonal and social problems. Critical life phases, such as puberty, are significant as these are stages of transition that are marked not only by biological changes but also major psychosocial stress.

Key skills required by medical practitioners include the ability to:

- Listen to and engage with children, adolescents and their families to discuss emotional and psychological issues in a comfortable manner.
- Manage common and less complex mental health problems either independently or in consultation with mental health professionals.
- Identify when mental health issues are serious, more complex and/or chronic in order to facilitate appropriate referral.

Approach to assessment of emotional, behavioural and mental health problems

History taking, interview and assessment

- Presenting problem: duration, severity, exacerbating and relieving factors, current sources of support, beliefs, concerns and expectations regarding the nature of the problem:
  - What are the parents' ideas about this problem?
  - In adolescents, what are their ideas about the problems?
- Impacts on: child, family, function at school, home and with peers. Why is this a problem for them? Why have they presented now?
- Perinatal history (including experience of the pregnancy, delivery and the child's early months).
- Medical history.
- Family history (medical and psychiatric).
- Friendships, relationships and dynamics within the family, resources, and sources of support.
- Developmental history.
- Educational and school history (including types of school, class sizes, academic performance now and previously, social relationships, attendance and behaviour in school, history of being bullied or bullying at school).
- Possible traumatic events and adverse childhood experiences (ACE's; see also Chapter 1, Communication in the paediatric consultation) at home and school (directly experienced or witnessed).
  Always consider physical or sexual abuse and ask sensitive questions directly where appropriate.
- The child's feeding, sleeping and toileting habits where appropriate.
- In adolescents also explore:
  - Substance use (type, amount, frequency, who with, motivation for change);
  - Sexual history;
  - Social relationships (including the type of peer group–related activities, closeness to peers, position in the peer group); and
  - Eating habits, patterns of exercise, self and body image in adolescents.
- Also look for self-harm and risk-taking behaviours.

Each interview of a child or adolescent and family should lead to an assessment and evaluation (including their strengths and difficulties) and the contributions of the family, peers and significant others to these difficulties and capacity to help overcome them. The child/adolescent and family should come to feel the problem is taken seriously and understood by the clinician.

The following points are general guidelines and must be applied according to individual situations:

- Interview itself can be an important part of the therapeutic process.
- See infants, preschool and early primary age children with their parents. See older children (7–11 years) with their parents initially but where possible, also interview and observe them in the room without their parents. Aim to speak with the child directly and engage other family members. This enables a therapeutic relationship to be established with the child.
- See adolescents both with their families and alone. This helps to give them a private space to discuss matters that they deem confidential. It also reinforces their efforts at separation from their parents and the developmental process of individuation. Inform them of your professional responsibility to keep matters discussed

with them confidential but also explain the exceptions to this rule where they may be at risk to their own self (suicidal ideas or plans, serious self-harm, sexual abuse) or pose a risk to others.

- Get the family/parents to identify and specify the main issue or two that they feel needs attention. At the conclusion of the assessment, come back to this and see if your assessment of the main issues to be addressed matches the family's view.
- Assess the presenting problem, noting the language and narrative used by the child/adolescent and family.
- Observe the verbal and non-verbal interaction between the child/adolescent and each parent and sibling present.

Aim to make a formulation of the problems based on the initial assessment, decide on an initial management plan and whether to refer for specialist mental health assessment.

- A clinician needs to be able to answer the following questions:
  - What is the problem now? Is the problem in the infant/child/adolescent or is the child a symptom bearer for family/parental psychological issues?
  - Why is the infant/child/adolescent presenting at this stage?
  - What is this infant/child/adolescent usually like?
  - In an adolescent, ascertain if the symptoms are part of an evolving major mental illness such as major depression, anxiety disorder or psychosis, the effects of psychoactive substances or a reaction to the psychosocial stressors that they are living with.
- Consider:
  - Stressors arising from family problems.
  - Inability of children and adolescents to cope with the demands of their developmental stage or phase of life.
  - Problems within the parental/carer support system including losses, conflicts, grief (e.g. death or illness in the family).
  - Bullying, academic and/or social difficulties in school.
  - In adolescents: conflict (e.g. victimisation by peers or arguments with parents) relationship breakdowns, problems with school work and a lack of emotional and interpersonal skills to deal with the developmental tasks of adolescence (e.g. initiating social contact, managing new sexual feelings and negotiating greater independence within the family) contribute to mental health problems.

Medical examination

- Perform a physical examination to rule out significant health problems (uncommon). In infants and toddlers, a thorough general examination is necessary and can have an important therapeutic role to addressing voiced or unvoiced concerns. In older children a more targeted examination is appropriate.
- Physical examination additionally provides an opportunity for some basic developmental screening through play in younger children, and additional developmental behavioural observations (remembering to interpret in the context of being an unfamiliar adult in a position of authority).

Mental state examination in children
Intervention

At the conclusion of the therapeutic assessment, the clinician should form a provisional diagnosis and assess the severity and urgency of the presenting problem. Options for intervention then include:

- Explanation and reassurance if the problem is transient or minor. Suggest further contact with primary care or community based counselling/ support services.
- Intervention through a paediatric or primary care service. Offer a follow-up appointment or telephone contact.
- Telephone consultation with/or referral to specialist mental health services.
- Psychiatric emergencies requiring emergency services

Available interventions in specialist child and youth mental health services

- Brief therapies – family or individual
- Crisis intervention
- Cognitive behavioural therapy (CBT)
- Interpersonal therapy in adolescents
- Acceptance and commitment therapy

- Dialectical behaviour therapy
- Psychodynamic psychotherapy
- Family and parent therapy incl. parent management training
- Supportive intervention for the child and family (clinic, school or home based)
- Psychopharmacology

When and how to make a mental health referral

Referral to mental health services should be discussed with families. The manner in which this is done can influence their engagement with these services, their expectations and understanding and even treatment outcome.

- Avoid coercion (unless the patient is at serious risk to themselves or others).
- Ensure an open and honest discussion about why you believe a mental health referral would be helpful.
- Explain what the child or adolescent and family should expect from an initial mental health consultation in clear and simple language.
- Where appropriate, continue your involvement and interest in a child and family.

Clinical Pearl: Clinician responses to mental health issues
Examine your own responses/feelings about mental health and ensure you do not impose these views on a child/adolescent or family (e.g. being sceptical about the usefulness of mental health services but referring anyway, or presenting the mental health clinician as the potential cure to all current and future difficulties).

Some children/adolescents and families accept mental health referral readily, whereas others are wary or even openly opposed to referral. In the latter, referral may be discussed over a period of weeks or months before being made. Stigma around mental health continues to be a powerful influence. Adolescents and families may interpret the suggestion of a referral as an indication that you think they are 'mad' or 'crazy'. Such beliefs may not necessarily be overt and reassurance is helpful.

Children who are hospitalised or have been subjected to significant medical interventions need to be reassured that the mental health clinician is a talking person (rather than someone who gives needles). In adolescents who are admitted to hospital with a medical illness and need to see a mental health clinician, it is important to reiterate that the role of this clinician is to assist them in coping with their condition and strengthen their resilience. Terms such as 'the talking doctor' can be useful. Similarly, talking to parents about mental health 'colleagues' as you would talk about other medical/surgical referrals can help reduce stigma or concerns.

Common emotional, behavioural and mental health problems in infancy, childhood and adolescence
Infant mental health

Infant mental health is an area of clinical work aimed at understanding the psychological and emotional development of infants from birth to 3 years and the particular difficulties that they and their families might face.

Babies come into the world with a range of capacities and vulnerabilities, and together with their parents negotiate their way through the next months and years. This process of attachment, growth and development may be challenged by a range of experiences that stress or interrupt this course. Examples include traumatic events, developmental concerns, hospitalisation of the infant or parent, prematurity, illness or disability, an experience of loss, changing family circumstances and/or postnatal depression.

Consider referral to a mental health clinician for:

- Persistent crying, irritability or 'colic'
- Gaze avoidance
- Bonding difficulties
- Slow weight gain
- Persistent feeding or sleeping difficulties
- Persistent behavioural symptoms, for example tantrums, nightmares, aggression
- Family relationship problems
- Infants with chronic ill health
- Premature babies and their families

Toddler independence

The developmental stage of toddlerhood, characterised by marked egocentricity and the growing need for autonomy, needs to be explained to the parents as the symptoms are often an expression of the child negotiating this stage.

Clinical Pearl: Supporting parent to manage typical toddler behaviours

It is normal for toddlers to try to control what they eat, to resist bedtime and to become frustrated if they do not get their way or fail in a task. In the process parents can sometimes feel that they are losing control, or are disempowered, or even defeated by a feisty toddler.

The doctor's role is to assist the parents to regain control, so that the toddler can develop a healthy sense of themselves without diminishing the parents' self-efficacy. Additionally, child behavioural problems can often generate or exacerbate conflict between parents. Calm and practical professional advice can help improve strained relationships.

There are three main types of problematic behaviour that often concerns parents of small children:
1. Sleep issues (see chapter 40 Sleep medicine)
2. Food issues
3. Tantrum behaviours

Food issues

Many parents worry that their toddlers do not eat enough, and mealtime battles often ensue. It is most unlikely that an otherwise healthy child will become significantly malnourished from poor eating. If the history does not indicate a structural or functional or a motor problem, a swallowing disorder or developmental disorder, the best approach is to reduce the stress around food:
• Plan a balanced toddler diet.
• Offer 3 meals and 3 snacks per day so that there is only about 2 hours between eating opportunities.
• Present the food/drink on a high chair tray or low table.
• Allow sufficient but limited time for finishing the meal (e.g. 20 minutes).
• Give the child a 5-minute warning before the food is taken away so that they can complete their meal.
• Take the unfinished food away until the next 'meal'.
• Offer no food in between the set meal and snack times so that the child develops an appetite.
• Try not to become upset if the child chooses not to eat.
Once again, phone contact during this process can be very reassuring and supportive, as it can be counterintuitive for a parent to resist 'feeding' their toddler.

Tantrum behaviours

Toddler tantrums are almost universal as an expression of frustration, and sometimes as a more controlled attention-seeking strategy. However, when frequent or intense, these behaviours can be very distressing and embarrassing for parents.

Tantrums can be minimised by applying some simple strategies:
• Try to prevent tantrums by distraction or avoidance of triggers.
• Ignore tantrums until they resolve.
• During a tantrum, avoid eye contact, say nothing and walk away. Try not to convey to the child that you are upset. Never engage a child who is having a tantrum, as it simply 'adds fuel to the fire'. This can be challenging in public places, such as supermarkets, but is important in order to reduce tantrums.
• Time out is a good strategy for more severe antisocial behaviours, such as physical aggression. Removing the child from the social group conveys the message that this behaviour is unacceptable. Place the child in an uninteresting place for a time-limited period, such as 1 minute per year of age. A corner, time out spot or separate room can be used, depending on the parent's preference. It is OK to close the door as long as the toddler can get out. If they come out, return them to the room or corner until they calm down. Once the tantrum is over, there is no need for discussion, simply re-engage with the child in enjoyable play.
Remember, toddlers respond well to positive reinforcement. Parents should be advised to 'catch the child being good' and reward them with praise, physical affection and/or a tangible reward, such as a sticker. This is important to promote more socially acceptable behaviours.

The objective of these behaviour strategies is not just to modify problematic behaviour and make the toddler comply with parental wishes, but also to help foster a loving relationship between the parent and child and reduce conflict. Sometimes, parental expectations of what is 'normal' may need to be addressed so that the toddler can be helped to develop strong self-esteem and reach their potential.

Preschool and school-aged behaviour problems

Challenging behaviour in preschool and primary school-aged children is common and lies on a spectrum from normal expression of emotion or autonomy, to a behaviour disorder. In the 2015 Australian Child and Adolescent Survey of Mental Health and Wellbeing (the most recent national data we have) the prevalence of Conduct Disorder in 4–11-year olds was 2.0%, and that of Oppositional Defiant Disorder was around 5.0%

The key to evaluating and managing behaviour problems is to remember that challenging behaviour is mostly a combination of emotional state and learned habits in the interaction between a child and those around them (whose behaviour is in turn driven by emotional state and learned habits). Being mindful of each part of that equation offers multiple avenues for intervention:

- Psychoeducation
- Situational factors and triggers
- Caregiver responses to behaviours
- Caregivers and other adults as role-models for behaviour and emotional regulation
- Caregiver-child relationships
- Child emotions and emotional coaching

Different levels of support may be needed based on child and family factors. Self-directed resources for families include books, websites, and more recently online course and programs. Group programs and workshops offer the additional benefit of peer support, whilst still offering some expert support/troubleshooting, whilst being more cost-effective than one-on-one support. One-on-one support offers more targeted intervention and GPs and paediatricians are well placed to provide this as trusted experts with experience in child development.

Table 14.3 General advice to parents for effective behaviour coaching.

1. Stabilise routines.

2. Make protected time for positive one-on-one time: effective coaching needs healthy relationships.

3. Know your child's physical and emotional needs and vulnerabilities. To be in control, kids need:
   - To be well-fed, well-rested and not over-stimulated
   - Feel safe, loved and worthy of love
   - Know what is expected of them, and believe that they can do it (remember to show that you believe in them). *Many kids and many adults find it hard to get into a calm, controlled state. It's a skill that needs practice and encouragement and they will make mistakes along the way*

4. Set consistent, realistic expectations that apply to everyone including adults: 'family rules'

5. Focus on the positive (and set the bar low enough to do so)
   - Actively acknowledge and reward acceptable behaviour
   - Challenge yourself to find and acknowledge acceptable behaviour three times as often as you have to step in for serious unacceptable behaviour.

6. Use rewards in short intense bursts and for one specific behaviour at a time.

7. Prioritise two or three more serious problem behaviours for which you provide consequences:
   - Immediate, calm, consistent, symbolic consequences that are within your control.
   - To avoid inadvertently reinforcing undesired behaviour, less is more: less talk, less emotion and less drama. And then move on.

8. Deal with all less serious problem behaviours by diversion, distraction and active ignoring.

9. Be a role-model and avoid escalation: "When they go fast you go slow" "Stay Out of the Jungle"
   - Take pride in keeping your emotions in check and not reinforcing provocative behaviour.
   - If you can't stay calm, learn to walk away.

10. When things are bad, first increase praise and rewards and look for a trigger (see point 3.)

Table 14.3 illustrates typical general advice that might be given for parents. One powerful strategy to identify priorities for more specific work with parents is to work through 1 or 2 specific instances of challenging behaviour, both working backwards to explore situational factors and triggers, and then forwards to explore adult responses and what whether these might be expected to reduce or reinforce such behaviour in the future.

Other professions who can offer one-on-one support include psychologists, occupational therapists, family therapists, and social workers (e.g. within family support services). Specialist supports where more intensive support is required include regional specialist child and youth mental health services.

Common childhood and adolescent mental health problems
Anxiety disorders

Common symptoms of anxiety disorders are listed in Table 14.4.

- In infants and toddlers, anxiety often manifests at separation from parents.

Clinical Pearl: Anxiety

Fear is a normal response to a frightful stimulus. Anxiety is a fear response that is abnormal in either context or extent. The cardinal symptom of anxiety is avoidance, which presents with distress and often other behavioural problems.

- Preschoolers and school-age children may be fearful of the dark or specific situations.
- Older children and adolescents may exhibit performance anxiety associated with exams, social situations, interpersonal relationship situations etc. Anxiety is most commonly experienced at times of transition (e.g. moving house, starting or changing schools).
- **Anxiety disorders** may be characterised by:
  - Persistent fears and/or developmentally inappropriate fears.
  - Irrational worries or avoidance of specific situations that trigger anxiety.
  - Impaired ability to perform normal activities (e.g. inability to attend school).

Table 14.4 Common symptoms of anxiety disorders in children.

Symptoms
Distress and agitation when separated from parents and home
School refusal
Pervasive worry and fearfulness
Restlessness and irritability
Timidity, shyness, social withdrawal
Terror of an object (e.g. dog)
Associated headache, stomach pain
Restless sleep and nightmares
Poor concentration, distractibility and learning problems
Reliving stressful event in repetitive play
Family factors
Parental anxiety, overprotection, separation difficulties
Parental (maternal) depression and agoraphobia
Family stress: marital conflict, parental illness, child abuse
Family history of anxiety

Source: Common child and adolescent psychiatric problems and their management in the community. *Medical Journal of Australia* 1998;168:241–248. (Tonge 1998. Reproduced with permission of AMPCo.) Reproduced with permission from the author.

- Anxiety disorders are common (4–9% in children and adolescents). This risk is greatly increased if a parent has/had an anxiety disorder or substance abuse disorder.
- Underlying neurodevelopmental problems such as Autism Spectrum Disorder or ADHD should be considered in children with marked anxiety or those in whom symptoms are more difficult to treat.
- Similarly, untreated anxiety disorders and substance use problems in parents are associated with reduced effectiveness of interventions for anxiety in children and adolescents.

General assessment and management principles
- A thorough history should include:
  - Details of baseline anxiety symptoms
  - Length of time anxiety has persisted
  - The degree to which the child is impaired in their day-to-day activities and their relationships.
- Behaviour: how does the problem manifest in their behaviour?
- Cognition: what are the thoughts and assumptions the child or young person has about the problem?
- Emotions: what are the emotions experienced by the child or young person with the problem?
- Family, school and developmental assessment.

Generalised anxiety disorder
Generalised anxiety disorder is persistent and pervasive anxiety that is not contextually based. This includes feeling 'on edge' at most times, with bodily symptoms such as tachycardia, palpitations, dizziness, headache and 'butterflies in the tummy'.

Management
- If symptoms are mild, explore behavioural and/or family support interventions with the child and family, then review.
- Cognitive behavioural therapy (CBT) techniques such as the F (Feelings), E (Expectation), A (Attitude/action), R (Reward) for generalised anxiety and systematic desensitisation and modelling for specific phobias are highly recommended. It is vital that the child practices the techniques between sessions.

Anxiety-based school refusal
School refusal is often an indicator of separation difficulties, where the child/adolescent is frightened to leave their parent or home. Children refusing to attend school often present with somatic complaints such as abdominal pain. In older children there is a predominance of social anxiety with concerns about negative evaluation by peers or teachers. Ascertain the basis of the child's/adolescent's anxiety. These may be related to factors at home, including a parent's physical or mental health, difficulties with parental or peer relationships, or school factors (such as bullying or academic performance).

Management
- Conduct a physical examination if the child/adolescent presents with somatic symptoms.
- Assess the source of the anxiety and consider whether further management is required (e.g. family therapy, school counsellor etc.).
- Returning to school is a high priority. If necessary, this can be done by gradually increasing the time at school over a short period of time.
- Evidence supports CBT in group settings and educational support therapy. The latter involves having a nominated teacher or aide support the child through participation in the therapeutic intervention and then assisting them practice the learnt strategies in school.

Obsessive-compulsive disorder
Obsessive-compulsive disorder (OCD) is one of the more severe forms of anxiety disorders. Although it is relatively rare (1–2% of children and adolescents, more commonly in males), OCD can be associated with other forms of childhood anxiety, as well as depressive and Autism Spectrum Disorders.

Symptoms include intrusive thoughts and a variety of compulsive/ritualistic behaviours. The condition does not tend to remit and can be present in other family members.

Management
- Provide support and explanation to the patient and family.
- Refer for assessment and management by a mental health specialist.

- Principles of treatment are symptom control, improvement and maintenance of function.
  - For mild symptoms; CBT is the treatment of choice.
  - For more severe symptoms; a combination of CBT and medication (SSRI – sertraline for >6yo and fluvoxamine for >8yo) in relatively higher doses is indicated. Clomipramine can be effective although it remains a second line due to adverse effect profile.
  - Treatments with medication should be for at least 6 months in most cases.

Post-traumatic stress disorder

Trauma can directly contribute to mental health difficulties and can manifest as post-traumatic stress disorder (PTSD, Table 14.5). Following traumatic experiences it is not uncommon to see features of anxiety disorders, depressive disorders and self-harm, substance use and aggression. *Immediate debriefing after traumatic events does not reduce the risk of subsequently developing PTSD.*

Background

- Children and adolescents show a variable response to trauma.
- PTSD is not an expected outcome of trauma.
- It is not strongly correlated to the perceived severity of the trauma.
- The triad of PTSD symptoms is intrusion or re-experiencing of the event/s, avoidance of situations associated with the event/s and persistent arousal.
- Diagnostic criteria for PTSD are not particularly sensitive to trauma effects in very young children.

Assessment

- PTSD can be diagnosed only when the traumatic event *precedes* the symptoms and symptoms are present for >1 month.
- When symptoms have persisted beyond a period of a few days or weeks, refer to mental health services for further assessment and management.

Management

- Trauma-focused CBT has been shown to be effective when delivered for over 12 sessions. Techniques include graded exposure, cognitive processing, psychoeducation, training in stress reduction, relaxation and positive self-talk.

Table 14.5 Common symptoms of post-traumatic stress disorder in children.

Intrusive thoughts and 're-experiencing' of the event(s) – may be demonstrated through play, enactment or drawings
Fear of the dark
Nightmares
Difficulties getting to sleep and/or nocturnal waking
Separation anxiety
Generalised anxiety or fears
Developmental regression, for example continence, language skills
Social withdrawal
Irritability
Aggressive behaviour
Attention and concentration difficulties
Memory problems
Heightened sensitivity to other traumatic events

Source: Common child and adolescent psychiatric problems and their management in the community. *Medical Journal of Australia* 1998;168:241–248. (Tonge 1998. Reproduced wtih permission of AMPCo.) Reproduced with permission from the author.

- Medication is not first-line treatment unless co-morbid conditions such as depression are present. In such circumstances alpha2 agonists (eg clonidine, guanfacine), dopamine antagonists (eg risperidone) or SSRIs (eg citalopram) can be helpful as an adjunct.

Paediatric medical trauma stress

Children, adolescents and families may experience a traumatic stress response as a result of their experiences associated with pain, injury, serious illness, medical procedures or invasive medical treatment. This cluster of symptoms has been referred to recently as paediatric medical trauma stress (PMTS). This trauma may be chronic, repetitive, predictable (such as associated with medical procedures), and involve interpersonal interaction. This is referred to as *complex trauma*.

Background

- The child, adolescent and/or family may experience symptoms of arousal, re-experiencing and avoidance in response to a medical event.
- Symptoms may vary in intensity but may impact on general functioning.
- Symptoms may not reach diagnostic criteria of PTSD or acute stress disorder (ASD) but can occur along a continuum of intensity (from normative stress reactions to persistent and distressing symptoms).
- *Subjective* appraisals of threat rather than *objective* disease/medical factors seem more predictive of stress responses.
- There is debate regarding the need to acknowledge complex trauma experienced by some children as a distinct form of trauma stress disorder.

Management

Prevention is the best cure. Health care providers are well placed to modify stress experiences of patients and families in the medical context, subsequently reducing the risk of persistent symptoms. This can be done by:

- Explaining procedures in a developmentally appropriate manner
- Checking their understanding of the explanation
- Teaching parents how to comfort and reassure their children
- Looking for opportunities for the child to make decisions in their management (e.g. in young children ask if they would prefer to sit up or lie down or if they would like for a parent to hold their hand during procedures; involving adolescents in the discussions regarding the diagnosis and treatment processes to give them a sense of ownership)
- Implementing good pain management practice (see Chapter 6, Pain management)
- Screening for persistent symptoms of distress post injury/illness

Depression

Child and adolescent depression is common. There is a 2% incidence in children with a cumulative incidence of 20% by 18 years of age. Whilst it is twice as common in females during adolescence, there is no gender bias in younger children. Depression is a chronic, frequently relapsing, and debilitating disorder.

Symptoms vary according to the age and developmental stage of the child.

- *Infants and younger children*: irritable mood, failure to gain weight and lack of enjoyment in play and other activities.
- *Children and younger teenagers* (Table 14.6): more symptoms of anxiety (e.g. phobias, separation anxiety), somatic complaints, irritability with temper tantrums and behavioural problems.
- *Older adolescents*: more 'adult like' symptoms of depression including insomnia, easy fatiguability, loss of interest in pleasurable activities and then in all activities, loss of appetite and weight, psychomotor slowing, in severe cases delusional thinking, self-harming and suicidal behaviours.

Co-morbidities of depression are common and include anxiety disorder, conduct disorder or attention deficit hyperactivity disorder (ADHD).

- Incidence of co-morbidities:
  - In patients with anxiety disorder, 10–20% have co-morbid depression.
  - In patients with depressive disorder, >50% have co-morbid anxiety.
  - In patients with disruptive behaviour disorders, 15–30% have co-morbid anxiety.

Table 14.6 Common symptoms of childhood depression.

Symptoms
Persistent depressed mood, unhappiness and irritability
Loss of interest in play and friends
Loss of energy and concentration
Deterioration in school work
Loss of appetite and no weight gain
Disturbed sleep
Thoughts of worthlessness and suicide (suicide attempts are rare before age 10 years, then increase)
Somatic complaints (headaches, abdominal pain)
Co-morbid anxiety, conduct disorder, ADHD, eating disorders or substance abuse
Family factors
Family stress (ill or deceased parent, family conflict, parental separation)
Repeated experience of failure or criticism
Family history of depression

Source: Common child and adolescent psychiatric problems and their management in the community. *Medical Journal of Australia* 1998;168:241–248. (Tonge 1998. Reproduced with permission of AMPCo.). Reproduced with permission from the author.

Assessment
- Recognition is important, as untreated childhood and adolescent depression increases the risk for depression in adulthood.
- Depression in childhood and particularly in adolescence increases the risk of suicide and self-harming behaviours.

Management
There are three phases of treatment:
1. Acute phase lasting 6–12 weeks (stages 1 and 2 of treatment)
2. Continuation phase 6–12 months (stage 3 of treatment)
3. Maintenance phase 1 year or more.
Most treatment effectiveness studies in children and teenagers have focused on the acute phase and some on the continuation phase and relatively few if any studies have focused on the maintenance phase.

Acute phase
Stage 1
- Form a therapeutic alliance to assist in making a thorough assessment (including biopsychosocial antecedents) and diagnosis.
- Psychoeducation can be particularly effective in involving the child and parents in this process.

Stage 2
- Target areas for intervention such as reduced self-care, social and occupational activity, ineffective coping with stressors, correcting the problem-solving deficits, reducing the social impairment and inadequate self-esteem.
- Psychotherapy is the first-line treatment for mild to moderate mood disorder. Effective psychotherapies include CBT and interpersonal therapy for adolescents.
- A combination of CBT and SSRI medication (fluoxetine, citalopram, escitalopram, sertraline) provides good outcomes. Fluoxetine appears to have the lowest number needed to treat. Fluoxetine is FDA approved in USA for the treatment of childhood depression. Fluoxetine and escitalopram are approved for adolescent depression.

Continuation phase
- Stage 3 focuses on relapse prevention. GPs can play an important role in this.
- Referral to local mental health services may also be required.
- Carefully monitor for self-harm, suicidal ideation and suicidal behaviour, ideas of hopelessness, deterioration in overall functioning.

Clinical Pearl: SSRIs and suicidality

Prescribers of SSRI's for depression in children and adolescents must be cognisant of the small but significant risk of activation and increases in suicidal thoughts in the initial 2–4 weeks following commencement of an SSRI.

The following guidelines should be adhered to when prescribing SSRI medications.
- Start with a low dose and increase slowly. Side effects are dose-dependent, but efficacy is not. Always use the lowest effective dose.
- Only use as an adjunct to psychotherapy.
- Explain to parents (and child if appropriate) about possible adverse effects of antidepressants. Discuss the issues of deliberate self-harm and suicidality and the need for close monitoring, especially in the first 2–4 weeks.
- Explain the discontinuation syndrome, which occurs when an SSRI is withdrawn abruptly. This can result in irritability, mood lability, insomnia, anxiety, vivid dreams, nausea, vomiting, headache, dizziness, tremor, dystonia, fatigue, myalgia, rhinorrhoea and chills.
- Monitor closely for adverse effects in the first 4 weeks; consider using structured rating instruments.

Psychosomatic problems
Somatic responses to stressful situations are common (e.g. sweating during a job interview or needing to go to the toilet before taking an exam). Somatic complaints in children are also relatively common and appear as physical sensations related to affective distress.

Somatisation disorders may present in children whose families have a history of illnesses or psychosomatic disorders. Such patterns may be evident at a multigenerational level where physical symptoms appear to be the 'currency' by which affective states are communicated. Possible family relationship difficulties (including sexual abuse) should be considered as part of a thorough assessment.

Somatic symptom disorders in DSM 5 (American Psychiatric Association. *Diagnostic and Statistical Manual of Mental Disorders Fifth ed. 2013)* include:
- Somatic symptom disorder
- Conversion disorder
- Illness anxiety disorder
- Psychological factors affecting other medical conditions
- Factitious disorder
- Other specified somatic symptom and related disorder
- Unspecified somatic symptom and related disorder

Psychosomatic or somatic symptom disorder
Refers to the presence of physical symptoms suggesting an underlying medical condition without such a condition being found, or where a medical problem cannot adequately account for the level of functional impairment.
- Common symptoms include:
  - Headache
  - Abdominal pain
  - Limb pain
  - Fatigue
  - Pain/soreness
  - Disturbance of vision
  - Symptoms suggestive of neurological disorders

Conversion disorder (functional neurological symptom disorder)
- May present with dramatic symptoms such as:
  - Gait disturbance
  - Paraesthesia
  - Paralysis
  - Pseudoseizures

In this situation, the onset of the symptom is closely associated to a psychological stressor. Conversion disorders are generally relatively short-lived. They are often alleviated by identification and management of the stressor(s) and in some instances, symptomatic treatment of the physical problem.

All somatisation disorders have the following in common:
- Noticeable bodily symptoms and signs.
- Undesirable thoughts, feelings, and behaviours about the body symptoms or signs.
- Significant distress associated with the body symptoms or signs.
- Impaired functioning due to the body symptoms or signs.
- Prevalence probably higher than reported, and more common in females
- Symptoms usually begin in childhood, adolescence or early adulthood
- Comorbidity common; depressive disorders, anxiety disorders, substance use, and personality disorders.
- Risk factors include:
  - An enhanced focus on physical sensations,
  - Persistent concerns about peer relationships
  - High achievement orientation.
  - Family history of physical/mental health problems,
  - Parental somatization and
  - Limitations in the ability to communicate about emotional stressors.
  - Life stressors including bullying, peer relationship breakdown, academic stress

Types of somatization seen in outpatient clinics
1. *Acute somatization:* temporary production of physical symptoms associated with transient stressors
2. *Relapsing somatization:* repeated episodes of physical symptoms associated with repetitive stressors and anxiety or depressive episodes
3. *Chronic somatization:* nearly continuous somatic focus, perception of ill health, and the development of disability

Identifying Somatic Symptom Disorder:
- Do a thorough history and detailed physical assessment
- Rule out medical illness
- Consider medication side effects
- Identify ability to meet basic needs
- Identify ability to communicate emotional needs
- Identify secondary gains
- Build therapeutic alliance with the patient
- Use screening tools appropriate for somatic symptom disorder (e.g. child somatization inventory, functional disability index, Chalder fatigue self report scale).

Management principles:
Always involves a central health professional that:
- Has patience and good interpersonal skills.
- Has established good rapport with the patient and family.
- Acts as an anchor person for the MDT.
- Follows-up the patient frequently.
- Always avoids habit forming drugs where possible.
- Always involves the search for comorbid mental illness that can be treated (e.g. anxiety and depression).

Schedule time-limited regular appointments (e.g. 4–6 weeks) to address complaints:
- Explain that although there may not be a reason for their symptoms, you will work together to improve their functioning as much as possible

- Educate patients how psychosocial stressors and symptoms interact
- Avoid comments like "your symptoms are all psychological." or "there is nothing wrong with you medically."
- Avoid the temptation to order unnecessary, repetitive, or invasive investigations
- Evaluate somatic symptom burden
- Collaborate with the patient in setting treatment goals
- Support the patient on how to cope with their symptoms instead of focusing on 'cure'.
- Case management to minimize economic impact
- Medications to treat anxiety and depression (SSRIs)
- Short term use of anxiety meds (dependence is a risk)
- Non-pharmacological treatments
  - CBT – Shows promising evidence
  - Psychodynamic therapy
  - Integrative therapy

Mental health problems associated with chronic illness

Children and adolescents with chronic illnesses may present with exacerbations of their physical symptoms that relate to their affective state. Such responses may be related to a precipitating stressor or may reflect the child's changing responses to their illness. Children and adolescents may be angry, resentful of the limitations their condition imposes, or be particularly sensitive to being different from their peers. Additionally, responses by their parents (e.g. over- or under-protectiveness) may contribute to adjustment problems. Along with somatisation, other difficulties may emerge, such as non-adherence with treatment and family relationship problems.

Management

Management depends on the nature, severity and duration of the problem. Some general principles include:

- Recognition that the physical symptoms as genuine and distressing.
- Thorough clinical examination, investigation and mental health assessment is usually required. Hospital admission may be required to facilitate this.
- Discussion of mind–body interactions can be useful. Discuss early on the possibility that psychological factors are contributing to symptoms or wellbeing. This may allow the patient and family to begin to discuss possible psychological stressors, reducing resistance to mental health input.
- Symptomatic treatment (e.g. heat packs, relaxation exercises, physiotherapy, mild analgesia) may be appropriate, along with supportive counselling and/or mental health referral.
- Avoid medical over-investigation based on the family's coercion or unwillingness to consider psychological factors.
- It is important that the patient and family do not feel they have 'wasted your time' if there is no evident medical problem. Maintain an interest in the patient and family with a review appointment or follow-up telephone enquiry as appropriate.

Developmental and family psychiatry
Family relationship difficulties

A family-sensitive approach is crucial to the assessment and management of childhood mental health issues. Behavioural and/or emotional difficulties in a child can occur in the context of chronic family dysfunction and interact with or compound those difficulties. Conversely, such difficulties can arise in the context of well-functioning families where the child's temperament, personality or precipitating stressors may lead to behavioural or emotional difficulties for the child and/or parent–child relationship difficulties. When a child is presenting with behavioural and/or emotional difficulties, assessment should include an understanding of the family dynamic and situation including:

- Family tree, living arrangements and caregiving roles
- Quality of family relationships
- Early attachments/relationships
- History of significant losses, stressors, and precipitating factors
- Social/family support networks
- Identifiable 'risk' factors such as poverty, substance use, illnesses, absent social supports

---

Clinical Pearl: The importance of understanding the family context

Children can be symptom-bearers for family dynamic and relationship difficulties. In such instances, treatment of the presenting symptom is unlikely to be successful in the long term without appropriate family and/or couple counselling.

When working with families

- Conduct at least one family interview when dealing with a child with significant behavioural or emotional difficulties.
- Interview all family members (including siblings, who are often insightful commentators on family life), and provide an empathic response to each member's point of view. In the case of young children, observing and commenting upon play themes is useful.
- Do not assume that different family members agree on what is the presenting problem. It is often useful to ask family members to rank their concerns such as
  o What is the problem you are most worried about today?
  o What is the number 1 worry you have at the moment … number 2 … number 3?
  o Who in the family is most worried about this problem? Who is the least worried?
- If family members are not present, seek further understanding by questions such as
  o If your husband were here today, what would he say about this problem?
  o Who else in the family has noticed the changes that you have described today?
- Encouraging and supporting families to find solutions to their difficulties is more likely to provide long-term change. This may involve helping families identify negative or unhelpful patterns of interaction, helping families identify strengths and resilience and noting small changes/improvements.

Grief and loss

Experiences of grief and loss are inevitable. Where losses are severe or traumatic or where a child has pre-existing vulnerabilities, these experiences can contribute to mental health problems or result in complicated grief reactions.

- Children may believe that they caused a loved one's death or illness.
- Adolescents may find it difficult to speak about the loss as it may be intricately linked in with their sense of self.
- Bereaved children or adolescents may feel different from others, thus feel isolated or have difficulty managing the reactions of their peers.

In most instances, the bereaved child or adolescent can be supported through family, school, community and religion. Where the loss is within the family, family-based counselling/therapy can be helpful to address the young person's grief in the context of other family members' reactions.

Grief and loss experiences for children or adolescents may also occur in situations other than bereavement (e.g. chronic illness, refugee status or having a parent with a mental illness). Parental divorce is a common source of grief and loss in young people. Grief associated with this situation can be complicated and often remains unacknowledged by significant adults. Young people may experience feelings of guilt and self-blame, harbour fantasies of a parental reunion, struggle with divided loyalties and feel anxious about their own future relationships. Feelings of anger, rejection and sadness may lead to behavioural or emotional manifestations of their grief.

Breaks ups with friends or the break up of a romantic relationship can be severely testing for adolescents, sometimes leading to depressed feelings, thoughts and acts of aggression or self-harm. There may be self-blame, an over focus on the importance of this lost relationship to their lives and catastrophising, and displacement of the negative feelings towards loved ones at home or authority figures such as parents and teachers. Help the young person see how such changes in relationships are common, that they can and will survive this and that they, as well as their lives, are bigger and more resilient than they may fear or imagine.

Management

- Acknowledge the child's loss in an empathic and appropriate manner. This can be helpful even when a loss is not recent.

- Where a grieving child presents with behavioural or emotional difficulties, gently probe their beliefs about why the loss occurred. This can help the clinician understand the child's predicament. For example:
  - "Sometimes, when I see young people who have lost their mum/brother, etc., they feel like it's their fault that they died or got sick. Does it ever feel like that for you?"
  - "How do you imagine your life would be different if your mum and dad were still together?"
  - "Why do you think people get cancer?" etc
- Assist the family in gaining access to appropriate support and counselling.
- Seek further specialist mental health services when a young person continues to exhibit extreme distress or prolonged behavioural or emotional difficulties.

Psychosis

The experience of hearing voices is relatively common in children and adolescents and it is important to distinguish these phenomena from a psychotic disorder through careful assessment. Similarly young people who have experienced traumatic events may describe periods of hallucinations in brief periods of extreme distress, often with features of dissociation.

Psychosis can be challenging to diagnose in children and young people due to frequent comorbidities and symptom overlap between schizophrenia, bipolar disorder, dissociative disorders, obsessive compulsive disorder and even Autism Spectrum Disorder and more transient conditions such as drug intoxication or drug-induced psychosis.

Psychotic disorders are very uncommon under the age of 13 years. Where a psychotic disorder develops under 13 years of age, it is often associated with strong genetic loading through family history, possible association with brain damage or neurodevelopmental problems such as Intellectual Disability or Autism Spectrum Disorder. Such cases are more likely to take a chronic course.

- The term 'First Episode Psychosis' is frequently used for young people presenting with a psychotic disorder, in recognition that the underlying process may be a primary psychotic condition or alternatively an initial presentation of a mood disorder such as Bipolar Disorder.
- There is usually a period of prodromal illness that precedes a psychotic disorder, characterized by a deterioration of functioning, withdrawal and transient or milder psychotic symptoms. This period can extend for up to 12–18 months.
- Psychotic disorders have the capacity to profoundly affect educational achievement, social functioning and identity formation in the developing young person. Effective treatments are available and therefore these disorders warrant prompt evaluation and assertive treatment.
- In some cases, there is an organic basis to a psychosis and it is vital to consider and exclude an acute and potentially-treatable condition. In the case of organic psychosis, there may also be a clouding of consciousness, confusion and disorientation, as well as perceptual disturbances.
- Symptoms consist of two main groups:
  1. *Positive symptoms*: reality testing and insight are lacking; delusions; hallucinations; incoherence; thought disorder and disorganised behaviour.
  2. *Negative symptoms*: inexpressive faces; blank looks; monotonous voice; reduced and monosyllabic speech; few gestures; seeming lack of interest in the world and other people; inability to feel pleasure and act spontaneously.
  Negative symptoms are much more pervasive and have a much greater effect on a patient's quality of life.

Management
- Admit to hospital for a full psychiatric and medical assessment to rule out an organic cause.
- The use of antipsychotic medications should be discussed with a child and adolescent psychiatrist.
- There are several RCTs for the use of Dopamine/Serotonin Antagonists in psychosis in young people, however each of these medications is associated with significant adverse effects including weight gain, hyperprolactinaemia and metabolic syndrome.
- Psychoeducation, social skills training, Cognitive Behaviour Therapy, family interventions, peer support programs, relapse prevention strategies and problem-solving interventions are effective in young people with a psychotic disorder.

Psychiatric emergencies

- The most common underlying problem that leads to psychiatric emergency presentations in children and adolescents is emotional (affective) dysregulation.
- Emotional dysregulation is a set of poorly modulated responses to a situation that are not socially acceptable or present apparent risks. They are characterised by verbal and/or physical aggression, threats and acts of self-harm, suicidal gestures, substance use, disinhibited sexualised behaviours and dissociation.
- Self-harm, aggression, substance use and dissociation may be means by which the patient avoids or distracts from internal psychological distress.
- Young people of all ages may have emotional dysregulation; however, it is more pronounced in adolescence. Possible associations include neurobiological vulnerability, attachment disorders, trauma, and experiences of abuse or victimisation and neglect.

Suicidality

After motor vehicle accidents, suicide is the next most common cause of death in 15–25 year olds in Australia. Children have a well-formed idea of death as being final from around the age of 9–10 years.

Factors most commonly associated with completed suicide are:
- History of suicidal gestures and/or deliberate self-harm
- Major depression
- Psychosis with command hallucinations
- Substance abuse
- Homelessness
- Antisocial behaviour

Adolescent suicide differs from adult suicide in that it is more likely to be:
- Motivated by revenge or a feeling of loss of peer supports
- Undertaken as an act of anger or irritation
- Impulsive
- Romantically and idealistically driven
- Related to low self-esteem

Clinical Pearl: Suicidal ideation and behaviour

Suicidal ideation and behavior in young people are typically unstable and can fluctuate within a day, meaning that assessments of risk are very much time-specific and often need to be reviewed frequently.

Assessment

Assess the patient's intentionality to end their life:
- Assess the risk of current and further suicidal behaviour, the precipitants and context of the suicide attempt, as well as the presence of coexisting psychopathology (e.g. depression, psychosis, bipolar disorder, severe anxiety).
- Enquire about past history of suicidal gestures including their circumstances and their lethality, and deliberate self-harm without suicidal intent.
- Ask about their expectations of death from this suicide attempt (e.g. there is life after death or that after punishing others by their suicide they can come back).
- Assess the 'finality' of their attempt (e.g. whether they left notes saying goodbye to loved ones, gave away possessions, completed commitments).
- When seeing the patient after a failed suicide attempt, check the individual's risk of trying other strategies to end their life.
- Assess the capacity of the patient to reflect on what effect their suicide might have on loved ones.
- Look for other relevant historical factors such as a history of the patient showing sudden changes in relationships, history of exhibiting violent and disruptive behaviour, withdrawing from friends and social involvements; look for episodic stressful precipitants, troubles with school authorities or police, feared pregnancy, major family dysfunction, recent break up with boyfriend or girlfriend, and refusal by significant others to provide anticipated help, support or love.
- It is helpful to distinguish static risk factors (from prior history) with dynamic risk factors (such as family relationship difficulties) which are open to interventions.

Immediate interventions
- Estimate immediate to short-term risk.
- Decide whether or not to hospitalise.
- Assess the availability of supports if the patient will not be hospitalised.
- If the patient can be managed at home, negotiate a management plan with the patient and family/caregivers.

Management plan
- Define the level of support to be provided by the family/carers and relevant services (e.g. parents to watch all the time or check in with the patient every few minutes/hours).
- Document a list of precipitating factors and early warning signs of another suicide attempt or escalating distress in the patient.
- Write a *crisis plan* that lists strategies on managing early warning signs and written information on how to seek further help.
- Follow-up is vital with young people with suicidal ideation and behaviour, and considerable efforts may need to be made to ensure this occurs.
- Provide a 24-hour telephone number and name of a contact person.
- Confirm a date and time for a reassessment.
- Convey this information to the mental health service/provider to whom the patient is referred for further care and treatment.

Medium term interventions
- Work with the young person.
- Develop a caring and empathic relationship.
- Instill hope for the future.
- Provide education to the patient and their family/carers about depression or other associated psychiatric condition.
- Provide advice on sleep, diet, hygiene and exercise where there are problems.
- Explore the incidents with the person, looking particularly at motivation and circumstances.
- Ensure the environment is safe.
- Increase support from family and friends.
- Contact the other professionals involved to ensure support is provided and coordinated.
- Ensure that basic needs are met (food, shelter).
- Identify individual risk and protective factors.
- Develop contingency and relapse plans.
- Arrange ongoing assessment of the capacity of the family to manage the young person's safety.

Psychoeducation
- Communication skills
- Conflict resolution
- Affect regulation within the family

Behaviour management
- Orientate the parents toward limit setting in a non-coercive way.
- Help the parents change their ways of interacting with the patient, improve cohesion and increase supportive gestures by the parents towards the adolescent.
- Reinforce non-suicidal, adaptive responses.
- Interventions in specialist mental health services would include:
  - CBT
  - Problem-solving therapy:
    - Social skills training
    - Effective communication
    - Affect management
    - Recognition and regulation of anger before it escalates to suicidal behaviour
    - Tension recognition (feeling thermometer)

- Interpersonal therapy
- Improvement of distress tolerance and mindfulness skills through dialectical behaviour therapy
- Relapse prevention
- Treatment of co-morbidities

Self-harm

Self-harm is more common than suicidal gestures in children and adolescents.

- Self-injury or self-harm may indicate anger, a response to perceived rejection by loved ones and peers, a coping mechanism to deal with states of internal distress or emptiness that may be associated with disturbed self-image.
- It may also be done as an alternative to suicidal gestures by those who are distressed by having suicidal urges.
- It may occur acutely at times of significant stress such as family and peer relationship problems, a loss of self-esteem through a break up of a relationship or failure in exams.
- Self-harm may also be a chronic problem in some adolescents with distressing and intrusive trauma-related images and memories or emerging borderline personality disorder.

Interventions

- Teaching emotional regulation skills
- Identifying emotions and obstacles to changing emotions
- Reducing vulnerability to stress
- Increasing positive emotional events
- Applying distress tolerance techniques
- Problem solving
- Identifying the current problem, and generating, evaluating and implementing alternative solutions that might have been used or could be used in the future
- Treatment of comorbid disorders (such as depression)
- Adolescents with chronic self-harm may benefit from highly specialised psychological therapies.

Acute behavioural disturbance

Challenging behaviours can occur in a number of settings with young people with conduct problems, with difficulties with emotion regulation and in children and young people with developmental disabilities such as Intellectual Disability and Autism Spectrum Disorder. In the latter group, sensory triggers and other environmental changes such as demands or restrictions placed on a young person can lead to aggressive behaviours. These are typically chronic but with acute events occurring as well.

- Understanding the purpose and the pattern of aggression is important to determine interventions, both immediately and in the medium term.
- Consideration should be given to the most suitable location to assess a young person, such as in a busy Emergency Department or clinic; including staff and carer safety and the availability of supports.
- As physical restraint and sedation deprives the patient of autonomy, it should only be contemplated as a last resort for safety and/or treatment.
- A patient who is 'acting out' and who does not need acute medical or psychiatric care should be discharged from hospital to a safe environment rather than be restrained.

Principles of calming/de-escalating a patient:

- Anticipate and identify early irritable behaviour (and past history).
- Involve mental health expertise early for assistance.
- Provide a safe 'containing' environment.
- Give a confident reassuring approach without added stimuli.
- Listen and talk simply and in a calm manner.
- Offer planned 'collaborative' sedation (e.g. ask the patient if they would take some oral medication to regain some control of their behaviour).
- When physical restraint is required, a coordinated team approach is essential, with roles clearly defined and swift action taken. Unless contraindicated, sedation should usually accompany physical restraint.

Indications for restraint
- Other methods to control the behaviour (such as de-escalation techniques) have failed.
- The patient displays aggressive or combative behaviour which arises from a medical or psychiatric condition (including intoxication).
- The patient requires urgent medical or psychiatric care.
- The behaviour involves a proximate risk of harm to the patient or others, or risk of significant destruction of property.

Contraindications to physical restraint and emergency sedation:
- Inadequate personnel/unsafe setting/inadequate equipment.
- Situation is judged as too dangerous (e.g. patient has a weapon).

Rapid tranquilisation
- There is limited evidence for interventions to achieve rapid tranquilisation (Figure 14.1) in children and young people; **If at all possible, the patient should be given the option of taking an oral medication.**

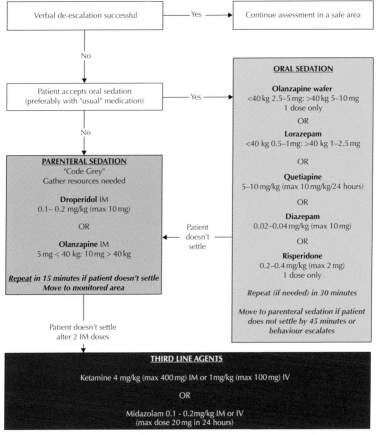

Figure 14.1 Acute behavioural disturbance management flowchart. *Source:* Royal Children's Hospital Clinical Practice Guidelines – Acute behavioural disturbance: Acute management. Reproduced with permission of the Royal Children's Hospital.

Table 14.7 Drug-specific information.

Drug	Time to review clinical effect before second med	Adverse effects
Midazolam	IM: 10–20 minutes IV: almost immediate	Respiratory depression[a] and airway compromise, paradoxical reactions.[d]
Olanzapine	Oral: 20–30 minutes IM: 15–30 minutes	Respiratory depression,[a] hypotension, ↑HR. Do not use if history suggestive of prolonged QTC, extrapyramidal reactions,[b] neuroleptic malignant syndrome,[c] may reduce seizure threshold.
Diazepam	Oral: 30–60 minutes	Respiratory depression[a] (unlikely to see immediate complications as longer half-lives) and paradoxical reactions.[d]
Lorazepam	Oral: 20–40 minutes	Respiratory depression[a] (unlikely to see immediate complications as longer half-lives) and paradoxical reactions.[d]

Notes:
[a] Respiratory depression – More commonly seen with benzodiazepines but can also occur with olanzapine and haloperidol.
[b] Extrapyramidal reactions – May be seen with olanzapine after only one dose. Reversible with benztropine.
[c] Neuroleptic malignant syndrome – A rare complication of typical and atypical antipsychotics. If suspected, get immediate help and check serum CK as it is invariably elevated.
[d] Paradoxical reactions – Administration of a benzodiazepine results in increasing agitation and anxiety as opposed to its normal sedating effect. This is more commonly seen in patients with developmental delay and/or a history of aggressive behaviour.

- Benzodiazepines are generally the medication of first choice, particularly in cases of known intoxication; medication naïve patients should generally be prescribed doses at the lower end of the range.
- If the patient has a known psychiatric disorder, consider using top-up doses of their regular medication.
- Give one option, wait for an effect and then consider further medication. If a drug from one group has had a poor therapeutic response after two doses, try a different drug and reconsider your diagnosis (e.g. underlying organic pathology) and indications for using emergency sedation (Table 14.7).
- Respiratory depression and acute dystonic reactions must be considered in monitoring and it is important to be prepared for such events should these arise.
- Similarly, if physical restraint is considered it is important both to reflect the legislative framework in place and to ensure that there are sufficient trained staff to execute the planned restraint safely.

If the patient can tolerate oral medications
- Diazepam (oral): 0.2–0.4 mg/kg (max 10 mg per dose if benzodiazepine naïve); OR
- Lorazepam (oral): 0.5–1 mg (if <40 kg); 1–2.5 mg (if >40 kg); OR
- Olanzapine wafer (sublingual): 2.5–5 mg (if <40 kg); 5–10 mg (if >40 kg).

If the patient cannot tolerate oral medications
- Midazolam IM/IV: 0.1–0.2 mg/kg (max 10 mg per dose); OR
- Olanzapine IM only: 5 mg (if <40 kg); 10 mg (if >40 kg); OR
The following antidotes should be readily available for reversal of potential side effects:
- Benztropine: 0.02 mg/kg (max 2 mg per dose) given IV/IM for reversal of dystonic reactions associated with haloperidol and olanzapine. Repeated doses may be needed.
- Flumazenil – 10 mcg/kg (max 200 mcg per dose) repeated at 1 minute intervals p.r.n. for up to five doses, to treat reversal of respiratory depression associated with benzodiazepines only. **Do not give unless you are sure the patient is not on long-term benzodiazepines.**

Psychotropic medications
Medication may be prescribed as part of the management plan for some children with development and mental health disorders, alongside behavioural and other therapies. Psychotropic medications can treat symptoms, improve function and quality of life for children with a range of disorders, including ADHD, anxiety disorders, OCD, Tourettes disorder, and moderate to severe depression. The target of medication is often a symptom rather than a diagnosis. For example, there is no medication to treat autism; however, children with autism often

Table 14.8 Psychotropic medications for children and adolescents.

Drug group	Indications	Common or serious side effects	Monitoring
Stimulants, e.g. methylphenidate	ADHD	Appetite suppression, anxiety, tics, emotional blunting	Exclude cardiac disease on personal and family history, examination Before prescribing; weight, height, blood pressure
Selective agonist of alpha 2 adrenoceptor e.g. guanfacine, clonidine	ADHD	Sedation, headache, abdominal pain, nausea, hypotension, dizziness	Exclude cardiac disease on personal and family history, examination Before prescribing; weight, height, blood pressure, heart rate
Noradrenergic agents, e.g. atomoxetine, tricyclic anti-depressants	ADHD, anxiety, sleep disturbance	Gastrointestinal upset, sedation, for tricyclics also look for urinary retention, constipation	Tricyclics – ECG at baseline and after some weeks on treatment
SSRI e.g. fluoxetine, sertraline	Anxiety, OCD, severe adolescent depression	agitation/increased self-harm or suicidality (soon after starting), GI upset, sleep disturbance;	Monitor closely in first weeks; avoid sudden cessation (discontinuation syndrome – flu-like symptoms)
Atypical antipsychotics e.g. risperidone, olanzapine, aripiprazole, quetiapine	Severe aggression, agitated behaviours esp. in children with autism spectrum disorder; Tourette's disorder; adolescent psychosis	Sedation, weight gain, metabolic syndrome, hyperprolactinaemia (particularly risperidone); QTc prolongation, acute dystonic reaction, chronic extrapyramidal symptoms	Weight/BMI, waist circumference during every clinic visit; fasting lipid profile, oral glucose tolerance test every 3 months, liver function tests if excessive weight gain; prolactin level only if symptoms
Mood stabilisers, e.g. valproate, lamotrigine	Irritability	Specific to drug used	Specific to drug used
Alpha-2 agonists, e.g. clonidine	Sleep disturbance, explosive aggression	Sedation	Heart rate, blood pressure

benefit from medications to treat symptoms such as anxiety, severe aggression or sleep disturbance (Table 14.8). Some conditions such as depression and oppositional defiant disorder do not respond as well to medications.

As with all therapies, the decision regarding prescribing psychotropics involves weighing up the potential benefits against potential harms. In general, medications should only be considered when the child has significant impairment which is not responding to non-pharmacological therapies. Where possible decisions to prescribe and target symptoms should be discussed with the child or adolescent in developmentally appropriate terms.

Principles of safe and effective prescribing of psychotropic medications
- Optimise non-pharmacological management.
- Be clear about a priori target, in order to evaluate effectiveness.
- Warn of common and serious side effects, provide clear written information on side effects in plain English/ language of the patient. Give written information in plain language from reputable sources (Choices UK, CMI from the TGA).
- Start with a low dose, and increase gradually until benefits are seen or unacceptable side effects restrict use.
- Avoid sedation, ensure adequate dose and duration of medication trial. This is particularly important for anti-depressants and atomoxetine.
- Be available for contact.
- Monitor regularly; phone contact is an efficient way to improve compliance and identify early response and adverse effects early.
- Consider a trial off treatment when symptoms are well controlled for a period of time.

USEFUL RESOURCES
- National Child Traumatic Stress Network *www.nctsnet.org*; excellent website containing practical resources for families and healthcare professionals.
- American Academy of Child & Adolescent Psychiatry *www.aacap.org*; contains useful practice parameters for doctors and information for families.
- National Institute of Mental Health in USA with parent information *www.nimh.nih.gov*; Health & Outreach > Topics > Children & Adolescents.
- Excellent resource for infant mental health *www.zerotothree.org*; Washington-based organisation.
- RCH clinical practice guideline on acute behavioural disturbance & verbal de-escalation https://www.rch.org.au/clinicalguide/guideline_index/Acute_Behavioural_Disturbance__Assessment_and_verbal_de-escalation/
- RCH clinical practice guideline on acute behavioural disturbance management https://www.rch.org.au/clinicalguide/guideline_index/Acute_behavioural_disturbance__Acute_management/
- E-headspace https://headspace.org.au/eheadspace/; a free national online counselling and support platform for 12–25yo young people.
- Raising Children Network https://raisingchildren.net.au; Australian parenting website.
- DSM-V reference: American Psychiatric Association. (2013). Diagnostic and statistical manual of mental disorders (5th ed.). https://doi.org/10.1176/appi.books.9780890425596.

CHAPTER 15

Cardiology

Remi Kowalski
Bryn Jones
Michael Cheung

Key Points
- At least 50% of school-age children have a murmur with no cardiac structural abnormality.
- Structural CHD should be considered in any unwell infant with cyanosis or features of poor peripheral perfusion, and prostin commenced.
- Cardiac failure in children presents with shortness of breath/tachypnoea and poor feeding, with a large heart on CXR, with a wide differential including myocardial, structural and arrhythmogenic aetiologies.
- Children with idiopathic pulmonary arterial hypertension have the potential to decompensate quickly and unpredictably, and should be managed in a specialist centre, even for simple interventions.
- Syncope in children is rarely related to a cardiac cause, but an ECG should be performed as a screening test in a first presentation with syncope.

Innocent murmur
At least 50% of school-age children have a systolic cardiac murmur with no structural or physiological cardiac abnormality (Table 15.1).

When to refer for investigation
A cardiac murmur associated with any of the following requires assessment by a specialist.

Concerning features in history
- Family history of cardiomyopathy or sudden unexplained death
- Chromosomal disorder
- Congenital malformation of other organs
- Maternal diabetes
- Exertional syncope or unexplained collapse
- Symptoms of cardiac failure

Concerning features on examination
- Cyanosis (Confirm on Saturation monitor), pallor, diaphoresis
- Signs of cardiac failure including breathlessness (tachypnoea), tachycardia, gallop rhythm, substernal heave, shifted apex, hepatomegaly
- Failure to thrive, not clearly due to other causes
- Unequal pulses
- Thrill associated
- Added cardiac sounds and clicks

Paediatric Handbook, Tenth Edition. Edited by Kate Harding, Daniel S. Mason and Daryl Efron.
© 2021 John Wiley & Sons Ltd. Published 2021 by John Wiley & Sons Ltd.

Table 15.1 Features of a physiological, functional or 'innocent' murmur.

History	Murmur	Other Examination
Asymptomatic	Soft Systolic murmur <3/6	Normal
Normal growth	May be continuous	
Benign family history	Usually varies with posture	
	Normal second heart sound	

Concerning murmur characteristics
- Diastolic murmur
- Continuous murmur (through systole and diastole) with no postural variation
- Pan-systolic murmur (obscures the second heart sound)
- Loud murmur (amplitude grade 3/6 or greater)

Concerning features on CXR
- Enlarged heart
- Abnormal cardiac contour
- Pulmonary plethora

Concerning features on ECG
- Abnormal QRS axis
- Increased voltages
- Abnormal intervals
- ST/T wave changes

See Basic ECG interpretation page 179 for reference ranges.

The neonate with symptomatic congenital heart disease
Critically obstructed systemic circulation (e.g. critical aortic stenosis, coarctation and hypoplastic left heart syndrome) can be indistinguishable from shock due to sepsis.

Clinical syndromes
Clinical syndromes of presentation with symptomatic CHD include:
- Shock due to low cardiac output, often with poor peripheral pulses and acidosis
- Persistent cyanosis
- Congestive cardiac failure with respiratory distress and hepatomegaly

Management
Use of prostaglandin (PGE$_1$)
Dose:
- Initial dose is 10 ng/kg/min IV; then increase to 20–100 ng/kg/min depending on response.
- Aim for saturations in the 80s and improving systemic perfusion.

Major side effects:
- Hypotension
- Apnoea

Contraindications:
- There are no congenital cardiac lesions for which PGE1 is absolutely contraindicated. The risk-benefit is in favour of PGE$_1$ infusion if:
  ○ Critically unwell
  ○ Cyanotic with a murmur
  ○ Poor peripheral pulses

Clinical Pearl: Symptomatic congenital heart disease in the neonate
- Congenital heart disease (CHD) should be considered in any unwell neonate, and prostaglandin may be lifesaving in duct-dependent lesions.
- Seek early advice from a specialist centre for support to arrange timely transfer for assessment.

Neonatal cyanosis

Cyanosis in any neonate must be investigated.

Clinical syndromes

- **Cyanotic CHD** is often more likely if there is persistent cyanosis with no respiratory distress and normal CO_2 clearance. The presence of a murmur increases the likelihood of a prostaglandin sensitive lesion.
- **Parenchymal lung disease** is likely if the infant has respiratory distress, elevated PCO2, lung field changes on CXR and a likely cause (e.g. meconium aspiration).
- **Persistent Pulmonary Hypertension of the Newborn (PPHN)** is difficult to distinguish clinically from cyanotic CHD.

Initial assessment

- **Examination:** respiratory rate and effort, abnormal pulses and presence of murmur.
- **Investigations**
  - Arterial blood gases: look for acidosis, PCO2.
  - CXR: look at cardiac silhouette, pulmonary vascularity and parenchymal lung disease.
  - 12-lead ECG: look at axis, rhythm, presence of sinus P waves, QRS complexes.
  - Echocardiography: diagnostic test of choice.
- **Hyperoxia test:** After 10 minutes of breathing 100% O_2, take right arm, preductal (radial artery) arterial blood gas.
  - A PaO2 <70 mmHg will occur with most major cyanotic defects.
  - A PaO2 >150 mmHg suggests cyanosis is not due to structural heart disease.
- **Trial of prostaglandin (PGE_1):** Will generally result in considerable improvement with duct-dependent CHD. Seek early advice from a specialist centre and neonatal transport service.

Hypercyanotic spells (tetralogy spells)

Severe cyanotic spells are a characteristic feature of Tetralogy of Fallot (TOF) but may occasionally occur with other cyanotic lesions. TOF consists of (1) over-riding aorta, (2) right ventricular outflow tract obstruction, (3) ventricular septal defect, with (4) right ventricular hypertrophy.

Clinical presentation

- Severe cyanosis with agitation and breathlessness.
- Often precipitated by exertion, feeding or crying, but can be spontaneous.
- The right ventricular outflow tract murmur becomes softer and may become inaudible.
- Most episodes are self-limiting, lasting 15–30 minutes, but can be prolonged or result in loss of consciousness.
- Mechanism probably involves acute reduction in pulmonary blood flow +/- peripheral vasodilatation.

Management

Initial

- Avoid exacerbating distress.
- Give high-flow oxygen via mask held close to face or head box.
- Morphine 0.2 mg/kg IM may help in severe cases to settle the infant and alleviate further distress as well as lower metabolic demand.
- Continuous ECG and oxygen saturation monitoring; frequent BP monitoring.
- Correct any underlying cause (e.g. arrhythmia, hypothermia, hypoglycaemia).

If prolonged

- IV/Intraosseous (IO) fluids: 0.9% normal saline 10 mL/kg bolus followed by maintenance fluids.
- Correct acidosis: sodium bicarbonate 1–2 mmol/kg IV.
- Beta-blocking drugs: IV esmolol 0.5 mg/kg over 1 minute, then 50–200 mcg/kg/min for up to 48 hours.
- Infusion of systemic vasoconstrictors may be considered in the form of metaraminol or noradrenaline infusion.
- Intubation and positive pressure ventilation may be required in extreme cases.

Longer term

- In most cases, hypercyanotic spells are an indication for palliative or corrective surgery.

- Oral propranolol may be given prophylactically to reduce the frequency of spells in a child awaiting surgery, but every potential cyanotic spell should be discussed with the child's cardiologist so that management can be altered accordingly.

Longer-term considerations in significant congenital heart disease
- Children undergoing major cardiac surgery in infancy are at risk of developmental delay and learning difficulties later in life. They should have ongoing neurodevelopmental assessment during childhood.
- RSV immunoprophylaxis should be offered to all children with significant left to right shunt or cyanotic CHD in the first year of life.

Heart failure after the neonatal period
Main causes
- Congenital heart defects with pressure or volume overload (±cyanosis)
- Myocardial dysfunction after repair or palliation of heart defects
- Cardiomyopathies and myocarditis
- Tachyarrhythmias
- Rheumatic heart disease (RHD), see Chapter 25, Infectious diseases.

Clinical features
- Infants and young children have non-specific symptoms and signs:
  - Dyspnoea, fatigue, feeding difficulties, increased sweating
  - Failure to thrive, poor exercise tolerance
  - Gallop rhythm, hepatomegaly, cardiomegaly
- Older children may have signs more like those in adults:
  - Breathlessness, fatigue, poor exercise tolerance, orthopnoea
  - Nocturnal dyspnoea, venous distension, peripheral oedema

Investigations and management principles
- Seek early advice from a specialist centre.
- An ECG can be helpful for diagnosis.
- Arrange urgent echocardiography to assess cardiac structure and function.
- Oxygen for hypoxia related to pulmonary congestion or respiratory infection.
- Reduce pulmonary and systemic venous congestion:
  - Frusemide: 1 mg/kg per dose (8, 12 or 24 hourly)
  - Spironolactone (dose by weight):
    - 0–10 kg = 6.25 mg/dose oral (12 or 24 hourly)
    - 11–20 kg = 12.5 mg/dose oral (12 or 24 hourly)
    - 21–40 kg = 25 mg/dose oral (12 or 24 hourly)
  - Monitor serum potassium if using spironolactone.
- Decrease afterload and commence neurohormonal blockade:
  - Captopril: 0.1–1 mg/kg per dose (max 50 mg) oral 8 hourly
  - Commence ACE inhibitor in hospital with blood pressure monitoring (every 30 minutes for 2–3 hours after dose)
  - Introduction of beta-blockade in a specialist centre
- Inotropes for acute, low-output cardiac failure:
  - Dobutamine: initially 5 mcg/kg/min IV
  - Dopamine: initially 5 mcg/kg/min IV
  - Milrinone: 50 mcg/kg over 10 minutes IV then 0.375–0.75 mcg/kg/min
- Positive pressure ventilation.
- Treat complications:
  - Infection
  - Anaemia
  - Arrhythmia
  - Malnutrition

Supraventricular tachycardia

Seek urgent specialist advice if any tachycardia is broad complex, is irregular or fails to respond to the management.

Definition

Supraventricular tachycardia (SVT) is usually a regular, narrow complex tachycardia, with a heart rate of between 160–300 beats/min.

Differential diagnosis

Sinus tachycardia up to 230 beats/min may occur in the neonate with:

- Hypovolaemia
- Hypoventilation
- Pain
- Fever

Note: Ventricular tachycardia in the neonate can have a relatively narrow QRS complex.

Clinical features

- In utero: may cause hydrops.
- Infancy: irritability, pallor, poor feeding and dyspnoea secondary to congestive cardiac failure though not usually with short episodes of tachycardia.
- Older children: palpitations, chest discomfort.
- Hypotension may be present at any age.

Initial assessment

- Physical examination:
  o Pulse, BP, temperature, heart murmur
  o Signs of cardiac failure (tachypnoea, increased work of breathing, hepatomegaly)
- 12-lead ECG to confirm a narrow complex tachycardia

Management

Child is normotensive and well perfused

Vagal manoeuvres

- Infant or young child:
  o Ice water in bag or icepack to face for a few seconds only (only try 2–3 times)
  o Oropharyngeal suctioning
  o Gag with spatula
- Older child:
  o Valsalva manoeuvre (e.g. forced blowing through a blocked straw, syringe, straight-leg raise)

IV adenosine (can be IO if IV access is unsuccessful)

- Full resuscitation facilities should be available.
- **IV access in a large, proximal vein.** This is important due to the very short half-life of adenosine in the circulation.
- Record a continuous ECG rhythm strip throughout administration, to monitor the pattern of reversal.
- Begin with adenosine 0.1 mg/kg as an initial bolus (max 6 mg):
  o Repeat doses can be given at 2 minute intervals, increasing by 0.05 mg/kg each dose, to maximum 0.3 mg/kg (18 mg)
- Dilute small doses of adenosine with saline to allow rapid infusion.
- Give adenosine quickly, followed immediately by a 5 mL normal saline flush.
- Check child's vital signs.
  o Rapid re-initiation of the tachycardia may occur due to premature atrial contractions, a repeated, and often lower, dose may be successful in this case.
  o A febrile child should be treated with antipyretics as the fever may make the tachyarrhythmia resistant to treatment.
- Side effects of adenosine: facial flush, chest pain, bronchospasm. It is helpful to warn older children of this prior to administration.

Child is shocked (hypotensive, poor perfusion, impaired mental state)
- This should be managed by cardioversion.
- Ensure child is given oxygen and has IV access.
- The airway should be managed by experienced staff.
- Administer midazolam 0.2 mg/kg (max. 10 mg) IV to minimise awareness and fentanyl 1–2 mcg/kg (max 50–100 mcg) if rapidly available for analgesia.
- DC revert using a **synchronised** shock of 1 J/kg.

Subsequent management
After stabilisation of SVT, specialist review is required for:
- 12-lead ECG in sinus rhythm (pre-excitation and other abnormality).
- Echocardiogram (structural associations of atrioventricular re-entry SVT, e.g. Ebstein's anomaly, cardiomyopathy).
- 24-hour Holter monitor (intermittent pre-excitation and initiating triggers such as premature atrial contractions).
- Consideration of electrophysiological study.
- Consideration of prophylaxis.

Infective endocarditis
Infective endocarditis is an infection of the endocardial surface of the heart. It is thought that for it to develop, two independent events are normally required: (i) a damaged area of endothelium and (ii) a bacteraemia.

Clinical features
- Usually insidious and non-specific presentation.
- Often suggestive of intercurrent viral illness.
- Fever, anorexia, myalgia, arthralgia, headache, general malaise.
- Splenomegaly, splinter haemorrhages, petechiae and other peripheral stigmata are rarely seen in children but do occur. Careful repeated examination for these signs is necessary as they may not develop until several days into the illness.
- Suspect endocarditis in any child with a structural cardiac anomaly and prolonged fever, or who develops fever and a new murmur.

Investigations
- Multiple blood cultures (≥3) at different times, before antibiotic administration.
- Full blood count.
- ESR and CRP.
- Echocardiogram.

Management
- Admission to hospital.
- Commence empiric antibiotics to cover endocarditis as well as other potentially serious causes for the presenting illness.
  - Native valve/homograft:
    - benzylpenicillin 60 mg/kg (max 2 g) IV 6 hourly **plus**;
    - flucloxacillin 50 mg/kg (max 2 g) IV 6 hourly **plus**;
    - gentamicin 2.5 mg/kg (max 240 mg, synergistic dose) IV 8 hourly.
  - Prosthetic valve:
    - vancomycin 15 mg/kg (max 500 mg) IV 6 hourly **plus**;
    - gentamicin 2.5 mg/kg (max 240 mg, synergistic dose) IV 8 hourly.
- Prolonged antibiotic treatment is required. Specialist consultation is recommended to tailor the antibiotic regimen to individual child and pathogens.
- Close monitoring of clinical and cardiovascular status including serial echocardiogram, blood cultures and inflammatory markers.
- Close monitoring for evidence of embolic phenomena including cerebral imaging for left-sided lesions.

Table 15.2 Cardiac conditions for which endocarditis prophylaxis with dental procedures is indicated.

Prosthetic cardiac valve or prosthetic valve material used for cardiac valve repair
Previous episode of infective endocarditis
Congenital heart disease (CHD) but only if it involves any of the following: Unrepaired cyanotic defects, including palliative shunts and conduits Repaired congenital heart defect with prosthetic material or device (surgical or catheter intervention) during the first 6 months after the procedure Repaired defects with residual defect at the site or adjacent to the sire of a prosthetic patch or prosthetic device
Cardiac transplantation recipients who develop cardiac valvulopathy
Rheumatic heart disease in indigenous Australians

Endocarditis prophylaxis
- Children at risk should establish and maintain the best possible oral health to reduce potential sources of bacteraemia which includes brushing and regular dental review.
- The following is a suggested guideline for prophylaxis.
  - Recommended only for children with the highest risk of adverse outcome of infective endocarditis (Table 15.2).
  - Give prior to at risk procedures, such as dental procedures involving dental manipulation of gingival tissue, the periapical region of teeth or perforation of the oral mucosa; invasive respiratory procedures (e.g. incision or biopsy of respiratory mucosa including tonsillectomy and adenoidectomy) and invasive genitourinary procedures (Table 15.2).
  - Give amoxicillin 50 mg/kg oral 1 hour preoperatively (max 2 g).
  - If unable to take oral medication, give amoxicillin 50 mg/kg IV at induction (max 2 g).
  - For penicillin allergy, see Appendix: Antimicrobial guidelines.

Clinical Controversy: Endocarditis
Recent evidence from the UK suggests that rates of endocarditis have increased since the major revision of guidelines in the mid 2000s. Accordingly, it is possible that these guidelines may be revised in the coming years as more evidence comes to hand.

Pulmonary hypertension
Pulmonary hypertension (PH) is more common in children than adults due to the relative frequency of children with CHD and lung problems secondary to prematurity and structural malformations. It is defined as a mean pulmonary artery pressure equal to or greater than 25 mmHg at rest and can be divided into idiopathic pulmonary arterial hypertension (iPAH) and associated pulmonary arterial hypertension (e.g. CHD, liver and lung disease and connective tissue disorders). Without treatment, survival is <12 months in iPAH.

Clinical features
Typical symptoms can be non-specific, but a diagnosis of PH should be considered in children with:
- Shortness of breath during mild physical exertion
- Syncope with exertion
- Chest pain

Examination
- Right ventricular heave
- Prominent pulmonary component of second heart sound
- Diastolic murmur of pulmonary regurgitation
- Signs of overt right heart failure are uncommon in children

Investigations
- CXR: enlarged central pulmonary artery arteries, 'oligaemic' lung fields
- ECG: Right atrial enlargement, RVH
- Echocardiogram: CHD, right ventricular function, estimate right ventricular and pulmonary arterial pressure

- Cardiac catheterization with pulmonary vasodilator challenge
- More specific tests may be required to determine any underlying aetiology before a diagnosis of iPAH is made.

Management
Treatment depends on aetiology and severity. The goal of medical treatment is to improve symptoms, quality of life and survival. There are multiple drugs that act to dilate the pulmonary vasculature dilatation and reverse remodeling.

Pharmacological treatment
Typical drugs used in Australia in children and routes of administration.
- Sildenafil, tadalfil (phosphodiesterase inhibitors)
  - Oral administration
  - Main side effect: systemic hypotension
- Bosentan, ambrisentan, macitentan (Endothelial receptor antagonists)
  - Oral administration
  - Side effect: elevation of liver enzymes and systemic hypotension
- Epoprostenol (prostacyclin)
  - Short half-life so requires a continuous intravenous infusion
  - Side effects: jaw pain, flushing and diarrhoea
  - Some countries use a nebulised or subcutaneous form of prostacyclin

Other
- Home oxygen (if desaturation during sleep)
- Anticoagulation (warfarin or aspirin to prevent thrombosis).
- Children with PH have markedly increased morbidity and mortality with anaesthesia and surgery and should have careful anaesthetic planning.

Cardiomyopathies
Cardiomyopathies are structural and functional abnormalities of the myocardium which can affect ventricular systolic and/or diastolic function. There can be both familial (genetic) and non-familial forms.
Subtypes include:
1. Dilated cardiomyopathy
2. Hypertrophic cardiomyopathy
3. Restrictive cardiomyopathy
4. Arrhythmogenic cardiomyopathy
5. Unclassified (including left ventricular non-compaction – LVNC)
Potential genetic and non-genetic causes of dilated and hypertrophic cardiomyopathy are listed in Tables 15.3. Features of dilated and hypertrophic cardiomyopathy are listed in Table 15.4.

Table 15.3 Aetiology of dilated and hypertrophic cardiomyopathy.

	Dilated cardiomyopathy	Hypertrophic cardiomyopathy
Familial	Sarcomeric protein mutations Cytoskeletal genes (Dystrophin, Desmin) Nuclear membrane Mitochondrial cytopathy	Sarcomeric protein disease Glycogen storage disease Lysosomal storage disease (Hurler's syndrome, Anderson-Fabry disease) Disorders of fatty acid oxidation Mitochondrial cytopathies Syndromic (Noonan, LEOPARD, Friedreich's ataxia, Beckwith-Wiedemann, Swyer)
Non-familial	Myocarditis (infective/toxic/immune) Kawasaki disease Eosinophilic (Churg Strauss syndrome) Drugs Endocrinological conditions Nutritional (thiamine, carnitine, selenium deficiencies) Tachyarrhythmia induced	Infant of diabetic mother Athletes heart Amyloidosis Obesity

Table 15.4 Dilated vs. hypertrophic cardiomyopathy.

	Dilated cardiomyopathy (50% of cardiomyopathies)	Hypertrophic cardiomyopathy (35% of cases)
Incidence	Estimated annual incidence 0.6 per 100,000 children.	3–5 per 1 000 000
Characterised by	Dilatation and impaired contractility of one or both ventricles	Myocardial hypertrophy in the absence of haemodynamic stress e.g. coarctation of the aorta, hypertension Commonest cause of sudden cardiac death (SCD) in children
Aetiology	25% are genetic (Table 15.3). Depends on age at presentation • <12 months: myocarditis and metabolic abnormalities more common • older children: familial forms more common	50% are genetic (Table 15.3)
Clinical Features	Few clinical signs until the degree of ventricular impairment is severe • Possible positive family history • Symptoms: chronic cough, poor feeding, failure to thrive, syncopal episodes, chest pain, decreased exercise tolerance, abdominal pain, palpitations, embolic phenomena. • Signs of heart failure	Infants: present with symptoms and signs of congestive heart failure Older children: usually asymptomatic, gallop rhythm ejection systolic murmur
Investigations	• Bloods: screen for general organ function, infective and metabolic cause, Brian Natriuretic Peptide (BNP) • CXR • Echo • Catheter	• Bloods: FBE, ESR, lactic acid, pyruvate, glucose, LFT's, carnitine and acylcarnitine profile, plasma amino acids • Urine: metabolic screen • ECG • 24-hour Holter monitor • Exercise test to assess blood pressure response • Echo
Management	• Stabilise heart failure: ACE-I, beta blockers, aldosterone antagonists • IV inotropes • Treat arrhythmias (medications, EP study, implantable defibrillators) • Anticoagulation (poor function or thrombus) • Heart transplantation • Screen family members	• Beta blockers: reduce heart rate. • Assessment of arrhythmia and SCD risk with implantation of implantable cardioverter defibrillator (ICD). • Relief of LVOT obstruction: Surgical resection, Cardiac pacing, Cardiac transplantation • Genetic review • Screen family members
Prognosis	14% mortality in 2 years post diagnosis	Mortality rate of 1% per year

The management of these children should be by specialist cardiac teams, including input from genetics, metabolic, neurology and developmental medicine. Medical and surgical options depend on the underlying aetiology for heart failure.

Syncope and fainting

Syncope is a brief, usually sudden loss of consciousness and muscle tone caused by inadequate oxygen or glucose supply to the brain.

Common causes

• Vasovagal: Usually associated with emotional or environmental stressors
• Orthostatic hypotension: Usually associated with a sudden change to upright posture

○ **Postural orthostatic tachycardia syndrome (POTS):** orthostatic intolerance presenting with symptoms including dizziness, pre-syncope, syncope and palpitations. Diagnosed in children where there is >40bpm elevation in heart rate when transitioning from lying to standing after several minutes in each position. There can be overlap with other dysautonomic symptoms and/or Chronic Fatigue (see Chapter 12, Adolescent medicine).

• Cardiac causes (only 2–6% of all cases of syncope)
   ○ Primary electrical: long QT syndrome, Brugada syndrome, catecholaminergic polymorphic ventricular tachycardia, short QT syndrome, pre-excitation syndromes.
   ○ Structural/functional: cardiomyopathy (dilated, hypertrophic, arrhythmogenic right ventricular dysplasia), coronary artery anomalies, aortic stenosis, pulmonary hypertension, acute myocarditis, CHD.

Concerning features on history
• Palpitations or chest pain
• Triggered by fright or auditory stimulus
• No identifiable prodrome
• Brief abnormal motor activity (rapid recovery)
• Syncope during exertion
• Syncope during swimming
• Requiring resuscitation
• History of CHD
• Family history (LQTS, cardiomyopathy, sudden cardiac death (SCD))

Investigations
All children presenting with syncope should have a 12-lead ECG performed.

Management
• Most children with vasovagal syncope or orthostatic intolerance can be managed effectively with simple lifestyle changes and avoidance strategies. This may simply include attention to fluid intake and diet.
   ○ Children with POTS may require more intensive lifestyle measures, physiotherapy input for rehabilitation and reduced pooling of venous blood in lower limbs. Occasionally pharmacological treatment is needed, in a specialist centre, to augment their blood pressure and manage symptoms. A range of drugs have been used including mineralocorticoids, peripheral vasopressors and beta-blockers.
• Any concerning features on history, examination or ECG should result in prompt specialist referral.

Basic ECG interpretation
ECG interpretation should include a systematic assessment of rate, rhythm, axis, P waves, QRS complex, ST segments, T waves and intervals (PR, QT and QTc). A normal ECG should have an appropriate rate for age and a P-wave, which should be upright in leads I and aVF, preceding each QRS complex (Figure 15.1). There are age-related normal values for axis, P waves, QRS complexes and all intervals on the 12-lead ECG (Table 15.5). For children >12 years, adult normals can be used as a guide.

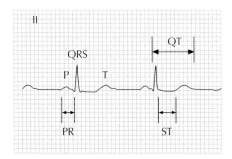

Figure 15.1 Normal ECG.

Table 15.5 Age-related ECG normal values.

	Neonate	Young child (1–2 years)	Older child (3–12 years)
Heart rate (per min)	107–182	89–151	62–130
QRS axis (°)	+65–+161	+7–+101	+9–+114
PR (s)	0.07–0.14	0.08–0.15	0.09–0.17
QRS (s)	0.03–0.08	0.04–0.08	0.04–0.09
R V$_1$ (mm)	3–21	2.5–17	0–12
S V$_1$ (mm)	0–11	0.5–21	0.3–25
R V$_6$ (mm)	2.5–16.5	6–22.5	9–25.5
S V$_6$ (mm)	0–10	0–6.5	0–4
Q V$_6$ (mm = 98th centile)	3	3	3

Rate
Calculate as 300/(number of big squares). At a normal paper speed of 25 mm/s, each small square represents 0.04 second, and each big square 0.20 second.

Rhythm
Sinus rhythm is present when there is a P wave with normal axis (upright in leads I and aVF) followed by a QRS complex. Alternatives include:
- Ectopic atrial rhythms: P wave with abnormal axis followed by QRS complex
- AV nodal or junctional rhythm: narrow QRS complexes unrelated to P waves
- Ventricular rhythms: broad often bizarre QRS complexes unrelated to P waves

QRS axis
Normal QRS axis values are listed in Table 15.5. An abnormal QRS axis can indicate ventricular hypertrophy (or hypoplasia with the larger ventricle contributing to relatively greater voltages) or be associated with anatomically abnormal conduction pathways in complex lesions.

P waves
The axis of a P wave arising from the normally located sino-atrial node is upright in leads I and aVF. Other appearances may result from ectopic atrial foci or structural congenital heart lesions. Tall P waves reflect RA enlargement (P pulmonale), broad bifid P waves LA enlargement (P mitrale). A prolonged PR interval occurs in first-degree heart block.

QRS complexes and T waves
The neonatal ECG shows right-sided dominance with large R waves and upright T waves in leads V1, V2, aVR and V4R. The T waves typically become inverted by about 1–2 weeks of age in the normal child. Persistence beyond this time indicates RVH. The T waves become upright in right-sided leads again in later childhood and the ECG takes on the adult appearance of dominant left-sided forces with small Q waves and large R waves in the lateral leads I, II, aVL, V5 and V6.

ST segments
Normal adolescents and young adults may have sloping elevation of the ST segment due to early repolarisation. Elevation or depression of >1 mm in limb leads and 2 mm in precordial leads is abnormal and occurs in pericarditis, ischaemia or infarction and with digoxin treatment.

Corrected QT interval
The QT interval can be corrected for heart rate by measuring the QT occurring after the shortest RR interval in sinus rhythm and applying Bazett's formula (all measurements in seconds). The QT interval is measured from the start of the Q wave to the point where a tangent to its down sloping portion crosses the baseline

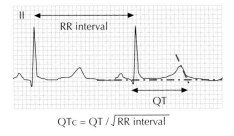

$$QTc = QT / \sqrt{RR\ interval}$$

Figure 15.2 Bazett's formula for calculating corrected QT interval (QTc).

(Figure 15.2). The QT interval may be prolonged in the setting of hypocalcaemia, hypothyroidism and hypothermia in addition to certain drugs. If there is intraventricular delay causing lengthening of the QRS duration, then this must be taken into account and measurement of the QTc interval with correction for heart rate should be considered instead.

USEFUL RESOURCES
- The RCH Cardiology Website www.rch.org.au/cardiology/heart defects/ includes resources with pictures and parent information regarding the major structural abnormalities.
- Howie's Place www.rch.org.au/cardiology/howie an interactive website to find out about cardiac procedures and tests that children may have.
- The RCH Supraventricular Tachycardia CPG www.rch.org.au/clinicalguide/guideline_index/Supraventricular_Tachycardia_SVT/
- HeartKids, www.heartkids.org.au parental support organisation

CHAPTER 16
Clinical genetics

Natasha J. Brown

Key Points

- In children with developmental delay, the probability of an underlying monogenic disorder is increased if there are associated neurological abnormalities (e.g. seizures, regression, hypo or hypertonia), growth anomalies (macro or microcephaly, short stature), structural organ malformation (e.g. congenital heart disease, polymicrogyria) or dysmorphic features.
- High resolution molecular karyotype (e.g. SNP microarray or array CGH) plus Fragile X analysis are recommended first tier diagnostic investigations for individuals with developmental delay and/or intellectual disability.
- Genomic sequencing (gene panel, exome or genome sequencing) is a powerful tool that allows confirmation of a specific molecular diagnosis in a significant proportion of individuals with suspected monogenic disorders. However, selection of individuals most likely to benefit from this technology, and of the appropriate test, can be complex, and is fundamentally reliant on accurate characterisation of the phenotype.
- In some individuals with developmental delay but no other specific neurological features, genomic sequencing may be a more informative diagnostic investigation than brain imaging.

Modes of inheritance
See Table 16.1.

Approach to the diagnosis of genetic syndromes
History
In addition to pregnancy, birth, neonatal and developmental histories, the following should be included:
- Family history: birth defects, stillbirth and miscarriage, neonatal death, consanguinity. Draw a family tree including minimum of three generations. Seek specific information if clinical suspicion for a particular diagnosis (e.g. if suspect congenital myotonic dystrophy ask about relatives with muscle problems/weakness, myotonia, diabetes, cataract, cardiac arrhythmia).
- Phenotypic information:
  - Organ malformation e.g. congenital heart disease, renal malformations, and medical problems e.g. seizures, recurrent infection, hip dysplasia etc.
  - Growth history/trajectory (explore similar patterns in the family) e.g. prenatal versus postnatal growth restriction.
  - Hearing and vision impairments
  - Development and intellect: Isolated or global delays; evidence of progression of symptoms or developmental regression; mild, moderate or severe intellectual disability.
  - Behavioural problems: autistic features, self-harm, aggression, sleep disturbance.
  - Other previous assessments e.g. echocardiogram, specialist consultation opinion, blood or urine test results.

Paediatric Handbook, Tenth Edition. Edited by Kate Harding, Daniel S. Mason and Daryl Efron.
© 2021 John Wiley & Sons Ltd. Published 2021 by John Wiley & Sons Ltd.

Table 16.1 Modes of inheritance.

Inheritance	Mechanism	Main features	Examples
Autosomal dominant	A mutation in one copy of a gene (located on an autosome) is sufficient to cause disease	• Male and females equally affected • A 50% chance that a child will inherit the gene mutation from a parent with the condition • There may be incomplete *penetrance*, variable *expressivity* • A single affected person in a family may have a *de-novo* mutation	Marfan syndrome Neurofibromatosis Tuberous sclerosis Achondroplasia
Autosomal recessive	Mutations in both copies of a gene (located on an autosome) are necessary to cause disease	• Male and females equally affected • Both parents almost always carry mutations in the same gene for their children to be at risk • If both parents carry a mutation, each child has a 25% chance of inheriting the disease • Increased risk of recessive conditions if parents consanguineous	Cystic fibrosis Thalassaemia Spinal muscular atrophy Phenylketonuria
X-linked	The disease gene is located on the X chromosome *X-linked recessive:* female carriers show no phenotype *X-linked dominant:* female carriers show a phenotype	• Affected males linked by unaffected/mildly affected females • *Transmission from female carrier:* 50% of sons will be affected; 50% of daughters will be carriers; 25% chance of an affected son each pregnancy • *Transmission from affected males:* 100% of daughters will be carriers; no sons will be affected	Duchenne muscular dystrophy Fragile X syndrome Haemophilia A G6PD deficiency
Polygenic	Multiple genes play an additive role in the development of a disease	• These conditions cluster in families but do not follow predictable inheritance patterns • Environmental factors often contribute to disease development	Non syndromic autism Hypertension Type 2 diabetes Schizophrenia
Mitochondrial	Mutations in the *mitochondrial* genome follow matrilineal inheritance	• Affected mothers pass on the mutation to all children, at differing levels • Males cannot pass on the disorder • Variable expressivity is common • Males and females affected equally	Leber hereditary optic neuropathy
Mosaicism	Mutations arise de novo in the individual, and are present in some but not all tissues	• No family history • Highly variable features • Clues may include patchy pigmentary skin features, syndactyly, segmental overgrowth	*PIK3CA* related overgrowth (PROS)

Examination

- Growth: height, weight, head circumference, relative proportions including trunk and limbs.
- Dysmorphic features: overall impression, specifically note head shape, hairline, ears, eyes, nose, philtrum, mouth, lips, tongue, palate, dentition, chin, morphology of hands and feet, chest wall. Compare to parents and siblings if available.
- Hands and feet: fingers and toes (number, size, shape). Note dermatoglyphics, palmar and plantar creases, nails.
- Skin abnormalities: birth marks, pigmentary abnormalities, neurocutaneous stigmata, skin texture, hair.
- Nervous system: gait, muscle tone (hypotonia, spasticity), reflexes, asymmetry, behaviour.
- Abdomen: hepatosplenomegaly, umbilical hernia, genitalia.
- Skeleton: scoliosis, joint mobility, limb proportions.
- Consider photographs, which can aid in diagnosis.

Investigations

1. **Chromosome analysis**. High resolution karyotyping i.e. Chromosome microarray (CMA) or array Comparative Genomic Hybridisation (CGH), has now replaced microscope chromosome analysis and fluorescence in situ hybridisation (FISH) testing for nearly all paediatric indications. CMA detects pathogenic abnormalities in approximately 15% of children with cognitive impairment, autism spectrum disorders or multiple congenital anomalies. However, CMA also detects chromosome variants of unknown significance, variants with incomplete penetrance, and incidental findings.
2. **Fragile X testing** should be undertaken in all males and females with cognitive impairment.
3. **Metabolic investigations** are especially important in the setting of developmental regression or progressive symptoms, seizures, hepatosplenomegaly, periodicity of symptoms, microcephaly or in the context of parental consanguinity (see Chapter 26, Metabolic medicine).
4. **Specific genetic tests** for individual syndromes may be utilised to diagnose certain disorders; however, broader genomic sequencing may be more appropriate in many cases.
5. **Genomic sequencing** is a new technology that allows the simultaneous and cost effective testing of large numbers of individual genes or even the whole genome. Various tests are currently available, including exome sequencing, limited exome sequencing (or virtual gene panels), and whole genome sequencing. Clinical utility is dependent on the phenotype (how likely is it that the child has a monogenic disorder) and the appropriateness of the specific test selected to the phenotype (Figure 16.1).
6. **Brain imaging** by MRI should be considered when developmental delay is associated with microcephaly, macrocephaly, seizures, focal neurological signs, or developmental regression.
7. **Skeletal survey** should be considered in the setting of short stature, disproportionate growth, bone malformations or fractures associated with minimal trauma.

Consider genetics consultation for the following reasons:

- To provide an accurate diagnosis
- To help understand aetiology
- To guide investigations, including screening for complications of a specific syndrome
- To advise about prognosis
- To guide management and possible therapeutic interventions
- To discuss recurrence risk in a future pregnancy
- To discuss options for prenatal diagnosis
- For clinical advice as to appropriate investigative pathways

---

Putting the Science into Practice: Diagnostic genomic sequencing

- New genetic technologies, such as massively parallel sequencing, have allowed children with suspected genetic disorders access to diagnostic genomic sequencing.
- Benefits of this technology include definitive molecular diagnosis, improved medical care through implementation of screening or intervention for specific complications, ending a potentially lengthy diagnostic odyssey, cascade testing for relatives who may be at risk of health complications, and more accurate genetic counselling regarding recurrence risks for parents and the wider family.
- However, many complexities exist, including appropriate selection of those most likely to benefit from this new technology, and accurate interpretation of results.
- Prior to ordering a genomic test, factors to consider include:
  - How likely is it that the child has a monogenic disorder and what is the differential diagnosis?
  - What is known about the genes and mutation types that cause the differential diagnoses?
  - Are those genes and mutation types readily identifiable by genomic sequencing? (Examples: Triplet repeat disorders such as Fragile X or myotonic dystrophy are not diagnosed routinely by exome sequencing and need to be specifically requested).
  - Would a targeted gene panel be better than a whole exome or genome? For example, conditions where the phenotype allows the clinician to make a definite diagnosis, but there are several possible causative genes to consider (e.g. isolated cystic kidney disease or Noonan syndrome) may be better investigated with a gene panel.
  - Has the child had a high resolution molecular karyotype prior to embarking on genomic sequencing?

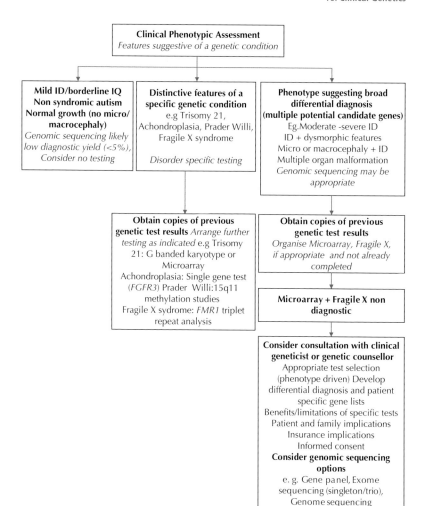

Figure 16.1 Genomics for Paediatricians Decision Aid. Courtesy of Zoe McCallum.

Common genetic syndromes
See Table 16.2.

Table 16.2 Common genetic syndromes.

Syndrome	Clinical features	Key management points	Genetics
Down syndrome	Hypotonia, small ears, upslanting palpebral fissures, flat facial profile, brachycephaly, congenital heart disease (40–50%), intellectual disability, hypothyroidism (20–40%), acute leukaemia (2%), dementia in 5th–6th decade	Early developmental intervention and educational support. Regular paediatric follow up and surveillance for complications (echocardiogram, thyroid function testing etc) Offer parental G banded karyotype to look for translocation	Additional chromosome 21, usually sporadic. 2% result from Robertsonian translocation of which 50% are familial. Mosaic Down syndrome accounts for ~2% of cases; typically less severe phenotype
Trisomy 18	Growth retardation, dysmorphism (prominent occiput, simple ears, overlapping fingers, rocker bottom feet, short sternum), congenital heart disease (>90%), short life expectancy, profound disability in survivors	Supportive care	Additional chromosome 18, usually sporadic
Trisomy 13	Growth retardation, holoprosencephaly, scalp defects, cleft lip/palate, congenital heart disease, polydactyly, short life expectancy, profound disability in survivors	Supportive care	Additional chromosome 13, usually sporadic
Klinefelter syndrome	Infertility, small testes, testosterone insufficiency, tall stature, learning difficulties in some	Testosterone replacement from around 10 years Monitor development and behaviour Assisted reproduction	Karyotype 47, XXY. Sporadic
Fragile X syndrome	Moderate intellectual disability in males; mild intellectual disability in females. Males may have a characteristic appearance (large head, long face, prominent forehead and chin, protruding ears), joint laxity, and large testes after puberty. Autistic features are common.	Early developmental intervention and educational support Offer testing to mother for future reproductive information, and cascade testing in the family	Expansion of CGG trinucleotide repeat in *FMR1* gene on the X chromosome. Fragile X full mutation is >200 repeats. Pre-mutation (55–200 repeats) has specific health risks for males and females, hence importance of cascade testing
Noonan syndrome	Early feeding difficulties, short stature, pulmonary stenosis (20–50%), hypertrophic cardiomyopathy (20–30%), variable developmental delay, webbed neck, sternum abnormality, cryptorchidism, characteristic facies	Treat cardiovascular complications, regular surveillance for risk of cardiomyopathy later in life Early developmental intervention and educational support	Heterozygous mutation (de novo or inherited) in one of >12 different genes including *PTPN11*, *SOS1*
Velocardiofacial syndrome (22q11.2 deletion syndrome, DiGeorge syndrome)	Highly variable, but include learning difficulties (70%), congenital heart disease (75%), cleft palate (10%), major immune dysfunction (1%), neonatal hypocalcaemia (60%), subtle dysmorphism (short palpebral fissures, prominent nasal bridge, rounded ears)	Early developmental intervention and educational support Surveillance for complications, including hypocalcaemia, immune dysregulation	Microdeletion at chromosome 22q11.2. Usually *de novo* but 7% inherited from a parent who may be mildly affected

Williams syndrome	Feeding difficulties in infancy, supravalvular aortic stenosis, distinctive facies, mild intellectual disability with unique personality characteristics, hypercalcaemia	Early developmental intervention and educational support; Surveillance for complications	Microdeletion at chromosome 7q11.2 (*de novo*)
Prader-Willi syndrome	Severe hypotonia and feeding difficulties in infancy, followed by excessive eating and development of morbid obesity (unless eating is controlled). Variable cognitive impairment and obsessive-compulsive characteristics, hypogonadism, incomplete pubertal development, short stature	Nutritional/feeding support in infancy; Strict supervision of daily food intake in older children; Early developmental intervention and educational support	Microdeletion at chromosome 15q11.2-q13 (*de novo* on paternal chromosome) or maternal UPD of chromosome 15, or imprinting defect
Angelman syndrome	Variable features including intellectual disability, severe speech impairment, gait ataxia, microcephaly, seizures, frequent laughing, smiling, and excitability	Early developmental intervention and educational support, seizure management	Microdeletion at chromosome 15q11.2-q13 (*de novo* on maternal chromosome) or paternal UPD of chromosome 15 or point mutation in the gene *UBE3A*
Beckwith-Wiedemann syndrome	Macrosomia, macroglossia, embryonal tumours (Wilms tumour, hepatoblastoma, neuroblastoma, and rhabdomyosarcoma), omphalocele, neonatal hypoglycaemia, ear creases/pits, hemihyperplasia	Tumour surveillance: abdominal ultrasound every 3 months until age 8 years. Serum alpha fetoprotein no longer recommended	Abnormal imprinting or UPD of chromosome 11p
Achondroplasia	Short (rhizomelic) limbs, macrocephaly, frontal bossing and midface retrusion, normal intelligence	Surveillance for complications, including cranio-cervical junction compression, obstructive sleep apnoea, middle ear dysfunction, bowed legs	Heterozygous mutation (*de novo* or inherited) in FGFR3 gene
Neurofibromatosis type 1 (NF1)	Multiple café au lait spots, axillary and inguinal freckling, multiple cutaneous neurofibromas, iris Lisch nodules, learning difficulties (50%)	Surveillance for complications including plexiform neurofibromas, optic nerve gliomas, central nervous system gliomas, malignant peripheral nerve sheath tumours, scoliosis	Heterozygous mutation (*de novo* or inherited) in *NF1* gene
Marfan syndrome	Skeletal: long limbs and fingers, scoliosis, sternum deformity, joint laxity; Eye manifestations: lens dislocation (60%), myopia; Cardiovascular: aortic dilatation, predisposition for aortic rupture, mitral valve and tricuspid valve prolapse.	Surveillance for eye and cardiac manifestations; Medications (e.g. angiotensin receptor blockers) proven to prevent progression of aortic dilatation; Surgical repair of aorta when maximum diameter reaches ~5cm; Avoid contact sports	Heterozygous mutation (*de novo* or inherited) in FBN1 gene

UPD = Uniparental disomy.

USEFUL RESOURCES
- The RCH Specimen Collection Handbook
- Genereviews www.ncbi.nlm.nih.gov/books/NBK1116/
- Unique Chromosome Disorders www.rarechromo.org
- The National Down Syndrome Society www.ndss.org/resources/healthcare-guidelines/ for management guidelines for individuals with Down syndrome

CHAPTER 17

Dentistry

Kerrod Hallett
Lochana Ramalingam

Key Points
- Good oral hygiene habits need to be implemented as soon as teeth erupt.
- See a dentist for a check-up 6 months after the eruption of the first tooth, 2 years of age, is too late.
- Avoid high frequency of sugar intake as it can cause dental decay.
- Stop night time bottle feeding habits from the age of 1 year old.
- In all cases of suspected dental trauma, lift the lips and look in the mouth.

Dental development
Primary dentition
Teeth start to form from the 5th week in utero and may continue until the late teens or early twenties. The first teeth to erupt are usually the lower central primary incisors at around 7 months of age. Table 17.1 summarises the eruption dates for primary teeth. **An infant who shows no sign of any primary teeth by the age of 18 months should be referred to a paediatric dentist.** By the age of 3 years, most children will have a complete primary dentition consisting of 20 teeth (8 incisors, 4 canines, 8 molars). In most cases, all primary or deciduous teeth are ultimately replaced, but 5% of children have one or more missing permanent teeth and primary teeth may be retained into adulthood.

Permanent dentition
At around the age of 6 years, the primary incisors become mobile and fall out. This process will continue for the next 6 years. The permanent dentition begins to develop, starting with the eruption of the lower first permanent incisors and molars (Table 17.2). Permanent teeth are much larger than the primary predecessors and often look more yellow or cream in colour. The period that follows, referred to as the mixed dentition phase, is highly variable. Some second primary molar teeth are replaced by the second premolars as late as 14 years of age. The simultaneous presence of primary and permanent teeth in the same site during the mixed dentition stage is common (known as the ugly duckling stage) and is not a cause for concern.

Dental caries
Dental caries (or tooth decay) remains one of the most common childhood diseases. In Australia, just over 60% of 5-year olds and 55% of 12-year olds are decay free. Unfortunately, 80% of the decay burden is experienced by approximately 20% of children. Of these, 10–15% have multiple decayed teeth requiring urgent surgical care. It is therefore important to identify children at high decay risk early (before 2 years of age) and specifically target them for prevention (Table 17.3).

    Dental decay can occur as soon as teeth erupt. Early childhood caries (ECC) is an aggressive form of dental decay that is seen in infants as young as 18 months of age. It affects >6% of Australian infants and has a characteristic appearance in which the upper front teeth are affected on their labial (or lip) surfaces.

Paediatric Handbook, Tenth Edition. Edited by Kate Harding, Daniel S. Mason and Daryl Efron.
© 2021 John Wiley & Sons Ltd. Published 2021 by John Wiley & Sons Ltd.

Table 17.1 Eruption sequence of primary dentition (months after birth).

Central incisors	Lateral incisors	Canines	First molars	Second molars
6–12	9–16	16–23	13–19	23–33

Table 17.2 Eruption sequence of permanent dentition (years of age).

Central incisor	Lateral incisor	Canine	First premolar	Second premolar	First molar	Second molar	Third molar Wisdom
6–8	7–8.	9–13	10–12	10–13	6–7.0	11–13	17+

Table 17.3 Dental caries: common risk factors assessable by medical practitioners.

Risk factor	Influence
Sugar exposure	Infant feeding habits are very important with frequency of exposure being most relevant. High risk behaviours such as prolonged on-demand night-time feeds and daytime grazing patterns
Family oral health history	Poor parental oral health places child at risk of decay, as cariogenic bacteria are transmitted from the primary caregiver
Fluoride exposure	Exposure to fluoridated water source and the regular use of fluoridated toothpaste are two key factors that reduce caries risk
Social and family practices	Low socio-economic status, indigenous and immigrant groups have higher levels of dental caries
Medical illness	Medically compromised children are more at risk of dental decay and are less likely to receive appropriate treatment

The cariogenic bacteria causing ECC are generally transmitted from primary caregiver to child, and decay is closely associated with inappropriate infant feeding habits such as bottle feeding with sweetened liquids and putting the child to sleep with a bottle.

Prevention

The prevention of dental decay should start as soon as the first tooth erupts. There are four aspects to preventing decay:

Diet

- Minimise the total intake and frequency of sugary foods and drinks.
- Limit sugary snacks to mealtimes with other noncariogenic solid and liquid foods, and when salivary flow is optimal.
- Minimise intake of drinks with high acidity (e.g. carbonated, fruit and sports drinks), as they cause erosion of the enamel tooth surface.
- Increase water intake.
- Encourage drinking from feeder cup from the age of 12 months.
- Avoid demand bottle-feeding at night-time and nursing during the night after 18 months.

Oral hygiene

- Tooth cleaning should commence following the eruption of the first tooth with a wet flannel.
- Start brushing with a soft children's toothbrush with a small head and a thin smear of paediatric fluoride toothpaste (400 ppm fluoride) at 18 months.
- Parents should supervise toothbrushing until around 8–10 years of age (when they can tie shoelaces).
- Use a soft toothbrush for children with a pea-sized amount of adult fluoride toothpaste (1000 ppm fluoride) after 6 years of age.
- Flossing should start once the child is proficient at toothbrushing.

Fluoride and amorphous calcium phosphate (ACP or tooth mousse)

- Fluoride enhances the ability of teeth to resist enamel demineralisation caused by sugar-related acids.
- Apart from systemic water fluoridation, the most common source of fluoride is toothpaste applied twice daily to the tooth surface.
- The preventive effect is dose-dependent (400, 1000 and 5000 ppm) and dental prescription is now based on perceived caries risk.
- ACP applied topically after toothbrushing can enhance enamel remineralisation for high risk children.
- Fluoride supplements in the form of tablets or drops are no longer available.

Regular dental check-ups

- A child should see a dental professional within 6 months of the eruption of the first tooth.
- The first visit is a 'well baby' visit and aimed at providing 'anticipatory guidance'.
- Children should have a dental check-up at least annually or sooner if risk is high.
- Developmental problems such as malocclusion should be identified early for interceptive treatment.

Dental emergencies

Toothache

- Assess level and nature of pain, for example sharp intermittent pain on eating or in response to hot/cold (pulpitis) or spontaneous dull pain (apical periodontitis) at night.
- Provide analgesia (paracetamol should be adequate in most cases).
- Refer to dentist for assessment and treatment of the affected tooth.

Dental abscess

Presentation

- History of spontaneous dull (usually constant) pain, particularly at night.
- Swelling or sinus evident intraorally near the diseased or carious tooth.
- Limited mouth opening and difficulty swallowing.
- Elevated temperature, enlarged lymph nodes and a generally unwell child.
- Teeth tender to palpation on side of the swelling.

Investigations

An orthopantomogram (OPG) will often show dental pathology, usually dental caries and pulpal pathology.

Management

- Consider oral amoxicillin for early infection.
- Admit to hospital if red swollen face, fever and generally unwell.
  - IV antibiotics (benzylpenicillin in the first instance).
  - IV fluids if dehydrated. Extraction of the tooth or intra canal drainage of the abscess is almost always indicated.
  - Occasionally, additional soft tissue drainage is required; however, dental abscesses in young children usually manifest with cellulitis rather than a collection of frank pus.

Clinical Pearl: Dental abscess
Red facial swelling, commonly unilateral and often spreading up under the orbit or under the mandible is consistent with facial cellulitis of dental origin.

Dental trauma

Traumatic injuries to the facial region can affect the teeth, soft tissues and jaw bones. **In all cases of dental trauma, lift the lips and look in the mouth.**

Primary teeth

Consider:

- How the injury occurred
- Other facial injuries or associated soft tissue (mucosal) injuries

- Time of the injury
- Where are the teeth or fragments of teeth?
- How much of the tooth is broken off or how far is the tooth displaced?
- Can the child bite their teeth together or does the displaced tooth get in the way?

Never replant a lost primary tooth. Injury (particularly intrusion) to a primary incisor can damage the permanent successor; therefore, dental review for all suspected intrusion injuries is important (Table 17.4).

Permanent teeth

Whenever possible, an OPG radiograph is useful as it allows a full examination of the jaws, temporomandibular joints and teeth (Table 17.5). A chest radiograph is useful if the tooth or fragments cannot be located. Many injuries can be managed under local anaesthesia, depending on the cooperation of the child and the presence of associated soft tissue or other injuries.

Locate all teeth or tooth fragments because:

- Most permanent teeth and tooth fragments can often be replaced or re-bonded.
- 'Missing' teeth may have been intruded (pushed in) rather than knocked out.
- Associated oral mucosal injuries may require suturing by the dentist.

Table 17.4 Dental trauma: Primary dentition.

Injury	Management
No tooth displacement	Non-urgent referral to dentist for review
Intrusion (tooth upwards and inwards)	Needs dental review within 24 hours to accurately locate the tooth. Likely that extraction will be required
Luxation (tooth palatal or sideways)	Needs dental review within 12 hours
Avulsion (knocked out completely)	**Do not** replant primary teeth

Table 17.5 Dental trauma: Permanent dentition.

Injury	Management
Fractures	
<1/3 crown	Non-urgent referral to dentist
>1/3 crown	Locate fragments, store in milk Needs dental review within 24 hours Some fragments can be reattached to broken teeth
Mobile but not displaced	Soft diet and analgesia
Displacements	Needs dental review within 12 hours May need dental splint
Intrusion (tooth upwards and inwards)	Locate teeth, using dental or OPG radiographs Tooth may re-erupt or require surgical/orthodontic repositioning Use gentle finger pressure to reposition teeth, if in doubt leave alone
Luxation (tooth pushed out/inwards or sideways)	Loose splinting can be achieved using aluminium foil until child sees dentist Urgent referral to dentist
Avulsion[a] (knocked out completely)	Urgent referral to dentist Replace tooth in socket if possible If not, store in milk at all times

[a]An avulsed permanent tooth is a genuine dental emergency.

- An avulsed permanent tooth is a genuine emergency. Try to replant the tooth or keep the tooth stored in milk until the dentist arrives. The longer the tooth is out of the mouth (>2 hours), the poorer the long term prognosis.
- The long-term psychosocial and economical impact on a young person of losing a front tooth should not be underestimated. Appropriate emergency management can make a significant difference to the prognosis of any injured tooth.

Mucosal lacerations

- Check carefully intraorally for degloving injuries (where the gum tissue around the teeth is stripped away from the underlying bone). Unless the lips are retracted, this injury can be easily missed. These injuries need suturing under general anaesthesia.
- Many superficial tongue and intraoral lip lacerations do not need suturing and heal well when left.
- Extraoral lacerations, particularly those crossing the vermilion border on to the skin, should be referred to a plastic surgeon.

Fractures to the jaw bones

- Whenever a jaw fracture is suspected, a maxillofacial surgeon should be called. If teeth are also obviously displaced or lost, a paediatric dentist should also be called.
- An OPG radiograph and a lateral skull examination and/or a variety of occipitomental/anteroposterior radiographic views can be useful to investigate the facial complex for fractures.
- Tetanus prophylaxis should be considered in any compound fractures opening to mouth or skin, and IV antibiotics commenced.

Bleeding from the mouth

- Rinse the mouth with cold water or saline and remove any debris, blood, tissue etc. from the teeth and gums.
- Identify the source of bleeding – usually an extraction socket.
- If the child has been bleeding for some time, assess haemodynamic status.
- Bleeding socket:
  - Compress the sides of the socket together using finger pressure.
  - If the child is cooperative, place a slightly damp gauze pack over the socket and have the child bite down on it for 20 minutes. Parents may be asked to assist. Do not pack foreign body into the socket.
  - Refer to dentist for further treatment if the bleeding has not stopped after 20 minutes.

USEFUL RESOURCES
- Spencer AJ. The use of fluorides in Australia: guidelines. *Australian Dental Journal* 2006; 51(2): 195–199.
- Dental trauma guide www.dentaltraumaguide.org/

CHAPTER 18

Dermatology

Rod Phillips
David Orchard

Key Points
- Do not underestimate the effect of skin problems. The morbidity from paediatric skin disease is as great as in any other paediatric speciality.
- Oral isotretinoin is the safest most effective treatment for acne.
- Do not stop a child with molluscum from swimming unless you actively treat the lesions to clear them rapidly.
- Corticosteroids used appropriately for eczema do not cause significant side effects.
- Flat red lesions on the face of infants can be developing segmental haemangiomas or (static) capillary malformations. Either refer urgently or monitor until you are certain which is the correct diagnosis.

Clinical approach to skin lesions
The key to accurate diagnosis and appropriate management of skin disorders in children is a careful history and astute observation of rashes, particularly focusing on their appearance, site and pattern of development. During the examination, consider a few key questions (Figure 18.1).
- Are there any vesicles, that is fluid-filled lesions? Finding these greatly narrows the range of possible diagnoses; small circular erosions may be the only signs of an underlying vesicular process.
- Is the rash raised (papular) or flat (macular)?
- Is the rash red? Redness is from haemoglobin. Most red rashes blanch, that is the redness disappears with pressure. If not, the haemoglobin is outside the blood vessels (purpura).
- Is the rash scaly? If so, the epidermis may be broken (eczematous) to give weeping, crusting or bleeding, or it may be intact (papulosquamous).

Vesiculobullous rashes
Vesicles are usually caused by infections (herpes simplex virus (HSV), varicella zoster virus (VZV), enterovirus, tinea, scabies or impetigo) or by contact dermatitis. Also, consider drug reactions, erythema multiforme and the immunobullous condition linear IgA disease. Larger blisters may be from staphylococcal infections, tinea, Stevens–Johnson syndrome, arthropod bites, contact dermatitis, burns or trauma.

Impetigo (school sores)
- Caused by *Staphylococcus aureus* or *Streptococcus pyogenes* (impetigo but not bullous lesions), or both.
- Presents as areas of ooze and honey-coloured crusts on the face, trunk or limbs.
- Occasionally the primary lesions are bullous but because the blisters are very superficial and break easily, one mostly only sees the 'peeling' edge of the blister. (Photo 18.1: A)
- Lesions are rounded and well demarcated and are most often grouped and asymmetrical but may be solitary and widespread.
- Their onset and spread may be acute or occur over days (subacute).
- In more chronic cases, there may be central healing with peripheral spread to give annular lesions.

Paediatric Handbook, Tenth Edition. Edited by Kate Harding, Daniel S. Mason and Daryl Efron.
© 2021 John Wiley & Sons Ltd. Published 2021 by John Wiley & Sons Ltd.

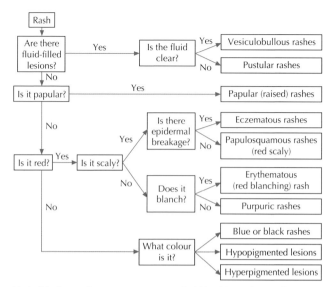

Figure 18.1 Algorithm for diagnosis of skin disorders in children.

Vesiculobullous rashes
- Impetigo (school sores)
- Eczema herpeticum
- Erythema multiforme
- Single blisters
- Stevens–Johnson syndrome/toxic epidermal necrolysis

Pustular rashes
- Acne

Papular (raised) rashes
- Scabies
- Urticaria/serum sickness
- Papular urticaria
- Keratosis pilaris
- Papular acrodermatitis
- Molluscum
- Warts

Eczematous rashes
- Atopic eczema

Red scaly rashes (papulosquamous)
- Seborrhoeic dermatitis
- Psoriasis
- Tinea corporis
- Pityriasis rosea

Red blanching rashes (erythematous)
- Fever and exanthem
- Erythema infectiosum

Red blanching rashes (erythematous)
- Roseola infantum
- Kawasaki disease

Purpuric rashes
- Enteroviral infection
- Septicaemia
- Leukaemia
- Henoch–Schoenlein purpura
- Child abuse
- Idiopathic thrombocytopenic purpura (ITP)
- Trauma and vasomotor straining

Blue or black rashes
- Vascular malformations
- Haemangiomas
- Mongolian spots

Hypopigmented lesions
- Tinea versicolor
- Pityriasis alba
- Vitiligo
- Post-inflammatory hypo- and hyperpigmentation

Hyperpigmented lesions
- Congenital pigmented naevi
- Acquired pigmented naevi

Management
- Bathe off crusts.
- Apply topical mupirocin 2% ointment 8 hourly if localised, or if more than one localised area cephalexin or flucloxacillin 25 mg/kg (max. 500 mg) orally QID for 7 days.
- Isolate the child from other children or from sick adults until all lesions are covered or treated.

- Treat any underlying condition such as scabies (a common cause of widespread impetigo).
- Treat coexistent eczema with topical corticosteroids.

Staphylococcal scalded skin syndrome

- Usually seen in younger children.
- Mediated by an epidermolytic toxin released from an often insignificant staphylococcal focus (e.g. eyes, nose or skin).
- Fever and tender erythematous skin are early features.
- Exudation and crusting develops, especially around the mouth.
- Wrinkling, flaccid bullae and exfoliation of the skin are seen – look for a positive Nikolsky sign ('normal' skin separates if rubbed).
- Blisters are very superficial and heal without scarring.

Management

- Flucloxacillin 50 mg/kg (max. 2 g) IV 6 hourly if there is any evidence of sepsis or systemic involvement.
- Look for a focus of infection and drain foci of pus if present.
- Monitor temperature, fluids and electrolytes if large areas are involved. Increased fluids will aid renal excretion of toxin.
- Handle skin carefully; use an emollient ointment
- Analgesia will often be required.

Erythema multiforme

- Occurs at any age.
- Lesions are usually symmetric and appear most commonly on the hands, feet and often the face. They can be found anywhere, including mucous membranes. They are not migratory.
- Typical *target lesions* have an inner zone of epidermal injury (purpura, necrosis or vesicle), an outer zone of erythema and sometimes a middle zone of pale oedema.
- Most cases are caused by herpes simplex, some by other infections. Drugs are an uncommon cause.

Management

- Ensure adequate fluid intake.
- Apply emollient ointment to the lips, if needed.
- If the condition is recurrent, it is highly likely to be related to HSV. Prophylactic aciclovir should be considered if recurrences are frequent and affecting the quality of life.

Stevens–Johnson syndrome/toxic epidermal necrolysis

Stevens–Johnson syndrome and toxic epidermal necrolysis are believed by many to be variants of the same condition.

- Characterised by widespread blisters on an erythematous or purpuric macular background, often with extensive mucous membrane haemorrhagic crusting.
- There may be tender erythematous areas with a positive Nikolsky sign ('normal' skin separates if rubbed).
- Conjunctivitis, corneal ulceration and blindness can occur. Some degree of permanent scarring around the conjunctivae is common even if eye symptoms are not severe.
- Anogenital lesions can lead to urinary retention.
- Fever, myalgia, arthralgia and other organ involvement can occur.
- Drugs, usually commenced a few weeks earlier, are the most common cause, occasionally caused by *Mycoplasma* infection.

Management

- Cease any drugs that may be the cause.
- Monitor temperature, fluids and electrolytes.
- Fluid maintenance.
- Apply emollient ointment to the skin, lips and anogenital areas – this may be required many times a day. Careful attention to emollients and/or dressing of the glans and undersurface of the foreskin may prevent secondary scarring, adhesions and phimosis.

- For eroded areas; dressings with or without silver impregnation (as per burns therapy) is appropriate.
- A regular opthalmology review for topical steroid drops if any eye involvement suspected.
- Pain management is essential; intermittent sedation to facilitate essential dressings and eye care may be required.
- IV gamma globulin is seen by many as standard therapy for cases threatening to become severe.
- Cyclosporin (5–6 mg/kg per day for a few days, then taper to 3–5 mg/kg per day for 2–3 weeks) commenced at diagnosis may prevent deterioration. Immunosuppression is controversial as sepsis is not uncommon but it is important to attempt to turn off the inflammatory process to limit skin loss.

Clinical Pearl: Stevens-Johnson syndrome and Erythema multiforme

Stevens–Johnson syndrome is *not* severe erythema multiforme (EM). They are distinct conditions with different aetiologies. Permanent sequelae are rarely seen in severe EM and concurrent drug use is unlikely to be the cause. Skin lesion morphology is the best discriminating factor. Classic target lesions are not seen in Stevens–Johnson syndrome. Mucous membrane involvement can be seen in both conditions but is usually localised in EM, and often confluent in Stevens–Johnson syndrome.

Eczema herpeticum

- HSV infection in children with eczema is common (Photo 18.1: B, C), but many cases are misdiagnosed as either an exacerbation of the eczema or bacterial infection.
- Grouped vesicles may be prominent, but more often vesicles are rudimentary or absent and the infection presents as a group of shallow 2–4 mm ulcers on an inflamed base.
- The infected area may not be painful or itchy and does not respond to standard eczema therapy.
- If untreated, resolution usually occurs in 1–4 weeks, but dissemination may occur.
- Recurrences may occur at different sites.

Management

- Collect epithelial cells from the base and roof of the vesicles for HSV PCR and culture.
- Mild cases demonstrating progression or facial involvement can be managed with oral aciclovir.
- A child with fever or multiple sites of cutaneous herpes infection may need admission to hospital and treatment with IV aciclovir.
- Eye involvement requires aciclovir and urgent review by an ophthalmologist.
- The underlying eczema can be treated with moisturisers, topical steroids and wet dressings. Topical corticosteroids can be used during the active infection phase.

Eczema coxsackium

Some coxsackie viruses (usually type A6) can give a widespread vesicular eruption with prominence around mouth, hands and feet in otherwise well children. Previous areas of eczema may be involved.

It can be differentiated from eczema herpeticum by the sudden symmetrical onset. Small, punched out erosions are not seen and the morphology is more of coalescing brownis crusts. Swab for both HSV and enterovirus if unsure.

Single blisters

When a child presents with a single blister as an isolated finding, consider impetigo, tinea, allergic contact dermatitis, mastocytoma, insect bite, cigarette burn or friction.

Pustular rashes

Consider acne, folliculitis, scabies, perioral dermatitis, acute generalised exanthematous pustulosis and rarely psoriasis.

Acne

- Mainly affects the forehead and face (Photo 18.1: D) but can involve other sebaceous areas (neck, shoulders, upper trunk).
- Early lesions include blackheads, whiteheads and papules. In more severe cases, there may be pustules or inflammatory cysts that can lead to extensive permanent scarring.

(A) (B)

(C) (D)

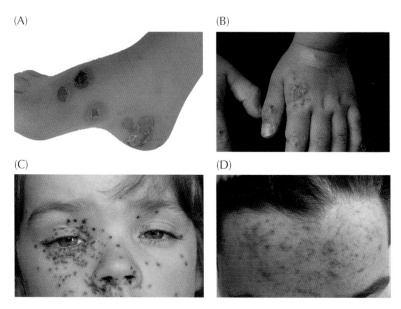

Photo 18.1 A = Bullous impetigo; B = Eczema herpeticum day 3, C = Eczema herpeticum day 7 (showing monomorphic & sometimes confluent lesions); D = Moderately severe acne warranting isotretinoin. *Source*: photos provided courtesy of Dr Rod Phillips and Dr David Orchard.

Clinical Pearl: Acne

Acne is treatable condition; no person with acne should just be told it is an inevitable part of adolescence. Undertreated acne is a cause of significant morbidity in adolescents and may be a factor in teenage suicide. Some skin types are particularly prone to scarring even from relatively mild acne. *Consider underlying endocrine disorders if acne begins before puberty.*

Management

- Effective acne therapies are available and should be used to control the disease.
- For mild disease, use topical benzoyl peroxide 2.5–5%.
  - Other topical agents include antibiotics (clindamycin, erythromycin or tetracycline), retinoids (Adapalene, Tretinoin and Isotretinoin) or azelaic acid.
  - These can be used singly or in combination and the main side effect is that of skin irritation.
  - Improvement occurs over 1–2 months, not within days.
- Treatment of moderate acne often involves the addition of oral antibiotic therapy (e.g. erythromycin 500 mg twice daily, doxycycline or Minocycline 50–200 mg per day) for 3–6 months.
- Oral hormone therapy can help female patients.
- Isotretinoin is indicated if:
  - Antibiotics and topical treatment have not resulted in considerable improvement within 3 months.
  - There is scarring or cyst formation.
  - An adolescent has significant acne and depression (concomitant assessment and treatment of depression is required).
  - Note that Isotretinoin prescription is limited mainly to dermatologists.
  - Provided pregnancy is avoided, even low dose isotretinoin (10-20mg daily, or less) is very safe and highly effective.

Papular (raised) rashes

If the child is itchy, consider scabies, urticaria, serum sickness, papular urticaria or molluscum. If not, consider urticaria, molluscum, warts, melanocytic naevi, keratosis pilaris and papular acrodermatitis. For vascular swellings, consider pyogenic granuloma.

Scabies

- An intensely itchy papular eruption develops 2–6 weeks after first exposure to the *Sarcoptes scabiei* mite or 1–4 days after subsequent reinfestation.
- The characteristic lesion is the burrow that is several millimetres in length. Burrows are best seen on the hands, especially between the fingers, and on the feet. Early burrows may be vesicular. There is varied morphology with papules, eczematous areas, excoriations, scabs and urticarial plaques.
- A clue to the diagnosis of scabies is the distribution of papules and pruritus; involvement of the palms, soles, axilla, umbilicus, groin and genitalia is common and the head is usually spared (Photo 18.2: E).

Management

- Treatment is expensive and upsetting. If diagnosis is unclear, confirm by scraping to find a mite, or refer before treating.
- Use permethrin 5% cream. An alternative for pregnant women or neonates is sulfur 2% in yellow soft paraffin.
- Oral ivermectin at the stat dose of 200 mcg/kg is effective and can be used particularly for more widespread or institutional breakouts.
- Note: **The following are not recommended:** lindane 1% (contraindicated in infants or women who are pregnant or breastfeeding) or benzyl benzoate 25% (too irritating for children and ineffective).
- Treat all household members and any other people who have close skin contact with the affected individuals.
- Apply to dry skin (not after a bath) from the neck down to all skin surfaces. For infants, apply to the scalp as well (not face). Use mittens if necessary to prevent finger sucking.
- Leave the cream on for at least 8 hours.
- Wash the cream off. Wash clothing, pyjamas and bed linen at this time.
- The itch takes a week or two to settle and can be treated with potent topical steroids.
- Reinfestation is common. The family should notify all social contacts (e.g. crèche, school or close friends) to ensure that all those infected receive treatment.

Urticaria

- See also Chapter 13, Allergy.
- Characterised by the rapid appearance and disappearance of multiple raised red wheals on any part of the body.
- Individual lesions are often itchy and clear within 1 day.
- There may be central clearing to give ring lesions (these are not the so-called target lesions of EM that persist for several days).
- The child is usually well.
- Urticarial episodes usually resolve over days or weeks and rarely last longer than 6 months.
- In most cases of short duration, the trigger is either a transient viral infection, allergic reaction or cannot be determined.
- Some children develop fever and arthralgias in association with urticarial lesions that are more fixed and may bruise or be tender (serum sickness-like reaction). This may commence a few days after commencing oral antibiotics, particularly cefaclor.

Management

- Urticaria may be the first sign of anaphylaxis. If there is associated wheeze, continued observation and appropriate treatment is required (see chapter 3 Resuscitation and Medical emergencies).
- Investigation is usually not required and is dictated by other symptoms rather than by severity of urticaria. The trigger is usually a previous viral illness.
- Ask about medications, new foods and environmental allergens. Consider food allergy testing only if urticaria starts suddenly, on the lips and face and within 1 hour of a newly introduced food.

- Treat the itch with oral antihistamine (see chapter 13 Allergy).
- Oral prednisolone (1 mg/kg per day, max 50 mg) for 2–5 days is beneficial in serum sickness and is warranted in urticaria when pruritus is severe.
- Urticaria can become chronic, and in the vast majority of cases, no underlying ongoing trigger is found. Consider investigating with a throat swab (for streptococcal carriage), FBE (for eosinophilia and anaemia), antinuclear antibodies, urine culture for bacteriuria, nocturnal check for threadworms and a possible challenge with any suspected agent. Adding cimetidine (10 mg/kg (max 200 mg) p.o. 6 hourly) to the antihistamine may help.
- If individual lesions last >2 days or are tender or purpuric, consider investigation for cutaneous vasculitis.

Papular urticaria
- This is a clinical hypersensitivity to insect bites.
- New bites appear as groups of small red papules, usually in warmer weather.
- Older bites appear as 1–5 mm papules, sometimes with surface scale or crust, or with surrounding urticaria.
- Vesicles or pustules may form.
- Individual lesions may resolve in a week or last for months and may repeatedly flare up after fresh bites elsewhere.
- The itch is often intense and secondary ulceration and/or infection.
- Many insect bites will only cause a reaction in a small proportion of the population and it is not uncommon to have papular urticaria presenting in only one member of a household.

Management
- Prevent bites (e.g. adequate clothing, modifying behaviours that leads to exposure, occasional repellent and the treatment of pets and house for fleas if necessary).
- Treat the itch with an agent such as aluminium sulfate 20% (Stingose), liquor picis carbonis 2% in calamine lotion, potent steroid ointment and/or antihistamines (see chapter 13 Allergy). Protective dressings (e.g. Duoderm) can speed the healing of lesions.
- Treat secondary infection with topical mupirocin ointment 2% or oral antibiotics.

Keratosis pilaris
- This is a rough, somewhat spiky papular rash on the upper outer arms, thighs, cheeks or all three areas, with variable erythema (Photo 18.3: F).
- It is common at all ages but commonly first presents as a toddler and most often is present in one or both parents to some degree.

Management
- Reassurrance; therapy is only needed for cosmetic appearance. Soap avoidance and moisturisers can improve the feel. Steroids do not help.
- Topical keratolytics (e.g. Dermadrate, Calmurid) can help the roughness.
- Older children with troublesome facial redness can be treated with vascular laser.

Papular acrodermatitis
- Characterised by the acute onset of monomorphic red or skin-coloured papules mainly on the arms, legs and face.
- Usually asymptomatic.
- Can be caused by coxsackie virus, echovirus, mycoplasma, EBV, adenovirus and others.
- **Management**
- Reassurance and advise that clearing can take several weeks

Molluscum
- Uncomplicated molluscum lesions are easily recognised as firm, pearly, dome-shaped papules with central umbilication (Photo 18.2: G).

- Presentation to a doctor is often prompted by the development of eczema in surrounding skin. In such cases, recognition can be difficult as eczematous changes can obscure the primary lesions. A careful history of the initial lesions is usually diagnostic.

Management
Education:

- Molluscum is caused by a virus and is very common. A child may develop a few, or a great many lesions and individual lesions may last for months. Complete resolution will not happen until an immune response develops, which may take from 3 weeks to 3 years.
- Children with molluscum should not share towels but should not be otherwise restricted in their activities.

Treatment:

- Depends on the age of the child, the location of the lesions and any secondary changes.
- Treatment of surrounding eczema with topical 0.1% methylprednisolone aceponate may be all that is required.
- Uncomplicated lesions not causing problems and not spreading can be left alone.
- Isolated or troublesome lesions (e.g. on the face) can be physically treated. One method is gentle cryotherapy or the use of topical Cantharadin.
- Rarely, children warrant curettage under topical anaesthesia. This is well tolerated and usually curative but can potentially scar.
- Alternatively, the stimulation of an immune response can be attempted with topical cantharadin, or with aluminium acetate solution (Burow solution 1:30) for large areas, or benzoyl peroxide 5% daily to small areas and covered with the adhesive part of a dressing.
- It is likely that molluscum spread more easily on moist skin such as via kickboards at swimming pools. However, swimming lessons are important for children. Generally children can cover lesions and should not be stopped from swimming. Any child stopped from swimming should have their molluscum treated intensively to clear them as rapidly as possible.
- Molluscum in the anogenital region are not an indicator of sexual abuse.

Warts

Many serotypes of the papilloma virus can cause warts. Different serotypes have a predilection for different areas of the skin. No treatment is necessary unless the warts are causing a problem to the child (e.g. social embarrassment, or pain from a plantar wart). Resistant warts on the limbs often respond to contact sensitisation (e.g. Diphenylcyclopropenone (DCP) 0.1% cream after sensitisation with 2% solution).

- **Ordinary warts:** if tolerated by the child, paring every 2–3 days with a razor blade or nail file will remove the surface horn. Apply a proprietary keratolytic agent that contains salicylic or lactic acid, or both, each day or two as directed.
- **Plantar warts:** these can be painful and can appear flat. Pare as for ordinary warts. Alternatively, place a small pad of cotton wool soaked in 3% formalin in a saucer on the floor. Rest the wart-affected sole on the pad/saucer for 30 minutes each night. Cryotherapy and surgery are often ineffective and can lead to painful keloid scarring.
- **Plane (flat) warts:** these are smooth, flat or slightly elevated, skin-coloured or pigmented lesions. They may occur in lines or coalesce to form plaque-like lesions. If treatment is needed for plane warts on the hands, apply a formalin solution as for ordinary warts. Lesions on the face are often subtle and may not need treatment. Topical retinoid creams can reduce the size of the warts whilst waiting for immune response but can be irritating for some.
- **Anogenital warts:** these are soft, fleshy warts that occur at the mucocutaneous junctions, especially around the anus. They may be isolated flesh-coloured nodules or may coalesce into large cauliflower-like masses. Management options include awaiting resolution, imiquimod, curettage and diathermy and carbon dioxide laser.

> **Clinical Pearl: Anogenital warts**
> *In isolation*, and without other red flags for abuse, the presence of genital warts in a young child is not a significant risk factor for sexual abuse and is not an indication for mandatory reporting to government protective services. Transmission is usually by normal close parent–child contact.

Eczematous rashes

Consider atopic eczema, allergic contact dermatitis, irritant contact dermatitis, photosensitivity eruptions, molluscum, tinea corporis and scabies.

Atopic eczema

- See also Chapter 13, Allergy.
- Eczema usually begins in infancy and can involve any part of the skin surface (Photo 18.2: H).
- Acute lesions: erythema, weeping, excoriation and rarely vesicles may be seen in.
- Chronic lesions may show scale and lichenification (Photo 18.3: L).
- In some children, the lesions are more clearly defined, thickened discoid areas that may intermittently be itchy.
- Weeping and yellow-crusted areas that do not respond to therapy may indicate secondary bacterial or herpetic infection.

Management

- **Education**: parents need to know the triggers and that treatments are effective in controlling the disease.
- **Avoid irritants** which may worsen eczema: soaps, bubble baths, prickly clothing, seams and labels on clothing, car seat covers, sand, carpets, overheating or contact with pets. Smooth cotton clothing is preferred.
- **Keep the skin moist:** use a plain moisturiser enough to prevent the skin from becoming dry.
- **Avoid overheating:** many babies and toddlers are overheated by overdressing. Emphasise this particularly if the flexures and other warmer areas are involved.
- **Treat inflammation:** an extremely important component of management as it is imperative to settle inflammation to enable the skin to heal and to relieve pruritus.
  - ○ Hydrocortisone may be used for the face and a more potent topical steroid for other areas; use until eczema is cleared completely.
  - ○ Oral steroids rarely indicated in eczema.
  - ○ Zinc and tar combinations are alternatives to steroids for chronic eczema on the limbs.
- **Treat itch** by effectively treating inflammation and by avoiding overheating; wet dressings can be helpful in some cases.
- **Treat infection if present**: take cultures and treat with simple wet dressings and oral antibiotics:
  - ○ Erythromycin, cephalexin or flucloxacillin.
  - ○ Consider if HSV is present.
  - ○ For recurrent bacterial infection, use antiseptic wash or 15-minute soak in salt/bleach baths (12 mL of standard household bleach per 10 litres of bath water).
- Diet: a normal diet is usually indicated. If a child has immediate urticarial reactions to a particular food, that food should be avoided. In difficult cases, consider a more formal allergy assessment.
- Hospitalisation: if a child is missing school because of eczema, they should generally be in hospital for intensive treatment or seen urgently in a specialist clinic for consideration of oral immunosuppressive agents.

> **Clinical Pearl: Eczema and food allergy**
> Whilst the majority of children with eczema *do not* have an underlying food allergy driving their eczematous flares; food allergy is more likely to be of relevance in a child less than 12 months of age with widespread eczema. Dietary restriction not generally recommended.

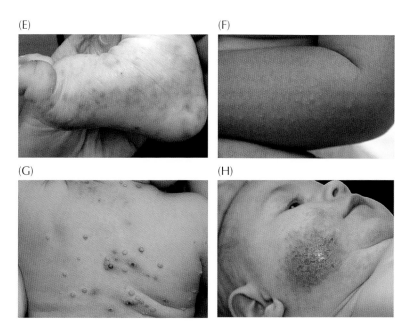

Photo 18.2 E = Scabies; F = Keratosis pilaris; G = Molluscum with mild secondary eczema; H = Infantile facial eczema.
Source: photos provided courtesy of Dr Rod Phillips and Dr David Orchard.

Red scaly rashes (papulosquamous)

Consider seborrhoeic dermatitis, psoriasis, tinea corporis, pityriasis rosea, pityriasis versicolor and atopic eczema. Ichthyosis vulgaris is a common cause of generalised scale without itch or redness.

Seborrhoeic dermatitis

- Presents in the first months of life, partly due to the activity of commensal yeasts and a dermatitis reaction to the flora overgrowth.
- Red or yellow/brown scaly areas will commonly affect the scalp and forehead and sometimes the upper chest and back.
- Dermatitis/eczema can be multifactorial in nature and if seen in areas outside the sebaceous gland zones, then it is best considered due to other causes such as atopic eczema or psoriasis.
- Resolution by the age of 4 months is usual.

Management

- Paraffin or olive oil applied to scalp to loosen scale.
- Imidazole creams with hydrocortisone 1% cream or with a mixture of salicylic acid (1%) and sulfur (1%) ointment, twice daily.
- Anti-yeast shampoos (e.g. selenium sulfide – Selsun) can be helpful; use carefully to avoid irritation or toxicity.

Psoriasis

- Occurs at any age.
- Lesions often begin as small red papules that develop into circular, sharply demarcated erythematous patches with prominent silvery scale.
- Common presentations include plaques on extensor surfaces, red anogenital rashes that can be moist or scaly (Photo 18.3: J), generalised guttate (small) lesions over the trunk and limbs, and thick scaly scalp lesions (Photo 18.3: I). Itch can be a variable feature.

- Nail changes are often seen in childhood.
- The distinction between psoriasis and eczema is often difficult in children.

Management

Treatment depends on the site and extent of disease, and the age of the child. Adolescents are less tolerant of tar creams. Psoriasis can be difficult to treat or control in some children and all therapy may be considered suppressive rather than curative.

- Isolated skin plaques: topical steroids (e.g. intermittent mometasone with clinical monitoring) or tar-based creams (e.g. liquor picis carbonis LPC 4%, salicylic acid 2% in sorbolene cream) or both. Generally, avoid tars on the face, flexures and genitalia.
- Face and anogenital region: Hydrocortisone 1% ointment and/or calcineurin inhibitors (tacrolimus, pimecrolimus). Topical steroids are not used for large areas in childhood psoriasis because of the possible development of rebound pustular disease.
- Widespread psoriasis: may benefit from oral therapy with one or more of etretinate, methotrexate or cyclosporin, or with ultraviolet therapy, all of which are variably effective.
- A number of new therapies may be of benefit for children whose severe psoriasis has not responded to topical, oral or UV therapy. These treatments include biologic agents such as etanercept, adalimumab and ustekinumab.

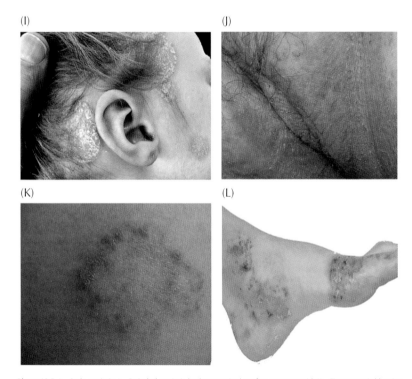

(I)   (J)

(K)   (L)

Photo 18.3 I = Scalp psoriasis; J = Perivulval psoriasis (under recognized as often asymptomatic); K = Tinea corporis (showing spreading annular accentuation) L = Chronic scaly, lichenified, eczematous plaques (given severe and localizing nature, allergic contact dermatitis & inflammatory tinea are differentials in the aetiology of this eczema presentation). *Source*: photos provided courtesy of Dr Rod Phillips and Dr David Orchard.

Tinea corporis
- The typical lesion is a slow-growing erythematous ring with a clear or scaly centre (Photo 18.3: K).
- However, tinea can present in a wide variety of ways, particularly if previous steroid treatment; eg. pustular, vesicular or bullous, and/or spread to many sites within days.
- Tinea should be considered in any red scaly rash where the diagnosis is unclear.

Management
- If diagnostic uncertainty confirm by scraping the scale from the expanding edge for microscopy and culture.
- Lesions are treated with terbinafine cream (twice daily for 1 week) or an imidazole cream (e.g. clotrimazole, miconazole or econazole 2–4 times daily, for 4 weeks).
- Oral griseofulvin (20–30 mg/kg per day in divided doses) or oral terbinafine is required for tinea capitis (for 6–8 weeks or for widespread lesions).

Pityriasis rosea
- Common between the ages of 1 and 10 years.
- Initially, a pink scaly patch appears, followed a few days later by many pink/red scaly oval macules mainly on the trunk. The pattern of the ovals on the back can resemble a fir tree.
- Usually asymptomatic but can be itchy.
- Management: reassure the patient; the condition can persist for weeks.

Red blanching rashes (erythematous)
Macular erythematous lesions are most commonly caused by viral infections (e.g. coxsackie, echovirus, Epstein–Barr virus, adenovirus, parainfluenza, influenza, parvovirus B19, human herpes virus 6, rubella and measles) or drug reactions. Consider also septicaemia, scarlet fever, Kawasaki disease (see Chapter 25, Infectious diseases) and *Mycoplasma* infection.

Fever and exanthem
The onset of fever and exanthem is usually due to a viral illness, often enterovirus. Some infections have specific clinical features that aid diagnosis; for example measles and erythema infectiosum. However, in most instances, a diagnosis cannot be made with certainty. To manage such a child, consider:
- Is the child sick? Is the child lethargic, not feeding well, cool peripherally or young? If yes to any – consider meningococcal disease, other bacterial sepsis, measles and Kawasaki disease. Investigate and treat.
- Are they taking any medication that could be responsible? Consider ceasing medication.
- Are there other people at risk? If relatives are immunosuppressed or pregnant, consider serology, viral PCR testing and viral culture. Advise the at-risk person to consult their own doctor.
- Is the rash papular and mainly on the limbs and face? Consider papular acrodermatitis.
  If the answer to all of the above is 'no', then reassurance and review is probably appropriate.

Erythema infectiosum and Kawasaki disease
See Chapter 25, Infectious diseases.

Roseola infantum
This condition is commonly seen in paediatric emergency departments. Typically, an infant has had a high fever for 2–4 days followed by a widespread erythematous macular rash when the temperature returns to normal. As many children with fever are commenced on antibiotics, it is difficult to determine whether an exanthem occurring in this setting is due to the infection or as a reaction to the antibiotic. There are no specific signs of the exanthem that can help determine this. The vast majority are due to the viral infection.

Purpuric rashes
Consider viral infections, meningococcal sepsis, other causes of septicaemia, platelet disorders, Henoch Schönlein purpura and less common causes of vasculiti, drug reactions and trauma.

Septicaemia
Suspect septicaemia (usually meningococcal) in a child with recent onset of fever and lethargy. Skin lesions may be erythematous macules progressing to extensive purple purpura. If you suspect meningococcal sepsis, take

blood cultures if possible rapidly, immediately give antibiotics and arrange admission (see also Chapters 3, Resuscitation and medical emergencies, and 25, Infectious diseases). Sepsis must be excluded in all children presenting with purpura.

Enteroviral infection
Scattered petechiae are common in children who have fever from enteroviral infections. These children are usually well. If in doubt, or if the child appears unwell, investigate and consider treatment for septicaemia.

Leukaemia
Suspect leukaemia in a child with generalised petechiae or purpura in the absence of trauma. Look for tiredness or pallor. Obtain an urgent full blood examination (see Chapter 30, Oncology).

Henoch–Schönlein purpura
Non-itchy, painless macules, papules or urticarial lesions with purpuric centres occur in a symmetrical distribution mainly on the buttocks and ankles, occasionally on the legs, arms and elsewhere. There may be associated abdominal pain, arthralgia, arthritis or haematuria. Renal involvement leading to chronic renal failure is rare, but can occur irrespective of the severity of the rash and other symptoms, and may be delayed until weeks or months after the onset of the illness. See detailed summary including Investigations and management in chapter 39 Rheumatology.

Idiopathic thrombocytopenic purpura
Bruises, petechiae or purpuric lesions appear over a period of days or weeks, mainly in sites of frequent mild trauma. The child is otherwise well. Full blood examination will show a low platelet count (see Chapter 23, Haematology).

Child abuse
Twisting, compression, pinching and hitting can all cause petechial or purpuric lesions. Look for bruises of bizarre shapes and different ages, evidence of bony fractures and an abnormal affect (see Chapter 20, Forensic medicine).

Trauma, dermatitis artefacta and vasomotor straining
- In some ethnic groups, it is common to treat a febrile or unwell child by rubbing or suctioning the skin with a variety of implements. This produces bizarre circular and linear patterns of petechiae that can alarm the unwary.
- Dermatitis artefacta refers to self-inflicted lesions, usually in older children or adolescents with some degree of psychosocial issues. Lesions usually appear rapidly, e.g. overnight, located at easily accessible parts of the body surface, and in often bizarre patterns difficult to attribute to other recognised diseases. Direct confrontation should usually be avoided and there is no need to prove self-infliction. Instead, create a supportive empathetic doctor-patient relationship and the children are usually content with accepting help for their stress/anxiety.
- Petechiae can appear around the head and neck in normal children after coughing or vomiting. Restraining a small child for a procedure such as a lumbar puncture or venepuncture can also lead to the development of petechiae on the upper body.

Blue or black rashes
Consider vascular malformations, haemangiomas, Mongolian spots, blue naevi and melanoma.

Vascular malformations
- These can be blue, red, purple or skin coloured. They are developmental defects and do not resolve.
- Such malformations can involve capillaries (e.g. port wine stain), veins, arteries (e.g. arteriovenous malformation) and lymphatics (e.g. cystic hygroma).
- Small vascular malformations may not cause any problems and do not require treatment.
- Extensive malformations can be associated with pain, soft tissue or bony hypertrophy, bone erosion, haemorrhage, thrombosis, infection, platelet trapping and death. No cure is available for most lesions. Troublesome or large lesions may benefit from anticoagulation, oral sirolimus, surgery or sclerotherapy. A multidisciplinary approach using expertise from surgical, paediatric, dermatological, radiological fields, orthopaedic, dental and other specialities is helpful.

Infantile haemangiomas (strawberry birthmarks)

- Superficial haemangiomas begin as flat red lesions in the first weeks of life and become soft, partly compressible, sharply defined, red or purple swellings that can occur anywhere on the body.
- Deeper haemangiomas may appear as blue or skin-coloured swellings.
- Most haemangiomas are not present at birth; they grow for several months and largely resolve over several years.

Management

Parents need reassurance about the inherently benign nature of these lesions. Most haemangiomas are best left alone and allowed to involute spontaneously. In some sites, haemangiomas can rapidly lead to problems such as permanent disfigurement, ulceration, blindness, destruction of cartilage, respiratory obstruction or death. For these lesions, treatment is necessary.

Urgent assessment by an experienced clinician is needed if any developing haemangioma:

- Is ulcerating and/or potentially disfiguring
- Is on the eyelid or adjacent to the globe of the eye
- Deforms structures such as the lip, ear cartilage or nasal cartilage
- Begins as an extensive macule that grows thicker, especially if on the face (Photo 18.4: M).
- Is associated with stridor

If treatment warranted:

- Topical timolol (for smaller flat lesions).
- Oral propranolol (e.g. increase dose upwards to 2 mg/kg per day given as divided doses).
- Oral prednisolone (3 mg/kg per day weaning over 6 weeks) can be used if propranolol is contraindicated.
- Vascular laser or early surgery may be used in certain circumstances.

Hypopigmented lesions

In hypopigmented lesions, look for a fine scale. If it is scaly, consider pityriasis versicolor or pityriasis alba. If it is not scaly, consider pityriasis versicolor, post-inflammatory loss of pigment, halo naevi or vitiligo.

Pityriasis versicolor

- This is common in adolescents and is caused by an increased activity of commensal yeasts. The yeast overgrows in an environment of sweat and sebum production, (therefore if the diagnosis is made in a younger child, consider the possibility of abnormal hormone production).
- Multiple oval macules, usually covered with fine scale, appear on the trunk or upper arms. The lesions may appear paler or darker than the surrounding skin.
- Treatment with anti-yeast shampoos is effective; eg. apply selenium sulfide 2% (Selsun shampoo), leave on for 5–10 minutes, rinse and treat weekly for 4 weeks and then monthly. The pigmentation takes weeks to resolve and relapses are common without ongoing maintenance.

Pityriasis alba

- Common in prepubertal children and represents post-inflammatory hypopigmentation secondary to mild eczema.
- Single or multiple, poorly demarcated hypopigmented 1–2 cm macules are seen on the face or upper body.
- Lesions are not itchy but often have a fine scale.
- Most families only need reassurance.
- If needed, treat with methylprednisolone 0.1% ointment once weekly for two months to active lesions and educate regarding skin care for eczema.
- Repigmentation takes months.

Vitiligo

This autoimmune condition is characterised by sharply demarcated, sometimes symmetrical areas of complete pigment loss. Eventual repigmentation in childhood vitiligo is common and is helped by topical corticosteroids or tacrolimus. Some children develop extensive areas of vitiligo that respond poorly.

Post-inflammatory pigmentation changes

This condition occurs particularly in dark-skinned people. Many inflammatory skin disorders may leave diffuse, hypo- or hyperpigmented macules after healing. No treatment makes much difference. Most lesions resolve over months or years.

Hyperpigmented lesions

If they are flat, consider junctional melanocytic naevi, café-au-lait spots (Photo 18.4: O), naevus spilus, pityriasis versicolor and post-inflammatory hyperpigmentation. If raised, consider compound melanocytic naevi, Spitz naevi and warts.

Congenital pigmented naevi

Congenital melanocytic naevi (Photo 18.4: N) that cover large areas or are likely to cause significant cosmetic concern need early assessment by a skin specialist and a plastic surgeon experienced in this area, for diagnosis, surgery, laser treatment and/or long-term follow up. Small congenital melanocytic naevi have no significant increased risk for the development of melanoma. Large ones do have an increased lifetime risk of melanoma, depending on their size.

Acquired pigmented naevi

During childhood, most children develop multiple pigmented lesions, which may be freckles, lentigines, naevus spilus, acquired melanocytic naevi or very rarely, melanoma. Immune-suppressed children and those who have had chemotherapy are at greater risk of skin malignancy.

Anogenital rashes

Anogenital rashes are common in children. Often, the anogenital rash is not mentioned during history-taking and is only discovered on examination. Parents and children may be unaware of anogenital rashes, sometimes because the changes are asymptomatic, or not recognised as abnormal, or not visible to the child or parent. For example, both vitiligo and psoriasis can be present in the anogenital area with no one in the family being aware of this.

- Most anogenital rashes seen in infants who wear nappies are primarily caused by reaction with urine or faeces (irritant napkin dermatitis). Soaps, detergents and secondary yeast infection may contribute.
- In older children, threadworms (*Enterobius vermicularis*) are a common cause of an itchy anogenital rash. Look for the worms at night and treat with mebendazole 50 mg (<10 kg), 100 mg (>10 kg) (not in pregnancy or <6 months) or pyrantel 10 mg/kg (max 500 mg) oral stat. A repeat dose 2 weeks later helps reduce the high rate of reinfestation.
- Consider also less common causes such as malabsorption syndromes (diarrhoea, erosive dermatitis and failure to thrive), zinc deficiency (a sharply defined anogenital rash with associated perioral, hand and foot 'eczema' and failure to thrive), Langerhans' cell histiocytosis, psoriasis and Crohn's disease. In all these cases, the rash will not respond to the simple measures outlined below.

Irritant napkin dermatitis

- The most common cause of napkin dermatitis in infants.
- Presents as confluent erythema that typically (but not always) spares the groin folds.
- Variant presentations include multiple erosions and ulcers, scaly or glazed erythema and satellite lesions at the periphery.
- Satellite lesions are suggestive of associated *Candida* infection.

Management

- Keeping the area clean and dry; leave the nappy off whenever possible.
- Use modern gel-based disposable nappies & avoid cloth nappies until the rash is clear.
- Topical zinc cream or paste for mild eruptions.
- Add hydrocortisone 1% cream if inflamed. Do not use stronger steroids.
- Consider mupirocin 2% cream if not settling.
- Antifungal therapy is often not needed, even if *Candida* is present.

Candida napkin dermatitis

This occurs secondary to irritant napkin dermatitis and antibiotic use. Swab to confirm and treat the underlying cause as above and use topical imidazole cream.

Perianal streptococcal dermatitis
- Due to Streptococcus pyogenes infection.
- A localised, well-demarcated erythema covers a circular area of 1–2 cm radius around the anus.
- Tenderness and painful defecation are typical.
- If not treated may persist for months.
- May have associated fissures and constipation.

Management
- Perianal and throat cultures to confirm the presence of *Streptococcus pyogenes*.
- Paraffin ointment three times daily to the perianal area for symptomatic relief.
- Oral phenoxymethylpenicillin 15 mg/kg (max. 500 mg) 6 hourly for a minimum of 2–4 weeks. Several weeks of therapy may be required. Intramuscular penicillin can be used if there are concerns about compliance.
- Keep stools soft with oral liquid paraffin for several weeks.

Lichen sclerosus
This condition usually presents as vulval itch in girls aged 3 or older (see also Chapter 22, Gynaecology). There may be an area of atrophy with white shiny skin, purpura or telangiectasia in the perivulvar region (Photo 18.4: P). Cases have been misdiagnosed as sexual abuse. Boys may have similar findings on the glans or foreskin.

(M)   (N)

(O)   (P)

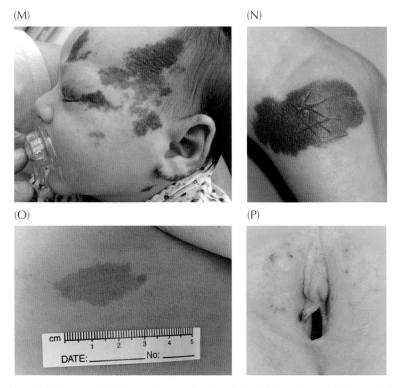

Photo 18.4 M = Segmental facial haemangioma (necessitates investigation for brain and chest arterial abnormalities); N = Congenital melanocytic nevus; O = Congenital café au lait macule; P = Lichen sclerosis with pallor and purpura. *Source*: Photos provided courtesy of Dr Rod Phillips and Dr David Orchard.

Management
- Avoidance of irritants, soaps, disinfectants and antibacterial washes, non-absorbent tight clothing.
- Treatment of any incontinence.
- Wash with water and use bland moisturisers.
- Potent topical steroid ointment to clear even if it takes months.
- Long term follow-up is required in all children given potential for recurrence and serious complications such as scarring, stenosis or cancer.

Hair problems
Consider alopecia areata, traction alopecia, tinea capitis, kerion and head lice.

Alopecia areata
- Typically, one or more oval patches of hair loss develop over a few days or weeks. Some hairs may remain within the patches but usually there is complete alopecia in the affected areas (rarely the hair loss is diffuse).
- Exclamation type broken hairs can be seen – thinner at the base.
- The scalp appears normal and does not show scaling, erythema or scarring.
- Most cases in childhood resolve spontaneously but progression to total scalp or body hair loss or recurrent alopecia can occur, even with treatment.

Management
- For isolated small patches present for weeks without further progression, no treatment is needed.
- Topical potent steroid ointment for a few months may minimise spread and may speed up regrowth.
- For progressive hair loss, treatment with intralesional steroids for a few weeks is beneficial.
- Other therapies including contact sensitisation, irritant agents, pulsed corticosteroids and other systemic immunosuppressive agents considered for resistant cases.

Traumatic alopecia
- This condition is usually caused by rubbing (as on the occiput of many babies), cosmetic practices (e.g. tight braiding) or hair tugging as a habit (trichotillomania - may be largely nocturnal and parents may be unaware of it).
- Affected areas are usually angular and on the anterior or lateral scalp.
- Affected areas contain hairs of different lengths and are never completely bald, unlike alopecia areata.
- Management includes recognition of the problem and a careful explanation to the family, with cessation of the precipitating behaviours.

Tinea capitis
- In Australia, tinea capitis is usually caused by *Microsporum canis* contracted from cats or dogs.
- Characterised by patches of hair loss with some short, dull, bent hairs a few millimetres in length.
- The scalp is usually red and scaly. Hair loss without any of these features is not likely to be fungal.

Management
- Confirming the diagnosis, if possible, by greenish fluorescence of the hair shafts with Wood light (not present with some fungi) or by microscopy and culture of hair and scale.
- Treatment with griseofulvin orally 20–30 mg/kg (max. 1 g) daily for 4–6 weeks or until non-fluorescent.
- Pulse therapy (1 week treatment, 3 weeks off, then repeat) with terbinafine or itraconazole may also be effective.
- Children may attend school, provided that they are being treated.

Kerion (inflammatory ringworm)
This represents an inflammatory scarring immune response to tinea. It is an erythematous, tender, boggy swelling that discharges pus from multiple points. The swellings appear fluctuant, but skin incision should be avoided. Treatment is with oral antifungals, often with antibiotics for secondary infection, and a brief course of oral steroids to suppress the immune response. Other inflammatory granulomas can mimic kerions.

Head lice
- Infestation of the scalp with *Pediculus capitis* is associated with itching.
- Eggs (nits) can be seen attached to the hairs just above the scalp surface.
- Epidemics of head lice regularly sweep through primary schools in all areas.

Management
- Pyrethrin 0.165% (e.g. Pyrifoam), or maldison 0.5% and permethrin 1% (e.g. Nix and Lyclear cream rinse). Resistance to all of these therapies has been reported.
- Wash the hair with soap and water. Thoroughly moisten the hair with the treatment and leave for 10 minutes. Rinse well and comb out with a fine-toothed comb. Reapply 1 week later to kill any eggs that have subsequently hatched.
- Re-infestation is common. A regular physical inspection, use of conditioner and combing of the hair are as important as chemical treatment.
- Children should continue to attend school whilst treatment is being undertaken.
- In very difficult cases, consider oral Bactrim for 2 weeks or single dose oral ivermectin.

Nail problems
- Congenitally abnormal nails are usually atrophic and can be the presenting feature of rare inherited conditions such as ectodermal dysplasias, dyskeratosis congenita, pachyonychia congenita, congenital malalignment of the great toenails and the nail–patella syndrome.
- Acquired nail disease is usually a result of fungal infection, psoriasis, ingrown toenails or 20-nail dystrophy. It may also be seen in association with diseases such as alopecia areata and lichen planus. Nail biting and picking can lead to marked deformity of involved nails.

Tinea unguium (onychomycosis, fungal nail infection)
- Dermatophyte infection may affect one or more nails, almost always toenails.
- White or yellow patches develop at the distal and lateral nail edges. The rest of the nail may become discoloured, friable and deformed with accumulation of subungual debris.
- Tinea is often also present on the adjacent skin, particularly in between the toes.

Management
- Confirm the diagnosis by microscopy and culture of nail clippings.
- Oral terbinafine (therapy of choice), taken daily for 12 weeks (<20 kg 62.5 mg, 20–40 kg 125 mg, >40 kg 250 mg).

USEFUL RESOURCES
Dermnet *www.dermnet.org.nz*; an excellent website with online courses (including pictures, investigations and management) and patient information.

CHAPTER 19

Endocrinology

Peter Simm
Fergus Cameron
Mary White
Margaret Zacharin
Jeff Kao
Michele O'Connell

Key Points

- To diagnose diabetes mellitus, an elevated BGL should be confirmed with a repeat test performed in a laboratory (as opposed to capillary blood test sampling only).
- Measurement of point of care ketones at the time of hypoglycaemia can greatly narrow the differential diagnosis in a timely manner (laboratory ketone/free fatty acid measurement may take several weeks).
- Rapid normalisation of thyroid hormone levels and maintenance of euthyroid state is essential to optimise neurodevelopment and growth outcomes in congenital hypothyroidism.
- All patients with adrenal insufficiency of any cause are at risk for adrenal crisis during periods of physiological stress. These patients require extra steroid cover during such periods to cover their endogenous deficiency.
- Precocious puberty is defined as the onset of pubertal changes under age of 8 years in girls and under 9 years in boys.
- Precocious puberty is more common in girls, most being functional, in contrast to boys where at least 70% have an organic cause.

Type 1 diabetes mellitus (T1DM)

Diagnosis is made by either:
- Random blood glucose level (BGL) ≥11.1 mmol/L in the presence of symptoms of diabetes; OR
- Fasting BGL ≥7.0 mmol/L.

Note:
- Hyperglycaemia detected incidentally, in the absence of symptoms, or under conditions of stress may be transient and should not in itself be regarded as diagnostic of diabetes.
- An elevated BGL should be confirmed with a repeat test performed in a laboratory (as opposed to capillary blood test sampling only).
- There is rarely a need for oral glucose tolerance testing to diagnose T1DM; symptomatic hyperglycaemia (± presence of ketones) is invariably present.
- Blood ketones can be tested on a bedside glucometer (Optium™), with a normal reading being <0.6 mmol/L. At diagnosis of T1DM, levels of >1.0 mmol/L are common.
- Any patient with ketone levels >1.0 mmol/L should have a blood gas assessment to check for acidosis. Serial monitoring of blood ketone levels in addition to capillary BGLs is very useful in assessing response to insulin therapy.

Paediatric Handbook, Tenth Edition. Edited by Kate Harding, Daniel S. Mason and Daryl Efron.
© 2021 John Wiley & Sons Ltd. Published 2021 by John Wiley & Sons Ltd.

Clinical features
Typical symptoms:
- Polyuria
- Polydipsia
- Lethargy
- Weight loss
- Glycosuria and ketonuria often present
- Family history of diabetes or other autoimmune disease (sometimes)
- T1DM presentation may range from being mildly unwell to severely unwell in diabetic ketoacidosis (DKA).

Differential diagnosis
Transient hyperglycaemia
- Transient hyperglycemia (+-glycosuria & ketonuria) may occur with intercurrent illness or medication such as glucocorticoids.
- This infers a higher risk of later developing diabetes (approximately 30%).
- Check HbA1c and diabetes-related autoimmune markers (antibodies against insulin, glutamic acid decarboxylase (GAD) and islet cells) and discuss with a specialist.

Type 2 diabetes mellitus (T2DM)
- Seen increasingly in children who are overweight/obese, specific ethnic groups, or family history T2DM.
- Oral glucose tolerance test is often required for diagnosis.

Monogenic diabetes
- Results from the inheritance of a mutation or mutations in a single gene.
- It may be dominantly or recessively inherited or may be a de novo mutation.
- Almost all paediatric monogenic diabetes results from mutations in genes that regulate beta cell function (very rarely it occurs from mutations resulting in very severe insulin resistance).
- Correct diagnosis can predict the clinical course, associated clinical features and most importantly guide the most appropriate treatment (eg. HNF1α mutations respond exceptionally well to oral sulfonylureas).

New presentation of T1DM, mildly unwell
(See also http://www.rch.org.au/clinicalguide/guideline index/Diabetes Mellitus/)

Assessment
<3% dehydration, no acidosis and not vomiting.

Management
Initial treatment
- 0.25 units/kg of quick-acting insulin s.c. stat (dose reduce if <4y or not ketotic).
- If within 2 hours prior to a meal defer and give mealtime dose only.

Ongoing treatment
Standard insulin regimes in newly diagnosed patients usually consist either of:
- Multiple daily injections (MDI) of insulin using a long-acting insulin analogue at night and pre-meal injections of rapid-acting insulin analogue.
- Twice daily injections of a mixture of short- and intermediate-acting insulins.
- In Australia, insulin pump therapy is uncommonly commenced at the time of diagnosis in children and adolescents, but may be an option at a later stage.

Established T1DM, hyperglycaemic and ketotic, mildly unwell
Patients with established T1DM who present with hyperglycaemia and ketosis but normal pH, will need additional s.c. insulin to clear their ketones.
- Patients on intermittent daily injections of insulin (MDI or BD)
  - Give 10% of the patient's total daily insulin dose (TDD) as an s.c. injection of rapid-acting insulin (in addition to the usual insulin regimen).
  - Monitor BGL and ketones 1–2 hourly. This dose of rapid-acting insulin can be repeated after 2–4 hours if blood ketones are not <1.0 mmol/L.

- Patients on insulin pump therapy
  - Need to assume line failure/blockage has interrupted insulin delivery. Give 20% of the patient's TDD as an s.c. injection of rapid-acting insulin. (This is a higher dose relative to the above patient group because there is no longer-acting insulin 'on board' in pump patients).
  - Once s.c. insulin has been given, ask the patient or family to resite the pump cannula and commence delivery at usual settings. Monitor BGL and ketones 1–2 hourly. For patients on pump therapy, ketones should clear to <0.6 mmol/L.

Diabetic ketoacidosis (DKA)

- Combination of hyperglycaemia, metabolic acidosis and ketonaemia.
- The biochemical criteria for DKA are:
  - Venous pH <7.3 or bicarbonate <15 mmol/L
  - Presence of blood or urinary ketones
- May be first presentation for a child with previously undiagnosed diabetes (>30% present in DKA at diagnosis) or precipitated by illness / poor compliance in established Type 1 diabetes.
- Rapid onset DKA more likely if poor underlying BGL control or on insulin pump.
- All patients with a BGL ≥11.1 mmol/L should have blood ketones tested on a capillary sample using a bedside OptiumTM meter.
  - If positive (ketones >0.6 mmol/L), assess for acidosis to determine further management (urinalysis can be used for initial ketones if blood ketone testing not available).

Causes

- Delayed diagnosis T1DM
- Omission of insulin in a patient with established diabetes
- Acute stress (infection, trauma, psychological)
- Poor management of intercurrent illness
- Mechanical factors obstructing insulin delivery by an insulin pump, (eg. line occlusion/failure)

Assessment of DKA

- Degree of dehydration (often overestimated)
  - None/mild (<4%): no clinical signs
  - Moderate (4–7%): easily detectable clinical signs of dehydration (eg. reduced skin turgor, poor capillary return)
  - Severe (>7%): poor perfusion, rapid pulse, hypotension, shock
- Level of consciousness – (Glasgow Coma Scale / AVPU)
- Investigations – Take venous blood sample & place IV line
  - FBC
  - BGL, UEC, CMP
  - Blood ketones (bedside test)
  - Venous blood gas (including HCO3)
  - Investigations for precipitating cause: if clinical signs of infection consider septic workup
  - For all newly diagnosed patients: insulin antibodies, GAD antibodies, coeliac screen (total IgA, anti-gliadin Ab, tissue transglutaminase Ab) and TFT's (TSH & FT_4)
- Urine:
  - Ketones (if capillary testing not available)
  - Culture (if clinical evidence of infection)
- Calculate:
  - Serum Osmolality = 2 x (serum Na^+ + serum K^+) + glucose + urea
  - Corrected serum Na^+ = [plasma Na^+ + 0.3 (plasma glucose − 5.5)]

Management of DKA

Fluids

Initial fluid requirements

- Not all patients in DKA require fluid boluses; remember, acidosis itself results in poor peripheral perfusion and confounds accurate assessment of dehydration.

- If hypoperfusion is present:
  - Give 10mL/kg 0.9% saline stat.
  - Repeat until perfusion re-established (warm, pink extremities with rapid capillary refill).
- Commence rehydration with 0.9% saline and potassium at rates determined by weight and degree of dehydration (Table 19.1).
- Keep nil by mouth (except ice to suck) until alert and stable.
- Insert a nasogastric tube & leave on free drainage if patient is comatose or has recurrent vomiting.

Subsequent fluid adjustments:
- Fluid replacement with 0.9% saline and potassium should continue for at least the first 6 hours.
- If the BGL falls very rapidly or reaches 12–15 mmol/L, change to 0.9% saline with 5% dextrose and potassium.
- Choice of fluid after the initial 6 hours will be influenced by the corrected serum sodium (see above for calculation) and the BGL; corrected sodium should remain stable or rise as BGL falls.
- Fluids with a tonicity of <0.45% saline should not be used.
  If a hypotonic solution is thought to be required this should be discussed with a paediatric endocrinologist.
- Aim to keep the BGL between 6 and 12 mmol/L.
- If the patient is still acidotic, and the BGL is <5.5 mmol/L or is falling rapidly within the range of 5.5–15 mmol/L, increase the dextrose concentration in the fluid to 10%.
  The insulin infusion rate should only be turned down if BGL continues to fall despite use of 10% dextrose. In such patients, reducing the rate of insulin to 0.05 unit/kg/h may be required, provided that metabolic acidosis continues to improve. In this circumstance please discuss with a paediatric endocrinologist.
- If the patient becomes hypoglycaemic, manage as per hypoglycaemia section below.
- Rehydration may be completed orally after the first 24–36 hours if the patient is metabolically stable, which usually coincides with insulin therapy being switched to s.c. injections.

Insulin
- Commence after initial fluid resuscitation.
- Add 50 units of clear/rapid-acting insulin (Actrapid or Humulin R) to 49.5 mL 0.9% saline (1 unit/mL solution).
- Ensure that the insulin is clearly labelled.
- Start insulin infusion rate at:
  - 0.1 unit/kg/h in newly diagnosed children, or those with established diabetes who have BGL >15 mmol/L.
  - 0.05 unit/kg/h for children with established diabetes who have had their usual insulin and whose BGL is <15 mmol/L, and should also be considered in young children or during inter-hospital transfer (accompanied by a doctor) when biochemical monitoring is more limited.
- Adequate insulin must be continued to clear ketones and correct acidosis.
- Insulin infusion can be discontinued when the child is alert and metabolically stable (pH >7.30 and HCO_3 >15 mmol/L). The best time to change to s.c. insulin is just before meal time.
- The insulin infusion should only be stopped 30 minutes after the first s.c. injection of insulin.

Potassium
- Potassium replacement therapy is required for treatment of DKA because a total body deficit of potassium occurs in DKA and correction of the acidosis in the absence of potassium therapy will usually rapidly result in hypokalaemia.
- Patients may have hyperkalaemia, hypokalaemia or normokalaemia at presentation, depending on the total body potassium deficit and degree of acidosis.

Management:
- Defer initial potassium replacement if serum K^+ is >5.5 mmol/L or the patient is anuric.
- Start potassium replacement if/once K^+ is <5.5 mmol/L and urine output documented.
- Start KCl at a concentration of 40 mmol/L if body weight <30 kg, or 60 mmol/L if ≥30 kg; subsequent replacement is based on serum potassium levels.
- Measure levels 1 hour after starting therapy and 2–4 hourly thereafter.
- Potassium replacement should continue throughout IV fluid rehydration and insulin infusion therapy period.

Table 19.1 Diabetic ketoacidosis rehydration fluid rates (mL/h), which include deficit and maintenance fluid requirements, to be given evenly over 48 hours.

Weight (kg)	Mild/nil dehydration	Moderate Dehydration	Severe Dehydration
5	24	27	31
7	33	38	43
8	38	43	50
10	48	54	62
12	53	60	70
14	60	65	80
16	65	75	85
18	70	80	95
20	75	85	105
22	80	90	110
24	80	95	115
26	85	100	120
28	85	105	125
30	90	110	135
32	90	110	140
34	95	115	145
36	100	120	150
38	100	125	155
40	105	130	160
42	105	135	170
44	110	135	175
46	115	140	180
48	115	145	185
50	120	150	190
52	120	155	195
54	125	160	205
56	125	160	210
58	130	165	215
60	133	171	220
62	136	175	226
64	139	179	232
66	140	185	240
68	145	185	245
70	150	190	250

Note: Fluids given as a bolus should be deducted from the ongoing rates.

Sodium

- Measured serum sodium is depressed by the dilutional effect of hyperglycaemia. To "correct" sodium concentration use the formula for corrected Na$^+$ above.
- Beware of falling adjusted sodium levels as glucose declines – hyponatraemia may herald cerebral oedema. If the sodium level falls, consider decreasing the rate of fluid administration to replace over 72–96 hours; see hypernatraemia section below.

Ongoing monitoring and management
Clinical
- Strict fluid balance
- Hourly observations: HR, BP, RR, and neurological observations
- 2–4 hourly temperature
Note: Any headache or altered behaviour may indicate impending cerebral oedema.
Biochemical
- Hourly capillary BGL and ketones (bedside meter) while on insulin infusion.
- Venous blood gas and laboratory BGLs, serum corrected sodium, potassium, chloride performed 2 hourly for the first 6 hours and 2–4 hourly thereafter. More frequent (hourly) measurements may be necessary if severe acidosis or as clinically indicated.

Bicarbonate

- Bicarbonate administration is <u>not</u> routinely recommended in DKA as it may cause paradoxical CNS acidosis.
- Continuing acidosis indicates insufficient fluid and insulin replacement – liaise with paediatric endocrinologist and/or paediatric intensive care unit in this circumstance.

Other considerations:

- Paediatric intensive care admission required if:
  - Age <2y
  - Cardiovascular compromise
  - Coma
  - Seizures
- Patient should remain nil orally until alert and stable.
- Nurse the patient in a head up position and in good light.

Complications of DKA
Hypernatraemia

- If Na$^+$ is >160 mmol/L, discuss with a specialist.
- Na$^+$ should rise as the glucose falls during treatment; if this does not happen or if **hyponatraemia** develops *it usually indicates overzealous volume correction and insufficient electrolyte replacement*, that may place the patient at risk of cerebral oedema (see below).

Hypoglycaemia

- If BGL falls below 4.0 mmol/L and patient still acidotic, give IV 10% dextrose 2–5 mL/kg as a bolus and use a 10% dextrose concentration for ongoing IV fluids (with 0.45% NaCl and K$^+$ supplements). Do not discontinue the insulin infusion.
- If hypoglycaemia occurred despite use of 10% dextrose in the preceding 2 or more hours, the rate of the insulin infusion may be decreased to 0.05 unit/kg/h as long as ketosis and acidosis are clearing. Continue with a 10% dextrose concentration in IV fluids until BGL stable.
- If BGL falls below 4.0 mmol/L and most recent pH is >7.30, oral treatment for hypoglycaemia (4–5 jelly beans followed by 15 g of complex carbohydrate) can be used instead of an IV bolus of dextrose 10%.

Hypokalaemia

- Monitor frequently and adjust the potassium concentration in the infusate.
- Children at highest risk are those with severe acidosis or low potassium levels at presentation.

Cerebral oedema
- This is an uncommon (0.5–3.0%) but extremely serious complication of DKA in children.
- Usually occurs 6–12 hours after commencement of therapy.
- *Mortality or severe morbidity is very high without early treatment.*

Prevention
- Slow & judicious correction of fluid and biochemical abnormalities.
- Optimally, the rate of fall of blood glucose and serum osmolality should not exceed 5 mmol/L/h, but in children there is often a quicker initial fall in glucose.
- Patients should be nursed head up.

Risk factors
- Newly diagnosed diabetes
- Young age (<5 y)
- Poorly controlled diabetes
- Excessive fluid rehydration, particularly with hypotonic fluids
- Severe initial acidosis
- Hyponatraemia or hypernatraemia and negative sodium trend during DKA treatment.

Clinical presentation
- Early: negative sodium trend, headache, behaviour change (sudden irritability, depression of conscious state), thermal instability and incontinence
- Late: bradycardia, elevated blood pressure and depressed respiration

Treatment
Cerebral oedema is a medical emergency.
- Administer 0.5 g/kg (2.5 mL/kg) of 20% mannitol IV as a bolus dose (range 0.25–1.0 g/kg). This can be repeated if the response is inadequate.
- Nurse the patient in a head up position, maintain the airway.
- Restrict fluids by reducing current fluid infusion rate by one third in the first instance and seek urgent intensivist support/advice.
- Transfer to an intensive care unit for further management.
- **Do not delay treatment for radiological confirmation – cerebral oedema is a clinical diagnosis.**

Hypoglycaemia in children with diabetes
Common causes
- Missed meal/snack
- Vigorous exercise (can be during exercise or hours afterwards)
- Alcohol
- Too much insulin

Management
See Table 19.2.

Sick day management (intercurrent illness) in the child with diabetes
Principles
- Frequent testing of blood glucose and ketones.
- The meal plan may temporarily be dropped – replace with fluids and easily digested carbohydrates.
- Ensure good fluid intake – alternate sugar and non-sugar-containing fluids depending on blood sugar levels (water is best if high).
- Insulin doses usually need to be increased, although additional doses of insulin may be needed if ketones are present. Never omit insulin.
- Keep in touch with diabetes team.

Testing ketones
- Blood ketone testing gives a more accurate picture of current ketone levels and is recommended for monitoring during sick days.

Table 19.2 Management of hypoglycaemia in children with diabetes.

Awake	• ~15 g of fast-acting carbohydrate e.g. 150–200 mL lemonade; 4–5 jelly beans; honey (1tbs); condensed milk in tube • Repeat in 10–15 minutes if no improvement • Follow with 'sustaining serve' ~15 g of complex carbohydrate, eg. bread, milk[a] ○ If awake and alert but unable to eat (e.g. vomiting due to viral illness), mini-dose glucagon rescue may be appropriate[b]
Drowsy / uncooperative / unconscious / fitting (at home)	○ Glucagon IM injection: 0.5 mg if <15 kg or <6y 1 mg (1 ampoule) if >15 kg or >6y ○ Blood glucose should rise in 5–10 minutes. Give sips of sugar-containing fluid when awake; contact diabetes team for advice
Uncooperative / unconscious / fitting (in hospital)	○ 10% dextrose 2–5 mL/kg IV over 2 minutes, then infuse 3–5 mg/kg/min until awake and able to eat/drink

[a]Sustaining serve not needed in patients using pump therapy.
[b]Mini-glucagon rescue is used when vomiting is associated with hypoglycaemia or for persistently low blood glucose levels resistant to oral therapy. The doses vary with age: ≤2 years 0.02 mg; 2–15 years 0.01 mg per year of age; >15 years 0.15 mg. These doses are given subcutaneously using an insulin syringe (0.01 mg of reconstituted glucagon = 1 'unit' on insulin syringe).
BGL should be checked 20–30 minutes later; if BGL is <5.5 mol/L, repeat mini-dose glucagon giving double the original dose.

Table 19.3 Sick day (intercurrent illness) diabetes management.

Blood glucose Blood ketones Urine ketones Vomiting	High 0.6–1.0 mmol/L 0–trace ±	High >1.0 mmol/L[a] >1+ none or occasional[b]	Normal/low <1.0 mmol/L 0–trace ±
Potential danger	Progress to DKA	DKA	Hypoglycaemia
Insulin	Increase normal dose by ~10% at next injection	Give rapid acting insulin at 10–20% total daily dose[c] Repeat 2–4 hourly if ketones persist	Reduce normal insulin by 10–25% in first instance
Monitor BGL and ketones	2–4 hourly	1–2 hourly until ketones clear	2–4 hourly
Further action	If ketones increasing, escalate care (see right)	If not improving admit	If BGL low, manage as hypoglycaemia If BGL high de-escalate care (see left)

Notes:
[a]A threshold of 0.6 mmol/L is used for those on insulin pump therapy (as ketosis develops more rapidly).
[b]If hyperglycaemic and ketotic with vomiting on >1 occasion, may require emergency department assessment (may be in DKA).
[c]Hyperglycaemia + blood ketone level >1.5 mmol/L likely to need 20% of total daily dose as extra rapid-acting insulin.

• Urinary ketone strips are cheaper and are adequate to use as an initial screen to check whether ketosis is present. If urinary ketones are present (1+ or more), blood ketone testing is advised for further monitoring.
• A 'normal' blood ketone level is 0–0.6 mmol/L.
• For children on injected insulin regimens, a level 0.6–1.0 mmol/L can generally be managed with additional insulin at the next dose. If ketones are >1.0 mmol/L, an additional injection of rapid acting insulin may be warranted (Table 19.3).

- For children using insulin pump therapy, ketosis may develop more quickly as there is no longer-acting insulin circulating. A blood ketone level of >0.6 mmol/L requires extra insulin.
  - If blood ketones 0.6–1.0 mmol/L, an insulin bolus is given through the pump: add 50% to the correction dose calculated by the pump.
  - If blood ketones are >1.0 mmol/L, the patient should assume a line failure/blockage and give rapid-acting insulin by a subcutaneous injection (20% of usual TDD). They should then resite their insulin pump cannula and recheck BGL and ketones in 1–2 hours.

Management of children with diabetes undergoing surgery or a procedure that requires fasting

The main aims are to prevent hypoglycaemia before, during and after surgery and to provide sufficient insulin to prevent the development of ketoacidosis. Factors that must be considered are:

- Time, duration and type of surgery
- Current insulin regimen
- Urgency of surgery; elective vs emergency
- Please refer to: https://www.rch.org.au/clinicalguide/guideline_index/Diabetes_mellitus_and_surgery/

Continuous subcutaneous insulin infusion use in children and adolescents

- Continuous subcutaneous insulin infusion (CSII), or insulin pump therapy, is increasingly used in the treatment of T1DM in children and adolescents.
- It relies on the continuous delivery of rapid-acting insulin into the subcutaneous tissues by an insulin pump, which is commonly worn on the belt/waistband or carried in a pocket.
- The insulin pump is connected to a subcutaneous cannula; the subcutaneous cannula is re-sited, and the pump reloaded with insulin every 3 days.
- Insulin pumps can be disconnected for 1–2 hours at a time for bathing, swimming or contact sports.
- CSII can either be used in isolation or in combination with continuous glucose monitoring systems (sensor-augmented pump therapy).
- The principle of sensor-augmented therapy is insulin delivery being driven in part by intercurrent glucose readings with insulin delivery increasing with increasing glucose levels and vice versa. Various sensor-augmented pump options are available with increasing degrees of pump autonomy/automation.

Indications

- CSII can be used at any age but in preschool and young children it requires adult supervision of the numerical data entered into the pump.
- Although it offers benefits in terms of reduction of hypoglycaemia, improved glycaemic stability and improved quality of life, it is not suitable for all patients.
- At a minimum, patients must do 4–6 finger-prick BGL's per day (or 3 per day if on a sensor-augmented pump), be able to carbohydrate count accurately and be cognitively able to cope with the challenges of operating the insulin pump.

Calculating dose

Insulin is delivered via the pump in two ways:

- A continuous background delivery; *basal delivery* which is preprogrammed for a given patient and delivered automatically.
- An intermittent meal or correction-based insulin delivery; *bolus delivery)* which is manually undertaken by the patient at the time of meals or when BGLs are to be corrected. Omission of bolus doses of insulin at meals or snacks will result in hyperglycaemia as there is no long-acting insulin to 'cover' food.
- Recurrent missed boluses or infrequent BGL testing are common reasons for failure to achieve good glucose control on CSII. Initial TDD calculation at commencement of CSII is derived from pre-existing insulin requirements or based on weight.
- 40–50% of the TDD is given as basal insulin and the remainder given as bolus insulin.
- In fully sensor augmented pump therapy, pump settings may be limited to just active insulin time and a carbohydrate ratio. The other dynamics affecting insulin delivery are all pre-set factory settings and not adjustable.

Table 19.4 Complications of CSII (insulin pump) use.

Complication	Causes	Management
Hyperglycaemia ±Ketosis ±Diabetic ketoacidosis	When insulin delivery is disrupted or when requirement increases, ketosis ensues within 2–3 hours; • Cannula dislodgement • Tube kinks • Pump malfunction • Infected insertion site • Intercurrent illness	All patients receiving CSII therapy should also carry a back-up insulin pen containing rapid-acting insulin. **Hyperglycaemia only:** • Give correction bolus using pump. • Recheck blood glucose in 1–2 hours. **Hyperglycaemia & ketones ≥0.6 mmol/L:** • Disconnect pump & give injection of rapid acting insulin (1/6 of usual pump TDD) using insulin pen. • Insert a new pump cannula. • Check BGL and ketones 1–2 hourly. **Hyperglycaemia, ketones ≥0.6 mmol/L & vomiting/abdo pain or otherwise unwell:** • Present to ED for assessment of DKA. • If >1h from hospital, can give NovoRapid injection as above (1/6 TDD) at home
Hypoglycaemia	• Excessive basal rate • Excessive bolus insulin • Increased physical activity	**Mild symptomatic hypoglycaemia:** • Give one serve (15g) of rapid acting carbohydrate **Severe hypoglycaemia:** • Give glucagon injection IM & call diabetes team; pump may be temporarily disconnected (e.g. for 20 minutes).

Complications
DKA is the most concerning acute complication of CSII use (Table 19.4). These patients are at higher risk of DKA because they do not use any long- or intermediate-acting insulin.

Hypoglycaemia
• The maintenance of a normal plasma glucose concentration depends upon:
  ○ A functional endocrine system.
  ○ Intact enzymatic function for glycogen synthesis, glycogenolysis, glycolysis, gluconeogenesis, and utilization of other metabolic fuels for oxidation and storage.
  ○ Adequate substrates.
• Clinical hypoglycaemia is defined as a blood glucose reading (BGL) low enough to cause symptoms and/or signs of impaired neurocognitive function.
• Generally accepted as a BGL <2.6–2.8mmol/l on a laboratory sample, and occurs when the normal physiological counter-regulatory responses to a falling blood sugar level are inadequate or impaired (Figure 19.1).
• Prolonged or recurrent hypoglycaemia can cause long term neurological damage or death, thus prompt recognition and treatment are essential.
• Hypoglycaemia in the context of T1DM is discussed in the previous section.

Symptoms: occur through autonomic or neuroglycopaenic pathways
• Autonomic symptoms (sympathetic activation) include tachycardia, anxiety, tremors, sweating, nausea/vomiting, and hypothermia.
• Neuroglycopaenic symptoms (decreased glucose availability to CNS) include lethargy, and motor/ sensory/ visual disturbance.
• Symptoms can be affected by clinical status, age, gender, and medication use.
• Blunting of counter-regulatory responses may occur with chronic hypoglycemia.

Neonatal Hypoglycaemia
See also Chapter 27, Neonatal medicine.

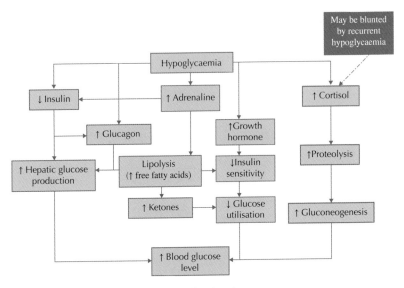

Figure 19.1 Physiological counter-regulatory responses to hypoglycaemia.

Clinical presentation
- Asymptomatic (most): detection is based on surveillance of at-risk infants.
- Mild/moderate: irritability, jitteriness, tremors, hypotonia, lethargy, temperature instability, high-pitched cry, tachypnoea, tachycardia, diaphoresis, poor feeding, vomiting.
- Severe: Eye-rolling, seizures – focal/generalised, hypoventilation, apnoea, cyanosis, pallor.
- Risk factors include:
  - Maternal factors: maternal diabetes, medication use (including beta blockers).
  - Iatrogenic: insufficient enteral / intravenous nutrition.
  - Perinatal factors: preterm birth, respiratory distress, hypoxic-ischaemic events.
    - Infant factors: Macrosomia, IUGR, sepsis, hypothermia, inborn errors of metabolism, hyperinsulinism (HI, transient or persistent), Beckwith-Wiedemann syndrome, congenital hypopituitarism, congenital adrenal hyperplasia.

Investigations
- Mild isolated episode of hypoglycaemia: should be treated and monitored with further investigation usually not required.
- Recurrent or refractory hypoglycaemia:
- **First line investigations ('critical screen'):** must be taken at time of hypoglycemia <2.6, prior to treatment
  - Bedside ketones
  - Glucose
  - Capillary/venous/arterial blood gas
  - Lactate, ketones (Beta hydroxybutyrate), free fatty acids, cortisol, insulin, growth hormone, UEC, LFT
- Further investigations if clinically indicated: C-peptide, ammonia, carnitine / acylcarnitine, amino acids, TSH/T4, LH/FSH, testosterone/oestradiol, 17-hydroxyprogesterone.
  All tests must go immediately to the laboratory on an ice pillow.

Management
- Glucose replacement may be enteral (enteral feed, Sucrose 33%) or intravenous (2–5ml/kg 10% dextrose bolus).
- For an isolated episode no further management required other than regular monitoring.

- Refractory or recurrent hypoglycaemia will require delivery of continuous enteral feeds, a 10% dextrose infusion and input from the Endocrinology +/- Metabolic teams.

Congenital Hyperinsulinism (CHI)

- Most frequent cause of severe, persistent hypoglycaemia in newborn babies.
- Pancreatic insulin secretion occurs autonomously and independent of BGL, such that hypoglycaemia can occur at any time (particularly when fasting) resulting in frequent, random episodes.
- Aim of management is to maintain BGL >3.5mmol/l to prevent short and long term morbidity.
- Can be transient or permanent, depending on aetiology (Table 19.5).

Work-up
Confirm diagnosis:
- Any infant with a glucose utilisation rate (GUR) >10mg/kg/minute should be investigated for HI; normal GUR is 4–8mg/kg/minute.
- Elevated insulin levels at the time of hypoglycaemia and the absence of ketones/free fatty acids are suggestive of hyperinsulinism. Conversely, the presence of ketones essentially excludes the diagnosis.
- A rise in BGL post glucagon administration at the time of hypoglycaemia is a sensitive marker for hyperinsulinism.
- A prolonged fasting study is sometimes required to provoke hypoglycaemia and confirm the diagnosis of HI.
- Specific gene testing: for causative mutations and/or to differentiate diffuse vs focal KATP-HI (see below).
- Imaging: The 6-[18F]-L-fluoro-L-3, 4-dihydroxyphenylalanine (F-DOPA) PET Scan is the most effective way to identify focal lesions.

Clinical Pearl: Hyperinsulinism diagnosis
Elevated insulin levels with hypoglycaemia and without ketones/free fatty acids are highly suggestive of hyperinsulinism. Conversely, the presence of ketones essentially excludes the diagnosis.

Latest / New Evidence: Focal vs diffuse KATP-HI
With the recent discovery of diffuse and focal KATP-HI, attempts to differentiate these two forms are clinically very significant. Surgical therapy can potentially cure focal K ATP-HI but not the diffuse form.

Management
Immediate management
- Mild: Enteral administration of fast-acting carbohydrate (fortified breast milk/formula if neonate).
- Severe:
  ○ Glucose IV 2–5ml/kg 10% dextrose bolus
  ○ Glucagon IM / IV/ subcutaneous (stimulates hepatic glucose release)

Table 19.5 Causes of Congenital Hyperinsulinism.

CHI type	Causes
Transient (days-months)	Small for gestational age neonate Premature neonate Foetal distress Neonatal surgery
Permanent	Potassium-ATP channel defects (KATP) Glutamate dehydrogenase mutations (GDH-HI) Glucokinase mutations (GCK) Short chain 3-hydroxacyl-CoA dehydrogenase mutations (SCHAD) Exercise induced hyperinsulinism Post-gastrointestinal surgery

Ongoing management for persistent and recurrent hypoglycaemia
Medical:
- Diazoxide: acts on the KATP channel to prevent insulin secretion.
  Dose: oral 5 to 20mg/kg/day p.o.
- Octreotide (somatostatin analogue): inhibits insulin secretion.
  Dose: subcutaneous frequent injection / infusion pump / monthly long acting.
  *note risk of necrotizing enterocolitis (NEC) in neonates.
- Nifedipine, Sirolimus, Glucagon-like peptide 1 (GLP-1) receptor antagonists have all been used with somewhat limited efficacy.

Surgical:
- Focal disease: In children with focal KATP channel HI, partial pancreatectomy is the procedure of choice.
- Diffuse disease: Children with diffuse disease may require a subtotal (95–99%) pancreatectomy (+- additional resections).

Hypoglycaemia beyond the neonatal period
- Any infant or child with first unexplained presentation, recurrent, or severe hypoglycaemia should be further investigated.
- Additional differential diagnoses to consider outside the neonatal period include:
  - Childhood: accelerated starvation ('ketotic hypoglycaemia'), hypopituitarism, altered metabolism (e.g. 6-mercaptupurine), adrenal insufficiency.
  - Adolescence: Insulinoma, adrenal insufficiency.

Accelerated starvation
- Accelerated starvation (previously "ketotic hypoglycaemia"): is the most common cause of hypoglycaemia beyond infancy, usually presenting between 18m and 5y age.
- Mechanism of hypoglycaemia not well understood; inappropriate gluconeogenesis in response to low BGL has been postulated.

Clinical presentation
- Occurs after a prolonged fast and is usually precipitated by a relatively mild vomiting illness.
- Most affected children have a slender build without malnutrition.
- Neuroglycopaenic symptoms: lethargy and malaise, unresponsiveness or seizures.
- Ketosis symptoms: anorexia, abdominal discomfort, nausea, vomiting.

Investigations and Diagnosis
- Diagnosis requires documenting a low blood glucose level in association with ketonuria and/or ketonaemia, but definitive diagnosis requires exclusion of other metabolic and endocrine causes.
- Biochemical findings include:
  - Elevated free fatty acids and ketones
  - Appropriately low/undetectable insulin levels
  - Appropriate cortisol and GH
  - Negative response to glucagon stimulation testing during fasting hypoglycaemia
  - Normal TFT
  - Reassuring metabolic screening

Management and Prognosis
- First episode: stabilisation of BGL as above with/without a short-stay or overnight admission.
- Prevention of further episodes: prevent prolonged fasts, ensure adequate carbohydrate intake particularly prior to bed when the child is unwell.
- Recurrent or severe episodes: may require parental education on self-monitoring BGL's after discussion with the Endocrinology team and exclusion of potential differential diagnoses.
- Families may be reassured that this is a self-limiting condition which will resolve over time; episodes of hypoglycaemia associated with accelerated starvation improve with age and the condition is rare in the second decade of life.

> **Clinical Pearl: Accelerated starvation (previously 'ketotic hypoglycemia')**
> Whilst a clinical diagnosis requires documenting a low BGL in association with ketonuria and/or ketonaemia, a true definitive diagnosis of this common condition requires the exclusion of other metabolic and endocrine causes of hypoglycemia.

Adrenal hypofunction causing hypoglyaemia
See Adrenal insufficiency section

Hypothyroidism
Congenital hypothyroidism
- 1 in 3–5000 births.

Causes
- Dysgenesis (absent or ectopic thyroid gland) – 75–85%
- Dyshormonogenesis (abnormal function) – 10–15%
- Transient (e.g. iodine exposure, maternal anti-thyroid antibodies) – 10%
- Central (pituitary, hypothalamic) – 5%

Clinical features
- Often asymptomatic at birth (protected by maternal thyroid hormone or some functioning thyroid tissue present)
- Lethargy with poor feeding
- Prolonged jaundice
- Constipation
- Large anterior fontanelle, persistent posterior fontanelle
- Coarse features
- Macroglassia
- Dry skin
- Umbilical hernia
- Harsh or hoarse cry
- Unossified distal femoral epiphysis

Investigations
- High TSH on newborn screening test (see also chapter 26 Metabolic medicine)
  Note: congenital hypothyroidism secondary to pituitary dysfunction / central cause will not be identified by TSH newborn screening.
- Confirmation of the diagnosis on whole blood TFTs is essential.
- Sodium pertechnetate technetium (Tc^{99}) scanning for position, function, size (presence of goitre, Tc^{99} uptake).
- Consider genetic studies if familial or syndromic (Table 19.6).

Management
Initial management
- Thyroxine 10–15 mcg/kg/day: start before 2 weeks of age (ideally <10 days) for better neurodevelopmental outcome.
- Retest 2–3 weeks after commencing therapy, aiming for:
  - FT$_4$ at / just above upper limit of normal range for age
  - Normalisation of TSH

Subsequent management
- Clinical review and TFTs (Table 19.7), targeting normal TSH
- For those with transient congenital hypothyroidism, re-evaluation of thyroxine requirement can be considered after 2–3 years of age.

Table 19.6 Genetic forms of congenital hypothyroidism.

Gene	Protein	Inheritance	Phenotype
SLC26A4	Pendrin	AR	"Pendred syndrome" – Childhood-onset goitre, congenital bilateral sensorineural hearing loss
PAX8	Paired box gene	AD	Thyroid hypoplasia, urogenital malformations
NKX2-1	Thyroid transcription factor 1	AD	Thyroid hypoplasia, benign hereditary chorea, lung abnormalities – "brain, thyroid, lung"
FOXE1	Thyroid transcription factor 2	AR	Athyreosis, cleft palate, choanal atresia, spiky hair – "Bamforth-Lazarus syndrome"
SLC5A5	NIS	AR	Goiter, low/absent radioiodine uptake
TSHR	TSH receptor	AR/AD	Variable resistance to TSH, normal thyroid to severe thyroid gland hypoplasia

Notes: AR = Autosomal recessive, AD = Autosomal dominant, NIS = Sodium iodide symporter

Table 19.7 Suggested frequency of clinical review and TFT's for babies with congenital hypothyroidism.

Age	Frequency
1st year of life	1–3 monthly
1–3 years of life	2–4 monthly
>3 years of life	4–6 monthly

Acquired hypothyroidism

Prevalence: 1–2% between 1 and 18 years of age; 4:1 female predominance.

Causes

- Autoimmune hypothyroidism (Hashimoto thyroiditis).
- Late appearing congenital dyshormonogenesis.
- Exogenous causes (radiation, amiodarone, severe iodine deficiency, high dose iodine exposure e.g. from surgical skin preparation).
- Central (pituitary or hypothalamic) hypothyroidism.

Clinical features

Hypothyroidism is often very difficult to detect clinically in children. Growth retardation may be the only sign, often with a *relative excess weight for height*. Hypothyroidism is rarely the cause of weight gain alone. The classical signs are usually absent when the cause is central.

- Growth retardation
- Lethargy
- Cold intolerance
- Constipation
- Weight gain (excess weight gain is associated with mild TSH elevation; see below)
- Menstrual irregularities
- Precocious or delayed puberty
- Goitre
- Dry cool skin, dry hair, myxedema of face/extremities
- Prolonged ankle-jerk relaxation time

> **Clinical Pearl: TSH elevation secondary to weight gain**
> Young people who have excess weight gain may also be noted to have a mild TSH elevation of between 5-10mIU/L, which is likely *secondary* to the weight gain, not the cause. It often normalises with weight loss.

Investigations
- FT_4 and TSH
- Thyroid autoantibodies (thyroid peroxidase, thyroglobulin)
- Technetium thyroid scan (if dyshormonogenesis suspected)
- Thyroid ultrasound where indicated (for assessment of gland structure)

Management
- Specialist management is required to ensure maintenance of biochemical euthyroidism and normal linear growth and development.
- Start thyroxine therapy (~100 $\mu g/m^2$/day) depending on degree of hypothyroidism and age (Table 19.8). Commence thyroxine at a low dose with slow titration if correcting prolonged profoundly hypothyroid patients to avoid precipitating cardiac complications.
- Recheck TFT's 6 weeks after commencing therapy and after each dose change.

Table 19.8 Thyroxine dose guide based on age.

Age (years)	Thyroxine dose ($\mu g/kg/day$)
1–3	4–6
3–10	3–5
10–16	2–4
>17	1.6

Hyperthyroidism
- Whilst hyperthyroidism can present in the neonatal period due to maternal Graves' disease it is almost always an event acquired later in life.
- Incidence: 0.1 to 3 cases per 100 000 children; 6:1 Female predominance.

Causes
- Autoimmune hyperthyroidism (Graves' disease, rarely a transient "toxic" phase of Hashimoto thyroiditis).
- Autonomously functioning thyroid nodule (i.e. "toxic" nodule).
- Genetic (e.g. TSHR mutation, McCune Albright syndrome).
- Infections (suppurative thyroiditis, subacute viral thyroiditis).
- Factitious (e.g. thyroxine consumption for weight loss).

Clinical features
- Diffuse goitre with bruit.
- Weight loss, heat intolerance, tiredness.
- Irritability and restlessness, behaviour issues, deterioration in academic performance.
- Menstrual irregularities.
- Warm sweaty hands, tremor, tachycardia, hypertension.
- Proximal muscle weakness and wasting.
- Accelerated ankle-jerk relaxation time.
- Thyroid ophthalmopathy (30% of cases): lid lag, lid retraction, chemosis, exophthalmos, ophthalmoplegia.
- Accelerated growth velocity.

Investigations
- FT_4, FT_3, TSH (low to undetectable).
- TSH receptor antibodies (or thyroid stimulating immunoglobulin).
- Thyroid peroxidase and thyroglobulin antibodies (can indicate toxic phase of Hashimoto's thyroiditis if TSH receptor antibodies negative).
- Bone age (usually advanced).
- Technetium thyroid scan – (if suspecting autonomous nodules; expect diffuse increased uptake in Grave's, variable uptake in Hashimoto's).
- Thyroid ultrasound only if thyroid nodule suspected.

Management
- Anti-thyroid drugs are used for long-term treatment of autoimmune hyperthyroidism in childhood and adolescence. Propylthiouracil is no longer used in childhood due to increased risk of drug-induced fulminant hepatic necrosis.
- The long-term remission rate in this age group is 35%. Management by a specialist is necessary.

Antithyroid drugs
- Carbimazole:
  - Dose: 0.2–0.5 mg/kg oral 8–12 hourly (up to 1 mg/kg/day or 30–60 mg/day depending on age, size) for 2 weeks.
  - Recheck TFTs 2–3 weeks after commencing therapy.
  - Continue at least 18–24 months.
  - If remission occurs; is usually after 24 months.
  - Warn patients regarding side effects: rash (e.g. urticaria) up to 20%, bone marrow suppression (agranulocytosis) & liver toxicity in <1% of patients (most common with high doses early in treatment).
- Consider cardioselective beta blockers (e.g. propranolol 0.5–1mg/kg/day q6–12H) if cardiac compromise suspected until symptoms resolve and/or TFT normalises. This is contraindicated in children with asthma.

Definitive therapy
- The aim of definitive therapy is to achieve permanent hypothyroidism using radioiodine ablation or total thyroidectomy, as thyroxine therapy is low risk and requires less frequent monitoring.
- Consider definitive therapy in those who:
  - Fail to achieve biochemical remission 3–5 years after initiation of antithyroid therapy.
  - Suffer from recalcitrant side effects of therapy.
  - Non-compliant with antithyroid therapy.

Adrenal hypofunction
Primary adrenal insufficiency
This is rare in childhood and adolescence, but should be considered in the presence of unexplained:
- Vomiting
- Weight loss
- Increasing pigmentation
- Chronic tiredness
- Low serum sodium
- High serum potassium

Autoimmune destruction (Addison disease)
- Autoimmunity is the most common cause of primary adrenal insufficiency in the developed world.
- This may present as part of the autoimmune polyglandular syndrome (APS 1/2) although it often can be the sole manifestation of the condition.
- APS 1 often presents as a triad; with history of mucocutaneous candidiasis, primary hypoparathyroidism and adrenal insufficiency (symptoms may appear at different time periods). It is due to variants of the AIRE gene (21q22). Ectodermal dystrophy and other auto-immune conditions may also be present.
- APS 2 is less well defined, with adrenal insufficiency associated with autoimmune thyroid disease, and/or other autoimmune conditions including T1DM / primary hypogonadism / myasthenia gravis / coeliac disease.

Infective
- Worldwide, the commonest cause of Adrenal insufficiency is TB, followed by HIV infection.

X-linked adrenoleukodystrophy
This rare condition manifests in boys from early childhood to late adolescence, and milder forms may not be detected until adulthood.

Clinical features
- Hyperpigmentation of the skin (ACTH-mediated).
- Tiredness, nausea, anorexia and weight loss.
- Adrenal features are usually, but not always, preceded by the development of a neurological disability (e.g. memory loss, sleep disturbance or ataxia). The absence of a recognised neurological phenotype does not preclude ALD however and its exclusion in boys with primary adrenal insufficiency is mandatory.

Investigation and management
- Test blood and skin fibroblasts for very-long-chain fatty acids (VLCFAs).
- Management of adrenal insufficiency as per usual hormone replacement regimens (see below).
- Dietary modification targeting VLCFA has been used, with variable / limited success.
- Bone marrow transplantation may be helpful in cases when repeated MRI evaluation demonstrates very early changes of leukodystrophy.

Congenital adrenal hyperplasia
- Due to 21-hydroxylase deficiency (95% of all congenital adrenal hyperplasia (CAH))
- Other rarer types

Clinical features
- Newborns may present with either atypical genitalia in a female infant (due to virilisation from androgen excess) or in a salt losing crisis (more common in males as androgen excess not clinically obvious).
- Non salt losing forms may present in early-mid childhood with clitoromegaly in girls or increasing penile size in boys, and premature pubarche with rapid/escalating linear growth in both sexes. Bone age can be very advanced in non-salt losing boys with adverse effects of final height.
- Non-classical forms of CAH present later with a milder phenotype, usually with signs of androgen excess such as hirsutism, significant acne and menstrual irregularity.

Investigations
- Serum electrolytes (low sodium and high potassium).
- Simultaneous serum cortisol and plasma ACTH.
- Specific investigations if CAH is suspected: 17-OH progesterone, urine steroid profile. Tandem mass spectrometry is also used.

Management
- Hydrocortisone 10–14 mg/m2 BSA per day in divided doses.
- Fludrocortisone 0.05–0.2 mg daily, orally.
- Steroid cover for stress (see below).
- NaCl tablets are useful to reduce salt loss in hot weather.

'Secondary' adrenal insufficiency (due to ACTH deficiency)
Causes
Hypothalamic pituitary failure due to tumour, trauma, post surgery, cranial irradiation (where it may be subtle) or Langerhan's histiocytosis.

Clinical features
- Not usually associated with salt-wasting
- No hyperpigmentation of the skin

Management
- Treat with hydrocortisone alone; fludrocortisone is unnecessary.
- Prednisolone may be used after growth is complete.

Steroid cover for stress in all patients with Adrenal insufficiency

> **Clinical Pearl: Steroid stress dosing**
> All patients with adrenal insufficiency of any cause are at risk for adrenal crisis during periods of physiological stress. These patients require extra steroid cover during such periods to cover their endogenous deficiency.

- In cases of acute medical illness (e.g. gastroenteritis, influenza), any surgery requiring general anaesthetic and any major fracture:
  - Hydrocortisone 2–3 mg/kg (usually 25–100 mg) IM/IV stat.
  - Repeat every 4–6 hours until recovery.
  - Follow by triple the usual daily doses of hydrocortisone for 2 days, then double the usual dose for 3 days.

Adrenal hyperfunction
Adrenocortical tumours
- May manifest as Cushing syndrome, virilisation, hypertension, abdominal mass or pain.
- These tumours are rare; Cushing disease in infancy or early childhood is usually due to an adrenal tumour, compared to older children where a secondary cause is far more common.

Adrenocortical hyperplasia
- This is usually secondary to a pituitary adenoma secreting ACTH (Cushing disease). Such lesions are usually very small (2–3 mm).
- A primary bilateral micronodular form (genetic cause: Carney complex) is rarely seen. A macronodular form is seen in patients with McCune Albright syndrome.

Clinical features
- Cortisol excess is more difficult to detect clinically in children than in adults.
- Symptoms include poor growth velocity and excessive weight gain. The child usually looks obese, but the clinical features of moon face, thin limbs and striae may be absent.
- Hypertension is also frequently absent.

Investigation
- 24 hours urinary free cortisol. Plasma cortisol is often abnormal in obesity and may give a spurious result. Loss of diurnal variation of plasma cortisol may be helpful.
- Overnight dexamethasone suppression (1 mg dexamethasone given at 2400 hours and a plasma cortisol at 0800 hours the following day) will differentiate Cushing syndrome from obesity.
- Further investigation for origin and type of cortisol excess is by a specialist; and treatment is surgical.

Adrenal medullary tumours
- **Neuroblastoma** (see Chapter 30 Oncology) usually occurs in very young children, but may present in adolescence.
- **Phaeochromocytoma** occurs in older children and causes hypertension.
  - May be associated with various genetic conditions – multiple endocrine neoplasia (MEN), neurofibromatosis, von Hippel Lindau, SDH mutations.
- **Paraganglioma** is increasingly recognised – mass occurs in the adrenal gland or anywhere along the aortic chain, without hypertension (SDH mutation).

Hypopituitarism
Presentations of hypopituitarism in paediatrics:
- Congenital conditions
  - All anterior pituitary hormones are absent resulting in emergency presentation in the neonate with hypoglycaemia on day 1 (plus microphallus & undescended testes in a male); due to pituitary hypoplasia secondary to one of many genetic causes.
  - Isolated deficiencies of one or two hormones and/or later presentation with short stature or pubertal delay.

- Acquired hypopituitarism
Secondary to:
  - Trauma, often after a contra coup head injury
  - Midline tumour
  - Treatment with cranial radiation
  - Infiltrative process

Clinical Presentation
- Acute onset diabetes insipidus or insidious growth failure and progressive loss of pituitary hormones.

Diagnosis
- History as above.
- Examination for midline defects (hypertelorism, central clefts, cardiac anomalies, malrotation of gut, micropenis).
- Growth chart showing deteriorating growth velocity.

Clinical Pearl: Hypopituitarism
The absence of cortisol and thyroxine in hypopituitarism can prevent free water excretion and mask diabetes insipidus in some patients.

Initial Investigation
- Morning cortisol, IGF1, free T4 – (if TSH is absent central hypothyroidism will be missed unless T4 is checked).
- Diabetes insipidus investigation is described as prior
- Infants 2–20 weeks should have FSH, LH, oestrogen or testosterone (absence of a normal mini-puberty at that age is informative).

Clinical Pearl: Investigation of growth hormone
Basal growth hormone level is entirely without value. If needed a formal growth hormone test with glucagon stimulation is required.

Management
- Commence cortisol at stress dosing 30–50 mg/m2/day of hydrocortisone, followed by maintenance 5–7 mg/m2/day (half primary adrenal insufficiency doses)
- After 24–48 hours add thyroxine 8–10mg/m2/day
- Growth hormone indicated in the first year of life if persistent hypoglycaemia despite adequate cortisol replacement. Application to national health department required & specialist input advised.
- Micropenis can be treated with 2–3 doses of testosterone ester, 3 weeks apart, each of 25mg. Alternative treatment with FSH and hCG very effective (requires specialist input).

Clinical Pearl: Panhypopituitarism hormone replacement
Cortisol should be commenced PRIOR to any other hormones. Failure to do so may result in collapse with adrenal insufficiency and shock.

Diabetes insipidus
- Central Diabetes insipidus (CDI) is an uncommon condition, where either relative or absolute lack of anti-diuretic hormone (ADH) leads to inability to concentrate urine.
- Increasing volume of free water is lost (polyuria), resulting in a clinical response of increased thirst (polydipsia). With uncontrolled loss of water, the serum becomes increasingly concentrated, manifested as a rising serum sodium and osmolality.
- Urinary loss of sodium is minimised, in order to try to conserve salt, so urine becomes dilute, with a low sodium level.
- When water losses exceed the capacity of the patient to replace them by increased intake, dehydration occurs.

Causes
- CDI must be distinguished from peripheral or renal DI, where the defect is solely in the ability of the kidney to concentrate urine, due to a lack of renal receptors for ADH.
- CDI occurring in children may be congenital (autosomal dominant inheritance).
  - This type usually does not manifest until age 15–18 months of age.
  - A family history is very important to suggest this diagnosis, confirmed by genetic analysis for the vasopressin gene.
- Acquired DI is never benign; all other causes indicate a severe problem, with an acute, radical change in fluid intake and associated polyuria.
  - Midline tumours, infiltrative or inflammatory conditions affecting the pituitary stalk or trauma, either via head injury or after neurosurgery are causative.

Clinical features
- When assessing a patient for possible CDI, the following features should be considered:
  - History of change in drinking habit, duration and volume of intake and output, where possible, together with evidence of fluid deficit – weight loss, dehydration.
  - History of familial CDI, trauma, symptoms to suggest intracranial lesion or surgery, renal disease or, in the young child, usually aged 2–4 years, a slow increase in oral intake over months, that might suggest a less serious problem of habit drinking.
  - Examination should confirm evidence to include hydration status, intercurrent illness such as urinary tract infection, plus any findings to indicate an underlying midline lesion.

Investigations
- Urea and electrolytes
  - Sodium is often elevated due to excess free water losses (only occurs once the patient is unable to keep up with losses by compensatory increase in water intake).
- Full ward test of urine to include specific gravity.
- Paired serum and urine osmolality and sodium level.
- Full pituitary function testing as indicated (remember that a lack of thyroxine or cortisol prevents free water clearance and will partially mask even severe DI).
- Formal water deprivation test requires inpatient admission, with hourly weighing, serum and urine osmolality, then challenge with desmopressin (DDAVP) at the end of the test.
  - Complete failure to respond to administered DDAVP may suggest a renal cause.
  - Habit drinking washes out renal receptors for vasopressin in a reversible fashion and thus may be difficult to distinguish from nephrogenic DI.

Clinical Pearl: Diabetes insipidus diagnosis

DI is likely when the serum osmolality is raised (>295 mOsmol/kg) with paired, inappropriately dilute urine (urine osmolality <700 mOsmol/kg); however very young children sometimes cannot concentrate urine above around 550mosol/kg.

If baseline tests are equivocal, the patient may require a formal water deprivation test to exclude DI. This should ONLY be performed as an inpatient in a controlled, well-monitored environment. Withholding fluids from a patient with DI can lead to rapid decompensation of fluid and electrolyte status; fluid restriction *should not* be commenced during nighttime hours for this reason.

Management
Rehydration
- Use the degree of dehydration and ongoing losses to calculate rehydration therapy.
- If the serum Na is >150 mmol/L, rehydration should occur over 48 hours (see chapter 7 Fluid and Electrolytes).
- If Na >170 mmol/L, contact the intensive care unit/specialist team. Excessively rapid rehydration can cause major fluid shifts, with changes in mentation.

Table 19.9 Formulation, dosage & administration of DDAVP.

DDAVP Formulation	Dosage	Practice Points
Intranasal Spray (10mcg/spray)	• <1y; d/w endocrinologist ~10% dose of older child • <2y; 2–5 mcg intranasal/d • ≥2y; 5–10 mcg intranasal/d (up to 30–40 mcg in some patients)	• Rapid onset & offset • Higher doses longer duration of action (NOT more efficacious)
Parenteral (IV/IM) (4 mcg/mL)	• 1mcg equivalent to 10mcg intranasal spray	• Short term post-operative (also infusion)
Oral (200 mcg / tablet)	• 200 mcg equivalent to 10 mcg intranasal	• Slow onset of action; (less suitable for initial DI control) • Most common long term therapy
Minirin wafer melts (60 or 120 mg)	• 120 mg equivalent to 10 mcg intranasal spray	

Initial administration practice points
- The following criteria should be met prior to dose administration:
  o Serum sodium is >145 mmol/L (reference range 135–145 mmol/L)
  o Urine output exceeds 4 mL/kg/h (calculated 6 hourly)
  o Urine specific gravity is 1.005 or less (dilute urine output)
- Careful fluid balance needs to be maintained to prevent fluid overload/hyponatraemia

Ongoing management principles
- Daily UEC, serum & urine osmolality until stable, and dosing regime established
- Once stable dosing regime, most patients do not require regular UEC testing

Desmopressin administration
- DDAVP (trade name: Minirin®) acts on the distal tubules and collecting ducts of the kidney, to increase water reabsorption. It is a long-acting analogue of ADH.
  o Discuss with an endocrinologist prior to commencement of DDAVP.
  o See Table 19.9 for dose & administration details.

Puberty: normal, delayed and precocious
Normal puberty
- On average puberty commences at around 10.5–11.5 years in girls, and 12.5–13 years in boys.
- The lower limit of normal pubertal onset is 8 years for girls, and 9 years for boys.
- The first sign of true puberty (gonadotropin-induced sex steroid production) is breast development in girls and testicular enlargement to ≥4 mL in boys.
  Adrenarche, a rise in adrenal DHEAS that normally precedes pubertal onset by about one year, results in pubic hair (pubarche) and is not a sign of true puberty.
- Accelerated growth begins at the onset of puberty in girls, and at mid-puberty in boys.
- Delayed puberty is equally common in both sexes but boys present for care more frequently.
- Precocious puberty is more common in girls (majority functional) than in boys (≥70% organic cause).

Delayed puberty
- Pubertal delay is defined as the absence of early pubertal changes:
  o By 13 years for girls
  o By 14.5 years for boys
- There is no absolute age for diagnosis of delayed puberty; later than average and inappropriately late compared with other family members are common red flags.

Causes
With normal or low serum gonadotropins (secondary hypogonadism)
- **Constitutional delay** (often familial) is the commonest cause. It is recognised with slow growth rate and delayed bone age in an otherwise completely healthy child.

- **Chronic illness/poor nutrition** (eg high cytokines: inflammatory bowel disease, JCA etc, coeliac disease, eating disorders, neuromuscular disorders/ cerebral palsy, chronic use of high dose glucocorticoid, cystic fibrosis).
- **Endocrine causes:**
  - ○ **Hypopituitarism;** may include growth hormone, TSH, ACTH deficiency plus central DI if there has been surgery, trauma, tumour, infiltration in the midline. Iron deposition with transfusion dependent conditions is commonly associated with hypogonadism.
  - ○ **Isolated gonadotropin deficiency** with or without with anosmia (including CHARGE syndrome and bilateral cleft lip/palate).
  - ○ **Hyperprolactinaemia:** structural with macro or micro-prolactinoma, or functional secondary to medication (e.g. antipsychotics)

With elevated serum gonadotropins (primary hypogonadism)

- **Gonadal dysgenesis:** including Turner, Klinefelter syndromes or more complex disorders of sex development, anorchia with prenatal testicular involution
- **Infiltration:** Galactosaemia, iron deposition (uncommon)
- **Gonadal Damage:** secondary to vascular injury, surgery, infection, radiation associated cancer treatment, chemotherapy alone in girls only

Assessment

- Detailed history to assess differential diagnosis.
- Auxology: height and weight, must be assessed in the context of expected family heights (eg. midparental height and target range).
- Growth velocity over as long a time period as is accessible– use maternal/child health record and any available measured heights and compare to siblings' growth rates.
- Pubertal stage – assessed using Tanner staging system and testicular volume in boys. Chest wall adiposity can mimic breast tissue in a prepubertal child and can be difficult to assess in an obese pubertal adolescent.

Investigations

- Bone age – may be the only test required if there is a family history of late puberty.
- Serum follicle-stimulating hormone (FSH), luteinising hormone (LH), testosterone or oestradiol, prolactin, IGF1. NB. basal growth hormone measurements are without any value – formal stimulation test is required for assessment (see Hypopituitarism section).
- FBE, ESR, CRP, ferritin
- Coeliac screen
- UEC, serum proteins
- TFT
- Karyotype for short girl and if suspicious for XXY or complex disorder in boys

Management

- Referral to a specialist is advised; a 'watch and wait' strategy may be reasonable in the first instance if the child is a <14.5y male or <13y female.
- If induction of puberty is thought desirable, an endocrinologist should be consulted. *Excess or early use of sex hormones for pubertal management will result in rapid advancement of bone age, epiphyseal fusion and stunting of final height in both sexes.*
- For girls, pubertal induction should use oral or transdermal oestrogen;
  - ○ Commence with low dose, increasing slowly over 2–3y to mimic normal pubertal progress, with addition of progestin at the end of that time.
- For boys;
  - ○ Primary hypogonadism; testosterone is commenced with incremental increases.
  - ○ Hypothalamic hypogonadism; may utilise hCG and FSH to achieve virilisation and maximise fertility (requires specialist management).
- Growth hormone therapy may also be offered to girls with Turner syndrome, if there is remaining growth potential on bone age assessment.

Precocious puberty

- Definition: precocious puberty is defined as the onset of pubertal changes;
  - <8y in girls
  - <9y in boys
- Prevalence: >10 times more common in girls than boys.
- Girls are less likely to have an underlying organic cause than boys.
- In girls, central puberty is accompanied by accelerated growth, breast and pubic hair development; breast development is usually seen first & vaginal bleeding may occur.
- In boys there is enlargement of both testes as well as accelerated linear and genital growth.

Causes
Gonadotropin dependent ('central' or 'true' precocious puberty [CPP])

- The majority of girls with CPP are not found to have a structural cause;
- 'Functional' CPP occurs spontaneously and is associated with a number of recognized genes; after head trauma; or with structural brain malformations and injury.
- The commonest organic cause is a midline lesion, most commonly glioma, germinoma (which may be very small) or hypothalamic hamartoma.
- After cranial irradiation, puberty occurs on average 2 years earlier in both boys and girls.

Gonadotropin independent ('pseudo' precocious puberty [GIPP])
Aetiology includes:

- Adrenal tumours (often secreting multiple hormones).
- Testicular or ovarian neoplasms.
- Tumours that secrete non-pituitary gonadotropin such as human chorionic gonadotropin (hCG) (eg. extra cranial germinoma or yolk sac tumour commonly seen in association with Klinefelter syndrome).
- Congenital adrenal hyperplasia with high androgens causing virilisation that may then prime the hypothalamus to produce secondary CPP.
- McCune–Albright syndrome: GNAS mutation in one or both ovaries or testes.
- Familial male precocious puberty (testotoxicosis).

Assessment
History should assess for symptoms associated with:

- Pubertal changes (linear growth acceleration, breast tenderness, vaginal discharge/bleeding, mood swings, enlargement of penis/testes/clitoris, voice change, acne), familial pattern of puberty.
- Features suggesting a possible aetiology: headaches, visual change, previous treatment such as irradiation, etc. *Examination* should include:
- Auxology.
- Careful assessment of pubertal staging (including testicular volume in boys and external genitalia in girls with apparent androgen excess).
- Breast texture (firm if oestrogen activity is present or very soft if switched off process).
- Blood pressure.
- Fundal and neurological exam.
- Skin for café au lait spots (NF1/McCune Albright syndrome).

Investigation of precocious puberty (both types)

- Baseline investigations:
  - Bone age.
  - Serum FSH and LH to define central activation or not.
  - GnRH stimulation test to confirm pubertal response (if basal levels not definitive).
  - Gonadal steroid (testosterone or oestradiol).
  - Tumour markers – αFP and βHCG where indicated.
  - Karyotype (XXY) if suspicious of hCG or yolk sac tumour, with rapid onset puberty.
  - TFTs (long-standing severe primary hypothyroidism can result in pseudo precocious puberty due to TSH interacting with the FSH receptor).

- Second line investigations:
  - MRI brain with targeted pituitary views if above tests indicate a central cause.
    - *>70% boys with central precocious puberty likely to have a structural cause.*
    - In girls MRI is less likely to yield an intracranial organic lesion but is still performed.
    - If germinoma suspected, MRI may need to be repeated at initially frequent intervals.
  - Pelvic ultrasound: if adrenal tumour suspected in either sex, or in girls for ovarian cyst or tumour.
  - Testicular ultrasound if indicated.

Management
- Primary goal of treatment is to preserve final height (aiming for a final height in the normal adult range and as close to MPH range as possible).
- Treatment may be required to also alleviate psychosocial distress relating to early puberty.
- An initial period of observation may be permissible to assess the tempo of pubertal change.

Treatment of CPP
- Endocrine referral should be made for management.
- Gonadotropin hormone releasing hormone (GnRH) agonist is the optimal choice for suppression of CPP; requiring 3 monthly IM or SC injections. Alternative options to suppress menses (less effect on bone age advance & final height) include medroxyprogesterone acetate or cyproterone acetate.
- Treatment continued until the child is comfortable with his or her peers, usually by age 11–12 years.

Treatment of GIPP
- Complex; requires blocking of peripheral hormone effect, often with multiple medications and frequently not very effective in preserving final height.

Conditions resembling precocious puberty
Premature thelarche
- Isolated breast development is common in girls <2 years of age, occurs in:
  - Infants of breast feeding mothers, in the early months of life.
  - Older children up to age 2; usually benign and seen in up to 50%.

Clinical Pearl: Premature thelarche in the infant and toddler

In older children up to 2y age, premature thelarche is common with spontaneous regression in the majority. Observation is usually sufficient, but if associated with rapid growth velocity one must consider true oestrogen excess of any cause and investigate as described.

Premature adrenarche and pubarche
- The isolated appearance of pubic hair (usually in a girl) under the age of 8 years may occasionally occur as a normal variant, but it can also signify non-classical congenital adrenal hyperplasia (NCCAH). If so, it will be associated with tall stature and rapid linear growth together with markedly advanced bone age (usually 3–4 years or more advanced).
- Premature adrenarche / pubarche is often observed together with mild bone age advance +/- prepubertal acne. Both this mild problem and NCCAH very frequently go on to polycystic ovary syndrome in adolescence. Families should be warned to seek advice in future should this pattern occur.

Investigations
- Bone age
- Basal serum dehydroepiandrosterone sulfate (DHEA-S), androstenedione, testosterone and 17-hydroxyprogesterone (17-OHP).
- The measurement of 17-OHP at 30 and 60 minutes after intramuscular Synacthen (synthetic adrenocorticotrophic hormone (ACTH)) is recommended to diagnose non-classical congenital adrenal hyperplasia.
- Referral to a specialist is recommended.

Disorders / differences of sex development (DSD)

A congenital condition in which:

* Development of chromosomal, gonadal or anatomical sex is atypical.
* A newborn's genital phenotype is not typically male or female.
* Chromosomal sex is inconsistent with phenotypic sex.

Terminology

There is no universally preferred term, and many patients choose to use their own diagnostic description.

Respect for an individual's preference is important.

* 'Intersex' and 'DSD' are umbrella terms for groups of conditions and are not entirely interchangeable (not all with DSD identify as intersex for example).
* 'Variations in sex characteristics' is also used in some context.
* *For the purposes of this text, DSD is used as it relates to a medical classification system.*

Typical sex development

* The typical developmental pathway is from a bipotential gonad to either a testis or ovary.
* Chromosomal/genetic influences are very important in **determining gonadal sex**.
* The Y chromosome is typically required for testicular development (however the presence of Y does not always equal functioning testis).
* The sex region of the Y chromosome (SRY) acts as a 'master-switch' that drives testis development, however numerous other genes play a role (including Sox-9) in a very tightly regulated process.
* Ovarian development lacks a single genetic 'switch', however a number of transcription factors are known to be essential.
* Once a gonad is determined, the secretion of sex-specific hormones influences further sexual differentiation beginning at week 7–9 of gestation.
* External genital development occurs in weeks 10–16 of pregnancy (midline fusion by ~12–14 weeks), with penile growth & testicular descent in the later half of pregnancy.
* *DSD can arise due to differences / variations at any point in this typical pathway of development, and is reflected by the specific phenotype noted.*

Common presentation

* Newborn with atypical genitalia;
  * Less androgen action than expected in XY (e.g. androgen insensitivity syndrome (AIS), gonadal dysgenesis, androgen biosynthetic defect).
  * More androgen than expected in XX (e.g. CAH).
* Newborn with phenotype that does not match known antenatal karyotype; increasingly recognised due to increased uptake of non-invasive pregnancy testing.
* Female with bilateral 'herniae' (46XY with inguinal testes, eg complete AIS).
* Absent secondary sex characteristics at puberty (e.g. 46 XY female with complete gonadal dysgenesis).
* Unexpected virilisation in puberty (e.g. 46 XY female with previously unrecognised testosterone biosynthetic defect).

Clinical assessment

* History:
  * Family history
  * Pregnancy history
  * Maternal: virilisation, known CAH, medications
  * Consanguinity
  * Previous stillbirth
  * Presentation in older childhood / puberty: timing of onset of any symptoms
* Examination:
  * Examination of the external genitalia can be very informative in a newborn but should be undertaken in older children/adolescents only after detailed explanation and clear consent is obtained.

- In a newborn, examination should note:
  - Size of phallus
  - ?Palpable gonad(s)
  - ?Midline fusion
  - Position of urethral opening
  - Pigmentation
- *Note; standardised assessment tools such as the Prader scale (for females with excessive androgen effect) and external masculinisation scores (EMS) are useful.*

Investigations
- Should be discussed with endocrinology team first (if able) to ensure appropriate investigations and sampling.

Ambiguous genitalia and/or bilateral impalpable gonads
- Karyotype and FISH for Y
- 17OHP, glucose, electrolytes
  - Most helpful on or after day 3 of life (late first week for UEC as this is when salt wasting begins).
- Urinary steroid profile (USP) – need timed specimen
- US – adrenals, pelvis, gonads, mullerian / internal structures, inguinal region
- **If 46XX karyotype:**
  - CAH most likely; add renin, timed USP
  - Other eg 11DOC if initial investigations not diagnostic
- **If karyotype other than 46XX:**
- 'Second tier' Ix really helpful
  - Anti-mullerian hormone (AMH) – indicates Sertoli cell function / likelihood of internal Mullerian structures
  - LH, FSH, T, E2
  - Additional androgens: DHT, androstenedione
  - +/- hCG stimulation testing and further imaging
  - Genetic testing, laparoscopy +/- gonadal biopsy may be indicated

Clinical clues
- **A palpable gonad is almost always testis;** this implies the presence of Y chromosome material (hence investigating for CAH less urgent).
- Two palpable testes indicate good testicular function (uterus is unlikely to be present).
- The presence of a uterus.
- External virilisation is proportional to androgen effect and hence the likely timing of androgen exposure can also be derived from clinical findings (eg midline fusion implies androgen effect at 8–12 weeks; androgen exposure after this time predominantly affects phallic growth).

46, XY DSD
- Disorders of testicular development:
  - Gonadal dysgenesis
  - Gonadal regression
  - Ovostesticular DSD
- Disorders of androgen synthesis or action:
  - Androgen biosynthesis defect
  - 5 alpha-reductase deficiency
  - 17-beta-hydroxylase deficiency
  - Defect in androgen action: CAIS, PAIS
- LH receptor defects
  - Disorders of AMH/AMH receptor (eg. persistent mullerian duct syndrome)
- Other
  - Severe hypospadias

Putting the science into practice: DSD

Improvements in knowledge of genetic variations underlying DSD and the availability of DSD gene panels has considerably improved molecular diagnostic rates in 46 XY DSD in recent years; however more than half remain without a molecular diagnosis.

---

46 XX DSD

- Disorders of ovarian development:
  - Ovotesticular DSD
  - Testicular DSD
  - Gonadal dysgenesis
- Androgen excess:
  - CAH (21 OH deficiency CAH is by far the most common 46 XX DSD)
- Maternal:
  - Iatrogenic (exogenous progestins or androgen exposure)
  - Tumour (maternal luteoma)
  - Placental aromatase enzyme deficiency (➔ maternal virilisation)

Clinical Pearl: Changing landscapes in DSD management and support

Management of a child/adolescent with a DSD should be undertaken in a tertiary centre with a specialist multi-disciplinary team. The treating team may include specialists from endocrinology, urology, gynaecology, neonatology, clinical ethics, genetics and psychology, with the support of a clinical co-ordinator.

Specific management depends on the underlying variation. Medical, surgical or no interventions may be appropriate, depending on the age of the child and the functional impact of the variation. *Urgent medical treatment in DSD is predominantly only indicated for 21-OH deficiency CAH in a female, to prevent a possible salt losing crisis.*

Clinical Controversy: The role & timing of genital/gonadal surgery in DSD

Where previously, genital or gonadal surgery may have been undertaken in children with DSD, an increasingly conservative approach is now more widely adopted. In particular, gonadectomy due to concern over future malignancy risks is now rarely indicated in childhood, except in complete gonadal dysgenesis where hormonal and fertility potential is absent, but a high malignancy risk (≥30% with presentation in the early years of life reported) is well documented.

Indications for and optimal timing of genital surgery remains a contentious issue with no evidence to support early or late surgery as optimal. Intersex advocates have been clear in their calls to abandon genital surgery on infants, except where medically necessary. Open discussion of potential interventions and their timing (including the option of no intervention as appropriate) along with shared decision making between a specialist DSD multi-disciplinary team and the family is important in each individual case. Psychological and peer group support for both the child/adolescent and their parents is also essential.

Disorders of calcium metabolism, Vitamin D, and bone health
hypocalcaemia

See Table 19.10.

Clinical features

- Rachitic changes in long bones (swollen wrists, etc.), rachitic rosary.
- Tetany (may be demonstrated using sphygmomanometer cuff above systolic pressure for up to 2 minutes – Trousseau sign).
- Facial nerve twitching when tapping over parotid gland – Chvostek sign.
- Laryngeal stridor.
- Seizure.
- Weakness, tiredness, irritability.

Note even extreme hypocalcaemia may be asymptomatic in an infant.

Table 19.10 Causes of hypocalcaemia.

Neonatal presentation	Infant/childhood presentation
Prematurity/IUGR/birth asphyxia	Vitamin D deficiency
Hypoparathyroidism ±	Hypoparathyroidism
Di George syndrome	A/w autoimmune polyglandular syndrome (look for mucocutaneous
Phosphate load (high phosphate milk)	candidiasis and/or Addison disease in a young child)
Low magnesium	Pseudohypoparathyroidism
Maternal gestational diabetes	Albright hereditary osteodystrophy
	Chronic renal failure
	Pancreatitis
	Organic acidaemia
	Critical illness
	1-α-hydroxylase deficiency (rare)
	Vitamin D resistant rickets (VDR receptor mutation)
	Post cardiac surgery (citrate binding during cardiac bypass)

Investigations
- Total and ionised calcium
- 25-OH vitamin D (1,25-diOH-vitamin D if non-vitamin D deficient rickets is suspected).
- UEC, lipase, albumin
- Mg, PO4
- ALP
- Parathyroid hormone (PTH)
- Radiographs of wrist, knee (metaphyseal splaying)
- Malabsorption studies
- Urinary calcium/creatinine ratio
- ECG (prolonged QTc interval)

Management
Emergency/symptomatic
Only use IV treatment if symptomatic (tetany, seizures) – ideally requires central access.
- IV calcium chloride 10% infusion – 1 mmol/kg per 24 hours in 5% dextrose. Monitor calcium levels 6 hourly.
- Occasionally IV calcium chloride 10% – 0.2 mL/kg stat may be required for severe tetany.
- Correct magnesium if low.
- Monitor ECG
- 25-OH-vitamin D if nutritional rickets is suspected – consider megadose therapy (100,000 to 150,000 units cholecalciferol stat) – careful with low calcium/hungry bones (see clinical pearl below).
- 1,25-diOH-vitamin D (calcitriol) if parathyroid disorders suspected or if severe vitamin D deficiency and waiting for 25OH vitamin D treatment to take effect: 0.01–0.02 mcg/kg per day starting dose (may need to be increased).
- Treatment of underlying condition.

> ### Clinical Pearl: Calcium supplementation in rickets
> In the first days to weeks after treatment is begun for rickets, bones are 'hungry'. Large doses of calcium supplements (and possibly calcitriol) may be required to maintain normocalcaemia and prevent carpopedal spasm once vitamin D is started.

Maintenance
- Adequate calcium intake, preferably as dairy products, 600–1500 mg per day depending on age.
- 25-OH-vitamin D for months to years depending on cause, dose will vary but often 400–1000 units per day.
- Stoss/megadose therapy is alternative method, using 100 000–150 000 units 25–OH-vitamin D at 0, 6–12 weeks then every 3–6 months as required, with appropriate monitoring – not for infants <3 months of age.
- 1,25-diOH-vitamin D for vitamin D resistant rickets, hypoparathyroidism

> **Clinical Controversy: Vitamin D deficiency without biochemical or clinical features of rickets**
> There are increasing numbers of young people found to be Vitamin D deficient on "routine" testing who have no current clinical sequelae. *Recommendations are that Vitamin D levels in young people should be maintained >50 nmol/L for optimal bone health.* The extra-skeletal role of Vitamin D remains controversial – there are many intriguing basic science/association studies that suggest further roles for Vitamin D on immune regulation and other cellular processes, but conclusive cause and effect remains elusive. Screening for Vitamin D deficiency in the absence of rickets/low bone mass is not recommended; supplementing high risk groups especially over April–October at higher southern latitudes is better clinical practice (see Chapter 35, Refugee health).

Hypercalcaemia
See Table 19.11.

Clinical features
- Polyuria, polydipsia
- Vomiting, dehydration
- Failure to thrive
- Abdominal pain (constipation, renal stones, pancreatitis)
- Confusion, apathy (if severe)

Investigation
- Total and ionised calcium, PO4
- Mg, albumin
- ALP
- PTH level
- 25-OH-vitamin D ± 1,25-diOH-vitamin D
- TFT
- Chest radiograph ± skeletal survey
- Parathyroid imaging
- Urinary calcium/creatinine ratio
- Renal ultrasound (nephrocalcinosis)
- ECG (short QTc interval)

Management
Severe
- Rehydration with 0.9% saline + 5% dextrose (Infants <2 years use 0.45% saline + 5% dextrose)
- Diuretics indicated in two situations:
  - Acute hypercalcaemia: frusemide given to reduce fluid overload while the patient is aggressively rehydrated.
  - Chronic hypercalcaemia with hypercalciuria (or normocalcaemia with hypercalciuria): thiazide diuretics are given to reduce oedema and prevent nephrocalcinosis (by decreasing urinary calcium excretion).

Table 19.11 Causes of hypercalcaemia.

Neonatal	Infant/childhood
Hyperparathyroidism (rare)	Primary hyperparathyroidism
Familial hypocalciuric hypercalcaemia – severe form	Familial hypocalciuric hypercalcaemia
Hypophosphatasia	1,25-diOH-D excess (nutritional, inflammatory disease, for example sarcoidosis, leukaemia)
William syndrome (elfin face, supravalvular aortic stenosis)	Vitamin D/Vitamin A intoxication
Subcutaneous fat necrosis	Neoplasia (lytic bone lesions or humoral hypercalcaemia PTHrP)
Iatrogenic	Immobilisation, for example burns (severe), quadriplegia – can be very severe and cause renal calculi, pancreatitis
	Drugs (lithium, thiazides)
	Endocrine disorders: hyperthyroidism (mild, usually asymptomatic), phaeochromocytoma, adrenal insufficiency

- Bisphosphonates, particularly for increased bone resorption (e.g. immobilisation).
- Glucocorticoid therapy for vitamin D excess (prednisolone 2 mg/kg per day, reducing).
- Low calcium diet – low calcium formula for infants.
- Surgery if indicated, treatment of underlying condition.

Paediatric bone health – fragility fractures

- A wide variety of conditions can lead to both primary and secondary issues with skeletal development.
- The effects on bone health of a number of chronic paediatric conditions is increasingly recognized (immobility, glucocorticoid use, chronic inflammation, poor nutrition, hypogonadism, etc.).
- While fractures are a relatively common part of childhood; recurrent fractures, fractures with low levels of force or fractures in clinical settings mentioned above should be further investigated.

Clinical features

The following factors should be considered during a bone health assessment:
- Number/type/mechanism/management of fractures.
- Ambulatory status/activity levels.
- Medication usage (i.e. glucocorticoids, anticonvulsants).
- Calcium intake/vitamin D levels.
- Pubertal status.
- Family history of fragility fractures (timing, number, mechanism).
- Presence of features suggesting collagen defects (ligamentous laxity, blue/grey sclerae, dental issues).

Investigations

- Blood tests: Ca, PO4, vitamin D, ALP, PTH, TFT, coeliac screen.
- Urine tests: Urine Ca, PO4, Creatinine (needs to be paired with serum to interpret).
- Plain X-rays – examine existing films looking at cortical width, general appearance/mineral content (can be difficult to judge), vertebral wedging/collapse if lateral spine X-ray performed.
- Bone density scanning; usually dual energy X-ray absorptiometry (DXA) scan:
  - Lumbar spine, hip and/or total body.
  - Paediatric software required to generate age matched Z score.
  - Remember confounders; short stature and maturational delay.

Management

- Optimisation of simple risk factors (calcium intake; vitamin D levels, activity levels, pubertal induction).
- If recurrent fragility fractures (especially vertebral), consider the use of intravenous bisphosphonates:
  - Prescribed by a specialist with experience in paediatric bone health disorders.
  - Dental review is required prior to commencement.
  - Monitoring for first dose effects of acute phase reaction and hypocalcaemia.
- Modification of environment to limit fracture risk.

USEFUL RESOURCES
- Australian Diabetes Society/Australasian Paediatric Endocrine Group (APEG) publication https://diabetessociety.com.au/documents/Type1guidelines14Nov2011.pdf; NHMRC evidence based guidelines for Type 1 diabetes in children, adolescents and adults (2011).
- International Society for Paediatric and Adolescent Diabetes (ISPAD) clinical practice guidelines (2018) https://www.ispad.org/page/ISPADGuidelines2018
- RCH Diabetes clinical practice guidelines and parent manual http://www.rch.org.au/diabetesmanual/
- Vitamin D guidelines:
  - **International:** Munns et al *2016 Global Consensus Recommendations on Prevention and Management of Nutritional Rickets.* JCEM 101(2) 394–415.
  - **Australian:** Paxton et al *2013 Vitamin D and health in pregnancy, infants, children and adolescents in Australia and New Zealand: a position statement.* MJA 198(3) 142–143.
- Bisphosphonate consensus guideline – Simm et al 2018 *Consensus guidelines on the use of bisphosphonate therapy in children and adolescents.* JPCH 45(3) 223–233.

CHAPTER 20

Forensic medicine

Anne Smith
Joanna Tully

Key Points

- Child abuse and neglect is so common we should think about it every time we interact with children.
- Interventions that aim to reduce vulnerability, modify risk factors and remediate harm require significant resources, but are not as costly as the lifelong consequences for the abused individual and the costs of intergenerational transmission of child maltreatment.
- Child abuse is easy to miss and easy to misdiagnose; diagnostic errors can have serious and sometimes fatal consequences.
- It is often possible to differentiate injuries and harms caused by abuse from accidents and medical mimics.
- Some injuries are sensitive and specific for assault, some injuries are less specific "red flags" for abuse, and some injuries are "sentinel injuries" indicative of a significant risk of serious injury in the future. We should understand the forensic significance of childhood injuries.

Background

The possibility of child abuse should always be considered when health professionals evaluate and treat injured children. Every interaction with children and their carers provides an opportunity to think about the child's vulnerability to harm from abuse and neglect, and the impact on the child of adverse childhood experiences. Whenever a child's living circumstances suggest the possibility of harm, a comprehensive psychosocial assessment should occur. Doctors who are unfamiliar with the processes of forensic interpretation of injury or the evaluation of vulnerability are encouraged to promptly consult with medical professionals who have expertise in this area.

The body of knowledge related to child abuse is increasing as is the demand for expert court testimony. Furthermore, there are expectations that doctors understand their legal obligations and demonstrate skill when providing evidence that will withstand the rigors of cross-examination in court.

Mandatory reporting

In most Australian states medical practitioners are legally required to notify the relevant statutory authorities of children who have experienced, or are likely to experience abuse. Thresholds and criteria for reporting vary across jurisdictions. Medical practitioners should be familiar with the relevant legislation and reporting procedures in their own state or territory.

Referral centres

Centres for the medical assessment and treatment of child abuse have been established in most tertiary paediatric hospitals. Paediatricians and other medical professionals working in these centres provide expert advice in relation to the assessment and management of suspected child abuse. Seek advice early.

Paediatric Handbook, Tenth Edition. Edited by Kate Harding, Daniel S. Mason and Daryl Efron.
© 2021 John Wiley & Sons Ltd. Published 2021 by John Wiley & Sons Ltd.

Definitions: types of child abuse and neglect

Child Abuse

- Child abuse is also termed child maltreatment.
- It encompasses words or actions that cause actual, threatened or potential harm (physically, emotionally or sexually), ill treatment, or neglect/deprivation (acts of omission) toward any child.

Physical Abuse

- Child physical abuse is physical trauma inflicted on a child.
- Objective evidence of this violence may include bruising, burns and scalds, head injuries, fractures, intra-abdominal and intra-thoracic trauma, suffocation and drowning.
- Injury can be caused by impact, penetration, heat, a caustic substance, a chemical or a drug.
- The definition also includes physical harm sustained as a result of fabricated or induced illness by the carer.

Child sexual abuse

- Child sexual abuse is the involvement of dependent, developmentally immature children and adolescents in sexual activities that they may not fully comprehend and to which they are unable to give consent.
- Sexual exploitation is included.

Child neglect

- Child neglect is the failure of caregivers to adequately provide for and safeguard the health, safety and well-being of the child *when resources are readily available to do so.*
- Applies to any situation in which the basic needs of a child are not met with respect to nutrition, hygiene, clothing or shelter.
- Also comprises the failure to provide access to adequate medical care, mental health care, dental care, education, stimulation to promote development, or failure to attend to a child's moral and spiritual care.

Psychological/Emotional maltreatment

- Psychological maltreatment consists of acts that are judged on the basis of a combination of community standards and professional expertise to be psychologically damaging.
- Such acts damage, immediately or ultimately, the behavioural, cognitive, affective or physical functioning of the child.
- Examples of psychological maltreatment include acts of spurning (hostility, rejecting or degrading), terrorising, isolating, exploiting or corrupting and denying emotional responsiveness.
- Exposure to interpersonal violence in the home is included in this definition.

Cumulative Harm

- Subtypes of child abuse and neglect often co-exist in children who are experiencing a range of adverse circumstances and events.
- The serious and pervasive harm that results from a number of episodes of maltreatment and/or a range of chronically harmful situations is recognised in (Victorian) legislation by the term 'cumulative harm' (see Clinical Pearl below: 'Adverse childhood experiences' [ACE's] and Chapter 1, Communication in the paediatric consultation).
- The Child Protection manual states: *"Cumulative harm refers to the effects of multiple adverse or harmful circumstances and events in a child's life. The unremitting daily impact of these experiences on the child can be profound and exponential, and diminish a child's sense of safety, stability and wellbeing."*

Consent for forensic medical procedures

Valid **informed consent** must be obtained:

- For the right procedure.
- From the right person;
    - Who *understands* the nature and purpose of the procedure.
    - Who has *considered the consequences* of going ahead or not going ahead with the procedure, which includes consideration of rare but important negative outcomes.
    - Who has the *capacity* to make a choice.

- Consent must be *freely given*.
- Consent *may be withdrawn* at any time during the procedure.

Consent for a forensic medical procedure occurs during a conversation. Documentation that includes a signed consent form is considered 'best practice' noting that consent should be specifically sought and provided for each aspect of the procedure. Consent should be obtained by the medical practitioner who will perform the procedure.

Capacity to consent

Jurisdictional differences affect the age at which mature minors may legally consent to medical procedures. In many jurisdictions assessment of a minor's capacity to consent involves consideration of *'Gillick competence'* (see chapter 2 Ethics) which includes evaluation of *maturity and understanding* as may be evidenced by a person's:

- Age
- Intelligence
- Capacity to make autonomous decisions (e.g. self-supporting, self-determining in daily life, financial independence, living independently)
- Factors that might impair capacity for decision making, both short-term and long-term.
- Capacity to make a choice.

The possibility of a guardian providing consent in the legal sense with the minor providing written verification of his/her assent. This approach often works well for forensic medical procedures.

It may be wise to defer forensic examination whenever situation-specific factors such as pain, fear, emotional upset, intoxication, being drug affected (or affected by drug withdrawal), tiredness, possible intimidation or coercion by others (including professionals) and an acute stress reaction are present, because these factors may also affect a person's capacity to assent.

Forensic Evaluation of Physical Injury

Aims of forensic assessment

The aim of a forensic assessment of injury is to determine, if possible, the cause (including mechanism), timing and consequences of injury. The overall aim is to diagnose or exclude the diagnosis of child abuse. The process aims to:

- Differentiate inflicted trauma from accidents and medical conditions confused with assault.
- Estimate time of injury.
- Consider a broad range of differential diagnoses.
- Determine the most likely cause(s) of the child's injuries or condition.
- Assess and manage the child's medical needs and plan ongoing care.
- Take action to protect the child or another child in the family from additional harm. This usually involves working in partnership with police, protective workers and support agencies. Discuss *all* situations of possible child abuse with a paediatrician or colleague with expertise in this field.

Interview techniques

Some health professionals prefer to interview parents separately when child abuse is suspected while others feel uncomfortable because such interviews may intrude into the territory of criminal investigators. There is insufficient evidence to recommend a specific interview process for health professionals to use. An independent observer and/or support person for the parents might be considered. In general terms it is good practice to:

- Ensure privacy.
- Allow adequate time.
- Use a non-judgmental, courteous and sensitive approach.
- Ask open, non-directive questions and encourage a free narrative.
- Listen.
- Record information sources and information provided, and use verbatim quotes whenever possible.
- Do not speculate or suggest possible mechanisms of injury.

History of Injury

A detailed account of the mechanism of injury should always be sought. Gather information about the possible mechanism, timing and circumstances of injury:

- Determine when, where and how the injury occurred (Table 20.1).
- Record
  - Who told the story
  - Where the information came from
  - Who (if anyone) witnessed the event(s) that caused the injury
  - The child's previous injuries, illnesses and emergency department presentations
- Assess the child's developmental capabilities

It is important to obtain details of the child's past medical, social and family history. Explore/investigate possible medical causes of easy bruising/excessive bleeding and bone fragility.

Examination

A thorough physical examination must be performed and recorded. A top-to-toe skin examination should be performed.

- See https://www.rch.org.au/vfpms/tools/ for standardised VFPMS evaluation forms to document clinical and examination findings.
- Describe injuries accurately, use body diagrams and photograph all visible injuries.
- Include details of the site, size, colour and shape of ALL injuries and skin lesions.

Search for:

- Skin injuries (bruises, petechiae, lacerations, abrasions, puncture wounds).
  - Note injuries that might have been inflicted by a human hand (slap, firm grip or fingertip pressure) or patterned bruising from impact with an implement.
- Intra-oral, intranasal and tympanic membrane injuries.
- Scalp injuries (inspect beneath the hair and palpate the scalp for swelling, bony steps).
- Eye injuries (examine from the lids to the retina).
- Internal injuries (organs in the thorax and abdomen).
- Genital injuries.

There are few examination findings that serve as definitive evidence of assault; *but*

there are many examination findings that should generate a strong suspicion about a non-accidental cause. These include:

- Bruising or fracture in infants and non-mobile children.
- Large numbers of bruises and bruises covering large areas of the body in the absence of a story of accidental trauma (medical conditions /coagulopathy require exclusion).
- Bruising in the TEN 4 FACES distribution (see clinical pearl below) and over soft parts of the body that are well protected from accidental trauma.
- Patterned bruising suggestive of human bite marks or forceful contact with an object.

Table 20.1 Features of 'the story' that should raise suspicion for a non-accidental cause.

- No story is offered to account for injuries
- No witnesses present to verify story
- Hypothesis regarding cause is based on minimal information or speculation
- The story offered by one individual changes over time
- The story offered by two individuals differs without apparent explanation
- The story is not in keeping with the child's developmental skills
- A young sibling or other child is blamed for causing the injury
- Injury sustained during an incident of family violence
- The story seems implausible or highly improbable
- An unexplained delay occurred between the alleged time of injury and the time when medical care was sought

- Extensive patterned bruising on both buttocks indicative of spanking.
- Clustered bruises.
- Intra-oral injury in young infants.
- Metaphyseal fractures (CML patterned fractures) at the ends of long bones.
- Postero-medial rib fractures in an infant.
- Fractures at varying stages of healing.
- Immersion-patterned scalds.
- Unexplained encephalopathy in a child aged less than 2 years (consider abusive head trauma).
- Unexplained intracranial bleeding in infants (particularly thin bilateral subdural haemorrhages over convexities and in the interhemispheric fissure).
- Retinal haemorrhages that are bilateral, too numerous to count, multilayered and may be associated with retinoschisis.

Medical investigation of suspicious injury

- **'Suspicious injury'** is a term commonly used to signify a possible non-accidental cause.
- The VFPMS website provides guidance in relation to the forensic investigation of particular types of suspicious injury (see https://www.rch.org.au/vfpms/guidelines/).
- A Free app produced by US Child Abuse Paediatricians (Child Protector) may assist with decision making (https://apps.apple.com/us/app/child-protector/id1019023917).
- **Investigations** in abused children are aimed at determining the extent of the injuries and identifying and/ or excluding possible medical causes or contributors.
  - A skeletal survey and bone scan, or two skeletal surveys two weeks apart may detect *occult fractures* in very young children.
  - Consider blood and imaging screening tests for *abdominal injury*.
  - Consider screening tests for possible *head injury* (abusive head trauma through shaking and/or impact) including imaging tests for cranio-spinal trauma.

Putting the Science into Practice: Algorithms to aid decisions regarding forensic medical investigation

Clinical decision rules and algorithms are currently being developed to guide decision-making in relation to investigating and diagnosing injuries caused by assault. Examples include the PediBIRN AHT probability calculator, and the PredAHT which offer tools to assist in the diagnosis of abusive head trauma.

Forensic investigation of bruising and bleeding

- Bruising is the commonest skin manifestation of abuse and may indicate that an infant or young child is at serious risk of harm (see https://www.rch.org.au/vfpms/guidelines/Bruising/).

Clinical Pearl: Forensic approach to bruising at a glance

Patterns of bruising that should raise concern for abuse are:
- Any bruise in infant <4-6 months of age.
- Bruising in TEN location (Torso, Ear, Neck) in child <4 years of age.
- Bruising to the buttocks and/or genitals.
- Bruising away from bony prominences or on posterior aspect of the body.
- Patterned or clustered bruising.
- Bruises containing petechiae.
- Injury to FACES (Frenulum, Angle of jaw, Cheek, Eyelid, Sclera) in a child of any age.

First line laboratory investigations to consider:
- FBE
- APTT, PT, INR
- Fibrinogen
- Calcium
- LFT, UEC
- Consider VWD screen and blood group and Factor VIII and IX levels.
- Additional investigations or consultation with a paediatric haematologist may be necessary.
- Remember that children with a coagulation disorder can also be abused – seek specialist advice in this circumstance.

Radiological investigation to consider
Infants and young children with concerning bruises are likely to need skeletal survey(s), +/- bone scan and cranial imaging.

Forensic investigation of fracture
- Fractures are the second commonest injury caused by physical abuse (after bruises).
- Many inflicted fractures are not clinically suspected because they occur in pre-verbal and non-ambulatory infants. *In infants, fractures are more commonly attributed to abuse than to accidents.*
- See https://www.rch.org.au/vfpms/guidelines/Fractures.

Clinical Pearl: Forensic approach to fractures at a glance

Features of fractures that should raise concern for abuse are:
- Fractures in infants and non-ambulatory children.
- Fractures in certain locations or of certain types eg posteromedial rib fractures, metaphyseal corner fractures.
- Multiple fractures or fractures of different ages.

In addition:
- No single fracture type is pathognomic for abuse.
- Dating of fractures is an inexact science and caution should be applied.
- Many children with fractures will have minimal or no external sign of injury – be vigilant to the need for additional investigations to screen for occult bony, cranial or intra-abdominal injury.

First line laboratory investigations to consider:
- FBE
- Serum Ca, PO4 & ALP
- LFT
- UEC
- If child is <6 months old or in the presence radiological evidence of osteopenia, consider 25OH vitamin D, PTH and urinary Ca excretion (eg. random urinary Ca:Cr ratio).
- Additional investigations may be necessary.

Radiological investigations to consider:
A skeletal survey and bone scan <u>or</u> two skeletal surveys performed 2 weeks apart are the investigations of choice depending on local availability and expertise.

Forensic investigation of intra-abdominal injury
- Abdominal injuries are a significant cause of morbidity and mortality in abused children and the diagnosis may be delayed due to the absence of external injury to the abdomen.
- Have a low threshold for considering and looking for intra-abdominal injury in abused children.
- See https://www.rch.org.au/vfpms/guidelines/Visceral_injury_including_abdominal_injury/

> **Clinical Pearl: Forensic approach to intra-abdominal injury at a glance**
> Features that should raise concern in relation to intra-abdominal trauma are:
> - Clinical pattern suggesting significant physical abuse
> - Abdominal or chest wall bruising, abdominal distension or tenderness
> - Clinical signs of paralytic ileus or intra-abdominal haemorrhage
> - AST or ALT > 80, elevated lipase/amylase
> - ≥2 abnormal abdominal laboratory results
>
> In addition:
> - Intra-abdominal injury in the absence of accidental trauma warrants serious consideration of abuse.
> - The signs and symptoms may be vague and non-specific so LOOK and FEEL.
> - CT is the investigation of choice for investigating suspected intra-abdominal injury.

Laboratory investigations to consider:
- Pancreatic enzymes (including amylase and lipase)
- Liver Function Tests
- Urine dipstick (for haematuria)
- FBE (for occult blood loss)
- Fibrinogen

Radiological investigations to consider:
- Abdominal X-rays (including erect and supine).
- Abdominal ultrasound.
- Abdominal CT Scan with contrast is the investigation of choice.

Forensic investigation of suspected abusive head trauma (including shaking)

Abusive head trauma (AHT) is the leading cause of mortality in abused infants. It is associated with high rates of long term neurodisability in survivors.
- Infants suffering AHT may present with non-specific signs and symptoms including irritability and vomiting; a history of apnoea is important.
- See https://www.rch.org.au/vfpms/guidelines/Head_injury/

> **Clinical Pearl: Abusive Head Trauma at a glance**
> Features that should raise concern for AHT are:
> - An infant with a history of being shaken, unexplained encephalopathy or subdural and/or retinal haemorrhages.
> - An infant with clinical and/or radiological signs of head trauma.
> - Bruising, especially in infants and especially to the head and neck is an important sentinel injury for later abusive head trauma.
>
> In addition:
> - Retinal haemorrhages are a cardinal feature of AHT and can resolve rapidly so an early eye examination by a consultant ophthalmologist is necessary.
> - Admission to ICU should be considered whenever an infant presents with altered conscious state and shaking is suspected because of the high risk of further neurological deterioration caused by progressive brain swelling.
> - Interpretation of findings in cases of suspected AHT can be challenging – seek advice.

- Laboratory investigations are aimed at identifying and excluding alternative medical causes. These may be extensive and include extending clotting profiles and tests for rare metabolic and genetic conditions – seek specialist advice.

Radiological investigations when AHT is suspected:

- Cranio-spinal imaging – A CT scan may be the investigation of choice in the initial stages in a sick infant.
- MRI brain and *whole* spine should be performed later. The correct sequences to identify ligamentous injury to the neck are important and should be requested.
- Serial imaging may be necessary.

Forensic investigation of burns and scalds

- If suspicion exists about intentional thermal injury such as scalds or contact burns in children aged <3 years, then skeletal survey and additional investigations for other forms of child abuse should be considered.
- See https://www.rch.org.au/vfpms/guidelines/Burns_including_scald_burns/

Toxicology

- When ingestion or poisoning is suspected, blood and/or urine samples for forensic drug analysis may be sent to both the hospital biochemistry laboratories (for an urgent result) and a forensic laboratory for a quantitative result.
- Collect blood and urine if ingestion or poisoning was within prior 24 hours, and urine alone if more than 24–48 hours. Samples should be sent to the forensic laboratory under Chain of Custody. Seek advice.
- See https://www.rch.org.au/vfpms/guidelines/Toxicological_testing/ and/or Chapter 4, Poisoning and envenomation).

Clinical photography

- Photographs augment, but should not replace a detailed written description of injuries and body diagrams.
- Photo-documentation should be obtained in all situations of visible injury likely to have been caused by assault.

Child sexual abuse

- Child sexual abuse affects approximately one in four girls, and one in seven boys before the age of 16 years.
- The nature of offending, types of sexual contact and types of harm are different to those associated with adult sexual assault.
- Health professionals are expected to have a good understanding of the dynamics of child sexual abuse as well as methods used by employers and statutory agencies to reduce the risk of sexual harm within organisations where children are present.
- Assessment of suspected sexual abuse (including sexualised behavior) should occur as a single assessment by a suitably trained medical practitioner who has expertise in interpreting genital injury, collection of forensic samples, production of medical reports and presentation of evidence in court.
- Doctors must ensure that all aspects of the examination and photo-documentation are in accordance with local policies, procedural guidelines and legislation.
- Proformas and medicolegal report templates may be useful for documenting the process and providing reports for police and statutory child protection professionals (see https://www.rch.org.au/vfpms/tools/)

Clinical Pearl: Child sexual abuse at a glance
- Child and adolescent victims of sexual assault are often very vulnerable; take a holistic approach to the child and family and maximise healthcare opportunities.
- Minimise the risk of DNA contamination.
- Protect forensic samples from tampering.
- Document the chain of custody.
- Collect samples in accordance with local recommended time frames and sampling techniques.
- Consider STI testing and prophylaxis, and post coital contraception.
- Ensure medical and psychological follow up.
- Implement strategies to minimise and remediate psychological trauma.

Child neglect and emotional maltreatment

The subtypes of child neglect and emotional maltreatment often coexist. Neglected and emotionally maltreated children may come to the attention of health professionals when the child's medical and developmental needs are neglected as evidenced by failure to attend scheduled appointments and/or failure to comply with recommended treatment or medical interventions when such interventions are unquestionably in the child's best interests. Emotional maltreatment is often manifest when the child's behaviour becomes of concern.

The hallmark of neglect is caregiver omission to provide for children's needs and of emotional maltreatment is the persistent, non-physical pattern of interaction with the child by the caregiver. Child neglect and emotional maltreatment are strongly associated with poverty, deprivation, adverse childhood experiences and inadequate social support for children at a neighbourhood and government level. These are forms of child maltreatment commonly transmitted to the next generation.

Assessment of neglect

- Involves assessment of the child's:
  - ○ General health, healthcare and dental care.
  - ○ Growth and development.
  - ○ Relationships and behaviour.
  - ○ Physical environment.
  - ○ Education, social and cultural engagement.
- A checklist approach to evaluating child neglect, similar to the HEADSS assessment of adolescents can be useful.
- See https://www.rch.org.au/Templates/intranet/RchContent.aspx?id=40474#neglecting
- The evaluation of the emotionally maltreated child can be approached in a similar manner (see VFPMS guidelines).

Putting the Science into Practice: Toxic stress and adverse childhood experiences
- Child abuse and neglect is a public health problem. The neuroscience around child maltreatment provides a powerful incentive for prevention. The negative effects of toxic stress and adverse childhood experiences are now well known.
- Most health organisations currently promote "trauma informed care" in which the 5 guiding principles as safety, choice, collaboration, trust-worthiness and empowerment.

Report writing

- At times medical professionals are required to explain medical information to a legal audience.
- Medical Report templates are available for use for a variety of presenting problems however health professionals are advised to use templates developed specifically for their jurisdiction in order to comply with local procedures and legislation.
- See https://www.rch.org.au/vfpms/tools/

Clinical Pearl: Forensic report writing
- Avoid bias; maintain an objective and impartial approach.
- Acknowledge uncertainty and known error rates.
- Consider a broad differential diagnosis.
- Clearly state your opinion in relation to the probability of the findings resulting from abuse and neglect.

Court testimony

- Medical evidence is heavily scrutinised in court, by the media, medical boards and by peers (particularly colleagues who provide opinion evidence for defence); thus high standards are expected.
- Colleagues familiar with working at the medicolegal interface provide useful advice and coaching; seek help early if required.

Clinical Pearl: Court testimony
- Be prepared: know your case details and know what to expect in court. Understand your role in providing testimony in court (different courts have differing requirements).
- Be pensive.
- Be painstakingly precise. Answer carefully and completely. Ask for questions to be repeated or reworded if you do not understand. Don't guess or speculate.
- Be patient. Be polite. Dress to impress.
- Don't panic.
- Don't be partisan – your evidence should assist the decision-makers, not advocate for a particular side in an adversarial situation.
- Don't talk about the case (particularly with other witnesses) prior to release of the judgement.
- Debrief with dignity.
- Don't feel responsibility for the outcome. You merely had a small part in the 'jigsaw'.

USEFUL RESOURCES
- Victorian forensic paediatric medical service (VFPMS) resources https://www.rch.org.au/vfpms/
- Royal Children's Hospital clinical practice guideline – Child Abuse https://www.rch.org.au/clinicalguide/guideline_index/Child_abuse/
- Resources relating to toxic stress and adverse childhood events (ACE's):
  - https://www.cdc.gov/violenceprevention/childabuseandneglect/acestudy/index.html
  - https://developingchild.harvard.edu/science/key-concepts/toxic-stress/
  - https://developingchild.harvard.edu/resources/aces-and-toxic-stress-frequently-asked-questions/
- Childsafe children's harm prevention charity website https://www.childsafe.org.au/; information and resources regarding children's harm prevention.

CHAPTER 21

Gastroenterology

Winita Hardikar
Liz Bannister
Susan Gibb

Key Points

- Children with moderate dehydration suffering from acute infectious gastroenteritis can usually be safely and effectively treated with rapid nasogastric rehydration, even in the presence of vomiting.
- Blood tests for coeliac disease are for screening, not diagnosis. Children should not be placed on a gluten free diet based on these tests alone.
- Inflammatory bowel disease is increasing in frequency worldwide. The goal of treatment is mucosal healing, which is superior to symptom control, for long term outcome.
- All infants with conjugated hyperbilirubinaemia require investigation. In infants under 10 weeks of age, this is urgent.
- Faecal Calprotectin should not be performed in children under 5 years of age or in children who have obvious blood in the stool.

Acute infectious gastroenteritis

Most cases of acute infectious gastroenteritis are caused by viruses. Since the introduction of the rotavirus vaccine into the National Immunisation Program in 2007, the incidence of rotavirus-induced gastroenteritis requiring GP/hospital presentation, and admission, has fallen dramatically. The most common presentation is diarrhoea, with or without vomiting or abdominal pain. The diarrhoea often follows poor feeding, vomiting and fever. Bacterial gastroenteritis is suggested by a history of frequent small-volume stools with passage of blood and mucus, and abdominal pain. Be wary of diagnosing gastroenteritis in the child with vomiting alone who is dehydrated or unwell. The two most important issues in the management of acute infectious diarrhoea are:

1. Exclusion of other important causes of vomiting and diarrhoea such as:
   - Appendicitis
   - Urinary tract infection
   - Other sites of infection (including meningitis, sepsis)
   - Surgical conditions including intussusception
   - Haemolytic uraemic syndrome
2. Adequate assessment and treatment of dehydration. See Chapter 7, Fluid and electrolytes.

Management

Many cases can be managed with oral rehydration, with enteral routes preferred over intravenous hydration. Children on fortified feeds need to have the fortification removed during the acute illness as it may drive the diarrhoea and dehydration. The risk of dehydration is increased with younger age, as infants (<6 months) have an increased surface area to body volume ratio. This results in increased insensible fluid losses. It is essential that all children with acute onset of vomiting, diarrhoea and fever are re-evaluated regularly to confirm the diagnosis of acute gastroenteritis and adequacy of rehydration therapy. See Table 21.1 for key features of acute infectious gastroenteritis.

Paediatric Handbook, Tenth Edition. Edited by Kate Harding, Daniel S. Mason and Daryl Efron.
© 2021 John Wiley & Sons Ltd. Published 2021 by John Wiley & Sons Ltd.

Table 21.1 Acute infectious gastroenteritis.

Aetiology	Viruses: rotavirus, adenovirus, enterovirus, norovirus Bacteria (5–10%): Salmonella spp., Campylobacter jejuni, Yersinia enterocolitica, Escherichia coli Parasites: Cryptosporidium (mostly in immunocompromised host)
Clinical presentation	Diarrhoea Poor feeding Fever Vomiting Cramping abdominal pain
Red flags	Severe abdominal pain or abdominal signs Persistent diarrhoea >10 days Blood in stool Isolated vomiting without diarrhoea Bilious vomiting Very unwell
Assessment of dehydration	See Chapter 7, Fluid and Electrolytes.
Investigations	In most children **none** are required Stool culture, consider if: • Blood or mucus in stool • Significant abdominal pain • Recent overseas travel • Prolonged diarrhoea (>7 days) • Sepsis suspected • Immunocompromised child Biochemical investigations (Glucose, electrolyte and acid-base) Consider if: • A history of prolonged diarrhoea with severe dehydration • Altered conscious state • Convulsions • Short-bowel syndrome, ileostomy, chronic cardiac, renal and metabolic disorders • Infants <6 months of age who are assessed to be dehydrated • Use of fortified feeds or recent hypertonic fluids (e.g. Lucozade) • Repeated presentations
Rehydration	See Chapter 7, Fluid and Electrolytes.
Pharmacotherapy	Anti-emetic: Ondansetron (sublingual wafer) • In hospital setting, for mild-moderate vomiting to aid oral rehydration • Not for children <6 months or <8 kg • Single dose only recommended • Dose: 8–15 kg 2 mg; 15–30 kg 4 mg; >30 kg 8 mg. Anti-diarrhoeal agents are **not recommended** Antibiotics • Most bacterial infections do not require antibiotics • Salmonella or Campylobacter gastroenteritis may require antibiotic treatment • Shigella dysentery does requires antibiotic treatment

Table 21.1 (*Continued*)

Complications	Hypernatraemic dehydration (Na >150 mmol/L)
	Hyponatraemic dehydration (Na <130 mmol/L)
	Lactose intolerance:
	• Uncommon
	• Usually infants <6 months
	• Temporary due to lactase deficiency
	• Clinical features: persistently fluid stool, excessive flatus, perineal excoriation, appear well
	• Diagnosis: ≥0.75% reducing substances in the stool
	• Treatment: breastfeeding should continue (unless persistent symptoms or failure to gain weight), formula-fed infants should be placed on a lactose-free formula for 3–4 weeks
	Monosaccharide malabsorption
	• Rare, in the setting of severe bowel damage
	• Specialist consultation required
Nutritional management	Aids mucosal recovery and reduces duration of diarrhoea
	• Breastfeeding should continue through rehydration and maintenance phases
	• Formula-fed infants and children should restart formula or food intake after rehydration is complete
	• Children can have complex carbohydrates (e.g. rice, wheat, bread and cereals), yoghurt, fruit and vegetables once rehydration is complete

Children requiring admission

- Children who have moderate or severe dehydration.
- Children at high risk of dehydration on the basis of young age (<6 months) with a high frequency of diarrhoea (8 per 24 hours) and vomiting (>4 per 24 hours) should be observed for 4–6 hours to ensure adequate maintenance of hydration.
- High-risk children (e.g. ileostomy, short gut, cyanotic heart disease, chronic renal disease, metabolic disorders and malnutrition).
- If the diagnosis is in doubt.

Chronic diarrhoea

An increase in stool frequency, change in consistency or colour is often of concern to parents, but does not necessarily imply significant organic disease, although this needs to be excluded. In every child who presents with chronic diarrhoea (considered chronic if lasting >2–3 weeks), the decision must be made as to whether further investigation is required. Figure 21.1 outlines an approach to the child with chronic diarrhoea.

Toddler's diarrhoea

This is a clinical syndrome characterised by chronic diarrhoea often with undigested food in the stools of a child who is otherwise well and growing well. Stools may contain mucus and are passed 3–6 times a day; they are often looser towards the end of the day. The onset is usually between 8 and 20 months of age and resolves around 3–4 years of age. The treatment consists of reassurance and explanation. No specific drug or dietary treatment has been shown to be of value in toddler diarrhoea. Some toddlers on a high-fructose intake (fruits juices, cordials) may responds to reduced fructose intake.

Constipation

Constipation is best characterised as difficulty passing bowel motions. The Rome IV criteria define functional constipation (Table 21.2).

In most children, chronic constipation is due to functional faecal retention. Painful or fear of painful defecation are the most common triggers, leading to apprehension and a cycle of withholding and passage of hard retained stool.

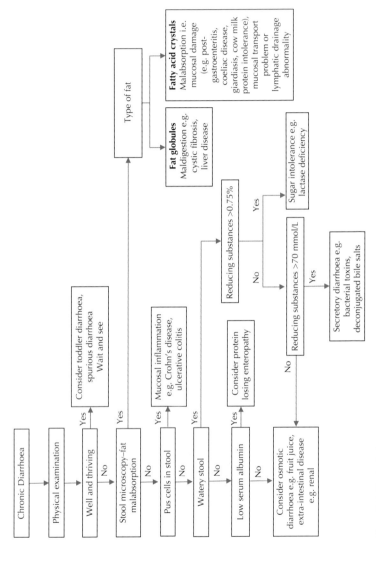

Figure 21.1 Chronic diarrhoea.

Table 21.2 Rome IV Criteria.

Rome IV criteria for functional constipation age 4 to 18 years
2 or more of the following at least once a week for a minimum of 1 months
• ≤2 stools/week
• History of painful or hard bowel movements
• History of large-diameter stools that can obstruct the toilet
• At least 1 episode per week of soiling after the acquisition of toileting skills
• History of retentive posturing or excessive volitional stool retention
• Presence of a large faecal mass in the rectum

Source: Hyams et al (2016). Childhood functional gastrointestinal disorders: child/adolescent. Gastroenterology 150: 1456–1468. Reprinted with permission of Elsevier.

Table 21.3 Organic causes of constipation.

Organic Causes Constipation	
Cow Milk Protein intolerance	Hypothyroidism
Hirschsprung disease	Hypercalcaemia
Coeliac Disease	Medications e.g. codeine
Spinal cord lesions	Anorectal malformations

Rarely (5% in some series) there is an organic cause (Table 21.3). The presence of "red flags" should prompt investigation or referral: delayed passage of meconium (beyond 48 hours), onset of constipation in the first month of life, the passage of ribbon stools, and vomiting. Low dietary fibre and poor fluid intake rarely contribute to childhood chronic constipation. Dyschezia (a healthy infant, straining and crying before passing soft stool) is normal but can be mistaken for constipation.

Faecal incontinence

Faecal incontinence (FI) or soiling is defined as the passage of stool in an inappropriate place in children over 4 years of age. In the majority it is associated with constipation.

Rarely there may be other explanations including functional nonretentive FI (i.e. not constipated), and organic causes such as neurological damage or anal sphincter anomalies.

Children with faecal incontinence may have co-morbidities including:

• Nocturnal enuresis and daytime detrusor overactivity: perhaps linked through pelvic floor dysfunction.
• Attention Deficit Hyperactivity Disorder or Autism Spectrum Disorder.
• Behavioural problems are common but may be secondary to FI rather than the cause.

The pathophysiology is likely withholding leading to chronic rectal dilatation, loss of the normal urge to pass stool and further retention. When stool leaks out with relaxation of the external anal sphincter, the child senses the passage of stool by its contact with external skin, initiating an urgent rush to the toilet and an impression that the child has 'waited until the last minute' leading to inappropriate blaming.

Assessment

A history (from both the child and parent) and examination should be performed to exclude organic causes.

• Try to identify possible precipitating event like anal fissures or other painful perianal conditions.
• Ask about soiling and associated evidence of bladder dysfunction: urinary incontinence and enuresis.

In the physical examination check lower limb motor function, abdominal examination, perianal inspection, and examination of the spine, lumbosacral region and gluteal muscles.

• Children with significant abdominal distension, neurological signs, lower back abnormalities (dimples, pigmented lesions, hair tufts), an abnormally appearing anus, or growth faltering warrant further assessment.

- Abnormal neurological findings are rare but must be investigated urgently.
- Digital rectal examination is not usually required as it will not change initial management.
- An abdominal X-ray is rarely required.
- The evidence for the role for bedside ultrasound is growing: an ultrasound rectal diameter >25–30 mm is thought to be indicative of rectal distension and retention of faeces.

Management

Management aims to keep the bowel empty and should be multimodal and maintained for a sufficient period for the child to overcome their apprehension about defecation, and for bowel sensation and function to improve. Children and their families need to understand the condition and treatment. A good therapeutic relationship with the child and their parent or carer is needed to enhance motivation, discuss ineffective interventions and provide alternatives.

Disimpaction

- Needed when there is a faecal mass unlikely to pass spontaneously.
- Initial treatment should be with a Macrogol 3350 (Movicol or Osmolax) disimpaction regime (Table 21.4).
- For children refusing oral medication: sodium sulfate (Colonlytely) 1–3 L per day, via nasogastric tube in hospital may be required. Rectal medication (suppositories or enemas) may add to the child's fearfulness.
- If using medications per rectum, consider sedation with nitrous oxide or midazolam.
- Surgical disimpaction can be considered if medical treatment fails.

Ongoing Management

A long-term approach is needed, often for months to years. The physician, child and family need to work together and design an individualised treatment plan.

Behaviour modification is the mainstay of treatment.

- This involves regular sitting on the toilet after meals up to three times a day for 3–5 minutes.
- Attention to the sitting position is important: feet supported, hips flexed and encourage 'bulging' of the abdomen.
- A diary should be kept, to record progress, with rewards focused upon effort, such as good compliance with sitting rather than clean pants.

Medications are an adjunct to a toileting regimen to facilitate passage of stools.

- Start with a single agent, either a lubricant (paraffin oil) or osmotic agents (macrogol or lactulose).
- Recommended initial doses are:
  ○ Paraffin oil 15–25 mL per day.
  ○ Movicol 1 sachet per day.
  ○ Lactulose: <12 months, 5 mL per day; 1–5 years, 10 mL per day; >5 years, 15 mL per day.
- Stimulants can be used as additional treatment: either Senokot or Bisacodyl: >4 years – 1 tablet per day (5 mg).

Long-term use of these medications does not render the bowel 'lazy' or make the child 'dependent'. Only when defecation has been effortless for months and toileting behaviour is consistent, should one try to gradually withdraw medications. Regular toileting is needed until there is return of sensation and spontaneous bowel actions. Consider referral to a sub-specialist continence clinic if combined faecal/urinary incontinence, suspected organic cause, complex or difficult cases.

Table 21.4 Dosage recommendations for disimpaction.

Age	Day 1	Day 2	Day 3	Day 4	Day 5	Day 6	Day 7
PEG 3350 + E (PAEDIATIC/JUNIOR formula – sachets)							
1–12 months	½ – 1	½ – 1	½ – 1	½ – 1	½ – 1	½ – 1	½ – 1
1–6 years	2	4	4	6	6	8	8
6–12 years	4	6	8	10	12	12	12

> **Clinical Pearl: Constipation**
> - Take time to design the regular toileting program with the child: it is the most important part of management.
> - Ask the child about their awareness of the need to defaecate and where they feel the sensation, as this may guide whether they still need active management.
> - The right laxative is the one the child will take.

Gastro-oesophageal reflux

Oesophageal reflux of gastric contents occurs normally and is more frequent after meals. Regurgitation of gastric contents is common in infancy. In most cases, this 'posseting' does not result in any adverse sequelae and the most appropriate treatment is parental reassurance. Reflux of gastric acid with heartburn may result in episodic irritability, but this is usually associated with obvious regurgitation and is rarely 'silent'. Although gastro-oesophageal reflux may cause infant distress, it is important to consider other possible causes. 'Physiological' gastro-oesophageal reflux with regurgitation usually resolves by the age of 9–15 months.

Gastro-oesophageal reflux is regarded as pathological if associated with any of the clinically significant adverse sequelae, listed below. It is important to recognise that vomiting may result from other causes, and these need to be excluded on the basis of history, physical examination and further tests if indicated. In selected cases investigations such as 24 hour oesophageal pH monitoring can be useful to correlate any episodes of reflux with irritability.

Complications

- Peptic oesophagitis: this usually correlates with an increase in the number and duration of reflux episodes. Blood-flecked vomitus and anaemia may result. May present as iron deficiency anaemia in children with developmental delay and no obvious vomiting.
- Peptic strictures: these are well recognised in childhood and present with dysphagia and failure to thrive.
- Growth failure: severe cases of gastro-oesophageal reflux may cause the loss of calories and anorexia.
- Pulmonary complications: recurrent or persistent cough and wheeze may be present and can occur without marked vomiting. These symptoms may result from aspiration of refluxed material (inhalation pneumonia) or through reflex bronchospasm. This mode of presentation requires a high degree of clinical suspicion to make the diagnosis.

Management

In the absence of signs of significant oesophagitis, aspiration or growth failure, the following should be suggested:
- Posture after feeds: the infant should be placed in a cot in the head-up position at or near 30 degrees.
- Thickened feeds: use a proprietary thickening agent or a pre-thickened formula if formula-fed.
- If cow's milk protein intolerance is considered a possible cause, a two week trial of maternal dairy exclusion or an extensively hydrolyzed formula may be indicated.

Medication

Medications are not indicated in otherwise healthy, thriving infants with frequent regurgitation. There is no conclusive evidence that antacids, alginates, H2 receptor blockers, proton pump inhibitors (PPI) or prokinetics improve symptoms in those with reflux without demonstrated complications. Medications are not without risk and if prescribed, should be given at the lowest dose for minimum intervals, given the mounting evidence of complications particularly from PPI use in adults.
- Mylanta (0.5–1.0 mL/kg per dose given 3–4 times a day). There are some concerns about its long-term use because of its mineral content.
- H_2 receptor antagonists such as ranitidine (2–3 mg/kg per dose given 2–3 times a day before meals) will reduce gastric acidity.
- Proton pump inhibitors: Omeprazole 1–4 mg/kg/day, Esomeprazole <20 kg 10 mg daily, >20 kg 20 mg daily are prescribed to infants and children with severe oesophagitis that is unresponsive to an H_2 receptor antagonist.

Surgery

A trial of post pyloric feeding may avoid the need for surgery cases where the main complication is one of growth failure. Laparoscopic fundoplication is indicated for reflux with complications when medical treatment has failed or is inappropriate. The indications include hiatal hernia, oesophageal stricture or Barrett's oesophagus, and life-threatening respiratory sequelae.

Clinical Pearl: Gastro-oesophageal reflux

Gastro-oesophageal reflux in infants is usually associated with obvious regurgitation and is rarely 'silent'. Pharmacological treatment should be reserved for those with complications such as erosive oesophagitis, growth failure, peptic strictures, or associated respiratory symptoms.

Eosinophilic oesophagitis

Eosinophilic oesophagitis (EoE) is a recently recognised eosinophilic gastrointestinal disorder affecting the oesophagus with unclear aetiology and is characterised by pan-oesophageal mucosal eosinophilia, peristaltic dysfunction (dysphagia), and progressive fibro-stenotic complications (oesophageal strictures). It is defined by histological evidence of at least 15 eosinophils per high power field on oesophageal histology, plus symptoms attributable to upper gastrointestinal dysfunction.

Clinical features

- Associated with other atopic disorders (asthma, eczema, allergic rhinitis), particularly both IgE- and non-IgE-mediated food allergies.
- Occurs in any age group, with a strong male preponderance.
- Infants/young children often present with reflux-like symptoms/regurgitation, food refusal, feeding difficulties, abdominal pain and persistent unsettled behaviour.
- Older children and adolescents typically experience dysphagia and recurrent food bolus obstruction.
- Natural history of EoE is not well documented, but generally follows a chronic relapsing course.

Diagnosis

- The diagnosis of EoE always requires a gastroscopy with multi-level oesophageal biopsies.
- A repeat biopsy after a trial of a proton pump inhibitor for 6–8 weeks is recommended to delineate EoE against so-called 'proton pump inhibitor-responsive oesophageal eosinophilia'.

Management

- Children with EoE often respond to elimination diets. Amino acid-based (elemental) diet is effective in over 90% of children, but poorly tolerated in the long term.
- Empirical elimination diets eliminate the most common food allergens in EoE (cow's milk, egg, wheat and soy). The diet is gradually liberalised, as tolerated, based on repeat gastroscopy after food challenges.
- Older children with EoE may require topical corticosteroids (swallowed fluticasone aerosol or viscous budesonide), due to high rates of dietary non-compliance.
- Newer biological agents are currently being trialed.
- In children with long-standing uncontrolled EoE, narrowing of the oesophageal lumen or strictures can develop requiring endoscopic management.

Non-IgE-mediated cow milk protein allergy

See Chapter 13, Allergy

Coeliac disease

Coeliac disease (CD) is an autoimmune enteropathy triggered by the ingestion of gluten in genetically susceptible individuals, with an approximate incidence of 1:100 in Australia. The prevalence of this disorder amongst first-degree relatives is approximately 10%. The clinical expression of this disorder is more heterogeneous than previously thought and onset may be at any time, after years without symptoms.

Screening tests

An IgA antibody to tissue transglutaminase (TTG-IgA), which is over 98% specific and sensitive, has replaced the anti-endomysial antibody test in many hospitals. False-negative results can occur with IgA-deficiency; hence, all children will require total IgA levels measured to interpret the results appropriately. At RCH, we now use the combination of the TTG-IgA and the Deamidated gliadin peptide IgG to screen for coeliac disease in suspected cases. Genetic susceptibility testing using HLA DQ2 and HLA DQ8 is best used for its negative predictive value for excluding CD, as while 50% of the population carry one or both of these genes only around 1 in 40 of these people will develop CD.

Diagnosis

A small-bowel biopsy remains the gold standard for diagnosis. Review by a paediatric gastroenterologist is recommended.

Management

A strict lifelong gluten-free diet is required. Long term outcome and avoidance of complications of coeliac disease is associated with a return of the mucosa to normal. This can be confirmed by return of both TTG-IgA and the Deamidated gliadin peptide IgG to the normal range. If this is not the case after 12 months on a strict gluten-free diet, then review and/or repeat endoscopy may be warranted.

Recurrent abdominal pain

Recurrent abdominal pain affects about 10% of school-age children. There is usually no specific identifiable cause. It is essential to take a careful history, including psychosocial details. It may be helpful to interview the parents alone, the child alone and the family together. Onset of pain after the consumption of dairy products in older children and young adolescents should be sought, as lactase deficiency can present in this manner. Constipation needs to be excluded. There may be a subgroup with migrainous abdominal pain (associated with pallor and a family history of migraine). Emotional factors, lifestyle and temperamental characteristics can modulate the child's response to pain, irrespective of its cause.

Recent evidence suggests 'Red flags' in the evaluation of chronic abdominal pain include pain localised away from the umbilicus, accompanying vomiting, diarrhoea, poor weight gain or linear growth, and pain awakening the child from sleep, PR bleeding. A thorough physical examination is essential.

Management

In the absence of an underlying cause being found, functional pain may be related to variation in the perception of visceral sensation. A detailed explanation to the child and family, and reassurance is often all that is required. Gut focused psychology or hypnotherapy by a qualified practitioner may also be of benefit.

Rectal bleeding

See Figure 21.2.

Inflammatory bowel disease (IBD)

This is a spectrum of disorders involving chronic inflammation of the entire GI tract (Crohn's disease) or restricted to the colon (Ulcerative colitis). The incidence of both these conditions has increased dramatically both worldwide and in Australian children since the 1970s.

Key features of IBD in children

- Crohn's disease can present in several ways including recurrent abdominal pain, weight loss, chronic diarrhoea, mouth ulcers and perianal disease. It may also present with isolated growth failure without any gastrointestinal symptoms.
- Ulcerative colitis is associated with bloody diarrhoea, which extends beyond the time frame of infective colitis.
- Extra-intestinal manifestations can occur in both disorders and include arthritis, erythema nodosum, hepatitis, sclerosing cholangitis and ophthalmological complications (uveitis and episcleritis).

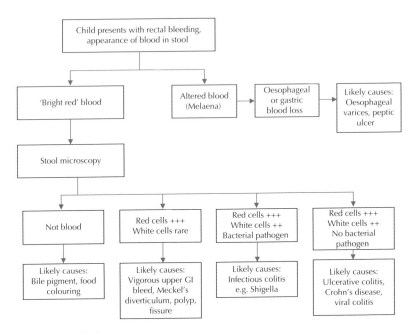

Figure 21.2 Rectal bleeding.

Diagnosis of IBD

Initial laboratory investigations should include:

- FBE (anaemia and thrombocytosis), ESR (often raised) and albumin level (low with active disease) and CRP.
- Stool microscopy (looking for WBC and RBC) and cultures for bacterial pathogens; Clostridium difficile and toxin should be collected.
- Stool calprotectin is a useful marker of gut inflammation. It **should not** be used in children under the age of 5 (as there are no robust normal levels) or when there is macroscopic blood in the stool (as calprotectin will be elevated in the presence of blood).

Management

Refer early for gastroenterological evaluation including endoscopy. Treatment paradigms including new medications and treatment targets have evolved considerably over the last 10 years. These include several new biological agents, so evaluation and management should occur under specialist guidance.

Liver disease

For causes see Table 21.5.

Liver disease in infants

There are a large number of significant and treatable conditions which present with jaundice in infancy. Successful management relies on a prompt diagnosis and early referral to a specialist.

Clinical presentation

- Jaundice (usually conjugated hyperbilirubinaemia).
- Passage of pale grey or white stools and dark tea-coloured urine.
- Hepatosplenomegaly.
- Failure to thrive.

Table 21.5 Causes of liver disease.

Mode of presentation	Time of presentation	
	Infancy	Older child
Acute	Infectious • Urinary tract infection • Bacterial sepsis • Congenital (TORCH) Biliary/obstructive • Inspissated bile • Cholelithiasis Metabolic • Galactosemia • Niemann-Pick C disease • Fatty acid oxidation defect • Mitochondrial disease Immunologic • Neonatal hemochromatosis	Infectious • Viral hepatitis (A–E) • Non A-E hepatitis Biliary/obstructive • Cholelithiasis Metabolic • Wilson disease (acute-on-chronic) Drug toxic • Paracetamol intoxication • Antibiotics, tuberculostatics, anticonvulsants, anticontraceptives
Chronic	Biliary/obstructive • Extrahepatic biliary atresia • Alagille syndrome Metabolic • α1-antitrypsin deficiency • Cystic fibrosis • Tyrosinemia type 1 • Glycogen storage disease	Biliary/obstructive • Sclerosing cholangitis (primary/secondary) Metabolic • α1-antitrypsin deficiency • Cystic fibrosis • Wilson disease • Non-alcoholic fatty liver disease Infectious • Chronic hepatitis B/C Drug toxic • Methotrexate (e.g. chemotherapy) Immunologic • Celiac disease • Autoimmune hepatitis

Source: South & Isaacs, Practical Paediatrics, 7th Edition, Elsevier: 2012. Reprinted with permission from Elsevier.

• Bleeding diathesis.
• Hypoglycaemia.
Biliary atresia is an important cause of conjugated hyperbilirubinaemia which presents with jaundice in the first 4–6 weeks of life. Infants may appear well on clinical examination, with conservation of growth. Stools are usually acholic (pale white). If untreated, biliary atresia is fatal, however, the natural history of this condition can be modified by early surgery (Kasai portoenterostomy). A rapid work up as per Figure 21.3 and urgent surgical referral is required so that surgery can occur as early as possible and preferably before 7 weeks of age.

Other important causes of conjugated hyperbilirubinaemia, many of which may have dire consequences if not recognised or treated adequately, include congenital infections, galactosaemia, tyrosinaemia, fructosaemia and hypothyroidism. Unconjugated hyperbilirubinaemia may be due to breast milk jaundice, haemolysis (immune or breakdown of a haematoma) or rare inherited conjugation defects (Figure 21.3).

Liver disease in children

Important causes of liver disease in children include autoimmune hepatitis, α1-antitrypsin deficiency, viral hepatitis (hepatitis A, B, C, EBV, CMV), non-alcoholic steatohepatitis, Wilson disease and drug-induced. Children may present with a history of jaundice, dark urine, pale stools, pruritus, abdominal pain or abnormal liver function

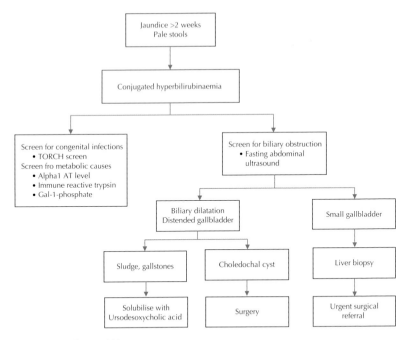

Figure 21.3 Liver disease in children.

tests found incidentally. The clinical signs of chronic liver disease include spider naevi, palmar erythema, dilated abdominal veins and splenomegaly.

Investigations
- Viral serology as above
- Autoantibodies (ANA, LKM, SMA)
- Serum copper and caeruloplasmin
- Iron studies
- α1-antitrypsin level and Pi type
- Liver ultrasound

In general, prompt specialist consultation is required, as both acute and chronic liver disease require urgent investigation and treatment.

Clinical Pearl: Conjugated hyperbilirubinaemia

Conjugated hyperbilirubinaemia in infancy requires close examination for pale stools. If present early referral and rapid evaluation for possible biliary atresia is essential, as early surgical intervention has been shown to improve outcome.

Pancreatitis

Acute pancreatitis has a variable presentation in children and symptoms may range from mild abdominal pain to severe systemic involvement with accompanying metabolic disturbances and shock. The pain is commonly in the epigastrium but may also be in the right and left upper quadrant. Back pain is an uncommon feature in children, unlike in adults. Other accompanying features may include vomiting, anorexia and nausea. Pancreatitis should be considered in children with complex disability, presenting with irritability. The aetiology of pancreatitis

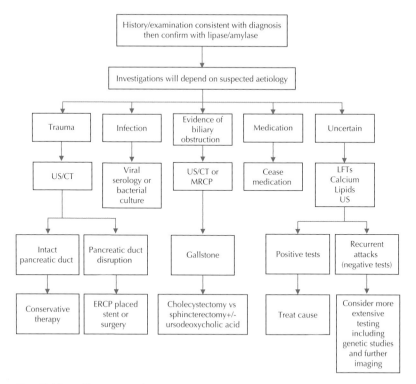

Figure 21.4 Pancreatitis assessment and management.

in children includes biliary disease, trauma, systemic disease and drug-induced, however up to 1/3 of cases are idiopathic. Genetic factors may contribute to acute recurrent presentations. The diagnosis is based on clinical symptoms and signs, accompanied by a threefold increase above the normal range, in either amylase or lipase – serum lipase having greater sensitivity and specificity (Figure 21.4).

Management
Is primarily supportive and aims at limiting exocrine pancreatic secretion and managing pain. Most mild to moderate cases will settle with bowel rest, IV fluids and analgesia, with early reintroduction of enteral nutrition depending on clinical progress. In children with recurrent attacks and/or a complicated course, specialist input is recommended.

Gastrostomy care and problems
Gastrostomies are now used frequently to nourish children who are either unable to eat or are at risk of aspiration from oral feeding. During a percutaneous endoscopically placed gastrostomy tubes (PEGs), the initial gastrostomy tube is usually long and is subsequently replaced by a low profile device or 'button'. If a gastrostomy is formed during a surgical procedure, a button is commonly placed initially. Most buttons require changing every 4 to 6 months and certain types may be replaced in an outpatient setting by suitably qualified staff or parents.

Common issues with gastrostomy tubes and their management are listed in the Table 21.6. It is best to consult with a gastroenterologist, surgeon or stoma nurse experienced in the care of these tubes as inappropriate management can be fatal.

Table 21.6 Gastrostomy tube management.

Problem	Causes	Clinical features	Management

Blocked tube	• Poorly crushed medications
	• Not flushing gastrostomy tube when feeds are completed
	• Feed too thick or containing lumps of powder
	• Vitamised food being put down tube
		Unable to pass feed	• Check device location
			• Flush with 10–20ml:
			  o Warm water
			  o Carbonated drink e.g. mineral water or diet cola
			• Try to aspirate blockage with a syringe

Peristomal skin excoriation	Leaking of gastric secretions	Erythematous, irritated, swollen, weeping skin around the gastrostomy	• Barrier ointment (do not use zinc-based product if fungal infection suspected) • Gastric acid suppression e.g. proton pump inhibitor Dressings: • Foam dressing, gauze or Sofwick to absorb ooze • Topical magnesium and aluminium hydroxide preparations (e.g. Mylanta) • Hydrocolloid powder to stop bleeding and absorb moisture • A thin hydrocolloid dressing to protect and aid skin healing
Infection at skin site	Usually staphylococcal infection, can be fungal (candida) or involve enteric organisms	Erythema, swelling, tenderness and weeping at insertion site	• Take swab if discharge present • If cellulitis present: oral or IV antibiotics e.g. flucloxacillin • Topical antifungal e.g. clotrimazole or nystatin
Granulation tissue	Tube movement may contribute, usually occurs around 6 weeks post-surgery	Vascular tissue growth at insertion site with bleeding	• Foam dressing to apply pressure • Silver nitrate application (to granulation only) • Kenacomb ointment • Review device for size and movement
Migration of tube out of stomach wall	Infection Trauma Pressure necrosis	Enlargement of entry site; visible retention device; pain, swelling, erythema, peristomal leak, and tenderness; peritonitis	Urgent Gastroenterology or Surgical referral
Migration of tube towards pylorus	Insertion site close to gastric outlet Scoliosis	Vomiting and gagging, feed intolerance, peristomal leak	Referral to Gastroenterology or Surgery Run feeds continuously

USEFUL RESOURCES
- The RCH Constipation clinical practice guideline www.rch.org.au/clinicalguide/guideline_index/Constipation/
- The Raising children network Encopresis http://raisingchildren.net.au/articles/encopresis.html
- The Raising children network Constipation http://raisingchildren.net.au/articles/constipation.html
- The RCH kids health info Constipation https://www.rch.org.au/kidsinfo/fact_sheets/Constipation/
- Australian Medicines Handbook (AMH) Children's Dosing Companion January 2018 https://childrens.amh.net.au

CHAPTER 22

Gynaecology

Sonia R. Grover
Charlotte V. Elder

Key Points

- Many gynaecological concerns relate to common physiological events and changes.
- Cyclical symptoms that impact on a young person's daily functioning and quality of life are not acceptable and need treatment even though they may be physiological. Missing school or activities because of pain, bleeding or fatigue on a regular basis is not appropriate.
- Whilst benign vulval conditions are common, sexual abuse should be considered and excluded in girls presenting with vulval conditions.
- Ovarian torsion needs to be considered and excluded in girls and adolescents presenting with acute lower abdominal pain (especially if associated with vomiting and dizziness).
- Hypothalamic hypogonadism due to low weight, excess exercise or stress is a common cause of irregular menses or amenorrhea in teens.

Paediatric conditions
Ovarian cysts
Ovarian cysts can be detected antenatally and are likely to be physiological. Follow-up ultrasounds postnatally usually demonstrate reduction in size and resolution. Torsion can occur and should be suspected if there is development of complex changes in a previously documented simple ovarian cyst, in the setting of an unsettled baby.

Labial adhesions
Usually occur in late infancy once the low childhood levels of oestrogens are achieved after mini-puberty. Often resolve by late childhood, may persist through to puberty, but will resolve around the time of menarche under the influence of oestrogen. The adhesions occur secondary to adherence of the atrophic surfaces of the labia minora, presumably as a result of irritation.
Management:
- Uncomplicated labial adhesions do not require any intervention
- Lateral traction to separate the labia is distressing and associated with recurrence, whilst treatment with topical oestrogen is unnecessary with associated risk of breast development secondary to systemic oestrogen absorption.
- Refer only if recurrent UTIs.

Vulvovaginitis
This is the most common gynaecological problem in prepubertal girls. The vagina is relatively atrophic due to the low oestrogen levels. The normal flora is bowel flora. Subtle overgrowth or alteration of this flora results in a discharge which is irritant to the atrophic labial skin causing a reddened appearance. The moist environment between the opposing skin surfaces may also be exacerbated by urine, particularly in obese girls.

Paediatric Handbook, Tenth Edition. Edited by Kate Harding, Daniel S. Mason and Daryl Efron.
© 2021 John Wiley & Sons Ltd. Published 2021 by John Wiley & Sons Ltd.

Presentation:
- Erythema/irritation of the contact skin between the labial surfaces, burning/pain with micturition, itch and offensive vaginal discharge.

Management:
- Simple measures – barrier creams to protect the atrophic skin.
- Bathing daily (with the addition of vinegar or bicarbonate of soda to change the vaginal pH and flora.
- Avoidance of irritants such as soaps.
- Do not take vaginal swabs – they are distressing and painful.
- Take an introital swab if there is profuse discharge when an overgrowth of one organism may be present (e.g. group A streptococcus).
- A vulval swab is appropriate where there is marked skin inflammation beyond the labial contact surfaces when likely to be a skin infection with streptococcus or staphylococcus.
- Thrush (candida infection) is rare in prepubertal girls as it thrives in an oestrogenised environment.
- Natural history: symptoms fluctuate over time – until the onset of puberty.

Vaginal bleeding
Causes in children include:
- Neonatal bleeding caused by the fall in maternal oestrogen levels.
- Vulvovaginitis.
- Trauma (including straddle injury and sexual assault).
- Vaginal foreign body; persistent vaginal discharge (often blood-stained)
- Urogenital tumours (vaginal bleeding or mass).
- Urethral prolapse may present as 'vaginal bleeding'. The red prolapsed tissue at the site of the urethra is diagnostic. Treatment is with topical oestrogen.
- Lichen sclerosis with skin splits can cause vulval bleeding.

Straddle Injury
Unfortunately, straddle or 'fall astride' injuries are fairly common.
Assessment:
- History – time, mechanism, blood loss, other injuries, witnesses, voiding since the accident
- Examination – aim to only do once, use sedation if required
- Minor injury – can visualise the complete wound, bleeding ceased, voiding successfully
Red flags for major injury:
- Unable to visualise the entire wound
- Expanding haematoma
- Anal or rectal involvement
- Ongoing bleeding despite ice and pressure with clean gauze
- Significant labia minora tear
Management:
- Minor; analgesia, salt baths, topical anaesthetic or barrier cream, avoid strenuous activity.
- Major; gynaecological referral, likely examination and repair under general anaesthetic, if anal or urethral involvement may required urology or general surgical input

Vulval itch
Causes include:
- Eczema. If this occurs elsewhere on the body, this can be superimposed on the symptoms of vulvovaginits. Treatment is then as for vulvovaginits + topical steroids.
- Threadworms (particularly if nocturnal itch).
- Lichen sclerosis. Whitened skin changes with associated splitting, blistering and resorption of labial skin. Referral to a specialist is appropriate, treatment is with topical steroids.

Vaginal pain
Nocturnal vaginal pain usually occurs due to 'lost' threadworms in the vagina. Movement of the worms on the sensitive hymen and introital area cause a shooting vaginal pain. Treatment includes repeated doses of pyrantel or mebendazole to ensure clearance of the worms and their eggs.

Vulval pain

Vulvodynia can occur in any age group and often does not have a precipitating cause. Allodynia of the vulva to light touch with a cotton bud is diagnostic and systemic or topical amytriptylline usually provides relief. Urinary urgency and frequency are often found in association with vulval pain, but also respond to systemic amytriptylline.

Clinical Pearl: A practical and sensitive approach to female genital examination
- Explain why the examination has to occur and ensure privacy and lighting prior to commencing
- For those in nappies, framing the examination as a nappy change with you standing beside the parent doing the nappy change is generally not distressing for the child or parent.
- For young children, ask the parent to get them undressed and then distract the child by letting them play with the bed controller or giving them a pair of gloves to put on. Often the examination is finished by the time the child has worked out how to put on one of the gloves!
- To examine the vulva, lateral traction on the buttocks or upper thighs generally gives a very good view of the vulva and lower vagina without needing to directly touch the genitals

---

Adolescent Conditions

Clinical Pearl: Puberty related medical exacerbations
The onset of puberty may be associated with the onset of a range of problems – often apparently not "gynaecological". These problems include migraines, mood disturbance, and cyclic exacerbations of pre-existing conditions such as poor diabetes control, seizure disorders, worsening of gastrointestinal conditions, POTS, chronic fatigue and chronic pain symptoms, and nausea/vomiting. These cyclical problems are often prostaglandin/cytokine mediated. Management should follow the same principles as management of other menstrual disorders, namely cyclic NSAIDs and/or menstrual suppression. Cyclical symptoms can commence prior to menarche.

Anatomy
Labia

There is a large variation in appearance of the post pubertal vulva, and the current fashion for pubic hair removal means that labial appearance is more noticeable than for previous generations. At puberty, the labia minora lengthen and darken first, followed by enlargement of the labia majora, then mons. In slim young women the labia majora and mons will often remain fairly flat for a number of years post menarche which can make the labia minora appear more prominent. Asymmetrical labia minora are common and not pathological. Young women who present with concerns about labial appearance can be reassured using the photographic resources from the online 'Labia Library'. It is important to respond sensitively to these concerns as issues regarding genital appearance can greatly impact on self-esteem. Labiaplasty is not indicated in the adolescent population.

Hymens

The majority of young women have a thin, stretchy fold of skin around the circumference of their vaginal entrance. Some young women will have thick, tight hymenal skin (annular hymen) or an obstructing mesh or band of tissue across the vaginal entrance. This may require surgical excision to allow passage of menses, tampon use and/or penetrative intercourse. Isolated hymenal bands often allow the introduction of a tampon, but removal of a full tampon is not possible due to the larger size. If a young woman presents with a retained tampon from a hymenal band, it should be managed with excision of the band (often under GA). Difficulty using tampons may reflect vestibulodynia (pain localised around the outer hymenal ring) or be a marker of more generalised vulval pain. The hymen does not particularly change appearance after penetrative intercourse in a post pubertal female. In general, hymenal skin does not tear or bleed with penetrative intercourse in the presence of adequate lubrication, pelvic floor relaxation and non-forceful penetration.

Ovarian Cysts

- Most ovarian cysts are physiological. Ultrasound report descriptions of physiological cysts include follicle, corpus luteum and simple cyst and these are mostly in in the 3–5 cm range. A simple cyst up to 8cm will likely spontaneously resolve and repeat scanning in 3 months can be performed for reassurance.
- Multifollicular ovarian morphology is normal in adolescence (up to 25 follicles).
- Ovarian dermoid cysts have a typical appearance on ultrasound and are non-malignant. Surgical excision (by ovarian cystectomy with conservation of the ovarian tissue) is indicated if they are larger than 3cm as there is a risk of ovarian torsion.
- Haemorrhagic cysts can cause pain but in general supportive management with analgesia and tranexamic acid is all that is required. Recurrent haemorrhagic corpus luteum cysts may indicate a bleeding diathesis.

Menstrual problems
Heavy menstrual bleeding

- Heavy menstrual bleeding is a common and often distressing symptom.
- It may occur as a result of anovulation (particularly in the first few years post menarche), anticoagulant use, or bleeding diatheses.
- Rarer causes include pregnancy related causes and endometritis secondary to chlamydia.

Assessment includes menstrual history:
- Date of menarche
- Frequency, regularity and length of periods
- Heaviness of loss (number of pads, passage and size of clots); heavy loss usually includes changing pads more frequently than 2 hourly, or overnight changes or overflow.
- Bleeding history (bruising, epistaxis, gum bleeds, painful ovulation/mittleschmertz, post-operative bleeding and family history of bleeding).
- Assess if sexually active (see HEADSS screening chapter 12 Adolescent medicine).

Investigations include:
- FBE
- Iron studies
- Consider further haematological testing for underlying bleeding disorder;
  - Coagulation studies, Von willebrand's screen, PFA-100 / platelet aggregometory,
- If sexually active β-HCG (for pregnancy-related heavy bleeding, ectopic pregnancy or miscarriage) and Chlamydia PCR urine

Management:
- Iron supplements if required.
- Non-steroidal anti-inflammatory drugs (reduce menstrual loss by 30%).
- Tranexamic acid (antifibrinolytic agent, reduce menstrual loss by 50%).
- Oral contraceptive pill. This can be used continuously to skip menses, or used cyclically with tranexamic acid.
- Depot medroxyprogesterone acetate.
- Continous or cyclical oral progestogens such as norethisterone or medroxyprogestone acetate.
- Levonorgestrel intrauterine system (reduces menstrual loss by 95% and requires a general anaesthetic for insertion in non-sexually active adolescents).

Irregular menses
- The interval between periods is accepted as normal if there are eight periods/year or the interval is between 21–35 days.
- In the first 1–4 years post menarche, it is within normal limits to have irregular periods due to anovulation and this is not an indication for further investigation.
- The normal range for period duration is 1–8 days.

Clinical Pearl: Common questions and answers about hormonal therapies

Is it safe or 'natural' to use the pill or other hormones to skip my periods?
Yes. Skipping periods is quite safe. Pregnant women do not have a period for nine months and breastfeeding women may not have a period for up to two years, depending on how often they breastfeed their baby. It is quite natural to **not** have a period every month. It is common for those who have many babies and who breastfeed their babies for extended lengths of time to have less than 50 periods in their lifetime. Some young women find they get break through bleeding with extended cycles, in which case having a bleed every 3–4 months might make the bleed more predictable. Trialling an alternate OCP may also work.

Will having a hormone secreting IUD make me not a virgin?
No, having sex is the only thing that can make someone 'not a virgin'(!). An IUD is inserted through the vagina and does not require any incisions.

Will the Pill give me cancer?
The rates of some cancers are lower, and some are higher in people who have used the OCP. Lifetime rates of ovarian and bowel cancer are lower in people who have used OCPs and rates of breast cancer are slightly higher in people *whilst* they are actively taking OCPs. Rates of cervical cancer are similar in OCP users and non-users – the main risk factor for cervical cancer is the HPV virus. Given the rate of breast cancer is very low in adolescents, from a cancer perspective, using the OCP during the teens or 20s is the optimal time.

Will the Pill give me a clot?
Deep Vein Thrombosis (DVT) rates are around 3:10,000 per year in the adult female population, around 6–7:10,000 in people on the OCP and around 30:10,000 in pregnancy; meaning that from a DVT perspective it is much less likely to occur whilst on the OCP than when pregnant. Most OCP related DVTs occur in the first six months. OCP users should be advised to present for care if they have shortness of breath, leg pain or leg swelling.

Amenorrhoea
Primary amenorrhoea
See Table 22.1.

Clinical Pearl: The adolescent with reproductive diagnoses
The management of adolescents with significant reproductive diagnoses (gonadal dysgenesis, ovarian insufficiency, uterovaginal agenesis, androgen insensitivity syndrome) requires a sensitive approach and recognition of the significant impact of the diagnosis on future fertility/infertility. Referral to a specialist familiar with these issues is recommended.

Secondary amenorrhoea
Causes of secondary amenorrhoea include:
- Hormonal causes – as listed above
- Overweight /obesity
- Pregnancy
- Strenuous exercise
- Stress (e.g. exams, social/family or travel)
- Polycystic ovary syndrome (PCOS)

Management involves treatment of symptoms as required:
- Amenorrhoea itself does not need treatment, but associated problems may require intervention.
- Oligomenorrhoea may require treatment on its own merits (heavy, painful, unpredictable).
- Eating disorder: diagnose and treat.
- Excess exercise/physical or psychological stress: advise on healthy exercise, manage underlying medical disorder, stress management strategies.

Paediatric Handbook

Table 22.1 Important causes & classifications of primary amenorrhoea.

WITH NO OR LIMITED SECONDARY SEXUAL CHARACTERISTICS

Central/hypothalamic causes	Underweight/over exercising	eg. Anorexia, elite athlete
	Secondary to a medical condition	eg Crohn's disease
Pituitary causes	Hyperprolactinaemia	
	Thyroid disease	
	Panhypopituitarism	
	Post irradiation	
Ovarian failure	Gonadal dysgenesis	Often XO or XY karyotype
	Premature ovarian insufficiency	Elevated FSH on two separate occasions

WITH NORMAL PUBERTAL PROGRESSION

Obstructive anomalies (Often cyclical pain)	Imperforate hymen	Bulging hymen should be visible with gentle suprapubic pressure
	Transverse septum	Often US diagnosis
	Obstructive cervical anomaly	Often US diagnosis
	Uterovaginal agenesis	Absent uterus on ultrasound, XX karyotype.

WITH ATYPICAL PUBERTAL PROGRESSION

Adrenal causes	Poorly controlled congenital adrenal hyperplasia (CAH)	Virilising features including excess hair, often early puberty, elevated 17-OH progesterone
	Late onset CAH	+/-Virilising features including excess hair, often early puberty, elevated 17-OH progesterone
Absent hormone receptor	Androgen insensitivity syndrome	XY karyotype, absent uterus on ultrasound, no/ minimal pubic & axillary hair

- Address obesity: this can significantly improve the irregular menses, and hirsutism.
- Hirsutism responds to the oral contraceptive pill due to improved oestrogen levels. This may be further aided by an oral contraceptive pill containing cyproterone acetate (an antiandrogen). This initiates withdrawal bleeds, which are lighter and more regular.
- Pregnancy: the identification of a pregnant adolescent should alert the clinician to other high risk behaviours associated with sexual activity in young people. A HEADSS screen should be performed and screening for chlamydia infection and other STIs. Appropriate referral for discussion of pregnancy options is required.
- Infertility: irregular ovulation may impede fertility. Specialist advice is recommended when planning conception.
- Osteopenia: prolonged amenorrhoea associated with low oestrogen levels can potentially lead to a negative effect on bone mineral density. The addition of hormonal treatment may then be indicated.

Clinical Controversy: Polycystic ovary syndrome (PCOS) in adolescence

The international diagnostic criteria were developed in adult women, not adolescents and require at least two of irregular menses, multiple follicles found on pelvic ultrasound, and signs of excess androgen (severe acne and/or hirstutism). The diagnosis of PCOS (particularly in adolescents) can be difficult as normal variants overlap. Many teenagers who have multiple follicles on pelvic ultrasound are inappropriately told they have PCOS. Multiple follicles (20–25 or "multifollicular" on ultrasound report) are completely normal in this age group and many adolescents have irregular menses in the first 1–3 years after menarche due to immaturity of the hypothalamic-pituitary–ovarian axis. There is little benefit from a label of PCOS and there is a risk of unplanned pregnancy when contraception is stopped or not used due to perceived infertility. Obesity is a common association with PCOS but should be treated on its own merits in adolescence.

Menstrual related pain/dysmenorrhea

Period pain is very common in adolescents. There are a number of potential causes:

- Prostaglandin-related dysmenorrhea
- Retrograde bleeding
- Congenital urogenital anomalies
- Endometriosis

Assessment: the pattern of pain may give clues to the underlying cause:

- Pain may begin a few days prior to menses (when the inflammatory processes associated with provoking endometrial shedding begin). Maximal pain is usually just before or on the first few days of menses.
- Pain may radiate to thighs and low back.
- Associated symptoms such as nausea, vomiting, diarrhoea, lethargy, fainting and dizziness may support a diagnosis of prostaglandin-related dysmenorrhea (predominantly a clinical diagnosis).
- Stress will often precipitate more severe episodes of dysmenorrhoea.
- Pain can also occur due to retrograde bleeding which occurs in >90% of menstruating women. Free fluid (blood) in the peritoneal cavity may cause symptoms of peritoneal irritation such as pain with movement, voiding and defecation.
- Pain due to an obstructive anomaly usually increases with each cycle and typically is worse towards the end of the period.
- Vaginal examination is not done if the young woman is not sexually active, and even then only with careful consent. Occasionally, vaginal examination in young women who are using tampons may be possible, but alternatives such as a transabdominal pelvic ultrasound examination will usually provide all the required information to diagnose an obstructive anomaly.

Management:

- Prophylactic non-steroidal anti-inflammatory drugs and/or tranexamic acid.
- The oral contraceptive pill will reduce menstrual loss and pain: can be used continuously to skip menses.
- If an obstructive anomaly is identified, corrective surgical intervention may be required.
- Other treatment options include:
  - Depot medroxyprogesterone acetate to suppress menses.
  - Levonorgestrel intrauterine system (Mirena IUS).
  - Etonorgestrel implant (may reduce menstrual loss, although may cause irregular bleeding in 30%).
  - Oral progestogens such as norethisterone or medroxyprogesterone acetate (non-contraceptive).

Endometriosis

Endometriosis is usually caused by retrograde bleeding and is more common in women with heavy menstrual loss. Reducing menstrual loss will reduce the amount of retrograde bleeding.
Management includes:

- Symptom management and menstrual suppression.
- Surgery is usually to be avoided; there is no evidence that an early laparoscopy will alter long-term outcome.

Sexual health

- Respectful inquiry about a young person's sexual health may identify individuals who are at risk because of unsafe sexual relationships and offers the opportunity for sexual health education.
- Adolescents, both male and female, who are sexually active at a young age are also more likely to be involved in other health risk behaviours and careful screening for these is appropriate. An initial screen can be done using HEADSS. Remind the young person that the discussion and any tests are confidential.
- It is important to understand the legal context of sexual intercourse in minors. For example, in Victoria, statutory rape refers to sexual intercourse when a person is under 16 years old and has sexual intercourse (consensual or not) with someone who is 2 years older.
- Do not assume knowledge regarding sexual activity, safe sex and contraception.
- Be opportunistic and discuss immunisation (e.g. HPV vaccine), contraceptive options, STI prevention and PAP smears.
- Chlamydia screening is recommended annually for sexually active young people.

Contraception

Clinical Pearl: Counselling on contraceptive options

Traditionally contraceptive counselling progressed from the simplest to the most complex option (condoms – OCP – implants – IUD) which meant that young people were presented with the least efficacious option first. Long Active Reversible Contraceptives (LARCs) are more effective that traditional contraception, easy to use, cheap, well tolerated and acceptable to young people. When contraceptives are offered from most to least effective, LARC is more likely to be used. Condom use should always be recommended together with LARCs as they provide superior STI protection.

Condoms
Condoms offer the advantage of protection from STIs, as well as fairly good contraception. They may not be a reliable form of contraception if alcohol and drug-taking are issues.

Long Acting Reversible Contraceptives
- Etonorgestrel implant: hormonal implant inserted under the skin in the upper arm. Very effective contraception that lasts 3 years. Often associated with a reduction in menstrual loss, although irregular periods occur in up to 30% of young women. Amenorrhoea occurs in 20%.
- Mirena IUD: very reliable, lasts 5 years. Associated with reduced menstrual loss and reduced period pain. May require a GA for insertion. Removal NOT required if infection with chlamydia occurs.
- Copper IUD: very reliable, lasts 5 or 10 years. Associated with increased menstrual loss and pain which can be reduced with strict regular NSAIDs during periods. Needs removal if infection with chlamydia occurs
- Depo Provera: a 150 mg, 3-monthly injection. This often causes irregular bleeding initially but amenorrhoea after 6–9 months. Very reliable contraception. Long-term usage in teenagers may have some impact on bone density although this appears to be reversible.

Oral Contraceptive Pill
Contraindications
- Thromboembolic disease
- Liver disease
- Oestrogen-dependent tumours
- Migraines with neurological signs
  Note: Migraines can be oestrogen-induced (onset with commencement of OCP) or secondary to oestrogen withdrawal (onset with menses) in which case menses should be avoided through continuous use of the OCP.

Short-term side effects
- Nausea; this tends to settle, although a lower oestrogen dose pill is an alternative option.
- Breast tenderness.
- Mood-related problems may relate to the type of progestagen. Altering the oral contraceptive pill to adjust the progestagenic component may help.
- Breakthrough bleeding (this should resolve with continuing usage or change of pill type).

Types
- Constant dose (e.g. Microgynon 30ED and Noramin): for the patient who suffers erratic, heavy periods, premenstrual moodiness or irregular lifestyle routines (greater leeway in the time of taking such pills).
- Higher oestrogen content: if using anticonvulsants or if there is persistent breakthrough bleeding.
- Progesterone-only pill: Not often used in adolescents as it is less reliable and must be taken at the same time every day to be effective.

Emergency Contraception
Prostinor 2 (levonorgestrel 75 mcg, 2 tablets).
- Take both tablets at once, as soon as possible after intercourse.
- Available over the counter.
- Can be used up to 72 hours after unprotected intercourse. Some evidence for use up to 5–7 days, although with reduced efficacy.

Ulipristal acetate
• Selective progesterone receptor modulator used for emergency contraception
• Requires doctor's prescription
• More effective than postinor if intercourse occurred very close to ovulation and in women with a high BMI

Copper IUD
• Insertion of a copper IUD within 5 days of unprotected intercourse will give both emergency and ongoing contraception but in practice is hard to access
• These treatments are >90% effective, but do not provide continuing contraception.
• It is essential to plan ongoing contraception, STI prevention, PAP smears and follow-up strategies to ensure that the emergency treatment has worked.

Pelvic Inflammatory disease
Common causative organisms of Pelvic Inflammatory disease (PID) include Neisseria gonorrhoea, chlamydia, coliforms, Gardnerella vaginalis, Haemophilus influenzae, group B Streptococcus and Bacteroides species.
Assessment:
• Consider PID in any sexually active young woman with pelvic pain.
• Often associated with vaginal discharge, dyspareunia and fever.
• Non-sexually acquired PID can occur in immunocompromised individuals or secondary to another pelvic source such as appendicitis.
Investigations:
• Endocervical and high vaginal swabs for culture and PCR. (Consider blood cultures if febrile).
• If unable to do speculum – urine PCR for chlamydia and gonorrhoea.
Management:
• Broad spectrum antibiotics
• Admission for IV antibiotics if febrile.

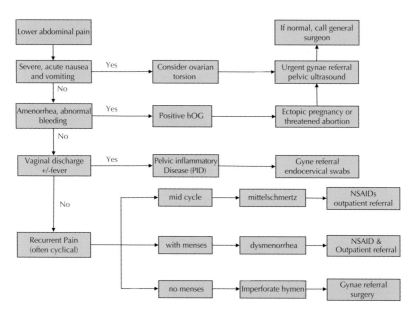

Figure 22.1 Diagnostic & treatment algorithm for acute gynaecological (lower abdominal) pain. *Source*: Royal Children's Hospital Clinical Practice Guidelines – Adolescent Gynaecology lower abdominal pain. Reproduced with the permission of the Royal Children's Hospital.

Acute Gynaecological Pain

Acute lower abdominal pain in an adolescent female may have a gynaecological, genitourinary, musculoskeletal or bowel cause (Figure 22.1).

- Ovarian torsion is the most important gynaecological cause of sudden onset acute lower abdominal pain and must be actively excluded.
- Surgical management for ovarian torsion involves laparoscopy, detorsion of the ovary and possibly removal of an ovarian cyst. Oophorectomy is NEVER indicated for ovarian torsion, regardless of ovarian appearance as functional recovery is possible even after many hours of torsion. (The rare exception to this is if the ovary is completely avulsed.)

USEFUL RESOURCES
- Royal Children's hospital clinical practice guideline on prepubescent gynaecology https://www.rch.org.au/clinicalguide/guideline_index/Prepubescent_gynaecology/
- Royal Children's hospital clinical practice guideline on menorrhagia https://www.rch.org.au/clinicalguide/guideline_index/Adolescent_Gynaecology_Menorrhagia/
- Royal Children's hospital clinical practice guideline on lower abdominal pain https://www.rch.org.au/clinicalguide/guideline_index/Adolescent_Gynaecology_Lower_Abdominal_Pain/
- Royal Children's hospital clinical practice guideline on sexually transmitted infections https://www.rch.org.au/clinicalguide/guideline_index/Sexually_transmitted_infections_STIs/
- Royal Children's hospital clinical practice guideline on vulval ulcers https://www.rch.org.au/clinicalguide/guideline_index/Vulval_ulcers/

CHAPTER 23

Haematology

Helen Savoia
Luisa Clucas
Gemma Crighton
Sally Campbell
Anthea Greenway
Paul Monagle

Key Points

- Iron deficiency (ID) is the most common cause of anaemia in children and serum ferritin is the most useful screening test for assessing iron stores. In most instances, iron deficiency anaemia and ID can be treated effectively with oral iron supplements.
- Consider B12 deficiency in any child with failure to thrive or neurodevelopmental abnormalities (particularly developmental regression) and an associated haematological abnormality (any cytopenia, macrocytosis or hypersegmented neutrophils). Urgent treatment may be required because of the potential for rapid neurological deterioration (seizures, apnoea, choreoathetosis) and the lack of reversibility if treatment is delayed.
- In children with haemophilia and suspected active bleeding, assessment and investigation should not delay factor replacement.
- ITP is characterised by an isolated low platelet count, in a well child with no concerning features on clinical history or examination and a normal FBE and film. Alternate causes for petechiae and purpura need to be excluded with a thorough history and examination. Most children who present with ITP, without moderate or severe bleeding, can be managed conservatively.
- The decision to give a RBC transfusion should not be dictated by Hb concentration alone, but on assessment of the child's underlying condition, signs and symptoms, cause of anaemia and consideration of the appropriateness of alternative therapies. A restrictive transfusion strategy is suggested, including in children who are critically ill.

Anaemia

Anaemia is a common blood condition where the body doesn't have enough red bloods cells or Haemoglobin (Hb). This is defined as a Hb level less than the 2.5th percentile for age (Table 23.1). In Australia, the prevalence of anaemia in children under the age of 5 years is between 5- 10%. Normal Hb values vary with age, ethnicity and sex, and results should be interpreted in relation to paediatric age and gender specific reference ranges.

Clinical features suggestive of anaemia

- Pale skin and pale conjunctivae
- Irritability
- Poor concentration
- Lethargy

Paediatric Handbook, Tenth Edition. Edited by Kate Harding, Daniel S. Mason and Daryl Efron.
© 2021 John Wiley & Sons Ltd. Published 2021 by John Wiley & Sons Ltd.

Table 23.1 Lower limit of normal Hb range by age.

Age	Lower limit of normal range Hb (g/L)	
2 months	90	
2 – 6 months	95	
6 – 24 months	105	
2 – 11 years	115	
> 12 years	Female 120	Male 130

- Reduced exercise tolerance
- Dizziness
- Shortness of breath
- Tachycardia, cardiac murmur or signs of cardiac failure
- Bleeding symptoms
- Signs of haemolysis – including jaundice, scleral icterus, splenomegaly and dark urine.
- In neonates, anaemia may be associated with poor weight gain, apnoea and respiratory distress.

The main causes of anaemia
- Loss of red blood cells from bleeding or iatrogenic causes
- Decreased red cell production
  - Haematinic deficiency such as iron, vitamin B12 or folate deficiency
  - Disorders of haemoglobin synthesis or structure e.g. thalassaemia or sickle cell disease
  - Chronic kidney disease due to decreased production of erythropoietin
  - Bone marrow infiltration due to tumour or leukaemia
  - Bone marrow failure due to genetic bone marrow failure syndromes, aplastic anaemia, transient erythro-blastopenia of childhood (TEC) or secondary to infection, metabolic disorders, chemotherapy, radiation or medications
  - Anaemia of prematurity
- Increased red blood cell destruction
  - Haemolysis
    - Red cell enzyme defects – e.g. G6PD deficiency
    - Red cell membrane defects – e.g. hereditary spherocytosis
    - Red cell alloimmunisation.
  - Mechanical destruction due to mechanical values or splenomegaly

History
The evaluation of a child with anaemia requires a detailed history outlining:
- Symptoms of anaemia
- Past medical history
- Family history
- Ethnicity
- Dietary history
- Medication history
- Developmental and growth history.

Investigations
If anaemia is suspected the initial investigations should include an FBE with review of the blood film, reticulocyte count and ferritin. Anaemia is usually classified based on the size of the red bloods cells as measured by the mean corpuscular volume (MCV) and is categorised as microcytic (small in size), normocytic (normal in size) or macrocytic (large in size). See Figure 23.1.

Treatment
Anaemia treatment should be directed to the specific cause.

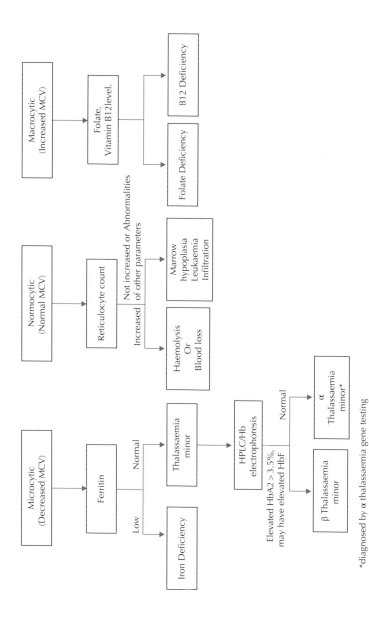

Figure 23.1 Approach to investigating the cause of anaemia. *Source:* The Royal Children's Hospital, Melbourne, Australia, Clinical Practice Guideline on Anaemia, 2019. Available from: www.rch.org.au/clinicalguide/.

Iron deficiency

Iron deficiency (ID) is the most common nutritional deficiency in children and ID is the most common cause of anaemia in children. It is highly prevalent in infants and toddlers, and rates are much higher in Aboriginal and Torres Strait Islander children. Most cases of Iron deficiency anaemia (IDA) in young children are due to inadequate dietary iron intake. Stages of iron deficiency are described in Table 23.2.

Assessment and management

Information regarding risk factors, assessment and management of iron deficiency is available in the RCH Iron deficiency CPG available at www.rch.org.au/clinicalguide/guideline_index/Iron_deficiency/.

Clinical Pearl: Iron deficiency

A reduce serum ferritin (<20ug/L) indicates borderline/low iron stores and requires treatment.

Vitamin B12 deficiency

B12 is essential for DNA synthesis in rapidly dividing cells such as bone marrow and neuronal tissue.

- Deficiency is associated with anaemia/cytopenias and neurological symptoms and most commonly presents during the first 2 years of life.
- Commonest cause is nutritional deficiency (undiagnosed maternal B12 deficiency in a fully breastfed infant)
- Dietary sources of B12 include animal protein such as meat, chicken, eggs and milk, therefore infants of vegan mothers or strict vegetarians with inadequate intake are most at risk.
- Earlier age of presentation, absence of proven maternal deficiency or failure to maintain B12 levels after initial replacement should trigger assessment for metabolic/syndromic/genetic causes.
- Consider B12 deficiency in any child with failure to thrive or neurodevelopmental abnormalities (particularly developmental regression) and an associated haematological abnormality (any cytopenia, macrocytosis or hypersegmented neutrophils).
- Urgent treatment may be required because of the potential for rapid neurological deterioration (seizures, apnoea, choreoathetosis) and the lack of reversibility if treatment is delayed.

Causes of vitamin B12 deficiency

See Table 23.3.

Initial assessment

- Dietary history, child and mother if a breast fed infant.
- Risk factors for malabsorption or symptoms of malabsorption.
- Neurological and developmental assessment.

Investigations

- FBE: macrocytic anaemia, neutropenia/pancytopenia, hypersegmented neutrophils.
- Active B12 level (if only serum B12 is available and the result is normal/borderline but clinical suspicion is high request active B12 level – active B12 levels may be low despite normal total B12).
- Serum homocysteine and urinary methylmalonic acid are essential to confirm cellular vitamin B12 deficiency and to allow monitoring of response to treatment.

Table 23.2 Stages of iron deficiency.

	Definition	Haemoglobin	MCV	Ferritin
Iron deficiency anaemia	Insufficient iron for physiological functions resulting in reduced production of Hb	Low	Low	Low
Iron deficiency	Insufficient iron for physiological function with mild impact on red blood cells, a precursor to IDA.	Normal	Low	Low
Iron depletion	Reduced iron stores but adequate for physiological functions.	Normal	Normal	Low

Hb – Haemoglobin, IDA – iron deficiency anaemia, MCV – mean corpuscular volume.

Table 23.3 Causes of vitamin B12 deficiency.

Causes of vitamin B12 deficiency	
Inadequate intake	Breast fed infants of B12 deficient mothers Vegan/strict vegetarian diet Highly restricted diet, food refusal

Impaired absorption	• Intrinsic factor deficiency
	  ○ Post gastric resection
	  ○ Autoimmune pernicious anaemia (consider in adolescents, adults)
	  ○ Juvenile pernicious anaemia
	• Decreased gastric acid (long term acid suppression)
	• Pancreatic insufficiency
	• Competition for B12 in intestine (parasite, bacterial overgrowth)
	• Impaired absorption in the ileum
	  ○ Crohn's disease
	  ○ Coeliac disease
	  ○ Surgical resection
	  ○ Abnormal ileal receptor (Imerslund-Grasbeck disease)

Inborn errors of B12 transport and metabolism	• Abnormal B12 transport
	  ○ Transcobalamin II (TCII) deficiency
	  ○ R-binder deficiency
	• Abnormal B12 metabolism – cobalamin disorders

- Further initial testing:
  - In breast fed infants, maternal investigations: FBE, active B12, serum homocysteine, urinary MMA.
  - In adolescents without a clear dietary cause investigate for pernicious anaemia: anti-parietal cell/intrinsic factor antibodies, fasting serum gastrin.
- Note: Some inborn errors of vitamin B12 metabolism will result in red cell macrocytosis despite normal serum active B12 levels on testing. If there is an unexplained macrocytosis, homocysteine and urinary MMA should be checked. If elevated may suggest tissue B12 deficiency, and metabolics referral is recommended.

Treatment

Initial treatment is with intramuscular vitamin B12 (hydroxycobalamin).
- An initial replacement dose of 3x IM 1000 micrograms of hydroxocobalamin over one week is often appropriate.
- If neurological features are present more intensive replacement with daily dosing may be recommended.
- Assessment of response should be performed after one week of treatment, including repeat FBE, active B12, homocysteine and urinary MMA.

If there has been a complete response (normalisation of all tests), with a clear dietary cause on history, ongoing oral supplementation may then be considered.
- If there are risk factors or clinical symptoms of malabsorption, ongoing parenteral replacement may be required.

In the setting of an incomplete response to initial supplementation, or where no clear cause has been identified, ongoing parenteral replacement should continue and referral to haematology and/or metabolics should be made for consideration of genetic or metabolic causes. Seek advice for frequency of treatment for metabolic causes. In all cases follow up testing to ensure stores remain replete is essential.

Haemoglobinopathies

Haemoglobinopathies are inherited disorders of globin, affecting haemoglobin synthesis or structure and are usually autosomal recessive. See Table 23.4 for normal adult haemoglobin levels. Disorders of *haemoglobin production* result in thalassaemia syndromes, whereas disorders of *haemoglobin structure*, cause variant haemoglobins.

Table 23.4 Normal adult haemoglobins.

Haemoglobin	Globin chains	% total of total haemoglobin in adult
Hb A (adult haemoglobin)	$(\alpha_2\beta_2)$	>95%
Hb A2	$\alpha_2\delta_2)$	<3.5%
Hb F (fetal haemoglobin)	$(\alpha_2\gamma_2)$	<1%

Table 23.5 Comparison of the laboratory parameters between IDA and β thalassaemia trait.

Red cell parameters	Iron deficiency anaemia	β thalassaemia trait
Hb	Reduced	Normal or mildly reduced
MCV	Reduced	Reduced
MCH	Reduced	Reduced
Red cell distribution width	Increased	Normal
Red cell count	Normal	Increased

β Thalassaemia

β thalassaemia minor/trait or carriers of β thalassaemia are frequently seen in children of whose families originate from Mediterranean, South East Asian and Middle Eastern regions.

- They are usually asymptomatic and there may be a family history.
- Red cells will be microcytic and hypochromic with a normal or mildly low haemoglobin, normal red cell distribution width and increased red cell count.
- See Table 23.5 to compare with findings for IDA. Usually the ferritin is normal, although it can be reduced if there is concurrent IDA.
- The diagnosis is confirmed by high performance liquid chromatography (HPLC); the HbA2 is >3.5% and there is often an elevated HbF. The HbA2 may not be elevated if there is concurrent IDA, and testing may need to be repeated after IDA has been treated.

β thalassaemia major typically results from mutations in both β globin genes resulting in reduced β-globin gene production.

- It is rarely seen in Australia today, due to the results of successful antenatal screening.
- It should be suspected when an infant presents with life-threatening anaemia in the first year of life, corresponding with the decline in HbF levels and inability to produce HbA.
- Clinically these children will have symptomatic anaemia (see Anaemia symptoms) and may shows signs of failure to thrive, jaundice, infection, hepatosplenomegaly and skeletal abnormalities of the face and long bones.
- Thalassaemia major is treated with regular blood transfusions and iron chelation; haematopoietic stem cell transplantation can be curative.

α Thalassaemia

α thalassaemia is due to impaired or absent α globin chain product, which leads to a relative excess of β globin chains in children.

- α thalassaemia carriers are frequently seen in Asian populations, Middle Eastern, Mediterranean, African, some European communities and Polynesians.
- Children with α thalassaemia trait (one or two-gene deletions) may have microcytic and hypochromic red cells since birth but will have normal or borderline low Haemoglobin (Table 23.6).
- They are asymptomatic throughout life (silent carriers).
- α thalassaemia trait may be suspected when a child has microcytic and hypochromic red cells, with or without anaemia, and have a normal ferritin and normal HbA2 and HbF (excluding β thalassaemia trait).
- α thalassaemia trait cannot be diagnosed by high performance liquid chromatography or Hb electrophoresis and α thalassaemia gene testing is required for formal diagnosis.
- Pre-pregnancy carrier testing of the partner is important.

Table 23.6 α thalassaemia genotypes and clinical and laboratory features.

α thalassaemia	Globin chains	Hb	MCV	MCH	Clinically
α (+) thalassaemia (α thalassaemia minor)	- α/ α α **Single gene α deletion**	Normal	Normal/ mildly ↓	Normal/ mildly ↓	Asymptomatic carrier
α (0) thalassaemia (α thalassaemia minor)	- -/ α α **Two gene α deletion**	Normal or mild anaemia	↓	↓	Asymptomatic carrier
Haemoglobin H disease	- -/ - α **Three gene α deletion**	Moderate anaemia	↓↓	↓↓	Moderate – severe lifelong haemolytic anaemia Splenomegaly Variable bony changes and iron overload
Barts Hydrops fetalis (Hb Bart's)	- -/ - - **No normal α genes**	Severe anaemia in utero			Incompatible with extra uterine life

Sickle cell disease

Sickle cell disease is caused by a structurally abnormal haemoglobin called HbS that polymerises when deoxygenated, changing the red cell shape. Sickle cell trait is a benign carrier condition, usually with none of the symptoms of sickle cell disease. It occurs when one of the β globin gene carries the sickle haemoglobin mutation and the other β globin gene is normal. Sickle cell carriers are often of African, Mediterranean or Middle Eastern descent. Pre-pregnancy carrier testing of the partner is important.

Homozygous (HbS/HbS) is the most severe form of SCD, but heterozygous combinations with other haemoglobinopathies can produced sickling syndromes of varying severity; Sickle/ β thalassaemia, HbS/C or HbS/E. Children with sickle cell disease may present with the following presentations:

- Anaemia (haemolysis or ineffective erythropoiesis)
- Vaso-occlusive crises (acute painful episodes)
- Dactylitis (bone and swelling of small joints of hand/foot seen in infants)
- Fever
- Sepsis, due to functional hyposplensim and an increased susceptibility to severe infection with encapsulated organisms *Streptococcus pneumoniae* and *Haemophilus influenzae*
- Acute chest syndrome (fever, chest pain, hypoxia, lower respiratory symptoms and a new infiltrate on chest x-ray)
- Acute ischaemic stroke.
- Acute splenic sequestration (a Hb drop of at least 20g/L below baseline with an acutely enlarged spleen)
- Priapism
- Asymptomatic when parents are known carriers

The FBE and blood film will show anaemia, polychromasia, nucleated red blood cells, sickle cells and hyposplenic features and HPLC and Hb electrophoresis will confirm the absence of HbA with elevated HbS levels (usually 70 – 90%).

Management

- Discuss acute sickle crisis management with specialist haematologist.
- Painful crises: intravenous hydration and analgesia (regular oral, may need IV morphine).
- Fever: broad spectrum antibiotics, third generation cephalosporin and consider cover for atypical organisms (Roxithromycin or Azithromycin) if significant respiratory component.
- Acute chest syndrome: oxygen and broad-spectrum antibiotics, third generation cephalosporin and consider coverage for atypical organisms (Roxithromycin or Azithromycin).
- Symptomatic anaemia: discuss blood transfusion with specialist.
- Stroke: transfusion support needed (usually simple transfusion followed by red cell exchange transfusion).
- Incentive spirometry to reduce the risk of acute chest syndrome during hospital admission.

Long term management involves:
- Folic acid supplementation.
- Penicillin prophylaxis starting in the newborn period.
- Routine and additional immunisations (pneumococcal, meningococcal, influenza) to prevent opportunistic infections.
- Hydroxyurea can reduce frequency of vaso-occlusive crises and prevent recurrent chest crises.
- Chronic red cell transfusion or exchange transfusion may be required for stroke prevention.
- Iron chelation for those receiving regular red cell transfusions.
- Stem cell transplantation.

Clinical Pearl: Sickle cell disease
- Sickle cell disease (SCD) is a chronic multisystem disorder.
- SCD should be identified in infancy, ideally through antenatal or newborn screening in order to commence penicillin prophylaxis which reduces mortality from hyposplenism related sepsis.
- All children with SCD will be asplenic with a risk of overwhelming infection. Broad spectrum antibiotics such as ceftriaxone should be commenced when there is fever with a temperature >38.5 degrees.
- Blood transfusion treatment, preferably red cell exchange is indicated for children with stroke.
- As transfusion is associated with a risk of hyperviscosity, specialist haematologist consultation should guide transfusion decisions in children with SCD.

Haemolytic anaemia

Haemolysis is the destruction of red blood cells, faster than the bone marrow can make them. Acute haemolysis in children is a life-threatening disorder, as severe anaemia can develop rapidly over hours. Children with haemolytic anaemia typically need hospital admission for observation, frequent heart rate assessment and close Hb monitoring every 6–12 hours to monitor for ongoing haemolysis and potential transfusion support.

Signs and symptoms associated with haemolytic anaemia
- Clinical features of anaemia, see Anaemia section above
- Jaundice, or yellowing of the skin and eyes
- Dark-coloured urine
- Fever
- Enlargement of the spleen and liver
- Tachycardia

History
- Dietary: fava beans in Glucose-6-phosphate dehydrogenase (G6PD) deficiency
- History of viral infection or illness
- Medication history
- Past medical history: need for phototherapy as a neonate, other autoimmune conditions
- Ethnicity
- Family history of jaundice or anaemia
- Travel history

Causes of haemolysis
See Figure 23.2.

Investigations
- FBE to assess the haemoglobin and platelet (microangiopathic haemolysis)
- Blood film examination to look for features of haemolysis
    - Polychromasia or nucleated red blood cells (immature red blood cells)
    - Spherocytes (hereditary spherocytosis or AIHA)
    - Red cell fragments (TTP/HUS, DIC, mechanical valves)
    - Bite and blister cells (oxidative haemolysis e.g. G6PD deficiency)

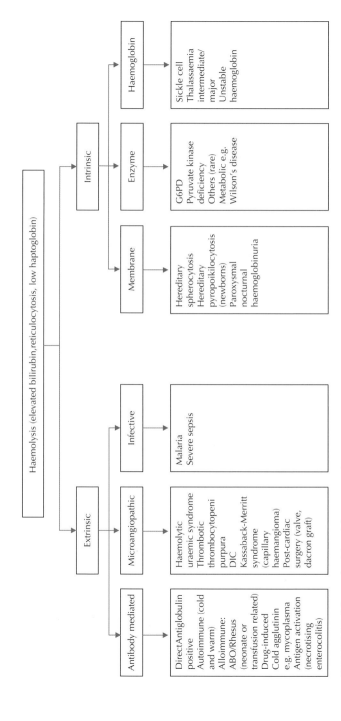

Figure 23.2 Potential causes of acute haemolysis.

- ○ Sickle cells in Sickle cell disease
- ○ Target cells in haemoglobinopathies
- ○ Red cell agglutination seen in cold agglutinin disease
- ○ Red cells with inclusions, seen in malaria
- Reticulocyte count indicates the bone marrow's response to anaemia and haemolysis
- Bilirubin (total and unconjugated)
- Lactate dehydrogenase (LDH)
- Haptoglobin is only useful in children >18 months, as hepatic synthesis is reduced in infants

Further investigations to establish the cause of haemolysis, based on blood film findings:

- Blood group and antibody screen looking for allo or auto-antibodies
- Direct Antiglobulin Test (Coombs) IgG and C3d
- G6PD assay
- Eosin 5 maleimide (E5M) flow cytometry testing for hereditary spherocytosis
- High performance liquid chromatography (HPLC) / Haemoglobin electrophoresis looking for Haemoglobinopathy or sickle cell disease
- Others e.g. rarer red cell enzyme analysis

Management

Haemolytic anaemia treatments vary depending on the type and cause for the haemolysis and how severe the anaemia is. Some children will not require any treatment.

For those that do require treatment, it may include:

- Blood transfusion support in those with severe uncompensated haemolysis
- Folic acid
- Corticosteroid
- Intravenous immunoglobulin (IVIg)
- Exchange transfusion
- Immunosuppressive treatments
- Antibiotics to treat infection or antimalarials
- Rarely, splenectomy or Rituximab (anti-CD20 monoclonal antibody)

Clinical Pearl: Haemolytic anaemia

- Acute haemolysis in children can be a medical emergency due to the rapid development of severe anaemia.
- The commonest causes are G6PD deficiency and cold antibody mediated haemolysis secondary to infection.

Transient erythroblastopenia of childhood

Transient erythroblastopenia of childhood (TEC) is an acquired, benign self-limiting condition that is characterised by a temporary suppression of erythropoiesis.

- It generally seen in children between the age of 1–4 years, and in half there will be a history of a viral illness in the preceding weeks.
- Children with TEC will have normal height, no splenomegaly or lymphadenopathy and no congenital abnormalities.
- The FBE will show a moderate to severe normochromic, normocytic anaemia with a low to normal reticulocyte count with normal white cell and platelet counts.
- During recovery, the reticulocyte count will be increased.
- Haematinic analysis e.g. iron, folic acid and vitamin B12 will be normal.
- A bone marrow aspirate is infrequently indicated, but if performed will show red cell aplasia with preservation of the other cell lines.
- Management is largely supportive; some children may require blood transfusion for symptomatic anaemia.
- In most cases there is spontaneous recovery within 2–8 weeks without any intervention.

- The main differential diagnoses are transient aplastic crisis due to parvovirus in children with a known haematological disorder or Diamond Blackfan Anaemia (DBA).
  - DBA is a congenital erythroid aplasia caused by genetic mutations affecting ribosome synthesis.
  - It typically presents within the first year of life, with a severe macrocytic anaemia, reticulocytopenia and many children will have associated congenital malformations.
  - The mainstays of treatment for DBA are corticosteroids and blood transfusions.

Coagulation abnormalities

The haemostatic system in neonates and children is physiologically different to that in adults, and these differences need to be considered when interpreting the results of testing. Severe inherited bleeding disorders can present at any age in childhood, however abnormal bleeding in the newborn period (such as bleeding from the umbilical stump or injection sites) should raise suspicions of an inherited disorder. In older children severe mucosal bleeding (such as epistaxis/menorrhagia) resulting in anaemia should prompt further investigation and consideration of specialist consultation. Family history (including consanguinity), drug history and response to previous surgical challenges (including tooth extraction) are important. Routine coagulation screening preoperatively in well children is rarely indicated and coagulation testing should be guided by the clinical history.

Investigation

First-line investigations of a suspected bleeding disorder include:
- FBE and blood film
- Activated partial thromboplastin time (APTT)
- Prothrombin time (PT) or international normalised ratio (INR)
- Fibrinogen

Interpretation of these investigations is shown in Table 23.7. Further investigations should usually be guided by consultation with a haematologist.
- Knowledge of the variation of reference range for age is essential to avoid unnecessary anxiety and investigation in a normal child.
- Fibrinogen is an acute-phase reactant. In severe sepsis, when fibrinogen should be elevated, a normal level is still consistent with disseminated intravascular coagulation (DIC).
- If the APTT or INR are prolonged a mixing study is performed. If full correction is seen a factor deficiency is likely and the appropriate factor assays should be performed.
- Incomplete correction suggests the presence of an inhibitor such as a transient lupus anticoagulant (which is not associated with bleeding or thrombosis and in children, is typically temporary in association with a viral illness).

Table 23.7 Investigation of coagulation abnormalities.

Screening test result	Causes
Low platelet count	Idiopathic thrombocytopenic purpura (ITP) Neonatal alloimmune thrombocytopenia Congenital thrombocytopenia syndromes Chemotherapy/marrow replacement
Isolated prolonged APTT	Factor XI, IX, VIII deficiency von Willebrand disease Heparin Factor XII (no clinical bleeding)
Isolated prolonged PT/INR	Factor VII deficiency Warfarin
Prolonged APTT, PT Low fibrinogen	Liver disease Disseminated intravascular coagulation (DIC) ± also low platelets Vitamin K deficiency, factor II, V, X deficiency (normal fibrinogen)

- If the investigations above are normal in the setting of clinically abnormal bleeding, consider factor XIII deficiency (AR), von Willebrand disease or platelet function defects. Specific investigations such as a PFA100, von Willebrand screen, platelet aggregometry may be required.
- In the setting of acute severe bleeding, if the diagnosis of a specific bleeding disorder is unclear, consider treatment with 10–20 mL/kg of fresh frozen plasma (FFP) ± platelets. If fulminant DIC is suspected with low fibrinogen (<1.0 g/dL) give cryoprecipitate (5–10 mL/kg) as well as FFP, platelets and red cells as above.
- Generally, children presenting acutely with a possible bleeding disorder should be discussed with a haematologist as specific treatment/factor replacement may be available/required.

General measures
These are applicable to all congenital bleeding disorders.
- RICES: Rest, Ice, Compression (gentle compression bandage), Elevation, Splinting
- Analgesia
  - Do not give aspirin or other NSAIDs.
  - Narcotic analgesics should only be given as part of a comprehensive pain management plan.
- Avoid intramuscular injections and arterial puncture.
- Lumbar punctures should only be done after haematological consultation and appropriate factor replacement.
- Splinting limbs reduces pain.
- Be aware of the risk of:
  - Compartment syndromes such as Volkmann's ischaemic contracture in forearm bleeds or with severe calf bleeds.
  - Femoral nerve palsies with retroperitoneal bleeds tracking underneath the inguinal ligament.
  - Potential for massive blood loss with shock due to psoas/retroperitoneal bleeding.
- Treatment options for children with haemophilia A and B is rapidly changing with a range of treatments now available. Plasma-derived and recombinant clotting factors, by-passing agents and more recently extended half-life clotting factors have improved quality of life in children with haemophilia. Gene therapy is likely to be a consideration in the near future.

Clinical Pearl: Coagulation abnormalities
- Coagulation test results in children should be interpreted in relation to age-appropriate paediatric reference ranges in order to reduce unnecessary investigations and over diagnosis.
- Minor abnormalities of coagulation tests should be interpreted along with clinical history and bleeding history.
- In a child under 9 months with unexplained bruising, Vitamin K deficiency must be considered as bleeding may progress rapidly and intracerebral bleeding rates are high.

Haemophilia A
X linked factor VIII deficiency: severe <1% FVIII, moderate 1–5% FVIII, mild 5–40% FVIII.

Management of bleeding
- Recombinant human factor VIII is used to treat all boys with haemophilia A. Dosage is usually 30–50 units/kg, which increases factor VIII levels by 60–100%. Note that 1 unit/kg of factor VIII raises levels by 2%. Repeat doses are usually required 8–12 hourly.
- Most bleeding can be controlled with one to two doses calculated to increase the factor VIII level to at least 50%. Higher doses are required for joint bleeding, major muscle bleeds, head injury with potential central nervous system (CNS) bleeding or prior to surgery where a continuous factor infusion may be required. A minor head injury can become serious; treatment with factor concentrate should not be delayed while waiting for diagnostic imaging if suspected bleeding of head/neck/chest or abdomen.
- Up to 30% of boys with severe haemophilia A may develop a factor VIII inhibitor, such that they will fail to respond to usual factor replacement. On demand treatment for bleeding episodes then requires recombinant factor VIIa (Novoseven) or a four factor concentrate (FEIBA). The usual dose of factor VIIa is 90–180 mcg repeated in 2 hours. Specialist consultation is required.

Mouth bleeding and epistaxis
Use tranexamic acid tablets (antifibrinolytic), which stabilizes clot formation (25 mg/kg TDS).

Haemophilia B
X linked factor IX deficiency: severe <1% FVIII, moderate 1–5% FVIII, mild 5–40% FVIII.

Management of bleeding
Bleeding is treated with recombinant factor IX concentrate.
- Dose: in general, 1 unit factor IX/kg increases levels by 1.6%.
- Frequency: injections at 24 hour intervals (the half-life for factor IX is 24 hours).
- Most bleeding can be controlled with levels of 50%, the standard dose for a minor muscle bleed is 50 IU/kg, which may require repeating on the following day.
- Discussion with haematologist about the nature of the injury and the dose required +/- continuous infusion is recommended.
- Head injuries can be serious, and treatment with factor replacement should not be delayed for imaging.

Mouth bleeding and epistaxis
Use tranexamic acid tablets (antifibrinolytic) which stabilizes clot formation (25 mg/kg TDS).

Von Willebrand disease
Von Willebrand disease is the commonest inherited bleeding disorder with clinical features of platelet-type bleeding including bruising, epistaxis, menorrhagia or bleeding with injury/trauma/surgery. Types, assessment and management is detailed in the RCH CPG www.rch.org.au/clinicalguide/guideline_index/Von_Willebrand_Disease_vWD/.

Vitamin K deficiency bleeding (VKDB)
Bleeding due to Vitamin K (VK) deficiency can be classified into three patterns based on the timing and type of complications (Table 23.8). Coagulation test results typically demonstrate a prolonged INR and APTT with normal fibrinogen and platelet count.

Treatment of vitamin K deficiency
- Any infant or child suspected to have VK deficiency should be treated immediately with VK while awaiting laboratory confirmation.
  - The route and specific type of treatment is dictated by the urgency of the clinical situation and potential side effects of treatment.
- VKDB should be treated with intravenous or subcutaneous VK at doses appropriate for age.
  - Depending on the severity of bleeding, 10 to 20 mL/kg of FFP should be given or alternatively 30 u/kg of a prothrombin complex concentrate.
  - In rare circumstances rVIIa may be warranted.

Prophylactic vitamin K administration
Current recommendations for VK prophylaxis in healthy newborns vary in different countries. Healthy newborns should receive either:
- 1 mg of vitamin K1 by intramuscular injection at birth
  or

Table 23.8 Vitamin K deficiency bleeding presentations.

Time of presentation	Presentation	Risk factors
Early First 24 hours of life	Serious bleeding, Intracranial haemorrhage, intra-thoracic/intra-abdominal bleeding	Mother on Vitamin K antagonist, certain anticonvulsants or anti tuberculous drugs
Classic Day 1–7	Nose, GI bleeding, bruising, bleeding from puncture sites, umbilical stump or following circumcision	Breast fed infant
Late Day 7–9 months	Bruising, GI bleeding, ICH	Diseases causing reduced Vitamin K absorption

- 3×2 mg vitamin K1 orally, at birth, at 4 to 6 days and at 4 to 6 weeks
  or
- 2 mg vitamin K1 orally at birth, and a weekly dose of 1 mg orally for 3 months

Intramuscular application is the preferred route for efficiency and reliability of administration. The oral route is not appropriate for preterm infants and for newborns who have cholestasis or impaired intestinal absorption, are too unwell to take oral vitamin K1, or those whose mothers have taken medications that interfere with vitamin K metabolism.

The frequency of VKDB is increasing in many westernised countries predominantly due to refusal of VK injections at birth. This practice is strongly linked to vaccine refusal. Appropriate education of parents, and/or documentation of reasons for refusal of VK is important. Parents who refuse VK for their infant should be given clear instructions about when to present urgently for medical attention as approximately 50% of children who present with late VKDB will have a signal bleed that gives an opportunity for early intervention.

Immune thrombocytopenia

Immune thrombocytopenia, commonly called ITP, is an acquired, isolated thrombocytopenia due to immune mediated destruction of platelets.

Presentation

- Common presenting features include petechiae, bruising, and in some cases mucosal bleeding such as epistaxis and oral bleeding. GI bleeding and haematuria are uncommon.
- There is often a history of a preceding viral infection.
- The most common age of presentation is 2–10 years, with a peak incidence in the preschool years.
- Presentation <12 months of age is rare and should prompt consideration for other diagnoses (congenital bone marrow disorders).
- A broader differential should also be considered in older children, including autoimmune conditions such as SLE, particularly in those with a family history or from high risk ethnic backgrounds.

Clinical assessment

Clinical assessment is required to exclude other causes of petechiae/purpura and thrombocytopenia such as malignancy, infection, consumptive coagulopathy and autoimmune conditions, and to assess for bleeding complications.

Bone marrow biopsy and other extensive investigations are not usually necessary where the clinical features are consistent with ITP. Features consistent with ITP include:

- A previously well child - absence of fever, loss of weight, bone pain
- Recent onset of symptoms
- No hepatosplenomegaly or lymphadenopathy
- FBE and blood film consistent with ITP – there should be no anaemia, neutropenia, or blasts.

Morbidity in ITP is usually minimal. Intracranial haemorrhage is the most concerning risk but the incidence is low (<1%). Evidence of mucosal bleeding may indicate an increased risk of serious bleeding associated with ITP. Children should be assessed for signs and symptoms of bleeding.

Management

Controversy surrounds the indications and best form of treatment for children with acute ITP. Common treatment modalities, including steroids and intravenous immunoglobulin (IVIg), have been shown to increase the platelet count more quickly but do not alter the natural history of the disease.

- In the absence of bleeding careful observation without specific treatment is appropriate.
- Children with active bleeding (e.g. mucosal, gastrointestinal, severe menorrhagia) should receive treatment to increase their platelet count.
- When treatment is indicated, corticosteroids are usually first-line treatment. Various steroid regimens have been used, most commonly prednisolone, with doses of 1-4 mg/kg per day. A recent international guideline suggests short courses (<7 days) rather than prolonged courses of steroids.
- IVIg may be an appropriate first line choice if there are concerns about steroid side effects, if more rapid improvement in platelet count is required or to avoid steroids if there is diagnostic uncertainty.

- Treatment may also be considered if there is a high risk of trauma (for example in younger children where activity modification is difficult).
- Modification of activity to avoid contact sports and rough physical activity should be discussed with the child and family. If there is any head injury, significant or persistent headache, families should be aware to seek medical review.
- Avoidance of aspirin/NSAIDs is recommended.
- Following recovery, relapse of thrombocytopenia may occur, particularly in the setting of intercurrent viral illnesses.

In the majority of children ITP will resolve, however some children will go on to develop chronic ITP. Chronic ITP (lasting >12 months) occurs in 13–36% and requires specialist management. The most commonly used second line treatment options include monoclonal anti-CD20 antibody (rituximab), splenectomy, azathioprine, and TPO receptor agonists. The risk–benefit ratio of these second-line treatments must be carefully considered.

Neutropenia

Neutropenia is defined as a neutrophil count below the reference range for age. Neutrophil count should be interpreted in relation to an age-appropriate reference range. Racial variation also occurs, with lower counts in African American and Middle Eastern populations.

General definitions regarding the severity of neutropenia are:
- Mild neutropenia >1.0 × 10^9/L
- Moderate 0.5–1.0 × 10^9/L
- Severe <0.5 × 10^9/L

Neutrophils are primarily involved in the body's response to bacterial infections, so the main risk associated with neutropenia is severe bacterial infection. Prolonged severe neutropenia is also associated with a risk of fungal infection.

Causes

Causes of neutropenia can be generally divided into two mechanisms: failure of production (bone marrow disorders) and immune-mediated peripheral destruction.

Causes to consider include:
- Transient neutropenia associated with viral or bacterial infection
- Immune neutropenia – NAIN (neonatal alloimmune neutropenia) or autoimmune neutropenia
- Drug induced
- Vitamin B12 or folate deficiency
- Splenic sequestration
- Cyclical neutropenia (may be familial)
- Bone marrow infiltration e.g. leukaemia/lymphoma, neuroblastoma
- Bone marrow aplasia
- Severe congenital neutropenia – Kostmann syndrome
- Inherited bone marrow failure syndromes including:
  - Schwachmann–Diamond syndrome (other features include FTT, exocrine pancreatic insufficiency)
  - Fanconi anaemia (other features may include congenital abnormalities including dysmorphic features, short stature, limb abnormalities, renal and cardiac anomalies, café au lait spots)
  - Dyskeratosis congenita (classic triad of nail dystrophy, oral leukoplakia, abnormal skin pigmentation)
  - Pearson syndrome (mitochondrial disorder)
- Associated with other conditions/syndromes including: Chediak–Higashi syndrome, reticular dysgenesis
- Associated with autoimmune disorders: SLE, IBD

Clinical assessment

- Early/unusual bacterial infections.
- Suspicious infections include chronic diarrhoea, recurrent sinopulmonary infections/pneumonia, periodontitis, cellulitis, bone/joint infections such as osteomyelitis.
- Poor growth/FTT, dysmorphic features.

- Family history.
- Periodic symptoms with fever, mouth ulcers, infections suggestive of cyclical neutropenia (cycles often occur every 3–4 weeks, lasting 3–6 days at a time).

Investigations
- FBE and blood film
- In neonates: maternal testing of FBE and neutrophil antibodies

Anticoagulation in children

Spontaneous thrombosis in children is rare, however it is occurring with increasing frequency as a secondary complication of complex treatments in sick children.

Common anticoagulants used in children:
- Unfractionated heparin
- Low molecular weight heparin (mostly enoxaparin, some centres use dalteparin or tinzaparin)
- Vitamin K antagonists (warfarin)

Each drug has different mechanisms of action and pharmacology, impacts on monitoring tests, side effect profile are all age and weight dependent. Using these drugs in children requires specific expertise and data supports that successful treatment and reduced adverse events are much more likely when anticoagulated children are being managed by a dedicated anticoagulation service. For outpatients, appropriate education and support are critical.

Bleeding is the most common side effect, although long term use impacts on bone density and rare other side effects are reported. Fatal bleeding secondary to unfractionated heparin in hospital inpatients is almost exclusively related to errors of dosing (confusing vial strength, incorrect infusion being made up) and can occur in children who are only meant to be receiving line flushes rather than formal anticoagulant treatment. In addition, particular care and the appropriate duration of cessation of treatment needs to be taken when performing invasive procedures for example lumbar puncture. Prior to performing a lumbar puncture on any hospitalised child, the medication chart should be reviewed to ensure no anticoagulation is being administered. Approximately 30% of teenage girls will have symptomatic heavy menstrual bleeding on anticoagulation and this requires specific (sometimes urgent) management.

DOACS (direct oral anticoagulants) are currently being trialled in children and will likely come into clinical use over the next few years. There are currently no readily available reversal agents for these drugs in children and currently they should not be used outside of formal paediatric studies, or without expert paediatric haematology involvement.

Antiplatelet treatment significantly increases the bleeding risk for children on anticoagulation. While they are used in specific circumstances in conjunction with anticoagulation, in general they should be avoided, and this includes the use of non-steroidal anti-inflammatory drugs (NSAIDS).

Transfusions in children

Blood transfusions have the potential to save lives when used appropriately and are common medical intervention in paediatrics. Australia's blood supply is very safe, but it still carries a not insignificant risk, and transfusion should only be given when the expected benefits outweigh any potential risks. Informed consent must be obtained from the child/parent and documented in the medical record. The consent discussion should include:
- The indication for the blood product transfusion and possible benefits.
- Risks of transfusion.
- Risks of not having the recommended transfusion.
- Potential alternative treatments.

Child and family information is available through the RCH website Kids Health information. The Australian Red Cross Blood Service has transfusion information for parents and children, see Useful resources below. This includes information in languages other than English.

Red cells

Red cells are transfused to increase oxygen carrying capacity and treat symptomatic anaemia. They can replace blood that is lost through surgery or trauma, or bone marrow suppression and suppress ineffective erythropoiesis in children with thalassaemia major or sickle cell disease.

Red cell transfusion indications
See Table 23.9.

Red cell transfusion volume
The desired red cell transfusion volume may be calculated from the following formula:

$$mL = weight \ (kg) \times Hb \ (g/L) \ rise \ (desired \ Hb - actual \ Hb) \times 0.5$$

- In neonates and children less than 20 kg, transfusion volume should be calculated based on weight and prescribed in mL.
- In children greater than 20 kg, prescribe a single red cell unit followed by clinical reassessment to determine additional transfusion requirements.

Platelets
Platelets are commonly transfused in children with low platelet counts as prophylactic transfusions to prevent bleeding or prior to procedures. They are also given to treat bleeding symptoms, where thrombocytopenia or platelet dysfunction is a significant contributing factor.

Platelet transfusion volume
The usual platelet dose for children less than 20 kg is 10 mL/kg. For children more than 20 kg a single adult unit may be prescribed.

The RCH guideline details clinical indications and platelet counts at which platelet transfusion should be considered in children, available at www.rch.org.au/bloodtrans/about_blood_products/Platelet_transfusion/

Fresh frozen plasma (FFP) and cryoprecipitate
FFP and cryoprecipitate transfusion indications
See Table 23.10 and Table 23.11.

FFP and cryoprecipitate transfusion volume
- The usual FFP dose for children is 10–15 mL/kg
- The usual cryoprecipitate dose is 5–10 mL/kg

Blood product modifications
- Irradiated blood products (to reduce the risk of graft vs. host disease)
  - Given to immunocompromised children, HLA matched products and directed donations
- CMV seronegative products
  - Leucocyte depleted blood products, are considered an acceptable alternative for the majority of children
- Phenotype matched red blood cells
  - Indicated for chronically transfused children or children with red cell alloantibodies
- HLA matched products
  - For children with immunological refractory thrombocytopenia

Table 23.9 Red cell transfusion indications.

Hb	Indication
Hb <70 g/L	Red cell transfusion is often indicated, however lower thresholds may be acceptable in children without symptomatic anaemia and where other specific treatment (e.g. iron) is appropriate.
Hb 70–90 g/L	RBC transfusion may be indicated, depending on the clinical setting e.g. presence of bleeding or haemolysis and clinical signs and symptoms of anaemia.
Hb >90 g/L	RBC transfusion is often unnecessary and may be inappropriate.

Transfusion may be indicated at higher thresholds for specific situations:
- Preterm neonates: Hb thresholds vary depending on post-natal age and respiratory support (See Neonatal Transfusion Recommendations at the RCH in Useful Resources below)
- Children with cyanotic congenital heart disease or on Extra Corporeal Life Support (ECLS)
- Children with haemoglobinopathies (thalassaemia or sickle cell disease) or congenital anaemia on a chronic transfusion program

Table 23.10 Fresh frozen plasma transfusion indications.

Fresh frozen plasma transfusion may be appropriate in the following settings
Acute bleeding in the setting of significant coagulopathy
Warfarin reversal, in the presence of significant or life-threatening bleeding or prior to emergency surgical procedures. Given in addition to vitamin K NOTE: Vitamin-K dependent clotting factor concentrates (e.g. prothrombinex) should be given instead of FFP for bleeding secondary to warfarin or emergency warfarin reversal
Liver disease, with clinically significant bleeding in the context of coagulopathy post liver transplantation
Acute disseminated intravascular coagulopathy (DIC) with bleeding and significant coagulopathy
During massive transfusion or cardiac bypass for the treatment of bleeding
Plasma exchange for the treatment of TTP
Specific factor deficiencies where a factor concentrate is not available

Table 23.11 Cryoprecipitate transfusion indications.

Cryoprecipitate transfusion may be appropriate in the following settings
Active bleeding and fibrinogen level <1.5 g/L
During massive transfusion or cardiac bypass, for the treatment bleeding when fibrinogen <1.5 g/L or there is hyperfibrinolysis
Acquired fibrinogen deficiency or acute DIC when there is significant bleeding and fibrinogen <1.0 g/L
Prior to an invasive procedure when the fibrinogen <1.0 g/L and there is a risk of significant bleeding associated with the surgery or it is at a critical site (e.g. neurosurgery or eye surgery)

Adverse reactions of blood transfusion

Each blood product transfused, carries a small risk of an adverse event. The most common reactions seen in children are fever, chills, urticaria and allergic reactions. Potentially significant and life-threatening reactions include acute and delayed haemolytic transfusions reactions, transfusion-transmitted infection, anaphylaxis, transfusion-related acute lung injury (TRALI) and transfusion-associated circulatory overload (TACO).

It is important to recognize, respond to and report any potential adverse reaction to a transfusion.

The RCH guideline details an approach to the assessment and immediate management of transfusion reactions, available at www.rch.org.au/bloodtrans/adverse_effects/Adverse_effects_of_transfusion/.

USEFUL RESOURCES
- The RCH Clinical practice guidelines
  - Anaemia www.rch.org.au/clinicalguide/guideline_index/Anaemia/
  - Iron Deficiency www.rch.org.au/clinicalguide/guideline_index/iron_deficiency/
- The RCH Blood transfusion resources www.rch.org.au/bloodtrans/
- Australian Red Cross Lifeblood https://mytransfusion.com.au/
- The RCH Kids Health info: IVIg www.rch.org.au/kidsinfo/fact_sheets/Intravenous_immunoglobulin_IVIg_infusion/
- The RCH Kids Health info: Blood product transfusions www.rch.org.au/kidsinfo/fact_sheets/Blood_product_transfusions/

CHAPTER 24

Immunology

Sharon Choo
Theresa Cole

Key Points

- Beware the infant with persistent lymphopenia (<2.5x10⁹/L), failure to thrive and/or persistent eczema – consider SCID.
- Any child with recurrent suppurative chest, ear and/or sinus infections should have immunoglobulins measured.
- Consider haemophagocytic lymphohistocytosis (HLH) and order a ferritin in any child with fever for more than 5 days, thrombocytopenia and transaminitis.
- Consider primary immunodeficiency in a child with an unusual infection.
- Recurrent infection at a single site is rarely a primary immunodeficiency.

Infections are common in immunocompetent children, who average 5–10 upper respiratory tract infections per year in the first few years of life (often more if the child attends childcare). Recurrent viral infections in a well, thriving child do not suggest immunodeficiency. Immunodeficiency should be suspected when there is a history of severe, recurrent or unusual infection and/or recurrent or severe autoimmunity or inflammation, particularly when more than one anatomical site is affected.

Primary immunodeficiencies (PID) are genetic disorders affecting the development and/or function of one or more components of the immune system. Excluding IgA deficiency, the prevalence of PID is 1 in 1200. There are more than 300 PID described to date, with more than 50 identified within the last 2 years.

Secondary immunodeficiencies arise from a range of medications and medical conditions such as prematurity, malnutrition, HIV infection, uraemia, liver failure, asplenia and malignancies.

Primary Immunodeficiencies
Combined Immunodeficiencies
Severe Combined immune deficiency (SCID)

SCID is an immunological emergency. It results from a range of genetic mutations causing defects in T cell development. Children can present with the classic SCID phenotype of failure to thrive with opportunistic or severe infection. However, they may also present with a severe "eczema" rash due to either maternally derived T cells (maternal engraftment) or autoreactive T cells (Omenn Syndrome). Persistent, severe eczema despite appropriate topical treatment, warrants investigation for SCID.

When to suspect SCID in an infant:

- Persistent lymphopaenia (<2.5x10⁹/L)
- Failure to thrive
- Persistent and severe "eczema"
- Persistent rotavirus positive diarrhoea after immunisation
- Unusual infection e.g. Pneumocystis jiroveci (PJP), or a severe course for a common infection e.g. CMV

Paediatric Handbook, Tenth Edition. Edited by Kate Harding, Daniel S. Mason and Daryl Efron.
© 2021 John Wiley & Sons Ltd. Published 2021 by John Wiley & Sons Ltd.

Investigations:
- A range of specialised functional tests of T cells are used to help in the diagnosis of SCID. Urgent referral to an immunologist is indicated if SCID is suspected.
- FBE, most (but not all) children with SCID with have a low lymphocyte count.
- Lymphocyte "subsets" for T cells (CD3, total T cells; CD4, T Helper cells, CD8, cytotoxic T cells), B cells (CD19), and NK cells (CD56).
- Naïve T cell (CD45RA+) evaluation is essential where a severe T cell defect is suspected as total lymphocyte count and CD4/CD8 T cell numbers may be within the normal range in SCID.
- Testing for HIV should be considered, particularly if there is hypergammaglobulinaemia.

Management when SCID suspected/confirmed:
- Isolate in a single room and only allow staff and visitors who are free from respiratory illness or cold sores to enter.
- Do not allow the child to wait in open waiting areas with other children.
- CMV can be transmitted through breast milk. If the infant is breast fed, check maternal CMV serological status urgently. If mother is CMV positive (IgG or IgM), breast feeding should stop, and a formula commenced.
- Commence PJP prophylaxis with cotrimoxazole (if acute PJP suspected, commence high dose cotrimoxazole until excluded).
- Blood products that contain cells (e.g. packed red cells or platelets) should be irradiated to prevent graft versus host disease. As CMV infection can be a significant problem in these children, CMV negative products should be given if available. If not available, the blood product should be filtered to remove contaminating white cells as it is delivered to the child. Note: In infants with SCID CMV PCR testing is required, as they cannot mount an antibody response to infection, CMV serology is not useful.
- All live viral vaccines should be avoided.
- Haematopoietic stem cell transplant (HSCT) is the definitive treatment for SCID. Donors may be HLA matched (related or unrelated) or haploidentical ("half matched"). The cure rate is approximately 80–90% if the child is in good clinical condition prior to HSCT.

Other Combined Immunodeficiencies (CID)

There are a range of combined (T and B cell) immunodeficiencies with syndromic features. The immunodeficiency ranges from severe and early onset (like SCID) to mild and later onset.
CID include:
- **Di George (22q11 deletion) syndrome (DGS):** DGS is a triad of immunodeficiency, hypoparathyroidism (resulting in hypocalcaemia) and cardiac defects. The immune defect is due to failure of thymic development. Most children with 22q11 deletion are immunocompetent, however a proportion have recurrent infections and rarely a SCID phenotype (called complete DGS). Some children with 22q11 deletion develop autoimmunity (e.g. ITP).
- **CHARGE syndrome:** The immune defect in CHARGE syndrome is similar to DGS, although antibody defects appear to be less common. Complete DGS phenotype can occur.
- **Wiskott-Aldrich syndrome:** An X-linked condition with the classical triad of thrombocytopenia, eczema and immunodeficiency. The diagnosis should be considered in a male infant with persistent thrombocytopenia. Although low platelet volume on FBE can be helpful, platelet size can be normal. Immunodeficiency and autoimmunity (e.g. vasculitis) generally occur in mid to late childhood.
- **Ataxia Telangiectasia:** An autosomal recessive condition that usually presents in early childhood with neurological symptoms. Children usually have a high alpha-fetoprotein and lymphopenia. Recurrent infection and antibody deficiency may develop in mid to late childhood. There is radiation sensitivity and predisposition to cancer.

There are a range of other immunodeficiencies with defective T and B cell function. Children with these disorders may present early in life with opportunistic infections, e.g. PJP, or later in life with recurrent or chronic infections, hypogammaglobulinaemia &/or autoimmunity. One example is HyperIgM syndrome (usually X-linked), which typically presents in early childhood with recurrent infection and hypogammaglobulinaemia, or severe unusual infections e.g. PJP, cryptosporidium. IgG and IgA levels are low, with normal or high IgM, and neutropenia is common.

Initial investigation for a CID should be similar to that used for suspected SCID, including:
- FBE
- Lymphocyte markers for T cells (CD4 and CD8), B cells and NK cells.
- Naïve T cells (CD45RA+)
- Immunoglobulins (IgG, IgA, IgM)

A range of specialised tests are available for specific CIDs. Referral to an immunologist and/or discussion with the diagnostic immunology laboratory is recommended.

Management:
- Children with CID may require cotrimoxazole prophylaxis and immunoglobulin replacement.
- Severe CID may require HSCT and severe thymic defects may require thymic transplant.
- Live vaccines can safely be given to many children with mild to moderate CID, under the direction of an immunologist.
- Other vaccines may be safely given but may not promote an adequate antibody response, depending on the severity of immunodeficiency.

Antibody deficiencies

Antibody deficiencies are defects of antibody production or function. They are the most common type of PID. Secondary antibody deficiencies are much more common than primary antibody defects. These can be iatrogenic (e.g. chemotherapy, immunosuppressants and B cell depleting therapies such as rituximab) or caused by disease (e.g. haematological malignancies, protein-losing states and asplenia).

B cell depleting therapies, given to patients with haematological malignancies and inflammatory/autoimmune conditions, can cause hypogammaglobulinaemia that may persist for years, with associated recurrent sinopulmonary infection. These treatments are given to children with haematological malignancies and inflammatory/autoimmune conditions. As some of these children have an underlying undiagnosed PID, the B cell depletion may "unmask" the antibody deficiency. Therefore, measurement of B cell numbers and IgG, IgA and IgM levels are recommended **prior** to initiation of B-cell depleting therapy (e.g. rituximab), with ongoing monitoring to demonstrate the return of B cells and adequate antibody production.

Primary antibody defects

- **X-linked agammaglobulinaemia (XLA):** Usually an X-linked condition that usually presents in the first 4 years of life with recurrent bacterial upper and lower respiratory tract and ear infections, with hypogammaglobulinemia and absent or very low B cells. There is a failure of differentiation into mature B cells. Children can also present with severe invasive infection e.g. bacterial meningitis. Children with XLA also have susceptibility to enteroviral meningitis.
- **Common Variable Immunodeficiency (CVID):** a descriptive term for hypogammaglobulinaemia with recurrent infection, with or without autoimmune/inflammatory manifestations. Children typically present in mid to late childhood with infections (usually recurrent respiratory infections), cytopenias, lymphoproliferation (e.g. splenomegaly) or enteropathy. There are an increasing number of genetic defects being identified that cause CVID. However, many cases remain genetically unidentified.
- **IgA deficiency:** defined as undetectable IgA with normal IgG and IgM in a child aged >4 years, is relatively common, affecting approximately 1:500 of healthy individuals. Young children commonly have low IgA levels that they outgrow. Although most children with IgA deficiency are asymptomatic, a small proportion develop recurrent sinopulmonary infection, and some of these will develop CVID with time. IgA deficient individuals are at increased risk of allergic disease and autoimmune disease (e.g. coeliac disease).

When to suspect an antibody deficiency

- Suppurative chest, ear and/or sinus infections, especially if due to encapsulated bacteria.
- Children with recurrent autoimmune cytopenias, in particular ITP.

Initial investigations

- FBE
- Immunoglobulins (IgG, IgA and IgM)
- Tetanus toxoid IgG
- Lymphocyte subsets (T, B and NK cells)

> **Clinical Pearl: Immunoglobulin levels**
> Immunoglobulin levels vary with age and are lower in infancy and early childhood. In the first few months of life, IgG levels reflect maternally acquired IgG.

Management

- Immunoglobulin replacement therapy (IRT): given when a significant deficiency of antibody production is demonstrated in a child with clinically significant infections (usually sinopulmonary). It is usually administered IV every 3–4 weeks or subcutaneously weekly. If commenced early, IRT usually results in good quality of life.
- Antibiotics: as IRT does not provide significant levels of IgA antibody (the mucosal surface antibody), aggressive treatment of respiratory infections in children with antibody deficiency is important in order to prevent bronchiectasis. In severe cases or those with end organ damage (e.g. bronchiectasis), long-term prophylactic antibiotics and regular chest physiotherapy are used to prevent recurrent severe sinopulmonary infections.
- Immunisations: although live vaccines can safely be given, they are unlikely to promote an adequate antibody response in children with significant antibody deficiency.

Complement defects

Complement deficiency

Deficiencies of individual complement components are individually rare. They can be autosomal recessive or X-linked. Classical complement pathway deficiencies typically present with recurrent respiratory and ear infections and/or severe invasive infection (e.g. pneumonia, sepsis or meningitis) with encapsulated organisms such as the pneumococcus, whereas alternative and terminal complement pathway deficiencies are more likely to present with Neisseria infection.
Initial investigations:

- C3 and C4
- Classical pathway activity (also known as total haemolytic complement or CH50)
- Alternative pathway activity (also known as AH50)

When interpreting the above results, it is important to keep in mind that plasma products, such as FFP and platelets, contain residual complement and can therefore falsely normalise the results.

Management: Children should receive Hib, pneumococcal and meningococcal vaccines, and may require antibiotic prophylaxis.

Hereditary Angioedema

This is an autosomal dominant condition in which C1 inhibitor (an inhibitor of the classical pathway of complement) is reduced or not functional, resulting in uninhibited activation of the complement, kinin and fibrinolytic cascade. This results in recurrent episodes of angio-oedema involving limbs, upper respiratory or gastrointestinal tract. The angio-oedema is typically painful (including abdominal pain due to intestinal oedema), without pruritus or urticaria. Laryngeal oedema may occur, and severe episodes can be fatal.
Initial investigations:

- C4
- C1 inhibitor function

Management:

- C1 inhibitor concentrate or icatibant (a bradykinin receptor antagonist) should be considered for emergency treatment of acute angioedema in children with hereditary angioedema.
- Adrenaline, antihistamines and corticosteroids have no role in management.

Phagocytic & Innate Defects

Phagocytic disorders comprise a range of diseases with abnormal number or function of phagocytic cells such as neutrophils. A number of genetic defects give rise to congenital neutropenia, but defects in ability for neutrophils to reach the site of infection, phagocytose or kill pathogens also result in serious infection and complications.

- **Chronic granulomatous disease (CGD):** caused by failure of the neutrophil oxidative burst, which results in defective killing of some types of bacteria and fungi. There are both X-linked and autosomal recessive forms. Children usually present in the first few years of life, but delayed diagnosis can occur, particularly in autosomal recessive cases. Children with CGD typically present with recurrent or severe infections due to

Staphylococcus aureus, Aspergillus, Nocardia, Burkholderia or Serratia, and pneumonia is the most common type of infection.
- **Leukocyte adhesion defects (LAD):** result in abnormal neutrophil trafficking to the site of infection. Children classically present early in life with high peripheral white cell counts, severe gingivitis, delayed umbilical stump separation, omphalitis and recurrent, severe, invasive bacterial infections.

There are other genetic defects of innate immunity. These can present with predisposition to a limited number of pathogens, for example mycobacteria (mendelian susceptibility to mycobacterial disease) or invasive pneumococcal and staphylococcal disease (due to toll like receptor defects).

When to suspect a phagocytic or innate defect
- Infection with unusual pathogens such as Burkholderia cepacia, Aspergillus and Nocardia (CGD).
- Delayed umbilical cord separation &/or omphalitis in a neonate with persistently high white cell count (LAD).
- Unusually severe, prolonged &/or recurrent infection with specific pathogens e.g. pneumococcus, staphylococcus, mycobacteria, salmonella, warts (HPV), candidiasis.
- Staphylococcal liver abscess is pathognomic of CGD.

Investigations
- Full blood count to identify neutropenia or leucocytosis.
- Specific tests are required for diagnosis e.g. neutrophil oxidative burst (DHR) for CGD and CD18 expression for LAD. These are specialised tests that can be organised with your local diagnostic immunology laboratory.
- Note: Phagocytic and innate defects will not be identified from lymphocyte subsets and immunoglobulins.

Management
- Identification and treatment of specific infections.
- Infections in CGD are slow to resolve. Repeated surgical intervention and drainage should be avoided. Corticosteroids may be commenced, but only in consultation with the immunologist.
- Phagocytic and innate defects range in severity. Those with a high risk of serious, life threatening infection can be treated with HSCT.

Immune Dysregulation
An increasing number of PID associated with immune dysregulation are being recognised. Haemophagocytic lymphohistiocytosis is the most severe form of immune dysregulation.

Haemophagocytic lymphohistiocytosis (HLH)
HLH is a rapidly progressive and life threating disease of severe hyperinflammation.
- Caused by uncontrolled activation of lymphocytes and macrophages (histiocytes), resulting in a cytokine storm, which drives the histiocytes to destroy red cells, white cells and platelets (haemophagocytosis).
- HLH occurs in children with predisposing genetic defects, but can also occur secondary to infection, malignancy or autoimmune disease in children without a known genetic predisposition.
- Some PID predispose to severe or chronic EBV infection, and the EBV infection may trigger HLH.
- HLH should be considered in any child with the combination of fever, cytopenias (a falling platelet count is an early warning sign) and hepatic dysfunction (typically an elevated ALT or AST). Other clinical features include lymphadenopathy, hepatosplenomegaly, neurological symptoms, coagulopathy and rash.
- If HLH is suspected, ferritin and fibrinogen should be performed urgently.
- A rising ferritin (often >2000 ng/mL) and falling fibrinogen (even if still within reference range), usually associated with falling ESR, is suggestive of HLH.
- Bone marrow haemophagocytosis is **not** required to make a diagnosis of HLH.

Initial investigations for suspected HLH:
- FBE
- U&E
- LFT
- Coagulation screen including fibrinogen
- Soluble CD25
- EBV IgG and IgM and EBV PCR

Management:
- HLH is an immunological emergency, often requiring aggressive immunosuppression and chemotherapy to achieve disease control.
- After this initial treatment, children with severe HLH usually require definitive treatment with HSCT. Despite progress in diagnostics and treatment, mortality is still above 30%.

Other immune regulatory disorders

These include an increasing number of identified defects of regulatory T cells (Treg) e.g. IPEX syndrome (X-linked), CTLA4 deficiency (autosomal dominant) and LRBA deficiency (autosomal recessive).

CHAPTER 25

Infectious diseases

Nigel Curtis
Mike Starr
Josh Osowicki

> **Key Points**
> - Choice of empiric antimicrobials should be based on thorough clinical evaluation, targeted investigations and local antimicrobial susceptibility patterns.
> - Serious bacterial infection is an uncommon cause of fever in fully immunised infants and children, and when it does occur, UTI is far more likely than bacteraemia or meningitis.
> - For suspected meningitis, antibiotics should be given immediately after the collection of appropriate cultures, but should not be delayed if lumbar puncture is deferred.

Approach to the febrile child

- Fever is the most common presenting symptom in children in the primary care setting.
- Definition: Core temperature (rectal or tympanic) >38.0 °C.
  Axillary and oral temperatures may underestimate body temperature by 0.5 °C or more.
- Measuring temperature
  - Babies <3 months: rectal thermometer (tympanic is not as accurate).
  - Immunocompromised: oral or axillary.
- Self-limiting viral infections are the most common cause of fever in children. The challenge to the clinician is to identify those children with a more serious cause.
- Fever in children may be classified into three groups:
  - Fever with localising signs.
  - Fever without focus.
  - Fever (or pyrexia) of unknown origin.

Fever with localising signs

A careful history and examination will identify the source of infection in many patients; manage according to the source of infection and its severity.

Fever without focus

In many children presenting with fever, no focus is found. The large majority will have a viral infection, but a more serious illness such as a urinary tract infection (5–8%) or meningitis may be present. Neonates and infants <3 months of age have a higher risk of serious bacterial infection.

Most children who present with fever and no identifiable focus do not appear unwell. History should include systems review and details about immunisation status, infectious contacts, travel, diet and contact with animals. Physical examination should pay particular attention to:

- General appearance: the level of activity and social interaction; peripheral perfusion and colour.
- Vital signs: pulse, respiratory rate, blood pressure and oxygen saturation.

Paediatric Handbook, Tenth Edition. Edited by Kate Harding, Daniel S. Mason and Daryl Efron.
© 2021 John Wiley & Sons Ltd. Published 2021 by John Wiley & Sons Ltd.

- Possible clues to source: full fontanelle, neck stiffness, photophobia; respiratory distress (tachypnoea; grunting; nasal flare; intercostal and subcostal retraction), abnormal chest signs; rhinitis, pharyngitis, otitis or mastoiditis; lymphadenopathy; abdominal distension, tenderness or masses; hepatosplenomegaly; bone and joint tenderness or swelling; skin rashes, petechiae or purpura, or skin infection.
- **Always consider Kawasaki disease in any child with a fever that persists for more than a few days**. Other classical signs may not be present. The disease requires urgent treatment to avoid long-term sequelae.

Children with unexplained fever in whom serious infection should be excluded (clinically and/or by investigation) include:

- Those <3 months of age.
- Those with seizure(s) (although febrile seizures secondary to viral infections are common).
- Immunocompromised patients.
- Asplenic children.
- Children with indwelling lines/devices.
- Sickle cell disease, cystic fibrosis or structural cardiac defects (risk of endocarditis).
- Children who appear toxic and unwell (Table 25.1; e.g. altered conscious state, decreased peripheral perfusion (check central (CRT) or purpuric rash).

These children may require admission to hospital, with septic screen including culture of blood, urine and consideration of cerebrospinal fluid (CSF) and chest x-ray if indicated. Antibiotic therapy should be based on the patient's clinical illness, local epidemiology and likely antibiotic susceptibility (see Antimicrobial guidelines).

In the absence of these risk factors, a febrile child >3 months of age without a focus of infection who appears well does not necessarily require laboratory testing or treatment, although urine microscopy, culture and sensitivities (MC&S) may be considered. Careful clinical assessment, scheduled early review and parental education are important (Table 25.2).

Table 25.1 Features suggestive of an unwell child.

Colour	Pallor* (including parent/carer report) Mottled Blue/Cyanosed
Activity	Lethargy or decreased activity* Not responding normally to social cues Does not wake or only with prolonged stimulation, or if roused, does not stay awake Weak, high-pitched or continuous cry
Respiratory	Grunting Tachypnoea Increased work of breathing Hypoxia
Circulation and Hydration	Poor feeding* Dry mucous membranes Persistent tachycardia Central CRT ≥3 seconds Reduced skin turgor Reduced urine output
Neurological	Bulging fontanelle Neck stiffness Focal neurological signs Focal, complex or prolonged seizures
Other	Non-blanching rash Fever for ≥5 days Swelling of a limb or joint Non-weight bearing/not using an extremity

Notes: *Pallor, poor feeding or decreased activity on their own may not suggest a seriously unwell child. *Source*: Adapted from: Feverish illness in children NICE guideline 2017.

Table 25.2 Advice for parents about fever.

When caring for your child:
- Make the child comfortable, for example dress in light clothing.
- Give small, frequent drinks of clear fluid, for example water or diluted juice.
- Fever does not necessarily require treatment with medication. Finding the cause and treating the cause is often more important.
- Paracetamol may be given if the child is irritable, miserable or appears to be in pain (15 mg/kg PO 4–6 hourly when required, to a maximum of 90 mg/kg per day).
- Giving paracetamol has **not** been shown to prevent febrile convulsions.
- Do not give regular paracetamol for more than 48 hours without having the child assessed by a doctor.
- Avoid aspirin due to risk of Reye syndrome. Caution with other non-steroidal anti-inflammatory drugs (NSAIDs).

Parents should seek immediate medical attention if there is no improvement in 48 hours or if their child:
- Looks 'sick': pale, lethargic and weak.
- Has severe headache, neck stiffness or complains of light hurting their eyes.
- Has breathing difficulties.
- Refuses to drink anything.
- Has persistent vomiting.
- Shows signs of drowsiness.
- Has a non-blanching petechial/purpuric rash.

Investigations and Management

- Any febrile child who appears seriously unwell should be admitted, investigated and treated, irrespective of the degree of fever.
- If clinically stable, it is preferable to complete investigations for an infective focus before commencing antibiotics.
- If clinically unstable, assess for signs of shock and manage as per sepsis.
- Do not accept apparent otitis media or upper respiratory symptoms as the source of infection in young infants or unwell children. These patients still require assessment for possible serious bacterial infection.
- In children from high-risk groups, have a lower threshold to investigate and treat.
- **Infants ≤ 28 days corrected gestational age**
  - Assess promptly and discuss with senior doctor
  - FBE, CRP, blood culture, urine (SPA), LP ± CXR
  - Admit for empiric antibiotics
- **Infants 29 days to 3 months corrected age** (Figure 25.1)
- **Children >3 months corrected age** (Figure 25.2)

Partially treated bacterial infection

Patients presenting with fever who have received prior antibiotics should be assessed carefully. Although the child may still have a viral illness, partial treatment with antibiotics may mask the typical clinical presentation of a serious bacterial infection, such as meningitis. A full septic screen should be considered, even if the child looks well. For this reason, neonates should almost never be treated with oral antibiotics in the community.

Pyrexia (fever) of unknown origin

Pyrexia of unknown origin (PUO) is defined as prolonged fever (usually defined as ≥2 weeks or longer) where history, examination and initial investigations have failed to reveal a cause.

- The term PUO is often *incorrectly* applied to patients with brief fever without source or children who have experienced multiple consecutive viral infections.
- In general, PUO in children is more likely to be due to chronic, non-infectious conditions, such as juvenile chronic arthritis and other collagen vascular diseases, inflammatory bowel disease or malignancy.
- Infectious causes include systemic viral syndromes (such as infectious mononucleosis) and occult bacterial infection including sinusitis, bone infection, TB, abscess (e.g. parameningeal, intra-abdominal) and endocarditis.

Febrile neutropenia

See Chapter 30, Oncology.

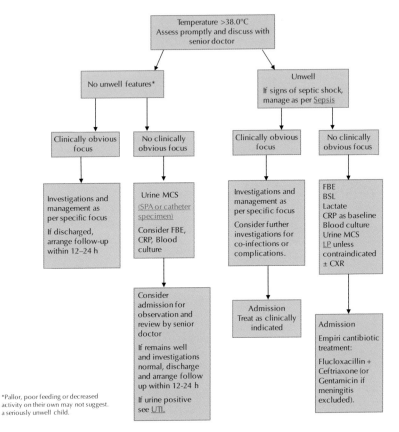

Figure 25.1 Treatment algorithm for infants 29 days to 3 months corrected age.

Toxic shock syndrome

Staphylococcus aureus and group A *Streptococcus* (GAS) can produce protein (superantigen) exotoxins causing a profound multisystem inflammatory syndrome.

Clinical features
- Fever, erythematous ('sunburn') rash, diarrhoea, vomiting, conjunctivitis, reddened mucous membranes, strawberry tongue and prolonged capillary refill time.
- A range of clinical presentations may be seen.
- At the most severe end of the spectrum, capillary leak leads to hypotension, shock and multi-organ failure (toxic shock syndrome).

Diagnosis
Early diagnosis depends on recognition of clinical features.
- A blood culture may be positive in ~30% of children with GAS, but in <5% of children with *S. aureus* toxic shock.

Management
- Remove any possible focus of infection (including retained tampon if present).
- Appropriate fluid management and intensive care support as required.

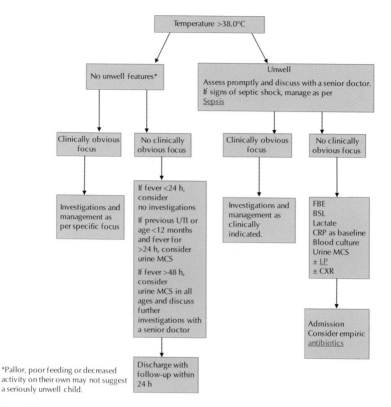

Figure 25.2 Treatment algorithm for infants and children >3 months corrected age.

- Antibiotics should include an anti-staphylococcal agent (e.g. flucloxacillin 50 mg/kg (max. 2 g) IV 4 hourly, see Antimicrobial guidelines).
- Clindamycin (to inhibit bacterial toxin and host cytokine production).
- IV immunoglobulin (2 g/kg) (as an immunomodulatory agent).

Rational antibiotic prescribing

- Unnecessary antibiotic use for viral illnesses contributes to the increasing problem of antibiotic-resistance.
- Most respiratory tract infections in children, including tonsillitis and otitis media, are self-limiting and do not require antibiotic therapy.
- If the diagnosis is unclear, it is preferable to repeat the clinical evaluation rather than use empiric antibiotic therapy 'just in case'.
- Antibiotics do not prevent secondary bacterial infection in viral illnesses.
- The use of antibiotics may make it more difficult to establish a definitive diagnosis and make rational decisions about management.
- Empiric antibiotics should be prescribed for suspected bacterial infection, based on the likely cause, local antibiotic-resistance patterns and individual host factors (e.g. immunocompromise), and in accordance with local guidelines.
- For mild infections, use the safest and best-tolerated antibiotic with the narrowest spectrum against the most likely pathogens (e.g. cefalexin for cellulitis).
- For serious infections use broad-spectrum antibiotics until the pathogen and its antibiotic susceptibility is available (e.g. third-generation cephalosporin for meningitis).

Antibiotic resistance

Antibiotic-resistant infections are an increasing problem worldwide. Risk factors include prolonged hospitalisation, overseas travel and prior colonisation with resistant organisms. Properly collected samples for culture (and molecular testing) prior to starting or changing antibiotics is important. Many resistant organisms are now routinely encountered in community-acquired infections in patients without risk factors, and should be suspected when initial empiric antibiotic therapy fails. Specialist consultation is strongly advised in managing infections caused by resistant organisms.

While many antibiotic-resistant bacteria are resistant to more than one antibiotic class, examples of particular clinical concern include:

- Penicillin (and cephalosporin) resistant *Streptococcus pneumoniae* (PRP)
- Methicillin resistant *Staphylococcus aureus* (MRSA)
- Glycopeptide (vancomycin, teicoplanin) heteroresistant, intermediate-resistant, and resistant *S. aureus* (hVISA, VISA, VRSA)
- Vancomycin-resistant *Enterococcus* (VRE)
- Multidrug-resistant (MDR) and extensively drug-resistant (XDR) *Mycobacterium tuberculosis* (TB)
- Gram-negative bacteria that produce extended-spectrum β-lactamases (ESBL), e.g. some *Escherichia coli* and *Klebsiella* spp. which are associated with third-generation cephalosporin resistance.

Kawasaki disease

Kawasaki disease (KD) is a systemic vasculitis that predominantly affects children under 5 years of age. Although the specific causal agent remains unknown, it is believed that KD is initiated by an infectious agent, although it is not transmitted from person to person. Early recognition and treatment are essential to reduce the risk of life-threatening complications.

Diagnosis

Diagnosis is often delayed as features are similar to many viral exanthems.

The features of KD can occur sequentially and may not all be present at the same time. The diagnostic criteria for KD are:

- Fever for ≥ 5 days (day of onset is first day); **plus**
- Four of the following five features:
  - Rash – maculopapular, diffuse erythematous or erythema multiforme-like.
  - Bilateral (non-purulent) bulbar conjunctival injection.
  - Mucous membrane changes; e.g. reddened or dry cracked lips, strawberry tongue, or diffuse redness of oral or pharyngeal mucosa.
  - Peripheral changes; e.g. erythema of palms or soles, oedema of hands or feet and desquamation *in convalescence*, particularly involving skin of hands, feet or perineal region.
  - Cervical lymphadenopathy (>15 mm in diameter, usually unilateral, single, non-purulent and painless).
- When four or more features are present (particularly erythema/oedema of the hands /feet), the diagnosis can be made with four days of fever.
- Exclusion of diseases with a similar presentation: staphylococcal infection (e.g. scalded skin syndrome and toxic shock syndrome), streptococcal infection (e.g. scarlet fever and toxic shock-like syndrome, but not just isolation from throat), measles, adenovirus, other viral exanthems, leptospirosis, rickettsial disease, Stevens–Johnson syndrome, drug reaction and juvenile chronic arthritis.
- Other relatively common features of KD include arthritis, diarrhoea and vomiting, coryza and cough, and hydropic gallbladder.

Clinical Pearl: Irritability in KD

Although irritability is not considered one of the diagnostic criteria, children with KD are frequently inconsolable and their fever is resistant to antipyretics.

Incomplete Kawasaki disease

- Clinical vigilance is needed to recognise patients with 'incomplete' or 'atypical' KD. These patients do not fulfil the formal diagnostic criteria, but are still at risk of developing coronary artery complications (see below).

- Incomplete KD can be diagnosed in infants with fever for 7 days of more without other explanation if they have raised acute phase markers plus ≥ 3 of: (1) anaemia for age; (2) platelets ≥450 after 7th day of fever; (3) albumin ≤30; (4) raised ALT; (5) WBC >15; (6) urine ≥10 WBC/hpf.

Investigations
Laboratory features may include:
- Neutrophilia
- Raised ESR and CRP
- Mild normochromic, normocytic anaemia
- Raised transaminases
- Hypoalbuminaemia
- Marked thrombocytosis in the second week of the illness

Complications
- Up to 30% of untreated children develop coronary artery dilation or aneurysm.
- Coronary artery aneurysms can be associated with early ischaemic heart disease.
- Can occur up to 6–8 weeks after onset of illness.
- Echocardiography should be done at least twice: at presentation and if negative, again at 6–8 weeks to exclude coronary artery involvement.

Management
Early (preferably within the first 10 days of the illness) administration of:
- IVIG (single dose of 2 g/kg IV over 10 hours)
  - IVIG is highly effective in preventing coronary artery complications in KD.
  - Treatment should still be undertaken in patients presenting after 10 days of illness if there is evidence of ongoing inflammation (fever, raised acute phase markers).
- Aspirin (3–5 mg/kg PO once a day (antiplatelet dose) for at least 6–8 weeks; maximum dose 150 mg).
  - There is no evidence that using high (anti-inflammatory) dose aspirin decreases the risk of aneurysm development above that prevented by IVIG. However, some guidelines suggest using high-dose aspirin (10 mg/kg PO tds) until defervescence.
- Paracetamol can be used for symptomatic relief; avoid NSAIDs (hinder the antiplatelet activity of aspirin).
- Repeat IVIG dosing (2 g/kg) given to patients who fail to defervesce within 24–36 hours after finishing first dose.
- Refractory cases with continuing fever and other signs of inflammation after IVIG need specialist advice for further treatment that may include high-dose steroids (e.g. methylprednisolone 30 mg/kg IV).

Common bacterial infections
Staphylococcus aureus
S. aureus is a Gram-positive coccus that causes a wide variety of invasive and non-invasive disease, and can also cause toxic shock syndrome (see section above).

Epidemiology
- Carried asymptomatically in the nose of about 1/3 individuals at any given time.
- Both hospital- and community-acquired methicillin-resistant *S. aureus* (MRSA) have emerged as a significant public health problem.

Clinical features
- Causes a variety of diseases including: impetigo, boils and abscesses, cellulitis (including periorbital cellulitis), osteomyelitis, septic arthritis, endocarditis, pneumonia, food poisoning, bacteraemia, toxic shock syndrome, and scalded skin syndrome in younger children.
- Staphylococcal infection may be accompanied by significant systemic symptoms (e.g. myalgia) in addition to localising features.

Diagnosis
- Infection (preferably from sterile site) confirmed by MC&S.
- Patients with *S. aureus* bacteraemia should undergo careful clinical examination to identify any focal infection.

Treatment
- Surgical drainage is often necessary for abscesses and other foci of infection (source control).
- *S. aureus* bacteraemia often needs prolonged treatment to prevent relapse.
- Anti-staphylococcal antibiotics include flucloxacillin, cefalexin, cefazolin and clindamycin.
- MRSA is resistant to all commonly used beta-lactam antibiotics (i.e. penicillins, 1st–4th generation cephalosporins, carbapenems).
  - MRSA can be susceptible to a wide range of antibiotics including clindamycin, cotrimoxazole, doxycycline, ciprofloxacin, vancomycin, teicoplanin, daptomycin, linezolid, rifampicin and fusidic acid.
  - Note ciprofloxacin, rifampicin or fusidic acid should never be used alone for *S. aureus*, as resistance develops rapidly.

Streptococcus pyogenes (Group A *Streptococcus*; 'Strep A'; GAS)
Group A β-haemolytic streptococci (*S. pyogenes*, GAS, 'Strep A') cause a variety of diseases including: pharyngo-tonsillitis (see chapter 33 Otolarnygology), impetigo, cellulitis, scarlet fever, otitis media, streptococcal toxic shock syndrome, necrotising fasciitis, glomerulonephritis and rheumatic fever.
- GAS pharyngitis is extremely uncommon in children <5 years of age.
- GAS is currently always sensitive to penicillin.

Scarlet fever
- Transmission: droplet, direct contact, with incubation period 2–5 days.
- Infectious period: 10–21 days (24 hours if adequate treatment).

Clinical features
- Prodrome: sudden-onset high fever, vomiting, malaise, headache and abdominal pain.
- Rash: appears during early prodrome; blanching, diffuse, erythematous, involving torso and skin folds.
- Associated features: circumoral pallor, strawberry tongue (initially white, then red day 4–5), pharyngotonsillitis and tender cervical/submaxillary nodes.
- Complications include: otitis media, retropharyngeal abscess, quinsy, rheumatic fever, glomerulonephritis and rarely meningitis.
- Differential diagnosis includes: viral infection, Kawasaki disease, streptococcal or staphylococcal toxic shock syndrome.

Diagnosis
- Throat swab MC&S may confirm clinical impression.

Treatment
- Phenoxymethylpenicillin (penicillin V) 250 mg PO (<10 years), 500 mg PO (>10 years) bd for 10 days.
- Once-daily amoxicillin is a reasonable alternative, and availability of a child-friendly formulation is assured across all settings.
- Control of case: exclude from school until treated for 24 hours.

Acute rheumatic fever
- Incubation period: 7–28 days after GAS infection.

Clinical features
- Specific criteria for diagnosis can be found at www.rhdaustralia.org.au.
- Diagnostic criteria are stratified according to risk.
- Carditis, polyarthritis and chorea are major manifestations for all risk groups.
- *Complications* include:
  - Heart valve damage: may be permanent (rheumatic heart disease), especially after severe or recurrent disease.
  - Increased risk of recurrent disease; particularly for first 5 years after an attack.

Diagnosis
- Clinical features, CRP, ESR, and culture/serology.
- Echocardiography may be useful in detecting and characterising subclinical lesions or typical rheumatic valvular involvement.

Treatment

- Admission to hospital.
- Oral phenoxymethylpenicillin (penicillin V) or a single IM injection of benzathine penicillin G.
- Non-steroidal anti-inflammatory drugs (e.g. naproxen) or aspirin for symptomatic relief of arthritis/ arthralgia.
- Corticosteroids are often used for management of severe carditis with cardiac failure, although they do not improve long-term outcome.
- For severe chorea; anticonvulsants, corticosteroids, and IVIG have been used with limited success.
- Follow-up and secondary prophylaxis is essential to prevent subsequent GAS infections, which may cause recurrences.
  - Intramuscular benzathine penicillin G every 21–28 days is preferred.
  - Oral penicillin is an alternative.
  - Long-term clinical and echocardiographic follow-up essential.

Acute Post Streptococcal Glomerulonephritis (APSGN)

See Chapter 37 Renal medicine.

Streptococcal toxic shock syndrome

GAS, like *S. aureus*, can cause toxic shock syndrome (see section above).

Streptococcus pneumoniae

S. pneumoniae (pneumococcus) is a Gram-positive coccus that it transmitted via droplet and causes a wide variety of infections including:

- Severe invasive disease (e.g. meningitis, pleural empyema, septic arthritis, peritonitis).
- Milder, sometimes self-limited disease (e.g. pneumonia, otitis media and sinusitis).

Epidemiology

This is changing as a result of the *routine* use of conjugate pneumococcal vaccines (7-valent and more recently 10-valent and 13-valent vaccines). Additional doses of conjugate pneumococcal vaccine are recommended for particular high-risk groups during infancy and early childhood (see chapter 9 Immunisation).

- Despite the decreasing incidence of pneumococcal disease, *S. pneumoniae* remains the most common bacterial cause of pneumonia, otitis media and meningitis in children.
- This is due in part to a rise in disease caused by non-vaccine serotypes (serotype replacement), some of which are resistant to penicillin and other antibiotics.

Clinical features

- Pneumonia, otitis media, meningitis.
- Bone and joint infections less common manifestations.

Diagnosis

- MC&S of appropriate sterile site specimens (eg. CSF).
- Blood culture positive in <10% of pneumococcal pneumonia cases.
- Polymerase chain reaction (PCR) based testing of blood, CSF and pleural fluid available (useful when specimens collected post antibiotic commencement).

Treatment

Penicillin (or ampicillin/amoxicillin) is the drug of choice, except in CNS infection with pneumococci that have reduced susceptibility to penicillin.

- For non-CNS invasive infection (eg. pneumonia): high-dose penicillin (benzylpenicillin 60 mg/kg (max. 2 g) IV 4–6 hourly.
- For otitis media or sinusitis: amoxicillin 30 mg/kg (1 g) PO bd.
- For CNS infection with third-generation cephalosporin-non-susceptible pneumococci: vancomycin or moxifloxacin in addition to third-generation cephalosporin and seek specialist advice (see bacterial meningitis below).
- Minimum duration of treatment: 10 days for meningitis, 10–21 days for bone and joint infections and 5–7 days for other infections.

Neisseria meningitidis

N. meningitidis (meningococcus) is a Gram-negative diplococcus that mainly causes meningitis and/or septicaemia (meningococcaemia). Less commonly, it may cause other infections including conjunctivitis, septic arthritis, pharyngitis and pneumonia. For recommendations specific to meningitis see section on Bacterial meningitis.

- Transmission is by droplet; incubation period is hours to 3 days; infectious period is as long as carried and may be months.
- Most meningococci are virulent within days of acquisition.

Epidemiology

- Peak age groups: <2 years and 15–24 years.
- Incidence of serogroup B and C infection have fallen in recent years since the introduction of conjugate vaccination, whilst serogroups W and Y have caused increased cases of invasive disease.
- Despite antibiotic treatment, overall case fatality in invasive disease remains high (5% for group B and 14% for group C infection).

Clinical features

- Meningitis – see section below (Bacterial meningitis).
- Septicaemia: often non-specific prodrome suggestive of viral illness, followed by rapid progression with any or all of the following:
  - Fever
  - Rash (classically purpuric or petechial, but can be less specific)
  - Malaise
  - Myalgia and arthralgia
  - Vomiting
  - Headache
  - Reduced conscious state
- Chronic meningococcaemia occurs rarely (consider terminal complement deficiency) and may be associated with progressive purpuric rash.

Diagnosis

- Diagnosis is initially based on clinical features, with confirmation by MC&S of blood and/or CSF, preferably collected before first dose of antibiotics.

Additional tests may include:

- Skin scrapings of purpuric skin lesions for MC&S
- PCR on blood and/or CSF

Clinical Pearl: Suspected meningococcal disease

Whilst confirmation of meningococcal disease via MCS or PCR is optimal, **under no circumstances should treatment be delayed while awaiting collection of clinical samples.** Treatment should always be commenced empirically if meningococcal disease is suspected clinically.

Treatment

- Manage septic shock appropriately (see Chapter 3, Resuscitation and medical emergencies).
- IV antibiotics:
  - Ceftriaxone 50 mg/kg (max. 2 g) IV 12 hourly or Cefotaxime 50 mg/kg per dose (max. 2 g) 6 hourly.
  - If unavailable give Benzylpenicillin 60 mg/kg (max. 2 g) IV 4–6 hourly.
  - *If IV access cannot be obtained, give antibiotics IM.*
- Change to IV benzylpenicillin when meningococcus is isolated and susceptibility confirmed.
- Duration of antibiotics is usually 5–7 days.
- Consider corticosteroids (hydrocortisone 1 mg/kg IV 6 hourly) in severe cases of meningococcaemia.
- All cases should be notified immediately to statutory health authorities.

Treatment of contacts of patients with meningococcal infection

Contacts should receive antibiotic prophylaxis (Table 25.4), and meningococcal vaccination should be considered for household and other higher-risk contacts. Patients with invasive disease who have received only penicillin should also receive treatment to eradicate carriage.

Meningococcal vaccines

Quadrivalent conjugate vaccine against groups A, C, W and Y has replaced group C vaccine in the routine NIP schedule (see chapter 9 Immunisation). This vaccine is also recommended for high-risk patients (e.g. asplenia), for travellers (e.g. to African 'meningitis belt' or attending the Haj), and for controlling outbreaks. Vaccines against group B are also available.

Mycoplasma pneumoniae

- *Mycoplasma pneumoniae* infection can affect children of all ages.
- Transmission via droplet; incubation period 1–4 weeks.
- Infectious period is unknown, likely to be months; typically infects all members of a family over a period of weeks/months although most are asymptomatic.

Clinical features

- Pneumonia: malaise, fever, headache, non-productive cough for 3–4 weeks (may become productive).
  - Bronchitis, pharyngitis, otitis media
  - Rash (10%; usually maculopapular)
  - CXR may show unilateral lobar or bilateral diffuse changes
- CNS manifestations (uncommon; likely post-infectious): aseptic meningitis, meningoencephalitis, encephalitis, polyradiculitis/Guillain–Barré syndrome, acute cerebellar ataxia, cranial nerve neuropathy, transverse myelitis, acute disseminated encephalomyelitis (ADEM) and choreoathetosis.

Diagnosis

- Serology: IgM poor specificity in acute setting (~30% of healthy preschoolers IgM+).
  - Current diagnostics cannot distinguish between asymptomatic carriage and symptomatic infection.
  - Infection diagnosed by fourfold rise in IgG over 2–4 weeks

Treatment

- Clarithromycin, azithromycin or doxycycline (although role of antibiotics uncertain).
- Suspected CNS disease: macrolides (e.g. IV azithromycin) recommended.

Localised bacterial infections
Cervical lymphadenitis

- Usually caused by infection or inflammation of the lymph nodes; malignancy is much less common.
- Infectious causes include:

Acute bilateral lymphadenitis

- Localised viral URTI.
- Systemic viral infection (e.g. EBV and CMV; +/- generalised lymphadenopathy and hepatosplenomegaly).
- Kawasaki disease: may present initially as cervical lymphadenitis alone (see KD section above).

Acute unilateral lymphadenitis

- GAS or *S. aureus*: 40–80% of acute unilateral lymphadenitis; occurs at 1–4 years of age with fever, tenderness, overlying erythema and may be associated with cellulitis.
- Anaerobic bacteria: older children with dental caries or periodontal disease.
- GBS: may have overlying cellulitis (neonates).

Subacute/chronic unilateral lymphadenitis

- *Bartonella henselae* (cat-scratch disease): occurs 2 weeks after a scratch or lick from a kitten or dog and usually involves axillary nodes; tender nodes +/- papule at infection site.
- *Mycobacterium avium complex* (MAC – formerly known as MAIS): patient usually 1–4 years of age, afebrile, systemically well and not immunocompromised; node usually unilateral, slightly fluctuant, non-tender, sometimes tethered to underlying structures and with violaceous hue to overlying skin.

- *Toxoplasma gondii*: systemic features (fatigue, myalgia), +/- generalised lymphadenopathy.
- *M. tuberculosis*: usually a contact history or relevant history of migration; affects older children; systemic symptoms (e.g. fever, malaise, weight loss), non-tender nodes.
- HIV.

Management
- Acute bilateral lymphadenitis without other signs (e.g. pallor, bruising or hepatosplenomegaly) is usually viral and does not need specific treatment or investigation.
- Acute unilateral lymphadenitis: oral cefalexin 33 mg/kg (max. 500 mg) PO tds for 7 days (see Appendix: Antimicrobial guidelines), with review in 48 hours.
  - If systemically unwell with large tender nodes, or failed oral treatment, admission for IV antibiotics may be required.
- Acute unilateral lymphadenitis with a fluctuant node may require incision and drainage (contra-indicated in suspected TB as may result in sinus formation).

Cellulitis
- Infection of cutaneous and subcutaneous tissue characterised by erythema, warmth, oedema and tenderness.
- Predisposing factors include a break in the skin (e.g. insect bite, trauma) or a pre-existing skin lesion.
- Usually caused by GAS or *S. aureus* (Hib uncommon, consider in unimmunised children <5 years age).
- May be associated with:
  - Regional lymphadenopathy
  - Systemic symptoms: fever, chills and malaise
  - Deeper involvement: including necrotising fasciitis (usually extremely painful), osteomyelitis, septic arthritis, or features of toxin-mediated illness (diffuse erythema, conjunctival injection and systemic features)

Diagnosis
- Primarily clinical - MC&S of blood, skin aspirate or skin biopsy unhelpful.

Management
- Cefalexin 33 mg/kg (max. 500 mg) PO tds
- IV antibiotics indicated if fever, rapid progression, lymphangitis or lymphadenitis:
  - Flucloxacillin 50 mg/kg (max. 2 g) IV 6 hourly
  - Add ceftriaxone 50 mg/kg (max. 1 g) IV 12 hourly or cefotaxime 50 mg/kg (max. 2 g) IV 6 hourly if non-immunised children <5 years with facial cellulitis
- Seek specialist advice if toxin-mediated disease suspected.

Central nervous system infections
Bacterial meningitis
Bacterial meningitis is a medical emergency.

Clinical features
- Infants: often non-specific, eg. fever, lethargy, irritability, high-pitched crying or vomiting.
- Older children: headache, vomiting, drowsiness, photophobia and neck stiffness may be present.
  Kernig sign (inability to extend the knee when the leg is flexed at the hip) and *Brudzinski sign* (bending the head forward produces flexion of the legs) may be positive.

Diagnosis
- Diagnosis is confirmed by examination of the CSF, however Lumbar puncture (LP) is contraindicated in certain situations (see chapter 5 Procedures).
- If LP is deferred or reveals no organism, identification of the pathogen may still be possible through:
  - Blood cultures – often positive where clinical signs of meningitis are present.
  - PCR on blood or CSF for *N. meningitidis*, *S. pneumoniae* and consider TB.
  - Skin scraping or aspirate of purpuric lesions for Gram stain, PCR or (less likely) culture.

Interpretation of CSF findings
CSF findings should always be interpreted in light of the clinical context (Table 25.3).

Table 25.3 Classical cerebrospinal fluid (CSF) findings.

	Neutrophils (×10⁶/L)	Lymphocytes (×10⁶/L)	Protein (g/L)	Glucose (CSF:blood ratio)
Normal <1 month of age	Higher than for older infant	<22	<1.0	≥0.6 (or ≥2.0 mmol/L)
Normal >1 month of age	0	≤5	<0.4	≥0.6 (or ≥2.5 mmol/L)
Bacterial meningitis	100–10,000 (but may be normal)	Usually <100	>1.0 (but may be normal)	<0.4 (but may be normal)
Viral meningitis	Usually <100	10–1000 (but may be normal)	0.4–1 (but may be normal)	Usually normal
TB meningitis	Usually <100	50–1000 (but may be normal)	1–5 (but may be normal)	<0.3 (but may be normal)
Encephalitis	Usually <100		0.4–1 (but may be normal)	Usually normal
Brain abscess	Usually 5–100		>1 (but may be normal)	Usually normal

Cell count
- **Perform microscopy without delay** (cell lysis begins shortly after collection and may affect cell count within 1 hour).
- The presence of neutrophils in the CSF should always raise concern for meningitis.
- In early bacterial meningitis there may be no increase in the CSF cell count (and may remain normal in up to 4% of young infants and up to 17% of neonates).
- In bacterial meningitis there can be a shift to a lymphocyte predominance after 48 hours of therapy.
- In viral (typically enteroviral) meningitis, the early CSF findings can mimic bacterial meningitis with a neutrophil predominance.
- Antibiotics usually prevent the culture of bacteria from the CSF, but they do not significantly alter the CSF cell count or biochemistry in samples taken early. In 'partially treated meningitis' the CSF should be interpreted like any other CSF.
- Seizures do *not* cause an increased CSF cell count.
- In neonates, interpretation of CSF may be difficult. Normal values for CSF cell counts and biochemistry differ from those of older infants (with typically higher cell count and protein and lower glucose; particularly in premature neonates).

Clinical Pearl: Interpretation of CSF contaminated by blood ('traumatic tap')
- CSF contaminated by blood can be difficult to interpret; whilst a ratio of one white blood cell to 500–700 red blood cells is sometimes used to correct for blood in CSF, this is unreliable.
- The safest way to interpret a 'traumatic tap' is to **count the total number of white cells, and disregard the red cell count**. If there are more white cells than the normal range for age, then the safest option is to treat.

Biochemistry
- CSF protein and glucose are unreliable markers in isolation:
  ○ CSF protein is normal in about 40% of school-age children with bacterial meningitis.
  ○ CSF glucose is normal in about 50% of school-age children with bacterial meningitis.

Adjunctive steroid treatment of meningitis
- Adjunctive steroid therapy should be given at the time of LP if there is strong clinical suspicion of bacterial meningitis in children >4 weeks old, as this can reduce the risk of hearing loss.
  ○ Antibiotics should *not* be delayed by any more than 30 minutes to administer steroids.

- Initial dose: dexamethasone 0.15 mg/kg IV ideally given 15 minutes before, but up to 1 hour after, the first dose of antibiotics.
- Ongoing dose: dexamethasone 0.15 mg/kg IV 6 hourly should be continued for 4 days (unless bacterial meningitis has been excluded).

Antibiotic treatment of meningitis
- Antibiotics must be given immediately after the collection of appropriate cultures, but should not be delayed if a LP is deferred.
- Antibiotics should only be rationalised when CSF or blood culture results are available.

Age >2 months
The incidence of bacterial meningitis has fallen dramatically since the introduction of conjugated *Haemophilus influenzae* type b (Hib) vaccine. The major pathogens are now *S. pneumoniae* and *N. meningitidis*.
- Initial therapy
  - Cefotaxime 50 mg/kg (max. 2 g) IV 6 hourly or Ceftriaxone 50 mg/kg (max.1 g) IV 12 hourly.
  - Pneumococci with reduced susceptibility to penicillin (and cephalosporins) should be considered (see Appendix: Antimicrobial guidelines for details).
- Continued therapy: IV antibiotics duration
  - 7 days for *N. meningitidis*
  - 10–14 days for *S. pneumoniae*
  - 7–10 days for Hib
- If there is prolonged or secondary fever, or where sensitivity testing indicates the pneumococcal isolate has reduced susceptibility to third-generation cephalosporins, LP should be repeated to detect treatment failure, and neuroimaging should be considered, looking for abscess or empyema.

Age <2 months
The most common organisms are neonatal pathogens (e.g. group B streptococcus (GBS), *E. coli* and other enteric Gram-negatives, and *Listeria monocytogenes*), or the same pathogens commonly detected in older children (e.g. *S. pneumoniae*, *N. meningitidis*, Hib).
- Initial therapy:
  - IV Benzylpenicillin and third-generation Cephalosporin (see Appendix: Antimicrobial guidelines).
- Continued therapy: treatment is adjusted according to culture and sensitivity results.

Meningitis associated with shunts, neurosurgery, head trauma and CSF leak
In addition to common pathogens causing meningitis, consider *S. aureus*, coagulase negative staphylococci and (especially with a ventriculoperitoneal shunt *in situ*) Gram-negative bacilli including *Pseudomonas aeruginosa* or anaerobes.
- Initial therapy: Vancomycin 15 mg/kg (max. 500 mg) IV 6 hourly **plus**:
  - *with* ventriculoperitoneal shunt: Ceftazidime 50 mg/kg (max. 2 g) IV 8 hourly
  - *without* ventriculoperitoneal shunt: Cefotaxime 50 mg/kg (max. 2 g) IV 6 hourly or Ceftriaxone 50 mg/kg (max. 1 g) IV 12 hourly

Antibiotic prophylaxis for contacts of meningitis cases
- Prophylaxis is required for confirmed cases of bacterial meningitis (Table 25.4).

General measures
Requirement for intensive care
Admission to ICU should be discussed with a specialist in the following circumstances:
- Age <2 years
- Coma
- Cardiovascular compromise
- Intractable seizures
- Hyponatraemia

Table 25.4 Prophylaxis regimens for contacts of meningitis cases.

Organism	Antibiotic	Those requiring prophylaxis
Haemophilus influenzae type b	Rifampicin 20 mg/kg (max. 600 mg) PO daily for 4 days *Infants <1 month:* Rifampicin 10 mg/kg PO daily for 4 days *Pregnancy/contraindication to rifampicin:* Ceftriaxone 250 mg IM daily for 2 days	Index case and all household contacts if household includes: • Any infants <12 months of age, regardless of immunisation status. • Other children <4 years of age who are not fully immunised. Index case and all room contacts, including staff, in a childcare group if index case attends >18 hours per week and any contacts <2 years of age who are inadequately immunised. **AND** children who are not up to date with Hib should be immunised.
N. meningitidis	Ciprofloxacin 500 mg (≥12 years) or 250 mg (5–12 years) PO as a single dose *Young children:* Rifampicin 5 mg/kg (<1 month) *or* 10 mg/kg (≥1 month) (max 600 mg) PO bd for 2 days *Pregnancy/contraindication to rifampicin:* Ceftriaxone 250 mg (≥12 years) or 125 mg (<12 years) IM as a single dose *or* Ciprofloxacin 500 mg (≥12 y) or 250 mg (5–12 years) PO as a single dose	Index case (if treated only with penicillin) and all intimate household or day care contacts who have been exposed to index case within 10 days of onset. Any person who gave mouth-to-mouth resuscitation to the index case
S. pneumoniae	Nil	No increased risk to contacts

Notes:
• Prophylaxis must be given early to both the index case and contacts, especially for *N. meningitidis* disease, because of the rapidity with which secondary cases may develop.
• Rifampicin interferes with the metabolism of several medications, including the oral contraceptive pill (alternative contraception should be instituted), anticonvulsants, warfarin and chloramphenicol.
• Rifampicin colours body fluids red, for example urine, saliva, tears (soft contact lenses may be damaged), sweat.

Fluid management
• Careful fluid management is important in the treatment of meningitis as many children develop the syndrome of 'inappropriately' increased antidiuretic hormone secretion (SIADH).
• The degree of fluid restriction varies with each patient according to their clinical state.
• Hypovolaemia should be corrected with 10 mL/kg of normal saline and repeated as required.
• A patient who is not in shock who has a normal serum sodium should initially be given 50% maintenance fluid requirements.
  ○ If the serum sodium is <135 mmol/L give 25–50% of maintenance requirements.
• Serum sodium (and clinical fluid status) should be measured every 6–12 hours for the first 48 hours and the total fluid intake adjusted accordingly.

Observations
• Neurological observations and blood pressure should be recorded every 15 minutes for the first 2 hours and then at intervals determined by the child's conscious state.
• Head circumference should be monitored daily in infants.
• Weight is measured daily or more frequently if required.

Seizures

- Exclude hypoglycaemia, electrolyte imbalance (especially hyponatraemia) and raised intracranial pressure before attributing seizures to the underlying infection or febrile convulsion.
- Control of seizures is vital and specialist consultation is advised.

Analgesia

- Ensure adequate analgesia; children in the recovery phase may have significant headache.

Fever persisting for >7 days

- May be due to nosocomial infection, subdural effusion or other foci of suppuration.
- Uncommon causes include inadequately treated meningitis, a parameningeal focus or drug related fever.

Outcome/follow-up

- All patients require a hearing assessment 6–8 weeks after discharge, or sooner if hearing loss is suspected.
- More than 25% of survivors have mild disabilities that adversely affect school performance and behaviour. Consequently, all children surviving bacterial meningitis should be regularly reviewed during their early school years.
- Less common sequelae include epilepsy, visual impairment and cerebral palsy.

Prevention

Many cases of meningitis are now preventable. All parents should be encouraged to have their children fully immunised.

Viral meningitis

Common pathogens include enterovirus (coxsackie and echoviruses), parechovirus and HHV-6 (see page 321).
- Clinical features: can mimic bacterial meningitis.
- Diagnosis: Enterovirus may be detected by PCR in CSF/throat swabs/stool.
- Natural History: most cases are self-limiting although severe life-threatening cases of meningoencephalitis due to enterovirus and parechovirus do occur.
- Treatment: support except in immunocompromised patients where IV immunoglobulin may be used (specialist advice is recommended).

Tuberculous meningitis

Tuberculous meningitis is uncommon in Australia, although it should be considered in children from countries where TB is more common.
- TB meningitis often presents in an insidious manner and can be difficult to recognise without a high index of suspicion.
- Large volumes of CSF are required (at least 10 mL) for diagnosis by microscopy and culture of mycobacteria, or molecular tests.
- Treatment with combination anti-tuberculous medications plus steroids should be started early and specialist advice is recommended.

Encephalitis

Most common pathogens: HSV-1 or 2, influenza virus, enterovirus, parechovirus, *M. pneumoniae,* adenovirus, EBV and VZV. Also consider non-infective causes of encephalitis (see chapter 29 Neurology).

Clinical features

- Usually presents with ≥1 of:
  - Fever
  - Headache
  - Vomiting
  - Change of behaviour
  - Drowsiness
  - Convulsions (particularly focal)

- ○ Focal neurological deficits
- ○ Signs of raised intracranial pressure
- Focal seizures and neurological signs are more typical of herpes encephalitis but clinical presentation, (especially early in the disease), is not specific to a particular pathogen.

Diagnosis
- CSF findings are non-specific (Table 25.3).
- MRI brain and EEG may show characteristic findings.

Treatment
- IV Aciclovir: commence in any child with encephalitis of uncertain aetiology (see Appendix: Antimicrobial guidelines).
- IV Aciclovir should be continued until
  - ○ An alternative diagnosis is reached; **or**
  - ○ Herpes encephalitis is excluded by
    - ▪ Absence of typical clinical features.
    - ▪ Normal serial MRI scans.
    - ▪ Normal serial EEG.
    - ▪ Negative PCR for HSV on CSF obtained >72 hours into the illness (this may necessitate a repeat LP).
- Macrolides (e.g. azithromycin) are sometimes used in encephalitis due to *M. pneumoniae* but their benefit is uncertain.

Brain abscess
Clinical features
- Classically presents with:
  - ○ Fever
  - ○ Headache
  - ○ Focal neurological deficit
- Although rare, early recognition important because most cases are readily treated and delayed diagnosis can lead to complications.

Diagnosis
- CT / MRI brain
- Neurosurgical intervention for diagnostics (aspiration for MC&S) and management is usually necessary.

Treatment
- Neurosurgical drainage (see above)
- Empiric treatment to cover the likely aetiological pathogens:
  - ○ Flucloxacillin 50 mg/kg (max. 2 g) IV 4 hourly; **and**
  - ○ Ceftriaxone 50 mg/kg (max. 1 g) iv 12H or Cefotaxime 50 mg/kg (max. 2 g) IV 6 hourly); **and**
  - ○ Metronidazole 15 mg/kg (max. 1 g) IV stat, then 7.5 mg/kg (max. 500 mg) IV 8 hourly (see Appendix: Antimicrobial guidelines).
- Treatment is usually continued for up to 6 weeks; specialist advice is recommended.

Common viral infections
Cytomegalovirus
Cytomegalovirus (CMV) is a ubiquitous herpes virus. It persists in latent form after primary infection and reactivation can occur years later, particularly with immunosuppression. The acquisition of CMV infection in early pregnancy may affect the unborn infant and lead to congenital CMV infection.

Transmission
- *Horizontal*: salivary contamination or sexual transmission; blood transfusion/organ transplantation.
- *Vertical*: transplacental, intrapartum (infected genital tract) and postnatal (ingestion of CMV-positive breast milk).

Incubation period
Unknown; symptoms usually develop 9–60 days after primary infection.

Clinical features
The presentation varies with age and immune status of child:
- Asymptomatic infection common.
- Symptomatic presentations include:
  ○ CMV mononucleosis, cervical lymphadenopathy, hepatosplenomegaly in children
  ○ Fever in adults
  ○ Note: clinical signs of CMV infection are similar to graft rejection in transplant patients.
- Congenital CMV may be asymptomatic (majority) or have clinical signs including:
  ○ Low birth weight
  ○ Microcephaly
  ○ Rash ('blueberry muffin')
  ○ Jaundice
  ○ Hepatosplenomegaly (see below)
  ○ Auditory brainstem evoked responses may show sensorineural hearing loss.

Diagnosis
- Congenital infection: urine or salivary viral PCR positive in the first 3 weeks of life is diagnostic.
  ○ After this period, positive results may represent postnatally acquired infection.
  ○ PCR of NST stored dried blood spots can confirm congenital CMV if suspected after 3 weeks of life (e.g. infants with sensorineural hearing loss that were asymptomatic at birth).
- Distinguishing past from active infection can be difficult; PCR of urine, saliva and even blood may be misleading as CMV can be excreted intermittently for life after primary infection (particularly if immunocompromised).

Complications
- Sepsis syndrome, colitis, pneumonitis, encephalitis, peripheral neuropathies, myocarditis, haemolytic anaemia, thrombocytopenia are rare manifestations.
- Pneumonia, retinitis, hepatitis and colitis occur more commonly in immunocompromised patients.
- Congenital infection:
  ○ >90% appear normal at birth.
  ○ 5% present early with petechiae, hepatosplenomegaly, microcephaly and thrombocytopenia – this group have high rates of neurological sequelae.
  ○ CNS sequelae in 10–20% (mainly sensorineural hearing loss, which may present in preschool or early school years).

Treatment
- Symptomatic congenital CMV: antiviral therapy (usually with oral Valganciclovir) reduces the risk of hearing loss and other neurological sequelae; specialist advice recommended.
- Immunocompromised active CMV: Ganciclovir or Valganciclovir (+/- consider CMV-specific cytotoxic lymphocytes).

Enterovirus (non-polio)
Coxsackie A, B, echoviruses and parechoviruses are important causes of childhood infections, especially in the summer months.
- These include a wide range of clinical presentations, including non-specific febrile illness; pharyngitis; herpangina; hand, foot and mouth disease; gastroenteritis; aseptic meningitis; encephalitis; myocarditis; pericarditis and several forms of viral exanthem (maculopapular, vesicular, petechial).
- Infection in agammaglobulinaemic patients can cause severe or persistent meningoencephalitis.
- In neonates, enteroviral infection may be difficult to distinguish from bacterial sepsis.

Hand, foot and mouth disease
- Cause: coxsackie A virus (usually A16).
- Transmission: direct contact/droplet.

- Incubation period: 3–6 days.
- Infectious period: until blisters have gone.

Clinical features
- Vesicles on cheeks, gums, sides of the tongue.
- Papulovesicular lesions of palms, fingers, toes, soles, buttocks, genitals, limbs (may look haemorrhagic).
- Fever, sore throat, anorexia.
- 'Eczema coxsackium': a more severe and atypical presentation of hand, foot and mouth with vesiculobullous eruptions.

Diagnosis
- Clinical diagnosis usually; tests are usually unnecessary.
- Enterovirus PCR may assist in atypical cases.

Treatment
- Symptomatic
- School/social exclusion not indicated and impractical as virus excreted in stool for weeks.

Epstein–Barr virus
- Incubation period: 30–50 days.
- Infectious period: unknown; viral excretion from oropharynx for months.

Clinical features
- Symptoms include:
  - Fever, malaise
  - Exudative tonsillopharyngitis
  - Generalised lymphadenopathy
  - Hepatosplenomegaly
- May be associated with hepatitis or CNS involvement.
- The acute phase lasts 2–4 weeks and convalescence may take weeks to months.
- In immunocompromised (particularly transplant); may be associated with the development of lymphoproliferative disease.

Diagnosis
- Serology is gold standard.
- Atypical lymphocytes in the peripheral blood.
- Monospot test (blood): good sensitivity (90%) in older children/adults, but poor sensitivity in younger children <4–5y age.
- PCR of blood or tissue can aid diagnosis of lymphoproliferative disease in immunocompromised (i.e. transplant) patients.

Complications
- Upper airway obstruction
- Dehydration from poor oral intake (uncommon)
- Chronic fatigue syndrome (uncommon)

Treatment
- Airway obstruction: Prednisolone 1–2 mg/kg (max. 50 mg) or dexamethasone 0.6 mg/kg PO daily.
- Splenomegaly: advise to avoid contact sports to prevent splenic rupture.
- Amoxicillin and Ampicillin can cause a florid rash in children with EBV infection.

Herpes simplex virus
Herpes simplex virus (HSV) infections can be primary (e.g. gingivostomatitis) or from a reactivation of the latent virus (e.g. cold sores). Manifestations of herpes simplex virus (HSV) infection include:
- Skin and mucous membrane involvement
- Gingivostomatitis (mainly HSV-1)

- Genital herpes (mainly HSV-2)
- Eczema herpeticum (see chapter 18 Dermatology)
- Herpetic whitlow
- Eye involvement
- HSV encephalitis (rare); important treatable condition presents with fever, encephalopathy and focal neurological signs or seizures.
- Perinatal infection
- Immunocompromised patients: pneumonia, hepatitis, and disseminated infection.

Primary herpes gingivostomatitis
- Transmission: droplet, direct contact
- Incubation period: 2–14 days
- Infectious period: indeterminate; virus excreted for ≥1 week and occasionally months after primary infection, and can be shed intermittently with or without symptoms (including cold sores) for years afterwards.

Clinical features
- Fever, irritability, cervical lymphadenopathy, halitosis, diffuse erythema and ulceration within the oral cavity (buccal mucosa, palate, gingiva and tongue) and mucocutaneous junction.
- Complications include: poor oral intake; autoinoculation resulting in herpetic whitlow, keratitis or genital herpes; eczema herpeticum; dissemination (particularly in immunocompromised).
- Lesions typically take 7–14 days to heal.

Diagnosis
- HSV PCR testing of vesicular fluid diagnostic

Treatment
- Symptomatic relief:
  - Topical anaesthesia (e.g. 1–2% lignocaine (lidocaine) gel, xylocaine viscous)
  - Analgesia (paracetamol)
  - Fluids and soft diet
- Antiviral medications:
  - Aciclovir, valaciclovir or famciclovir considered in immunocompromised patients.
  - May be used to suppress recurrent HSV in certain patients.

HSV in pregnancy
- Primary infection during the first 20 weeks of gestation associated with increased risk of spontaneous abortion, stillbirth and congenital disease.
- Primary infection beyond 20 weeks gestation; premature labour and growth retardation are more common.
- Primary infection after 34 weeks associated with high rates of neonatal HSV disease.

Neonatal HSV
- Transmission: most commonly acquired perinatally:
  - Intrapartum (70%–85%): perinatal acquisition from maternal genital tract.
  - Postnatal (10%)
  - Intrauterine (5%): transplacental.
- Transmission is 10 times more likely to occur with primary infection than with recurrent infection.
- Both primary and recurrent infection may be asymptomatic in women – >70% of women who give birth to infants with neonatal HSV infection give no history of genital HSV in themselves or their partners.
- The risk of HSV infection in a baby of an asymptomatic woman with a history of recurrent genital herpes is <3%.

Clinical features
Neonatal infection presents in three ways:
- Localised skin, eye and/or mouth (SEM) disease (20-45%)
  - CSF examination reveals CNS involvement in ≥30% (i.e. disseminated disease).
  - Death is rare.

- CNS disease (30-35%)
  - Mortality 15%
  - High long-term morbidity; CNS sequelae (50-60%): developmental delay, +/-microcephaly, spasticity, blindness, etc.
- Disseminated disease (25%)
  - Involves any organ; primarily liver, adrenal glands, brain (encephalitis ≥ 70%)
  - Presentation includes irritability, seizures, respiratory distress, jaundice, coagulopathy, shock and characteristic vesicular rash (20% of babies never have skin lesions).
  - High mortality (50–60%) and morbidity (CNS sequelae 40%) even with appropriate treatment.
- Symptoms presents most commonly within the first month of life (0–6 weeks); disseminated disease and SEM typically occur at an earlier age than CNS disease.

Diagnosis
- HSV PCR testing from all potentially infected sites: vesicular fluid, mouth/conjunctival swabs, blood, CSF, stool, urine, maternal genital tract.
- Serology often not helpful as maternal IgG (which crosses the placenta) confounds interpretation in the neonate, and IgM may not be produced until 2 weeks after the onset of illness.
- MRI brain and EEG may show characteristic findings.

Treatment
- Aciclovir 20 mg/kg IV 8 hourly for at least 14 (SEM disease)–21 days (CNS or disseminated disease) (see Appendix: Antimicrobial guidelines).
- Aciclovir suppressive treatment for ≥ 6 months in infants with disseminated disease may improve developmental outcomes.
- Prevention: antiviral prophylaxis for pregnant women with a history of recurrent HSV (from 35 weeks gestation) can reduce congenital infection rates.

HSV encephalitis
See Encephalitis section (above), and Chapter 29, Neurology.

Human herpes virus 6 (roseola infantum)
Human herpes virus 6 (HHV-6) has infected 95% of children by the age of 2 years. Up to 30% will present with clinical features of roseola; in others it will present as an acute febrile illness without a rash.
- Transmission: direct contact/droplet (asymptomatically shed).
- Incubation period: 9–10 days.
- Infectious period: unknown (most infectious during period of rash).

Clinical features
- Fever with occipital lymphadenopathy; then rapid defervescence corresponding with appearance of red, maculopapular rash over trunk and arms lasting 1–2 days.
- *Note*: Many children are started on antibiotics during febrile period and subsequently misdiagnosed as having a drug reaction when the rash appears.
- Complications include:
  - Febrile convulsions (may cause of up to 1/3 febrile convulsions in children <2y)
  - Aseptic meningitis, encephalitis (rare), hepatitis
  - Severe disease in immunocompromised patients; meningoencephalitis, bone marrow failure, hepatitis and severe colitis.

Diagnosis
- Serology and PCR available; usually only helpful in immunocompromised patients

Treatment
- Symptomatic management in immunocompetent children.
- Antiviral medication considered in immunocompromised patients; specialist advice recommended.

Influenza virus
- Cause: influenza A or B virus.
- Transmission: direct contact/droplet.

- Incubation period: 1–4 days.
- Infectious period: 3–7 days after symptom onset (longer if immunocompromised).

Epidemiology

Continuous genetic reassortment of influenza A viruses can lead to epidemics (and pandemics); the degree of cross-immunity from previously circulating strains and vaccines determines whether epidemics occur. Although the virus may cause disease at any time, seasonal epidemics occur during winter.

Clinical features

Variable; severity of illness is dependent on partial immunity from previous exposure to related influenza viruses and vaccines.

- May be asymptomatic.
- Commonly presents with:
  - Fever and rigors
  - Respiratory symptoms: coryza, pharyngitis, cough, pneumonia, wheeze, croup
  - Headache, myalgia, fatigue
  - Vomiting and diarrhoea (less common)
- Complications include:
  - Bacterial superinfection causing pneumonia (especially *S. aureus*), otitis media or sinusitis
  - Neurological (encephalitis, meningitis, encephalopathy)
  - Myositis
  - Cardiomyopathy
  - Death in ~1% of hospitalised children.

Diagnosis

- PCR on respiratory specimens (nasal swab or NPA) may allow early treatment.

Treatment

- **Routine treatment of influenza in immunocompetent patients is not recommended**.
- Neuraminidase inhibitors (oseltamivir, zanamivir): considered in children with laboratory-confirmed influenza who are severely unwell, immunocompromised or who have chronic medical conditions.
  - May reduce severity and length of illness by up to 36 hours if started within 48 hours; earlier initiation is associated with better outcome.
- School exclusion until symptoms resolved.

Prevention

- Vaccines can be used to prevent influenza in children.
  - Quadrivalent inactivated intramuscular vaccine is ~65% protective against influenza and prevents ~30% of influenza-like illnesses, but efficacy varies from year to year (see chapter 9 Immunisation).
- Neuraminidase inhibitors may be used to prevent influenza in children at higher risk of complications.

Measles

Measles is now uncommon as a result of widespread measles immunisation; however, outbreaks continue to occur in most parts of the world.

- Transmission: droplet, direct contact.
- Incubation period: 7–18 days (usually 14 days) prior to the appearance of a rash.
- Infectious period: 1–2 days prior to symptom onset to 4 days after the onset of rash. *Measles is highly infectious.*

Clinical features

- Prodrome: fever, conjunctivitis, coryza, cough and Koplik spots (white spots on a bright red buccal mucosa).
- Rash: appears 3–4 days later; erythematous and blotchy; starting at hairline and moving down the body, before becoming confluent; lasts 4–7 days and may desquamate in the second week.
- Complications include:
  - Otitis media (1 in 4)
  - Pneumonia (1 in 20)
  - Encephalitis (1 in 2000)
  - Subacute sclerosing panencephalitis (SSPE; 1 in 25 000).

Diagnosis
- Serology: IgM usually detectable 1–2 days after onset of rash, and almost always 4 days after.
- PCR on nose/throat swab.

Treatment
- Predominantly symptomatic
- Observation for complications
- Vitamin A: consider in young infants with severe measles, immunocompromised patients and those with vitamin A deficiency.
- School exclusion for at least 5 days from the appearance of rash.

Contacts of confirmed measles cases
- Measles, mumps, rubella (MMR) vaccine within 72 hours of exposure to unimmunised children >9 months of age (another dose should be given at 12 months of age or 4 weeks after the first dose, whichever is later).
- Normal human immunoglobulin (NHIG) should be given IM within 7 days if:
  - MMR contraindicated, or if >72 hours since exposure
  - Exposed pregnant women have had only 1 dose of MMR

Parvovirus B19 (erythema infectiosum, slapped cheek disease, fifth disease)
- Transmission: droplet, direct contact.
- Incubation period: 4–21 days.
- Infectious period: highly infectious until rash appears (50% of adults immune).

Clinical features
- Non-specific febrile prodrome in 15–30%.
- Rash has three stages:
  - 'Slapped cheek' appearance (1–3 days).
  - Maculopapular rash: on proximal extensor surfaces, flexor surfaces and trunk; fades over days, then central clearing to form a reticular pattern (after 7 days).
  - Reticular rash: reappears with heat, cold and friction (weeks/months).
- Complications include:
  - Arthritis
  - Aplastic crisis in children with chronic haemolytic anaemia
  - Bone marrow suppression
  - Fetal hydrops in newborns

Diagnosis
- Primarily clinical diagnosis.
- PCR on blood and serology may be helpful but rarely required.

Treatment
- Predominantly symptomatic.
- Blood transfusions may be required in certain patients (eg. severe haemolytic anaemia, *in utero* hydrops).
- School exclusion inappropriate as no longer infectious once rash appears.
- Pregnant contacts should seek advice regarding the unlikely possibility of intrauterine infection (as treatment of foetal infection may prevent sequelae i.e. hydrops).

Rubella virus
- Transmission: droplet, direct contact.
- Incubation period: 14–21 days.
- Infectious period: 5 days before to 7 days after rash.

Clinical features
- Asymptomatic: 25–50%.
- Prodrome: (1–5 days) low-grade fever, malaise, headache, coryza, conjunctivitis (more common in adults), postauricular/occipital/posterior triangle lymphadenopathy precedes rash by 5–10 days.

- Rash: small, fine, discrete pink maculopapules; starts on face and spreads to chest and upper arms, abdomen and thighs within 24 hours.
- Congenital rubella syndrome:
  - ~50% Infants affected if maternal infection during first trimester
  - 10–20% have single congenital defect if infection at 16–40 weeks
  - Clinical manifestations include deafness, neurological abnormalities, cataracts, retinopathy, tooth defects and growth retardation.

Diagnosis
- Serology
- PCR on urine or throat swab may be helpful (negative result does not exclude infection).

Treatment
- Symptomatic
- Exclude from school for at least 5 days from the onset of the rash.
- Pregnant contacts: If unimmunised, immunoglobulin after exposure in early pregnancy may modify risk of abnormalities in the baby.

Varicella zoster virus (chickenpox, shingles)
- Transmission: Droplet from respiratory secretions and/or direct contact with vesicle fluid from skin lesions. Highly contagious.
- Incubation period: 10–21 days (shorter in immunocompromised patients and prolonged if prior Zoster immune globulin (ZIG)).
- Infectious period: 1–2 days before appearance of the rash until skin lesions fully crusted.

Clinical features
- Fever, irritability, anorexia and lymphadenopathy.
- Pruritic rash develops over 3–5 days, with progress from maculopapular to vesicular, followed by crusting within 5–10 days.
- Lesions appear in crops with a central distribution; may affect scalp, face, trunk, mouth, conjunctivae and extremities.
- Complications occur in ~1% of cases and include:
  - Secondary bacterial infection of skin lesions (usually GAS or *S. aureus*).
  - Bacterial pneumonia.
  - Neurological complications (cerebellitis, transverse myelitis, Guillain–Barré syndrome).
  - Rarely dissemination (pneumonitis, hepatitis, encephalitis), particularly in patients with abnormal T-cell immunity.
  - Herpes zoster (shingles), results from reactivation of latent virus and post-herpetic neuralgia is less common in children than in adults.

Diagnosis
- Clinical diagnosis usually sufficient.
- PCR of vesicular fluid.
- Varicella serology may be helpful.

Treatment
- Antiviral treatment is **not** indicated in the immunocompetent child.
- Antiviral treatment: Aciclovir, famciclovir or valaciclovir in patients with impaired T-cell immunity.
- Antibiotics: for secondary bacterial skin infection (e.g. cefalexin).
- Symptomatic treatment:
  - Paracetamol
  - Aspirin (Reye's syndrome) and other NSAIDS (risk of invasive GAS) should be avoided

Prevention
- Live attenuated varicella vaccine is available as a monovalent vaccine and as a quadrivalent vaccine combined with the MMR vaccine (see chapter 9 Immunisation).

- Zoster Immunoglobulin (ZIG) indicated post varicella exposure (or direct contact with shingles) for:
  - Immunocompromised children
  - Newborns whose mothers develop chickenpox from ≤7 days before until 2 days after delivery.
  - Newborns <7 days of age if mother seronegative / has no history of chickenpox.
  - Hospitalised premature infants with no maternal history of varicella.
  - Hospitalised premature infants <28 weeks gestation or <1000 g (regardless of maternal history or varicella).
- ZIG:
  - Should be administered ≤ 96 hours post exposure but may have some efficacy up to 10 days.
  - Dose based on weight: 600 IU for >30 kg, 400 IU for 11–30 kg and 200 IU for 0–10 kg).

Viral hepatitis
See also Chapter 21, Gastroenterology.

Hepatitis A
Hepatitis A virus (HAV) is the most common viral hepatitis; and is particularly prevalent in developing countries.
- Transmission: faecal–oral route.
- Incubation period: mean of 4 weeks (2–7 weeks).
- Infectious period: viral shedding 1–3 weeks; the highest viral load/transmission risk is 1–2 weeks before the onset of illness; lowest risk is after onset of jaundice.

Clinical features
Either asymptomatic or associated with an acute self-limited illness:
- Infants and preschoolers: mild, non-specific symptoms without jaundice
- Older children and adults:
  - Fever, malaise
  - Jaundice
  - Nausea, anorexia
- The presence of dark urine may precede the onset of jaundice.
- Complications are uncommon and include relapse (unusual) and fulminant hepatitis (rare). *Hepatitis A does not cause chronic liver disease.*

Diagnosis
- Serology for HAV-specific IgM and IgG.
- Abnormal LFT's usually normalise within 4 weeks.

Treatment
- Supportive only
- Exclusion from childcare/school for 7 days from the onset of illness.
- Contacts can be given post exposure prophylaxis with hepatitis A vaccine.

Prevention
- Inactivated HAV vaccine is recommended for travellers to endemic areas, and patients with chronic liver disease (e.g. hepatitis B or C infection) or transfusion-dependent illness.
- Several monovalent HAV vaccines are available as well as HAV-containing combination vaccines.

Hepatitis B
Hepatitis B virus (HBV) infection is endemic in Africa and south Asia. The carriage rate is about 0.2% in Australians of European origin, and >10% in some indigenous and migrant populations. Rates are highest in those born in Asian, sub-Saharan Africa or Mediterranean countries. Immunisation against hepatitis B is part of the Australian Immunisation Schedule and is a priority in non-immune children and adolescents in high-prevalence subgroups, and household contacts of people with hepatitis B.
- Transmission: blood or body fluids that are hepatitis B surface antigen (HBsAg) positive.
  - Vertical transmission can occur in infants born to HBsAg-positive mothers.

- ○ Horizontal transmission is highest in the first years of life.
- ○ Can also occur through needle-stick injury in health care setting.
- Incubation period: 7 weeks–6 months
- Infectious period: from weeks before onset until documented clearance of virus.

Clinical features
- Asymptomatic (usually) in young children, particularly in vertically acquired infection.
- Symptomatic acute hepatitis: jaundice, anorexia, malaise and nausea in adults.
- Complications include: fulminant hepatitis (rare), and chronic HBV infection.
- Chronic HBV infection:
  - ○ Results in chronic hepatitis, cirrhosis (1/3) and increased risk of hepatocellular carcinoma (HCC), with 25% mortality from HCC or liver disease.
  - ○ Is most likely after exposure in early life; 70–90% of infants infected at birth develop chronic HBV.
  - ○ People who clear the infection generally have no long-term effects.

Diagnosis
- Test for HBV serology:
  - ○ HBsAg (active disease or if detectable >6 months = chronic carrier).
  - ○ HBsAb (protective immunity due to either past infection or immunisation). HBsAb >10 IU/L indicates adequate immunity.
  - ○ HBcAb (past or present HBV infection).
- If HBsAg positive need further testing:
  LFTs, HBcAb, HBeAg, HBeAb, HBV PCR (increased infectivity and risk of sequelae); and screen for hepatitis A,C,D and HIV.
- STI screening may be needed depending on age and history.
- Hepatitis B is a notifiable disease.

Treatment
- There is no specific therapy for HBV; α-interferon and nucleoside analogues may suppress chronic infection but are less effective for infection acquired during childhood.
- Hepatitis A vaccination is recommended.
- All acute cases of hepatitis with clinical illness need immediate discussion with a specialist and children with hepatitis B infection and abnormal liver function tests require specialist review.
- All patients with chronic hepatitis B should have explanation/education/counselling about:
  - ○ Blood spills and infection risk.
  - ○ Not sharing toothbrushes (or razors where relevant).
  - ○ The need to notify other treating doctors when starting medications, and to commence hepatotoxic drugs cautiously – particularly anti-TB therapy.
  - ○ Avoiding excess alcohol consumption.
  - ○ Using barrier contraception and sexual health in adolescents.
  - ○ The need to screen household contacts for hepatitis B and vaccinate those who are non-immune (check post-immunisation serology to confirm immunity).
- Other management depends on serology, LFTs and clinical status; with the primary goal of therapeutic management to eliminate or suppress hepatitis B.

Prevention
- In Australia, recombinant HBV vaccine is currently recommended for all infants from birth.
- Infants born to HBsAg-positive mothers should be given HBV-specific immunoglobulin in addition to HBV vaccination.
  - ○ They should be tested at 12–18 months with HBsAg and HBsAb.
- See Needle-stick injuries (below) for management of exposure to infected blood or body fluid.

Hepatitis C
Hepatitis C virus (HCV) causes acute and chronic hepatitis. The carriage rate is ~0.3% in apparently healthy new blood donors in Australia, but this probably underestimates the prevalence in the population, which may be around 1%.

Transmission
- Parenteral exposure to HCV-infected blood and blood products.
- Vertical transmission occurs in ~6% of HCV-positive mothers (higher if mother co-infected with HIV); avoid use of fetal scalp electrodes; breastfeeding is not contraindicated but should be avoided if the mother has bleeding or cracked nipples; sexual transmission is rare.
  - Incubation period: 6–7 weeks (range 2 weeks to 6 months).

Clinical features
- Mild, insidious hepatitis; usually asymptomatic in children.
- Complications include:
  - Persistent infection (>85%); most asymptomatic
  - Chronic hepatitis (65–70%)
  - Cirrhosis (20%)
  - Uncommonly HCC may develop in the absence of chronic hepatitis.

Diagnosis
- Serology: current or past infection (anti-HCV antibodies)
- PCR for HCV RNA: current infection

Treatment
- Monitor patients for chronic hepatitis, cirrhosis and hepatocellular carcinoma.
- Hepatitis A and B vaccination is recommended.
- Provide advice on avoiding transmission (see hepatitis B above).
- Optimal paediatric treatment regimes are under investigation and specialist advice should be sought.

Hepatitis E
Hepatitis E virus (HEV) is an uncommon cause of hepatitis, which occurs predominantly in tropical countries, especially in parts of India. Cases have been reported in travellers returning from these regions.
- HEV is transmitted by the faecal oral route.
- The clinical features are similar to HAV infection.

Gastrointestinal infections
Infectious diarrhoea (see also Chapter 21, Gastroenterology) continues to cause significant morbidity in children from developed and developing countries. Aside from rotavirus, other important pathogens include norovirus, enteric adenoviruses, astroviruses, *Salmonella* spp., *Campylobacter jejuni*, *Giardia intestinalis (lamblia)*, *Cryptosporidium parvum*, enteropathogenic (and other) *Escherichia coli*, *Shigella* spp. and *Yersinia enterocolitica* and *Clostridium* spp.
- Most bacterial causes of diarrhoea are self-limiting and do not usually require antibiotic therapy; antibiotics should be considered for the immunocompromised, neonates and in those with persistent symptoms.
- Repeat stool examination and culture are not helpful except in patients with chronic diarrhoea, suspected *Salmonella* carriage or suspected parasitic infection.
- Nosocomial infection is common. Hence, adequate infection control measures established by the hospital are essential in preventing spread.
- It is unusual to find a protozoal parasite in the setting of acute diarrhoea.

Rotavirus
- Incubation period: illness usually begins 12 hours to 4 days after exposure.
- Infectious period: most children shed the virus in the stools for up to 10 days.
- Prior to the introduction of routine vaccine (see chapter 9 Immunisation) this was the major cause (>50%) of diarrhoea in children <5 years of age admitted with acute gastroenteritis, and a common cause of nosocomial infection.
- Annual peak period of infection occurs in the winter–spring period.

Clinical features
- Symptoms generally last up to 7 days, and commonly include:
  - Vomiting (may precede diarrhoea)
  - Diarrhoea

- ○ Respiratory symptoms
- ○ Fever in the first few days
- Complications include: dehydration, electrolyte imbalance and acidosis.

Diagnosis
- PCR, enzyme immunoassay (EIA) and latex agglutination assay can confirm diagnosis but rarely influence management so are rarely necessary.

Treatment
- Supportive treatment
- Fluid rehydration (see Chapter 7, Fluid and electrolytes)
- Prevention: Safe and efficacious rotavirus vaccines are available.
  There is evidence that intussusception is not associated with these new vaccines (a concern with previous vaccines).

Adenovirus diarrhoea
Similar clinical presentation to rotavirus, but no seasonality and infection more common < 12 months of age.
- Diarrhoea and vomiting may persist for longer and high fever is less common.
- May be associated with prolonged diarrhoea and other manifestations in immunocompromised children.

Salmonella (non-Typhi) gastroenteritis
- Transmission: faecal–oral route from person to person or animal to person; ingestion of contaminated or improperly cooked foods.
- Incubation period: 6–72 hours.

Clinical features
Non-typhoidal salmonella (NTS) may be associated with a broad spectrum of clinical features including:
- Asymptomatic carriage
- Gastroenteritis: cramping abdominal pain and loose stools
- Bacteraemia +/- focal infections (e.g. bone and joint)
- Invasive infections and mortality are more common in infants, the elderly and those with underlying diseases (e.g. sickle cell, HIV, immunocompromise).

Diagnosis
- Culture from stool, blood or other clinical specimens.
- PCR is also available.

Treatment
- Antibiotic treatment is not usually indicated for uncomplicated gastroenteritis (symptoms usually resolve within 7 days) *as may prolong excretion.*
- Antibiotic treatment indicated for:
  - ○ Bacteraemia
  - ○ Systemic involvement
  - ○ Infants <3 months of age
  - ○ Patients with underlying disease (e.g. immunocompromised)
- The choice and duration of treatment depends on the clinical manifestation and antibiotic susceptibility.

Campylobacter jejuni
Transmission
Ingestion of contaminated food or water or undercooked poultry.

Clinical features
- More common in children >5 years of age.
- Diarrhoea with visible or occult blood, abdominal pain, malaise and fever.

Diagnosis
- Stool culture is diagnostic.
- Serology available but not routinely recommended.

Treatment
- Antibiotic treatment is not usually necessary (majority symptoms improve within 7 days); except in circumstances where elimination of carriage important, e.g. food handlers.

Giardia intestinalis (lamblia)
Transmission
- Major reservoir and means of spread is contaminated water and to a lesser extent, food.
- Person-to-person spread may occur and the infective dose is low in humans.
- Giardia is the most common parasite identified in stool specimens from children.

Clinical features
Broad spectrum of clinical manifestations, but most commonly:
- Diarrhoea (persistent and non-bloody)
- Abdominal distension
- Flatulence
- Abdominal cramping
- Weight loss/failure to thrive

Diagnosis
- Confirmation by stool microscopy (usually no blood, mucus or leucocytes). Repeat specimens may be necessary over a week to increase detection rate.
- Stool antigen testing and PCR available but are not routinely recommended.

Treatment
- Metronidazole 30 mg/kg (max. 2 g) PO daily for 3 days **or** tinidazole 50 mg/kg (max. 2 g) PO as a single dose.
- Additional treatment regimens available for difficult cases.

Dientamoeba fragilis and Blastocystis hominis
Transmission
Dientamoeba fragilis is thought to be transmitted with the eggs of *Enterobius vermicularis* (pinworm).

Clinical features
- Both organisms are of uncertain clinical significance as they can be part of the colonising flora and are present in asymptomatic children.
- Symptoms that have been associated include acute or chronic diarrhoea and abdominal pain.

Diagnosis
- Stool PCR (often incidental findings)

Treatment
- Asymptomatic patients in whom the organism is found incidentally do not need treatment.
- If another cause for gastrointestinal symptoms not identified, then a trial of metronidazole (dose as above) may be considered.

Escherichia coli
There are at least five categories of diarrhoea-producing *E. coli*:
- Enterohaemorrhagic *E. coli* (EHEC): haemolytic uraemic syndrome (HUS), haemorrhagic colitis.
- Enteropathogenic *E. coli* (EPEC): watery diarrhoea in children <2 years of age in developing countries.
- Enterotoxigenic *E. coli* (ETEC): the major cause of traveller's diarrhoea (usually self-limiting).
- Enteroinvasive *E. coli* (EIEC): usually watery diarrhoea, but may cause dysentery.
- Enteroaggregative *E. coli* (EAEC): chronic diarrhoea in infants and young children.

Treatment
- Antibiotic treatment is not usually indicated for diarrhoea caused by *E. coli* (may be associated with increased rates of HUS in EHEC infection).

Clostridioides difficile (Clostridium difficile)
Transmission
Acquired from the environment or faecal–oral transmission from colonised host.

Up to 50% of healthy neonates and infants <2 years of age colonised (usually asymptomatic), compared to 5% of children >2 years of age.

Clinical features
- Rare cause of diarrhoea in infants <12 months of age.
- May cause diarrhoea in older children.
- Pseudomembranous colitis usually occurs only in patients on antibiotics (particularly penicillins, clindamycin and cephalosporins).

Diagnosis
- Stool culture.
- Stool cytotoxin, EIA and PCR tests also available.

Treatment
- Cessation of antibiotics if possible; **and**
- Oral metronidazole 10 mg/kg (max. 400 mg) PO tds for 10 days
- Severe disease: vancomycin 10 mg/kg (max. 125 mg) PO (not i.v.) qid for 10 days
- Treatment failure or relapse (~25%) due to reinfection, non-compliance, continued antibiotic use, or, rarely, a metronidazole-resistant organism: vancomycin as above.

Enterobius vermicularis (threadworm, pinworm)
Pinworm is the most common worm infection in Australia, with highest rate of infection occurring in school-age children.

Transmission
- Eggs survive for up to 2 weeks on clothing, bedding or other objects and can remain under the fingernails; reinfection by autoinfection is common.
- Infection often occurs in more than one family member.
- Incubation period: At least 1–2 months from the ingestion of eggs until adult female migrates to the perianal region to deposit eggs.
- Infectious period: Eggs are infective within a few hours of being deposited on the perianal skin.

Clinical features
- Pruritus ani and vulvae
- Perineal pain in females (occasionally)

Diagnosis
- Visualisation of worms in the perianal region (at night); *or*
- Microscopy of eggs collected on sticky tape from perianal skin in the morning.

Treatment
- Mebendazole 50 mg (<10 kg), 100 mg (>10 kg) PO (not in pregnancy or in those <6 months of age) or pyrantel 10 mg/kg (max. 750 mg) PO as a single dose, followed by a second dose 2 weeks later.
- Wash bedding in hot water, avoid sharing towels, and cut fingernails.
- Treat all family members.

Uncommon but serious infections
Tuberculosis
Up to 1/3 of the world's population is infected with *M. tuberculosis*; the majority will remain well and not go on to develop tuberculosis (TB) disease.

Transmission
- Human-to-human transmission through infected droplets.
- Infectiousness is related to burden of disease:
  - Smear-positive individuals are highly infectious.
  - Only cases with pulmonary TB can transmit the organism to others.
  - Children less infectious than adults, as generally they have paucibacillary disease and do not develop cavitatory TB.
  - A new presentation of TB disease in a child should lead to a search for the index (adult) case.

Risk factors for progression to active TB disease
- Age <3 years
- Immunosuppression (e.g. HIV infection or immune-modulating medications)
- Malnutrition
- Low body weight
- Migration within 5 years from a high TB prevalence area (recently infected)

Clinical features
Infection with *M. tuberculosis* is associated with a wide variety of clinical presentations from asymptomatic latent TB infection (LTBI) to invasive TB disease.
- Pulmonary TB disease:
  - Chronic cough
  - Weight loss
  - Night sweats
  - Non-specific signs and symptoms including fatigue
- Extra-pulmonary TB disease:
  - Lymphadenopathy: enlarged cervical or axillary lymph nodes, usually painless (although symptoms will reflect site of infection)
- TB meningitis: infants/children may present with:
  - Lethargy, decreased feeds, headache
  - Photophobia, neck stiffness
  - Focal seizures
  - Coma

Diagnosis
The diagnosis of LTBI relies on detection of an immune response to *M. tuberculosis* using either the tuberculin skin test (TST) or an interferon gamma release assay (IGRA) blood test. Although more specific than the TST, an IGRA is not recommended as the sole test for identifying children with LTBI as false negative results occur, particularly in children under 5 years of age.
- Asymptomatic children: with normal examination and CXR who have either a positive TST and/or IGRA have LTBI.
- Symptomatic children: require appropriate clinical specimens (sputum/gastric aspirates/lymph node/CSF) to be sent for culture (gold standard – can take up to 6 weeks for the organism to grow in the laboratory).
- Culture of *M. tuberculosis* allows for drug susceptibility testing to guide treatment and identify multidrug resistant (MDR) TB.
- New molecular assays (e.g. PCR, *GeneXpert*) can detect *M. tuberculosis* DNA within 2 hours in appropriate clinical specimens.

Treatment
- LTBI: Preventive therapy with isoniazid for 6 months, rifampicin for 4 months, or a combination of isoniazid and rifampicin for 3 months.
- TB disease: Treatment with several TB medications for at least 6 months.
- Specialist advice should be sought.

Screening

- Refugee and asylum seeker children and adolescents (as well as adults) should have TST (and/or IGRA in older children) testing for LTBI or TB disease as part of routine post-arrival refugee health screening (see chapter 35 Refugee Health).
- TB screening should also be completed in any child migrating from a country with a high prevalence of TB.

Prevention

- Bacillus Calmette–Guérin (BCG) vaccine is highly effective in preventing severe forms of TB (e.g. disseminated or military TB, and TB meningitis) that more commonly affect infants and young children.
- BCG immunisation is recommended for infants and children (particularly <5y age) travelling to high TB incidence countries; and also for Aboriginal and Torres Strait Islander neonates living in certain regions.

HIV infection

HIV infection causes acquired immunodeficiency syndrome (AIDS).

Transmission

- Blood and body fluids.
  - Perinatal mother-to-child (vertical) transmission is the most common mechanism of paediatric HIV infection.
  - Horizontal transmission is the main means of transmission in adolescents and adults.
- Incubation period: must distinguish between HIV infection (may be asymptomatic during a variable latent period) and the progressive immunological derangement that leads to AIDS (increasingly uncommon in children).
- Perinatally infected infants may be asymptomatic for months or years.

High-risk groups

- Infants of mothers who are known to be HIV positive or who are members of a high-risk group (e.g. IV drug users, sex workers, and those with bisexual partners).
- Intravenous drug users (HIV prevalence ~3% in Australia).
- Men who have sex with men (HIV prevalence 5–10%).
- Sexual contacts (including sexually abused children) of individuals with HIV.
- Individuals from countries with a high prevalence of HIV infection.

Clinical features

- Symptomatic clinical presentations of HIV infection include:
  - Prolonged fever
  - Failure to thrive or weight loss
  - Generalised lymphadenopathy, hepatosplenomegaly, parotitis, tonsillitis
  - Chronic or recurrent diarrhoea
  - Chronic candidiasis and/or chronic eczematous rash
- The indicator diseases for the diagnosis of AIDS in children include:
  - Oesophageal candidiasis
  - Lymphocytic interstitial pneumonitis
  - Recurrent episodes of serious bacterial infection
  - Opportunistic infection (e.g. *Pneumocystis jiroveci* pneumonia and disseminated *Mycobacterium avium complex* disease)
  - CMV retinitis
  - Cerebral toxoplasmosis, progressive neurological disease and malignancy (e.g. primary brain lymphoma)

Diagnosis

- Patients (± parents) require counselling and informed consent before testing for HIV.
- Suggestive blood test results include:
  - Lymphopenia
  - Abnormal T-cell subsets
  - Hypergammaglobulinaemia

- Specific antibody detection: sensitive indicator of HIV infection in older children, but confounded by passively transferred maternal antibodies up to 18–21 months age.
- HIV ultrasensitive viral load (PCR): can detect actively replicating HIV infection (consider in < 18 months age group).
- Disease monitoring: combination of absolute CD4+ T-cell count and HIV PCR (viral load) quantification.

Management
A multidisciplinary approach by a specialised team is required to manage the unique needs of these patients and their families. Medical management of HIV-positive patients includes:
- Combination anti-retroviral treatment.
- Prevention of opportunistic and other infections:
  - Children should be routinely immunised unless CD4 count is <200 in which case specialist advice should be sought for live vaccines.
  - CD4 <200 also warrants PJP prophylaxis with co-trimoxazole.
- Early diagnosis and aggressive management of opportunistic infections.

Prevention
Antenatal testing of pregnant women to detect HIV infection is critical:
- Without treatment, HIV-infected mothers will pass infection to the neonate in up to 30% of cases.
- With preventative mother-to-child treatment (PMTCT), including complete avoidance of breastfeeding (where formula available and safe), transmission is approximately 0.1%.
- Potential HIV exposures (including sexual assault): post-exposure prophylaxis can be started within 72 hours, *specialist advice should be sought*.
- Antiretroviral therapy and other interventions (e.g. immunisation, pneumocystis prophylaxis) means AIDS is now a preventable disease syndrome in HIV-infected individuals.

Needle-stick injury
Community-acquired needle-stick injuries
- The risk of seroconversion to HIV, HBV or HCV from a community-acquired needle-stick injury is very low; exposed individuals should be reassured.
- Immunity to hepatitis B should be confirmed, and if incomplete, hepatitis B vaccine should be given.
- Unless the injury is considered to be particularly high-risk, no further management is required at the time.
- Follow-up should be arranged for counselling and serology.
- Tetanus toxoid ± immunoglobulin should be considered.

Occupational needle-stick injuries
Standard precautions
It is recommended that all health care workers are aware of their hepatitis B immune status and are appropriately vaccinated.
- All sharp objects and body fluids should be considered as potentially contaminated.
- Avoid contact with blood and other body fluids by
  - Using protective barriers (e.g. gloves).
  - Immediately cleaning up accidental spills.

Management
Managing needle-stick injury or exposure to blood/blood-stained body fluid:
- Squeeze the puncture wound.
- Wash blood off the skin with soap and water.
- Rinse blood from the eyes and mouth with running water.
- Document the date and time of exposure, details of incident, names of the source and exposed individuals.
- Inform source individual of exposure.
- Assess the risk of HIV, HBV and HCV in the source individual (Table 25.5).
- If indicated, test known source (after consent) for HBV surface antigen (HBsAg), HCV antibody (anti-HCV Ab) and HIV serology/viral load.

Table 25.5 Evaluation of needle-stick injury sources.

High-risk of HIV and HBV	High-risk of HCV
• Unsafe sex, particularly with multiple (or homosexual) partners • Intravenous drug users (IVDU) (particularly if they share equipment) and their sexual partners • Family members of an infected person • Individuals from communities with high HIV prevalence	• Recipients of blood products prior to 1985 • IVDU past or current (particularly if they share equipment)

Table 25.6 Management of needle-stick injury.

Exposure	Virus	Bloods from exposed	Bloods from source	What to give the exposed individual
High-risk	Hepatitis B	Anti-HBsAb (urgent)	HBsAg (urgent)	HBV immune: Nil
				HBV non-immune: -Source HBsAg positive/unknown: give HBV immunoglobulin (within 48 hours)[a] + HBV vaccine -Source HBsAg negative: give HBV vaccine
	Hepatitis C	Hold serum	Anti-HCV Ab (urgent)	Nil
	HIV	Hold serum	HIV viral load (urgent)	HIV prophylaxis[b] if source is HIV positive and/or risk of transmission is significant
Low-risk	All viruses	Anti-HBsAb (if unsure of immunity) Hold serum	HBsAg	HBV immune: Nil HBV non-immune: HBV vaccine

[a] HBV immunoglobulin should be given as soon as possible, but can be deferred for 48 hours, while awaiting results of serology to confirm affected individual's immunity (when checking whether a vaccinated individual has maintained immunity or whether the individual is immune from previous infection).
[b] Urgent expert advice should be sought.

- Even if the source individual is not infected with a blood-borne pathogen, storage of a serum specimen from the exposed person is recommended.
- Follow-up should be arranged for counselling (of exposed person).
- Give HBV-specific immunoglobulin ± HBV vaccine if appropriate (Table 25.6).
- HIV post-exposure prophylaxis is only required if source is HIV Ab positive, or if the source is unknown and HIV is considered likely.

Assessing risk

A significant exposure is considered to have occurred if there has been:
- An injection of blood/body fluid (particularly if >1 mL).
- A skin-penetrating injury with a sharp that is contaminated with blood/body fluid.
- A laceration from a contaminated instrument.
- A direct inoculation in the laboratory with contaminated material.
- A contaminated wound or skin lesion.
- Mucous membrane/conjunctival contact with blood/body fluid.
- The incidence of HBV, HCV and HIV in Victorian IV drug users is 1.8, 10.7 and 0.2 per 100 person-years, respectively.
- The estimated risk of virus transmission from an occupational needle-stick injury from a *known positive donor* (e.g. in Victoria) is
  ○ HBV: 6–30%
  ○ HCV: 0–7%
  ○ HIV: ~0.4%
  Note: These figures are for needle-stick injury from a positive source. When the source is unknown, the actual risk of infection for the affected individual depends on the probability of infection in the source population.

Acknowledgements

We thank Dr. Josh Wolf for his contribution to the previous version of this chapter.

USEFUL RESOURCES

- The Department of Human Services "Blue book" *http://www.health.vic.gov.au/ideas/bluebook/* has detailed information on most infections.
- The US Centers for Disease Control and Prevention *www.cdc.gov* has information on infectious diseases and travel medicine.
- Royal Children's Hospital Antibiotic Clinical Practice Guideline *https://www.rch.org.au/clinicalguide/guideline_index/Antibiotics/* provides recommended antibiotic regimens for many infections.

CHAPTER 26

Metabolic medicine

Joy Lee
Heidi Peters

Key Points
- Metabolic disorders are inherited disorders with abnormalities of a specific enzyme or transport protein.
- Clinical manifestations can be non-specific; symptoms may present at any age and therefore a high index of suspicion is required for diagnosis.
- Detailed history taking and physical examination remains the cornerstone of diagnosis.
- Urine and blood samples should be collected during acute presentation when possible for improved diagnostic yield; proper collection and handling of samples are important to avoid erroneous results and collection of excess samples for storage is helpful.
- Once a metabolic condition is suspected, stop the intake of potentially toxic compound (e.g. protein, galactose) and start intravenous glucose. Consultation with specialist metabolic service should be undertaken as soon as possible.

Metabolic disorders

Metabolic disorders, while individually rare, collectively represent an important cause of paediatric morbidity and mortality. The majority of metabolic disorders are inherited in an autosomal recessive manner. There are a small number of disorders (such as the urea cycle disorder e.g. Ornithine transcarbamylase deficiency) that are inherited in an X linked manner with females at risk of disease due to lyonisation. The clinical presentations can be easily confused with common acquired conditions. A high index of suspicion is therefore important for diagnosis.

Approach to the diagnosis of a metabolic disorder
History
In addition to pregnancy, birth, neonatal and developmental history, the following should be included:
- Maternal history: e.g. HELLP syndrome (fetus may have a fatty acid oxidation disorder), diet and nutritional status (vegetarian/vegan diet causing low carnitine or vitamin B12 levels).
- Family history; consanguinity, ethnicity, sudden infant death syndrome (SIDS), unexplained deaths.
- Dietary; aversions, food intake in relation to onset of symptoms.
- Review of organ systems.
- Progression and evolution of symptomology; developmental regression, diurnal patterns, recurrent unexplained symptoms (vomiting, ataxia, respiratory symptoms), presence of precipitating factors (infection, prolonged fasting, surgery, or certain medications), unusual smell or urine colour e.g. black urine in alkaptonuria.

Clinical Presentation
Metabolic disorders can present for the first time at any age. The presentation may be non-specific and there is often variability in presentations, even within families. A review of organ systems is important since most

---

Paediatric Handbook, Tenth Edition. Edited by Kate Harding, Daniel S. Mason and Daryl Efron.
© 2021 John Wiley & Sons Ltd. Published 2021 by John Wiley & Sons Ltd.

Table 26.1 Clinical features suggestive of a metabolic disease.

Age	Clinical Symptoms and Signs	Possible Diagnosis
Neonatal to Infancy	Acute encephalopathy[a] Vomiting, feeding refusal, lethargy or irritability Changes in respiration Hypo/hypertonia, seizures Altered conscious state	Aminoacidopathies e.g. Maple Syrup Urine Disease (MSUD) Organic Acidurias (OA) Urea Cycle Disorders (UCD) Fatty Acid Oxidation Disorders (FAOD) Mitochondrial disorders
	Liver dysfunction, prolonged cholestatic jaundice, hepatomegaly, hypoglycaemia +/− renal dysfunction	Galactosaemia Tyrosinaemia I Hereditary fructose intolerance Glycogen Storage Disorders (GSD) Certain FAOD Disorders in ketogenesis Bile acid defects Mitochondrial disorders
	Seizures as a predominant feature	Pyridoxine Responsive Seizures Pyridoxal 5 phosphate responsive seizures Glucose Transporter Defect I Biotinidase deficiency Nonketotic Hyperglycinaemia
Early to late childhood	Developmental delay, regression, seizures behavioural problems, learning difficulties Psychiatric symptoms, ataxia Stroke-like episodes, movement disorder	Aminoacidopathies e.g. classic homocystinuria Organic Acidurias (OA) Urea cycle disorders (UCD) Lysosomal Storage disorders e.g. Mucopolysaccharidosis Disorders of Creatine Metabolism Disorders of Purine and Pyrimidine X-linked adrenoleukodystrophy Mitochondrial disorders Congenital disorders of glycosylation
	Cardiac (conduction defects Cardiomyopathy) +/− rhabdomyolysis, muscle pain	Certain GSD e.g. GSD III or GSD V Pompe Disease Certain FAOD Mitochondrial disorders
	Dysmorphism, progressive symptoms +/− other systems: hepatomegaly, splenomegaly, cherry red spot, obstructive sleep apnoea, hair, skin and skeletal changes	Biosynthetic defects e.g. Smith-Lemli-Opitz Peroxisomal Disorders Lysosomal Storage Disorders e.g. Mucopolysaccharidosis

[a] Can present at ANY AGE and usually precipitated by infections, prolonged fasting, large protein meal or changes in diet.

metabolic disorders involve more than one organ system. The pattern of abnormalities and degree of organ involvement may suggest a specific metabolic disorder. Common clinical presentations of some metabolic disorders are shown (Table 26.1).

Investigations
Metabolites indicative of a metabolic diagnosis are best detected at the time of the acute presentation and may normalise between events in some disorders. Therefore blood, urine and CSF samples collected *at the time of presentation* are most valuable. Proper collection and handling of these samples is important, however collection of samples should not delay management of patients in critical situations.

Table 26.2 Interpretation of first line metabolic results.

Metabolic Condition	Glucose	Lactate	Metabolic Acidosis[a]	Ammonia	Anion Gap[b]	Urine ketones
Mitochondrial disorder	N	very high	present	N	increased	negative
MSUD	low or N	N	variably present	N	may be increased	positive
OA	low or N	may be high	very acidotic	may be high	usually increased	positive
FAOD	low or N	may be high	variably present	may be high	may be increased	negative or low[c]
UCD	N	N	N	high	N	negative

N – normal; MSUD – Maple Syrup Urine Disease; OA – Organic Acidurias; FAOD – Fatty Acid Oxidation Disorders; UCD – Urea Cycle Disorders.
[a] Serves as a guide. Secondary factors (dehydration/poor perfusion/sepsis) can affect interpretation.
[b] Compute by using Na – (Chloride + Bicarbonate). Normal < 16 mmol/L.
[c] Inappropriately low.

The first line metabolic investigations include:

- Blood – acid base, glucose, lactate, ammonia, plasma amino acids (AA), FBE, LFT, U&E, CK, Uric acid, cholesterol, triglycerides, carnitine level, Guthrie card acylcarnitine (do not put in a plastic specimen bag – check local collection requirements).
- Urine – smell, pH, glucose, ketones, urine reducing substances, amino acids, organic acids and glycosaminoglycans (GAG) screen
- Note: collect and freeze extra urine and plasma samples for storage.
  Interpretation of some common metabolic tests are shown below (Table 26.2).

Second tier of metabolic investigations include:

- Paired blood/CSF for: glucose, AA, lactate, pyruvate (Lumbar puncture should be done in fasting state and blood should be collected first to avoid stress related hyperglycaemia.)
- CSF Neurotransmitters
- Serum transferrin isoforms
- Biotinidase testing
- Galactoscreen
- Lysosomal enzymes testing
- Very long chain fatty acids and phytanic acid
- Urine for bile acids, creatine and guanidinoacetic acid
- Urine for purines and pyrimidines
- Urine for mucopolysaccharide testing.

Expanded newborn screening (NST) by tandem mass spectrometry
The sample is collected on day 2 to 3 of life and screens for more than 20 metabolic conditions (e.g. aminoacidopathies, fatty acid oxidation disorders and organic acidurias).

- This is a screening test, not a diagnostic test; if abnormal then further follow-up and confirmatory testing are required.
- Newborn screening does not detect all disorders reliably and will miss certain disorders (e.g. certain urea cycle disorders, Tyrosinaemia I).

Clinical Pearl: Newborn screening for metabolic disorders
Certain metabolic disorders are well detected in newborn screening, but other conditions can be missed. Classical galactosaemia is not included in the newborn screening in Victoria.

Post mortem samples

- Collect samples as soon as possible after death, preferably within 2 hours.
- Note the time between death and freezing or collection of the samples.
- Obtain blood, urine, CSF and bile samples if possible for further metabolic analysis. A vitreous humour specimen should be obtained if urine is unavailable.
- Collect blood on Guthrie cards (1 to 2) for biochemical testing and source of DNA.
- Obtain a skin biopsy for fibroblast culture (one piece of full-thickness skin, 2–3 mm surface diameter, in a tissue culture medium bottle, or a viral medium bottle or sterile container with normal saline without preservatives). Store in a refrigerator at 4 °C. *Do not freeze this sample.*
- Tissue biopsies for enzyme testing, light microscopy and electron microscopy.
- Blood for DNA testing

Clinical Pearl: Post mortem sampling for suspected metabolic disease
Urgent tissue collection after death for suspected metabolic disease is not a replacement for full autopsy (if indicated). It can however help with diagnostics, and hence inform risk for future pregnancies / family planning.

Management of Metabolic Disorders (always consult a metabolic physician)

Treatment Principles

1. In the acute setting, stop the intake of potentially toxic compounds (e.g. protein, galactose, fructose).
2. Avoid catabolism, which can lead to further accumulation of toxic metabolites, by providing sufficient calories in the form of glucose and/or fat. Do not use more than 5% dextrose for suspected mitochondrial disorders to prevent exacerbation of lactic acidosis.
3. Increase the disposal of toxic metabolites by giving certain medications, or by haemofiltration in severe cases e.g. rapid neurological deterioration.
4. Enhance enzymatic activity by providing vitamins and cofactors.
5. Management should also include:
   - Good hydration
   - Treatment of any precipitating events
   - Antibiotic cover as needed
   - Avoidance of certain medications (e.g. phenylalanine containing containing for PKU; valproic acid for urea cycle disorders, fatty acid oxidation disorders and mitochondrial disorders).

Specific Metabolic Conditions

Classical Galactosaemia

- Due to severe deficiency of galactose-1- phosphate uridyl transferase (GALT) enzyme
- Clinical features: Onset within first few days of life after intake of lactose (galactose is one of the sugar molecules in lactose) containing milk with progressive symptoms of; feeding difficulties, poor weight gain, vomiting, diarrhoea, liver dysfunction, prolonged jaundice, coagulopathy, gram negative sepsis e.g. E.coli, renal tubular dysfunction, development of cataracts.
- Diagnostic: Galactoscreen (measurement of GALT enzyme)*.
  *False negative result can occur due to packed red cell blood transfusion.
- Initial Management: lactose/galactose free formula (start as soon as galactosaemia is suspected).

Pompe Disease (Infantile form)

- Due to deficiency of alpha glucosidase enzyme involved in breakdown of glycogen in lysosomes, particularly involving muscle cells.
- Clinical Features: failure to thrive, feeding difficulties, severe head lag, hypotonia, muscle weakness, severe cardiomyopathy, typical ECG (P wave, massive QRS wave and shortened PR interval), elevated creatine kinase.
- Diagnosis: urine tetrasaccharides, dried blood spot alpha glucosidase enzyme testing** (urgent testing to avoid delay in diagnosis and treatment).
- Therapy: Enzyme replacement therapy.

Mucopolysaccharidosis (MPS)

- Due to a defect in a specific enzyme involved in the breakdown of glycosaminoglycans e.g. dermatan sulphate, keratan sulphate.
- Clinical Features: variable age of onset and severity, progressive symptoms, coarse features, global developmental delay, frequent ear or chest infections, hernias, organomegaly, obstructive sleep and behavioural problems, joint contractures, skeletal abnormalities.
- Diagnosis: urine glycosaminoglycan screen and electrophoresis* (can miss certain types of MPS) *and* specific enzyme testing
- Therapy: Enzyme replacement therapy or bone marrow transplantation depending on type of MPS. Gene therapy trials for specific MPS disorders.

Urea Cycle Disorders (except arginase deficiency)

- Due to deficiency of a specific enzyme in the urea cycle.
- Autosomal recessive conditions (except ornithine transcarbamylase (OTC) deficiency which is X-linked, carrier OTC females at risk of hyperammonaemia of variable severity).
- Clinical features: variable age of onset from neonatal to adulthood; acute or recurrent vomiting episodes, feeding difficulties, neurological or psychiatric symptoms, *protein aversion*.
- Diagnostic: ammonia, plasma amino acids, urine orotic acid.
  Blood gas shows respiratory alkalosis due to hyperammonaemia
- Initial Management: stop protein and start glucose containing fluids.

Organic acidurias e.g. methymalonic aciduria, propionic aciduria, isovaleric aciduria)

- Due to specific enzyme defects
- Clinical features: vomiting, feeding difficulties, respiratory distress, neurological symptoms
- Diagnostic: urine organic acids and plasma or dried blood spot acylcarnitine
- Initial Management: stop protein and start glucose containing fluids

Fatty Acid Oxidations Disorders (FAOD); e.g. Medium Chain Acyl-Co A Dehydrogenase (MCAD) deficiency, Long chain fatty acid disorders

- Clinical manifestations:
  - Hypoketotic hypoglycaemia in both MCAD deficiency and Long Chain FAOD.
  - Rhabdomyolysis, cardiomyopathy and cardiac conduction defects in Long Chain FAOD.
- Investigations: urine organic acids, plasma or dried blood spot acylcarnitine profile
- Management: avoidance of fasting, glucose containing fluids (orally or intravenous)

USEFUL RESOURCES
- Victorian Clinical Genetics Service (VCGS) website https://www.vcgs.org.au/tests/metabolic; information on metabolic screening, tests and collection.
- Inherited Metabolic Diseases: A Clinical Approach (textbook); Hoffmann G, Zschocke and Nyhan W (eds).
- Inborn Metabolic Diseases: Diagnosis and Treatment 5th edition (textbook); Saudubray, van den Berghe and Walter (eds).
- A Clinical Guide to Inherited Metabolic Diseases, 3rd edition (textbook), J.T.R Clarke.

CHAPTER 27

Neonatal medicine

Leah Hickey
Ruth Armstrong
Warwick Teague

Key Points

- If ongoing neonatal hospitalisation is required, great effort should be made to engage parents in the care of their baby as this is a critical time for infant-parent bonding and attachment.
- Survival of extremely preterm infants (EP; < 28 weeks PMA) has improved dramatically but minimising long-term morbidities remains an ongoing challenge.
- If neonatal sepsis is suspected, investigate and treat with empirical antibiotics while awaiting results and evolution of clinical picture.
- Conjugated hyperbilirubinemia in a neonate requires urgent assessment and investigation to exclude serious diagnoses including biliary atresia.
- All bilious vomits must be referred to a neonatal surgical centre for urgent assessment.

Resuscitation, stabilisation and transport

Neonatal resuscitation

The neonatal period is defined as the first 28 days of life for a term-born infant, or 44 weeks post-menstrual age (PMA) for a preterm infant (born before 37 weeks completed gestation).

Most newborn babies do not require resuscitation following birth, however basic resuscitation equipment and appropriately trained staff should be available at every birth in case immediate action is required. Predictors that action may be required include:

- Neonates who are preterm
- Neonates who are small or large-for-dates
- The presence of antepartum haemorrhage
- The presence of meconium-stained liquor
- The presence of prolonged rupture of membranes (>18 hours)
- Known congenital anomalies, e.g. congenital diaphragmatic hernia
- Other causes of acute fetal compromise, e.g. cord prolapse or shoulder dystocia

Airway and breathing

Lung aeration and ventilation using PEEP and/or Intermittent Positive Pressure Ventilation (IPPV) are the main priorities in newborn resuscitation. If the lungs are adequately aerated such that foetal lung fluid is shifted out of the alveoli, gas exchange will occur and improved oxygenation will lead to an increase in heart rate and optimal conditions for transition to extra-uterine life. The Australian and New Zealand Council on Resuscitation (ANZCOR) treatment algorithm for newborn life support reflects this practice (Figure 27.1).

Paediatric Handbook, Tenth Edition. Edited by Kate Harding, Daniel S. Mason and Daryl Efron.
© 2021 John Wiley & Sons Ltd. Published 2021 by John Wiley & Sons Ltd.

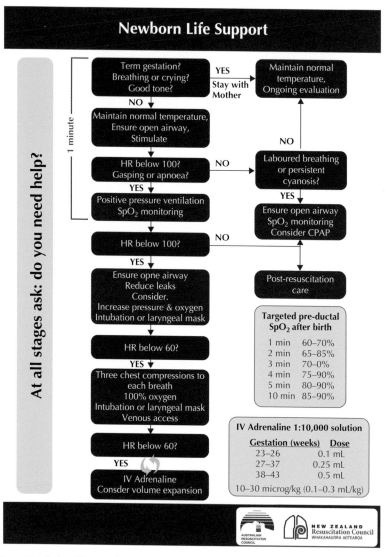

Newborn Life Support

At all stages ask: do you need help?

1 minute

Term gestation?
Breathing or crying?
Good tone?

YES → Stay with Mother → Maintain normal temperature, Ongoing evaluation

NO ↓

Maintain normal temperature, Ensure open airway, Stimulate

HR below 100? Gasping or apnoea?

NO → Laboured breathing or persistent cyanosis?

YES ↓

Positive pressure ventilation SpO₂ monitoring

NO ↑

Laboured breathing or persistent cyanosis?

YES ↓

Ensure open airway SpO₂ monitoring Consider CPAP

HR below 100?

NO →

YES ↓

Ensure opne airway
Reduce leaks
Consider.
Increase pressure & oxygen
Intubation or laryngeal mask

Post-resuscitation care

HR below 60?

YES ↓

Three chest compressions to each breath
100% oxygen
Intubation or laryngeal mask
Venous access

Targeted pre-ductal SpO₂ after birth

1 min	60–70%
2 min	65–85%
3 min	70–0%
4 min	75–90%
5 min	80–90%
10 min	85–90%

HR below 60?

YES ↓

IV Adrenaline
Consder volume expansion

IV Adrenaline 1:10,000 solution

Gestation (weeks)	Dose
23–26	0.1 mL
27–37	0.25 mL
38–43	0.5 mL

10–30 microg/kg (0.1–0.3 mL/kg)

AUSTRALIAN RESUSCITATION COUNCIL

NEW ZEALAND Resuscitation Council WHAKAHAUORA AOTEAROA

Figure 27.1 Newborn life support flowchart. *Source*: Australian & New Zealand committee on Resuscitation (ANZCOR); permission to reproduce obtained.

In order to avoid hyperoxia, which may be harmful, the current guidelines recommend
- Commencing resuscitation for term and near-term infants using air and increasing the oxygen concentration only if the infant does not respond to effective ventilation.
- Commencing resuscitation for preterm babies in 30% oxygen.
- Pulse oximetry should be available and applied as soon as possible to the right hand or wrist to allow titration of oxygen delivery according to the saturation targets listed in the flowchart (vary with age).

Table 27.1 ETT tube size and length by corrected gestation and weight.

Corrected gestation(weeks)	Weight(kg)	ETT sizeID (mm)	Depth of insertion at the lip (cm)	Depth of insertion at the nare (cm)
23–24	0.5–0.6	2.5mm	5.5	6.5
25–26	0.7–0.8		6.0	7.0
27–29	0.9–1.0		6.5	7.5
30–32	1.1–1.4	3.0mm	7.0	8.0
33–34	1.5–1.8		7.5	8.5
35–37	1.9–2.4	3.5mm	8.0	9.0
38–40	2.5–3.1		8.5	9.5
41–43	3.2–4.2		9.0	10.0

Circulation

Infants whose heart rate remains below 60 beats per minute despite effective ventilation, should receive:

- Chest compressions and IPPV with a ratio of 3 compressions to 1 breath.
- May require IV adrenaline and fluid resuscitation with 10ml/kg boluses of 0.9% Sodium Chloride.
- May require Intubation with an appropriately sized endotracheal tube (Table 27.1) if appropriately skilled personnel are present.

*An alternative method of **estimating** ETT insertion depth is:*
Oral ETT depth at lips (cm) = Weight [kg] + 6cm

Clinical Pearl: Newborn resuscitation: airway and venous access

- IPPV is the mainstay of early newborn resuscitation. If considering intubation and a skilled intubator is not available or if intubation attempts fail, consider the use of Guedel or laryngeal mask airways. Recurrent unsuccessful attempts will prolong exposure to hypoxia. IPPV with or without oxygen should be provided between attempts, guided by the saturation targets listed in the algorithm.
- The easiest way to gain IV access in the newborn is via the umbilical vein (see Chapter 5, Procedures).

Temperature

It is very important to maintain normothermia during resuscitation as temperatures above or below the normal range (36.5–37.5 °C) can exacerbate hypoxaemia and acidosis. The best way to prevent hypothermia is to place the infant skin-to-skin on their mother's chest with a blanket or towel covering their back. If this is not possible:

- Term infants should be dried, wrapped in a blanket and a hat placed on their head.
- Preterm infants should be placed in a polyethylene bag or wrapped with a polyethylene sheet without being dried, and have a hat placed on their head.
- Radiant warmers or incubators can be used to assist with ongoing thermoregulation.

Latest Evidence: Neonatal stabilisation & resuscitation

- Delayed cord clamping (DCC) is beneficial for infants born at any gestation, including term newborns who require resuscitation; evidence of safety of DCC for preterm infants requiring resuscitation at birth is currently awaited from ongoing trials.
- Tracheal suctioning in the setting of meconium-stained liquor is no longer recommended as it delays lung aeration and adequate ventilation.
- Sustained inflations, e.g. PPV of up to 25cm H_2O for up to 30 seconds to establish functional residual capacity(FRC), have been recently shown to increase mortality at seven days in preterm infants and are not recommended.
- Since the introduction of non-invasive ventilation (NIV) modes, far fewer infants require intubation and this has affected the ability to teach intubation skills to new medical staff. Video-laryngoscopy improves rates of successful endotracheal intubation in training and in practice.

Table 27.2 The Apgar score.

Sign	0 (absent)	1 (present)	2 (normal)
Heart rate	Absent	<100	≥100
Respiratory effort	Absent	Slow, irregular	Good, crying
Muscle tone	Limp	Some flexion	Active
Response to stimulation	No response	Grimace	Cry
Colour	Pale, blue	Centrally pink, blue periphery	Pink

Apgar score

The Apgar score is routinely used to assess newborn infants at 1, 5 and 10 minutes of life (Table 27.2). A total score of:

- ≥7 indicates the infant is well
- 4 – 7 indicates the infant requires assistance
- <4 indicates severe cardiorespiratory compromise and the need for urgent resuscitation.

Although persistently low scores are associated with poor neurological outcome, observer subjectivity means scores should not be relied upon as the sole assessment of the newborn. A full examination (detailed below) should be undertaken within the first 24 – 48 hours of life.

Stabilisation

Any newborn infant requiring resuscitation beyond the first few minutes of life to establish spontaneous breathing requires ongoing monitoring and transfer to a special care nursery (SCN) or Newborn Intensive Care Unit (NICU). Table 27.3 summarises some considerations for stabilisation and/or retrieval following initial resuscitation.

Transport

If appropriate level of care cannot be delivered locally, then the newborn should be referred to the local neonatal retrieval service for consultation and transport (PIPER 1300 137 650 in Victoria, Australia). Appropriate documentation and antenatal/perinatal/postnatal information should be available. The process should be explained to the parents and they should be asked to provide their written consent for retrieval.

Routine care for the term newborn

Newborn examination

Newborn infants should have a thorough assessment performed by trained personnel within the first 48 hours of life (Table 27.4). A full history should be taken from the parents or the medical records, including any relevant maternal diseases or social issues, pregnancy or birth-related issues, feeding and general behaviour since birth. Consent should be sought from parents before a physical exam is performed.

Early postnatal care

- For healthy term newborns the family should be supported to provide most of their baby's care themselves on the postnatal ward or at home if early discharge (from 6 hours after birth) can be safely facilitated.
- Feed establishment is a major focus of the first few days of life
  - Maternal breastfeeding support.
  - If not possible, formula feeds or intravenous fluids may be required (see below).
- In hospital routine observations taken and documented on an appropriate chart.
- Educate parents about **safe sleeping practices.**
- Routine injections of **Hepatitis B vaccine and Vitamin K** (to prevent Haemorrhagic Disease of the Newborn) should be administered once parental consent obtained.

Table 27.3 Stabilisation of the sick newborn.

Airway and breathing	• Monitor RR and work of breathing • Target SaO2 based on gestation & pathology • Assess level of breathing support required: LFO2, HFO2, CPAP, mechanical ventilation with ETT if indicated • Consider surfactant • Caffeine if preterm • Check blood gas and CXR if respiratory support required • Insert oro/nasogastric tube if respiratory support required
Circulation	• Monitor HR, BP, CRT, lactate • Access: consider PIVC, UVC +- UAC or PAL • Ensure adequate fluid resuscitation: 2 x 10ml/kg boluses 0.9% NaCl +/- blood • Consider inotropes if MAP below targets for gestational age
Disability	• Sucrose & non-nutritive sucking to reduce procedural pain • Minimise handling once procedures completed • Ventilated infants may require opiates analgesia +/- sedation
Examination	• A full physical examination to assess condition & congenital anomalies
Fluids	• 10% Dextrose infusion at 60mls/Kg/day (unless fluid restriction for suspected encephalopathy) • Monitor blood glucose as required (see Hypoglycaemia section)
Sepsis	• Take blood for culture & give empirical antibiotics (see Neonatal Infection section)
General	• Maintain normothermia • Facilitate parent-infant bonding where possible • Plan further care according to local capabilities and transfer guidelines

- In Australia, several newborn screening programs (see additional resources) exist to facilitate early diagnosis and treatment of a variety of serious conditions, undertaken within 72 hours of birth, including:
  - **Inborn Errors of Metabolism** (Newborn Bloodspot screening, NST; see chapter 26 Metabolic medicine).
  - **Hearing Deficits** (Newborn Hearing screening).
  - **Critical Congenital Heart Disease** (Oxygen saturation screening).
- Before discharge the family should be provided with their baby's birth record, an electronic or written child health record, details of any follow-up investigations or treatment required and an appointment to have the infant assessed and weighed again within the first week of life.

Feeds and fluids

The newborn baby's body is largely composed of water, with the extracellular fluid (ECF) comprising 40% of body weight at term. After birth there is a rapid loss of the interstitial fluid through diuresis and subsequent weight loss of 5 – 15% of body weight in the first week of life. Newborns also have relatively high insensible water losses (IWL) via their immature skin and their respiratory tracts. Humidification of ambient air via a double-walled incubator reduces IWL via the skin, whilst humidification of inhaled gases, if receiving respiratory support reduces IWL via the respiratory tract.

Feeds

- Breast milk is the best possible food for infants due to the many health benefits of the milk itself and the physiologic process on both mother and baby.
- If breast milk is not available, commercial infant formula is the only other suitable and safe feed to ensure optimal newborn growth and development. Sterile ready to feed infant formula that should be used in hospitals instead of powdered infant formula due to the risk of bacterial sepsis from non-sterile powdered infant formula in the hospital setting.

Table 27.4 Approach to newborn examination.

	Examine	Abnormalities
General Observation / Neurological assessment	Colour	Jaundice, cyanosis, pallor
	Tone and posture	Limbs not held in flexion
	Spontaneous movement	Limbs not moving equally or spontaneously
	Level of alertness	Irritable or lethargic
	Cry	May indicate upper airway or neurological problem
Head and face requires: Tape measure Opthalmoscope Tongue depressor	Measure head circumference	Micro/macrocephaly
	Head shape	Caput, cephalhaematoma, subgaleal haemorrhage, encephalo / myelomeningocoele, Brachy/plagio/scapho/turricephaly
	Fontanelles and sutures	Splayed, fused, bulging, sunken
	Eyes and pupils	Conjunctivitis, haemorrhage, unequal/unreactive pupils, absent red reflex, yellow or blue sclera
	Ears	Low set, small or absent, skin tags
	Nose	Any level of atresia or stenosis
	Mouth and palate	Lip, soft or hard palate cleft, asymmetry with crying, poor suck/latch
	Mandible	Micro/retrognathia
	Dysmorphic features	
	Primitive reflexes: Root, Suck, Gag, Asymmetric tonic neck reflex	
Upper limbs Requires: Tendon hammer	Active and passive movement	Asymmetry may indicate fractured clavicle or brachial plexus injury, e.g. Erb's Palsy
	Tone	Hypo/hypertonia
	Digits	Fused, too many/too few, contractures, malpositioned
	Palmar creases	Single crease may indicate Trisomy 21 (also a common normal variant)
	Primitive reflexes: Grasp, Moro	
	Deep tendon reflexes	
Neck and chest Requires: Stethoscope Pulse oximeter	Neck	Masses may be cystic hygroma or lymphangioma Neck oedema or webbing (syndromic)
	Chest shape	Bell or barrel-shaped
	Heart sounds	Murmur, arrhythmia
	Heart rate, pulses and oxygen saturations	Low saturations may indicate cyanotic heart disease
	Breathing effort and rate	Tachypnoea, nasal flaring, grunting, stridor, tracheal tug, recession
	Breath sounds	Uneven chest rise or sounds (PTX / CDH)
	Nipples/breasts	
Abdomen and pelvis	Feeding and/or vomiting	*Bilious vomiting requires urgent assessment at surgical centre*
	Stool output	*Delayed passage of stool > 48hrs may indicate Hirschsprung's Disease*
	Urinary output	*Delayed passage of urine >24 hrs may indicate renal tract obstruction*
	Antenatal renal tract dilatation	
	Abdominal wall	Organomegaly (liver, kidneys, spleen), bowel distension, pneumoperitoneum Scaphoid may indicate CDH Gastroschisis, exomphalos, venous congestion
	Umbilicus	Omphalitis, number of cord vessels
	Anus	Anorectal malformation +/- fistula, patulous tone may indicate neural tube defect
	Genitalia	Ambiguous Male: undescended or torted testes, hydrocoele, hypo/epispadias, inguinal hernia Female: vaginal discharge (usually normal), inguinal hernia

Table 27.4 (*Continued*)

	Examine	Abnormalities

Hips	*Enquire about DDH risk factors*
	Breech position after 36 wks,
	   Family history in first-degree
	   relative
	Abnormal clinical exam
	Barlow Manoeuver
	Ortolani Manoeuver
		The presence of a risk factor should trigger referral for
		Hip Ultrasound at 6 weeks of age (or 6 weeks CGA
		for preterm infants)
		
		Positive if femoral head is dislocatable
		Positive if femoral head is dislocated and can be
		   returned to the acetabulum

Lower limbs
Requires:
Tendon hammer
	Movement, tone, posture
	
	Digits
	Feet
	Primitive Reflexes: Place, Step
	Deep tendon reflexes including
	   Babinski
		Abnormalities may indicate CNS or PNS injury or
		   disorder
		Fused, too many/too few, contractures, malpositioned
		Talipes, fixed or positional
		
		Positive Babinski (i.e. upgoing toes) normal < 2y

Back	Spine and sacrum
	
	Buttocks
	
	Primitive reflexes: Gallant
		Overt or occult neural tube defect (abnormal skin/hair,
		   baseless sacral dimple)
		Wasting may indicate sacral agenesis or Neural Tube
		   Defect

Skin and hair	See www.dermnetnz.org for
	   information & images
		Many rashes in infancy are benign e.g. erythema
		   toxicum, neonatal milia

Weight/length	Measure using standardised
	   neonatal equipment;
	Plot on growth chart with head
	   circumference
		Small/Large for gestational age infants require
		additional monitoring & investigations, e.g. testing
		for common congenital infections (SGA) and/or
		blood glucose level checks (LGA)

Note: Abnormal findings should be discussed with an experienced paediatrician or neonatologist to ensure that timely & appropriate management can be enacted.

Clinical Pearl: Breastfeeding support

Every effort should be made by the clinical teams involved in routine care to encourage and support every mother to breastfeed their baby starting as soon as possible after birth if mother and baby are well enough. Additional support with feeding and growth may be provided by lactation consultants, dieticians, speech or pathologists. *Exclusive breastfeeding is recommended for the first 4–6 months of life.* Extensive breastfeeding information & support is available online and within the community (see useful resources).

Clinical Controversy: Donor breast milk

Whilst some tertiary centres offer pasteurised donor breast milk (PDM) services for vulnerable (e.g. premature) newborns, *informal breast milk sharing arrangements without medical oversight are not recommended.* Unscreened and unpasteurised donor breast milk poses significant risks to infant health, including the transmission of harmful bacteria or communicable diseases. Additionally, raw unpasteurised milk from lactating animals is unsafe due to the high risk of bacterial contamination and should NEVER be given to human infants.

Introducing enteral feeding

Neonates who show readiness to feed but who cannot commence with full demand breast feeding may require an incremental introduction to enteral feeds (Table 27.5). Start feeds, **ideally expressed breast milk,** as soon as possible via suck, oro/nasogastric tube or bottle.

Table 27.5 Recommended total daily fluid intake (ml/kg/day) of enteral feeds.

Age (hours)	Term Infant (ml/kg/day)	Preterm Infant (ml/kg/day)
<24	30	60
24 – 48	60	60
48 – 72	80	80
72 – 96	100	100
96 – 120	120	120
120 – 144	150	150
>144 (Day 6 life)	Demand feed to minimum 150	Demand feed to minimum 180

Note: Small-for-Gestational-Age (SGA) infants should be closely observed for signs of feed intolerance (see below) and feed volumes adjusted accordingly.

Growth monitoring

Weight, length and head circumference should be measured as soon as possible after birth and stabilisation for infants of all gestations. Thereafter, regular checks plotted on appropriate centile charts is necessary to ensure growth is progressing and to support assessment of fluid balance/hydration.

- Whilst newborn infants are expected to lose 5–15% of body weight in the first week of life, they **should regain their birth weight by day 7–10 of life**. Medical review is recommended if weight loss >10% is noted.

Considerations for preterm infants:

- **Breast milk:** reduces the risks of feed intolerance and necrotising enterocolitis (NEC), and improves long-term neurodevelopmental outcomes when compared with infant formula. It may be appropriate to delay enteral feeding until the mother's EBM is available.
- **Donor milk:** when the mother's own milk is not available, pasteurised donor milk, if available, is the next best option, particularly for unwell or high-risk infants.
- **Breast milk fortification:** combining breast milk with commercial breast milk fortifier can be considered in babies with birth weight < 1500 g or born < 30 weeks gestation once tolerating adequate enteral feed volumes. Human milk fortifier provides increased protein, energy and minerals for the breast milk fed preterm infant.
- **Infant formula:** preterm formula (85 kCal/100mL) may be used for infants less than 1500 grams and/or less than 30 weeks gestation and can be used from birth.
- **Skin-to-skin care:** promotes the development and maturation of infant feeding behaviours and enhances breast milk production. Close contact also triggers the entero-mammary pathway by which a mother produces antibodies in response to antigens in the infant's environment. *Always encourage and facilitate early, frequent and extended skin-to-skin care.*
- **Feeding method:** preterm infants who are not mature enough to suck feed (<32-34 weeks) are exclusively fed via oro/nasogastric tube as they cannot safely coordinate their suck / swallow / breathe sequence. Thereafter, the infant may be offered suck feeds once displaying signs that they are ready to suck, including:
  - Alert & looking for feed
  - Rooting reflex, mouthing, swallowing saliva
  - Sucking on feeding tube, fingers, dummy
  - Fighting feeding tube

  Breastfeeding in combination with skin-to-skin care is the optimal way to introduce suck feeds.
- **Feeding frequency:** Enteral feeds are commenced when the infant's condition has stabilised, with a preference for all feeds to be commenced as bolus feeds. Feeding frequency depends upon birth weight (Table 27.6).
- **Feed intolerance:** can indicate inappropriate feeding volumes / frequency, or more significant pathology. Signs of feed intolerance can include:
  - Positing or vomiting
  - Abdominal distension and/or discolouration
  - Increased respiratory effort
  - Apnoea and/or bradycardia

Table 27.6 Feeding frequency based on weight.

Weight	Frequency
< 1000 g	1–2 Hourly
1000–1500 g	2-hourly
> 1500 g	3-hourly

Table 27.7 Intravenous fluid recommendations.

Age (hours)	Fluid type (500ml premade bags)	Fluid volume per day (mls/kg/day)	Fluid Volume per hour (mls/hour infusion rate)
0–24	10% Glucose	60	Birth weight x 2.5
25–48	10% Glucose	60	Birth weight x 2.5
49–72	10% Glucose + 19 mmol NaCl + 10 mmol KCl	72	Birth weight x 3
72–96	10% Glucose + 19 mmol NaCl + 10 mmol KCl	96	Birth weight x 4
96–120	10% Glucose + 19 mmol NaCl + 10 mmol KCl	120	Birth weight x 5

Notes:
- Birth weight should be used for calculations until current weight surpasses birth weight (usually D5–10 life)
- The values in the table are recommendations for infants with anticipated normal renal function (if abnormal seek specialist opinion).

- Absolute indications to withhold feeds include suspected or diagnosed NEC, significant abdominal distension / discoloration or other suspected bowel pathology, blood in stools, or blood / bile stained vomiting.

Intravenous Fluids
- Neonates that cannot commence feeds immediately after birth, such as extremely preterm or sick term neonates, must be commenced on intravenous fluid (IVF) to maintain hydration, maintain normoglycemia and to avoid biochemical disturbances.
- Neonates who need to fast for more than 4 hours, e.g. for surgical procedures, should also be commenced on appropriate IVF.
- IVF is usually commenced at a rate calculated from anticipated water, glucose and electrolyte requirements, and estimated renal and insensible losses.
- These requirements change with the newborns day of life (Table 27.7).
- Fluids should be reviewed daily and adjusted accordingly (e.g. balanced with enteral intake).
- Although enteral feeding targets may exceed 150 mls/kg/day;
  IVF should not be increased above 120 mls/kg/day due to the risks of pulmonary and cerebral oedema secondary to excess water administration.
- **We strongly recommend the use of pre-manufactured neonatal-specific fluid bags for IVF in all neonates; this reduces the risk of iatrogenic harm.**

Clinical Pearl: Parental nutrition
Consideration should be given to commencing parental nutrition solutions (see chapter 10 Nutrition) for newborn infants who are not anticipated to receive adequate enteral feed volumes by Day 5 of life, or who may undergo a prolonged fasting period (>3 days). This is to provide adequate *nutrition* in addition to hydration, glucose and electrolytes.

Weaning from IVF to feeds

- Neonates receiving IVF who show a readiness to feed will require IVF weaning while grading-up on enteral feeds, and in doing so maintaining an appropriate combined total fluid intake (TFI; ml/kg/day).
- Enteral feeds should be introduced via breast (demand feed or use EBM as per table below), bottle or tube (start at 30mls/kg/day) and subsequently increase in similar increments each day as tolerated.
- Reduce IV infusion rate each day or according to rate of feed increases (may be twice daily) to maintain TFI within suggested range for enteral intake.
- **If neonates have previously been receiving full enteral feed volumes but have been fasted due to illness or surgery, they may be able to restart at half or full volume enteral feeds and not require such incremental grading up.**

For example, if a 33 week gestation infant weighing 1.3kg has had respiratory distress and been receiving only IVF until 48 hours of life, but is ready to commence feeds from 48 hours, their suggested fluid regime for the first week of life would be:

Age (hours)	TFI (mls/kg/day)	IVF (mls/kg/day)	Feeds (mls/kg/day)
<24	60	60	0
24–48	60	60	0
48–72	80	50	30
72–96	100	40	60
96–120	120	30	90
120–144	150	0	150
>144 (D6 of life)	Minimum 150	0	Demand feed to minimum 150

Monitoring & safety considerations for neonates receiving IVF

- Frequent (at least daily) examination for signs of fluid overload (oedema, tachypnoea) or dehydration (blood pressure below expected target, CRT > 2s, reduced skin turgor, dry mucous membranes, sunken fontanelle).
- Frequent clinical review of IV insertion sites for signs of extravasation, phlebitis or infection, as per local policies.
- Daily BSL and UEC for the first 48 hours, or longer if levels abnormal.
- Urine output: newborns should pass urine by 24 hours of age, failure to do so should prompt clinical review.
- IVF and feeding orders should be reviewed at least once per day by an appropriate prescriber.

Glucose requirements
- The neonatal liver normally produces 6–8mg/kg/min of glucose – this is the approximate basal requirement of a newborn neonate.
- 10% Glucose (10mg glucose per 100mls water) is the standard basic component of neonatal IVF.

Clinical Pearl: Glucose delivery rate (mg/kg/min)
The formula to calculate glucose delivery rate (i.e. intake) or glucose utilisation rate (GUR) is:

$$\text{Glucose delivery rate (mg/kg/min)} = \frac{\%\text{Glucose} \times \text{hourly rate (ml/hr)}}{\text{Weight (Kg)} \times 6}$$

Several different digital calculators are easily accessible online and within apps (e.g. NICU TOOLS) that can assist with calculating glucose delivery rates.
A neonate requiring >12.5% glucose to maintain normoglycaemia should prompt discussion with a neonatologist or neonatal retrieval service (see hypoglycaemia section below).

Table 27.8 Causes of low or high serum sodium levels in a neonate.

Hyponatraemia	Hypernatraemia

• Excessive administration of fluid (most common)
• Inadequate excretion of water or excess excretion of sodium due to renal immaturity
• Inadequate intake of sodium
• GIT losses
• *Rare causes in neonates:*
  ○ SIADH
  ○ Renal tubule disorders
  ○ Adrenal insufficiency
	• Insufficient administration of fluid
	• Excess free water loss
	• Excess sodium administration

Electrolyte requirements (see also Chapter 7, Fluid and Electrolytes)
- Once the transitional fluid shifts have occurred in the first 48 hours after birth, the newborns requirement for both sodium and potassium is 2–4 mmol/kg/24 hours.
- An unexpectedly abnormal electrolyte result in a well, asymptomatic infant may be due to sampling (eg. haemolysed sample) or laboratory error. Prompt repeat testing to re-check the level is advised before correction of the electrolyte imbalance.

Hyponatraemia and hypernatremia
See Table 27.8.
- A sodium (Na^+) value of 135–145 mmol/L is indicative of appropriate total body water and sodium balance.
- Changes in Na^+ concentration need to be assessed in the context of total body weight, and any recent increase or decrease in weight.

Clinical Pearl: Hyponatremia in the early neonatal period
Hyponatraemia in the first 48–72 hours of life is likely to be due to excess water. This should be managed with fluid restriction and NOT with administration of additional sodium as there is a risk that hypernatraemia will occur when normal postnatal fluid shifts and diuresis occur.

Treatment of hyponatraemia if Na+ <130mmol/L:
- **Refer immediately for tertiary care if serum Na^+ <125 mmol/L or infant is symptomatic with Na^+ <130mmol/L.**
- Review fluid administration orders (may require fluid restriction), monitor weight and urine output.
- The serum Na^+ should never be increased faster than 0.5mmol/L/hour as rapid or over correction can cause neurological complications such as cerebral oedema, demyelination, and seizures.

Treatment of hypernatraemia if serum Na+ >145mmol/L:
- Refer immediately for tertiary care if serum Na^+ >150 mmol/L
- If due to net loss of water AND associated with circulatory compromise, give 10ml/kg 0.9% NaCl bolus IV initially and reassess.
- If due to net loss of water but not associated with circulatory compromise, increase maintenance fluids by 10–20mls/kg/day with the goal of rehydrating slowly over 24–48 hours, guided by repeated measurements of serum Na^+.
- If due to excess Na^+ administration, check amount of sodium administered and consider reducing.
- Review fluid administration orders, monitor weight and urine output.

Hypokalemia and hyperkalemia
Corrections of hypo/hyperkalaemia (see also Chapter 7, Fluid and Electrolytes) in neonatal patients is not recommended in non-tertiary centres. Management may be initiated under the guidance of a neonatologist or neonatal retrieval service while awaiting the arrival of a retrieval team and transfer to a tertiary centre for ongoing care.

Neonatal medical conditions

Neurological Problems

Neonatal seizures

The brain of a newborn is more prone to seizures than an adult brain, and neonatal seizures affect 3–12/1000 term babies (more common in preterm babies but harder to detect). Seizures are rarely idiopathic and are a major predictor of adverse outcome in the newborn.

Causes include:

- Hypoxic ischaemic encephalopathy (HIE)
- Cerebral infarction: stroke, venous sinus thrombosis
- Intracranial haemorrhage (Intraventricular, parenchymal, subarachnoid, subdural)
- Infection: bacterial or viral meningitis / encephalitis
- Electrolyte disturbance: hypoglycaemia, hypocalcaemia, hypomagnesaemia, hypo- / hypernatraemia,
- Less common causes include developmental brain abnormalities, inborn errors of metabolism, drug withdrawal (maternal or infant), 'day 5 fits' (benign nonfamilial), autosomal dominant neonatal seizures

Clinical features are often subtle and varied (Table 27.9).

Investigations:

- Blood: BGL, electrolytes (Na+, Ca2+, Mg2+), FBC, CRP, culture, ABG or CBG
- CSF: MCS, glucose, PCR for HSV, enterovirus, parechovirus (delay if unstable)
- Urine: metabolic screen (amino and organic acids), CMV PCR
- Neuro-imaging:
  - Cranial ultrasound: IVH, hydrocephalus, gross white matter changes.
  - MRI: Modality of choice. Exclude infarction or developmental brain abnormality, determine extent of injury in HIE. (CT scanning: rarely indicated unless concern for hemorrhage needing neurosurgical intervention, or traumatic bony injury).

Second line investigations should include:

- Blood: TORCH screen, metabolic investigations (ammonia, amino acids, carnitine. Lactate and pyruvate may be paired with CSF samples)
- Urine: ketones, reducing substances and toxicology
- EEG: detects seizure activity and aids prognosis.
- Bedside amplitude integrated EEG (aEEG) useful in detection & monitoring of some seizures.

Table 27.9 Clinical features of neonatal seizures.

	Clinical manifestation	Comment
Subtle	*Oculo-orofacial deviation:* rolling of eyes, staring, abnormal sucking, lip smacking *Central/autonomic:* apnoea, desaturation, altered breathing, tachy/bradycardia.	Difficult to differentiate from normal neonatal behaviours; seizures more likely repeated, stereotypical movements.
Tonic	Sustained stiffening of limbs or trunk, deviation of head usually symmetric, +/- apnoea & eye deviation.	Only 30% have EEG correlates.
Clonic	Usually unilateral, may be bilateral. Rhythmic jerking 1–4/second. Cycling/boxing limb movements. Persists despite holding the limb.	May indicate focal intracranial pathology.
Myoclonic jerks	Fast flexor muscle movement. Focal or multifocal.	Seen in drug withdrawal (opiates), encephalopathy.
Benign sleep myoclonus	Neurologically normal infants. Occur only during sleep.	EEG normal; No treatment required. Resolves within 2 months; may worsen with benzodiazepines

Table 27.10 Anticonvulsants.

First line	**Phenobarbitone** full loading dose 20mg/kg IV (ceases 50–70%) If seizures continue after 30 minutes give a half loading dose (10mg/kg) If seizures continue give a further half loading dose or add another anticonvulsant
Second line	*Phenytoin* loading dose 20mg/kg IV *(ceases a further 15%)* Give a second dose if seizures continue
Third Line	*Midazolam bolus* (200mcg/kg IV). Consider intravenous infusion (1–5 mcg/kg/min) *Clonazepam* (250mcg (not per kg)). Reduce to 125mcg in preterm infants. *Levetiracetam* (20mg/kg IV)
Fourth Line	Consider *Pyridoxine* 1 week trial (50–100mg IV or PO) for intractable seizures.
Maintenance	Indication: severe neonatal encephalopathy or brain injury, duration 6-8 weeks. *Phenobarbitone* (3-5mg/kg/day in divided doses), or *levetiracetam* (10mg/kg BD) Underlying seizure disorder may require ongoing treatment by Neurologist.

Management:
- Admit to a neonatal intensive care unit
- Identify and treat underlying reversible causes
- Support airway, breathing and circulation if compromised
- Anticonvulsant therapy (Table 27.10) indicated if: prolonged >3m, recurrent >3/hr, or associated with cardiorespiratory compromise
- Anticonvulsants may cause respiratory depression and apnoea; ensure monitoring and ventilator support available

> **Clinical Controversy: Seizure treatment goals & duration**
> Large doses of anticonvulsants may have deleterious effects on the developing brain, and should be used discerningly. It remains unclear whether the goal of treatment should be the elimination of abnormal EEG activity or the resolution of clinical seizures. It is also unclear how long to continue treatment after the initial seizures, as there is currently no evidence that prolonged treatment reduces the risk of subsequent epilepsy

Neonatal encephalopathy
Clinically defined as disturbed neurological function in the early newborn period of infants ≥35 weeks' gestation and manifest by lower than normal conscious level or seizures.
- Associated features may be difficulty with breathing, and reduced tone and reflexes.
- Neurological assessment at 2 weeks of age can help predict outcome.
- MRI with spectroscopy can refine the prognosis by providing further information about cause and injury timing.
Causes include:
- Perinatal hypoxia or ischaemia
- Infection (sepsis or meningitis)
- Intracranial haemorrhage or cerebral infarction
- Metabolic disturbance
- Structural brain anomalies
- Genetic syndromes

Investigations depend on likely aetiology and include
- Blood: FBC, UEC, Ca, Mg, BGL, ABG, lactate, CRP, LFT, Coagulation profile, blood culture
- Blood: ammonia, amino acids, chromosomal analysis
- Lumbar puncture: MCS, virology, specialist metabolic testing
- Urine amino and organic acids, ketones, reducing substances

Hypoxic ischaemic encephalopathy
The most commonly presenting encephalopathy is in the infant who is exposed to perinatal hypoxia. Moderate to severe hypoxic-ischaemic encephalopathy (HIE) occurs in 0.5- 1 per 1000 live births. Up to 60% of these die as neonates and 25% survive with major neurodevelopmental problems.

Clinical features:
- Reduced conscious level +/- seizures
- Hypoxic injury to all end organ systems:
  - Cardiac; hypotension, reduced function
  - Respiratory; apnoea, bradypnoea, or tachypnoea despite low pCO2
  - Renal; anuria, oliguria followed by polyuria
  - Hepatic; deranged LFT, coagulopathy
  - Bowel; NEC

Management:
- Resuscitation & stabilisation at delivery, consider transfer to tertiary centre
- Ongoing management to reduce impact of primary insult and protect from secondary injury:
  - Intubate and ventilate if: respiratory depression and acidosis, frequent seizures, encephalopathy, and post anticonvulsant medication
  - Restrict maintenance fluids to 40mL/kg/day 10% glucose (to reduce incidence of cerebral oedema and hyponatraemia; may cause hypoglycaemia requiring increased glucose concentration)
  - Manage hypotension and perfusion with cautious fluid boluses and inotropic support
- Treat seizures (Table 27.10)
- **Therapeutic Hypothermia**: Lowering the temperature of vulnerable deep brain structures to 33.0°C–34.0°C has a neuroprotective effect. Due to risks of therapeutic hypothermia it should only be undertaken in a tertiary centre. It is reasonable to not actively warm an infant with HIE whilst awaiting transfer to a tertiary hospital provided the rectal temperature is closely monitored.
  Eligibility criteria for therapeutic hypothermia:
  - ≥ 35/40 gestational age *and* < 6hrs of life; AND
  - Acute perinatal event that may result in HIE *with* evidence of asphyxia defined by presence of ≥ 2 of:
    - Apgar ≤5 at 10 min
    - Ongoing resuscitation with IPPV +/- chest compressions at 10 min age
    - Cord pH <7.0 (or ABG pH <7.0 or base deficit of ≥12mmol/L within 1 hour of birth);
    AND
  - Moderate/severe HIE (stage 2/3 based on modified Sarnat Classification): defined as seizures (clinical/aEEG) OR the presence of signs in ≥ 3 of the 6 categories below (Table 27.11).

Neonatal abstinence syndrome (NAS)
Neonatal abstinence syndrome occurs in babies born to chemically dependent women, who may use multiple substances. These babies exhibit signs of withdrawal, which are assessed using a standardised scoring system (commonly adapted from one devised by Finnegan). Onset of withdrawal symptoms is dependent on drug, can be variable and may be less evident in preterm babies.

Table 27.11 Characteristics of moderate and severe encephalopathy.

Parameter	Moderate encephalopathy	Severe encephalopathy
Level of consciousness	Lethargic – reduced response to non-painful stimulus	Stupor (response to painful stimulus) or Coma (no response to painful stimulus)
Spontaneous activity	Decreased	None
Posture	Distal flexion, full extension	Decerebrate (arms and legs extended)
Tone	Hypotonia reduced trunk or extremity tone or both	Flaccid – no tone
Primitive reflexes	Weak suck, incomplete Moro	Absent suck, absent Moro
Autonomic system Pupil Heart rate Respirations	 Constricted Bradycardia Periodic breathing	 Dilated/non-reactive Variable heart rate Apnoea

Clinical features:
- Heroin: onset from 48–72 hours
- Methadone: onset may be delayed for up to 1–2 weeks
- Neurological signs:
  - Hypertonia, tremors, hyperreflexia
  - Myoclonic jerks, seizures (1–2% heroin, 7% methadone)
  - Irritability, restlessness, high-pitched cry
  - Sleep disturbance
- Autonomic system dysfunction:
  - Nasal stuffiness, sneezing, yawning
  - Low grade fever, sweating
  - Skin mottling
- Gastrointestinal abnormalities: regurgitation, vomiting, diarrhoea
- Feeding issues: poor feeding, immature swallowing, failure to thrive
- Respiratory symptoms: tachypnoea, apnoea
- Excoriations (especially perianal)

Management:
- **Do not use Naloxone in these babies, as can precipitate acute withdrawal associated with seizures.**
- Consider administration of morphine (opiate withdrawal) or phenobarbitone (other forms of withdrawal) to assist gradual withdrawal.
- Breastfeeding; *seek specialist advice:*
  - If women are stable on methadone or buprenorphine and not using any other drugs, breastfeeding is encouraged.
  - If women are dependent on heroin, methamphetamine, alcohol and most other illicit drugs, breastfeeding is actively discouraged.

The 'floppy' baby
Common causes of hypotonia include prematurity, neonatal encephalopathy and drugs (maternal or newborn). Rarer causes include central neurological conditions, peripheral neurological and neuromuscular conditions (often congenital), and metabolic conditions (congenital & acquired).
Seek specialty Neurology input; assessment & management approach includes:
- Differentiating central from peripheral hypotonia (Table 27.12).
- Exclude and/or treat acute reversible causes such as sepsis and hypoglycaemia.
- Cranial ultrasound (exclude haemorrhage) and consider MRI.
- Blood: FBC, UEC, Ca, Mg, CRP, glucose, ABG, TFT, culture, TORCH screen, creatinine kinase (CPK).
- Metabolic screen: lactate, ammonia, amino acids, urine organic acids.
- Genetics: chromosomal analysis, karyotype, cytogenetics particularly if dysmorphic features (trisomy 21, Prader-Willi, Zellweger syndrome or congenital myotonic dystrophy).
- Consider maternal and baby ACh receptor antibodies if Myasthenia suspected (+/- Tensilon test).
- Electrophysiology: EMG and nerve conduction studies.

Table 27.12 Central & peripheral hypotonia.

Hypotonia Aetiology	Muscle strength	Deep tendon reflexes
Central Cause	Good	Present/increased
Peripheral cause	Weak – more marked distally	Decreased /absent
Muscular cause	Weak – more marked proximally	Decreased /absent
Neuromuscular	Ptosis, bulbar weakness	Present
Spinal muscular atrophy	Weak – tongue fasciculations	Variable /decreased

- Muscle biopsy: if results will alter acute management then performed in neonatal period (may be easier to interpret when the baby is a few months old).
- Assess the need for ventilation support.
- Facilitate feeding with OGT/NGT if necessary.

Prognosis is dependent upon the underlying cause.

Neurodevelopmental follow-up
Despite advances in neonatal care, admission to a NICU continues to place a baby at higher risk of impaired neurodevelopment. The greatest risks are seen in those with moderate to severe encephalopathy and the very preterm infant. Possible sequelae include cerebral palsy, sensorineural deafness, visual impairment, feeding & growth impairment, developmental delay and other neurocognitive / neurobehavioural vulnerabilities. Close follow-up after discharge is recommended (until at least 2 y corrected age if high risk), and may involve a multi-disciplinary team (MDT) with a view to engaging local community services where indicated.

Cardiovascular & haematological disorders
See also Chapters 15, Cardiology, and 23, Haematology.

Blood pressure ranges in neonates
Blood pressure increases with gestation, birthweight and postnatal age (especially in the first 72 hours of life).

- In clinical practice, the infant's blood pressure is generally considered to be adequate as long as urine output (> 1 mL/kg/hr) and capillary refill (< 3 seconds) are within normal limits and there is no metabolic acidosis.
- **These findings usually correlate with a mean blood pressure that is the same as the infants gestational age in weeks except for extremely preterm infants** who should have a mean blood pressure above 30 mmHg after 72 hours of age.
- See https://www.bettersafercare.vic.gov.au/resources/clinical-guidance/maternity-and-newborn-clinical-network/blood-pressure-disorders for blood pressure ranges by birth weight, gestation and age.

Hypotension
The recognition and treatment of hypotension is particularly important to avoid complications such as cerebral ischaemic injury or intraventricular haemorrhage (IVH). Hypotension is often multifactorial.

- Major causes include: intravascular hypovolaemia (blood loss, third space losses), infection with septic shock, cardiogenic shock (congenital heart disease, myocarditis, cardiomyopathy), asphyxia, air leak (pneumothorax) and drug effects (induction agents, anticonvulsants).

Clinical features include:
- Tachycardia
- Bradycardia
- Tachypnoea
- Mottling of the skin
- Prolonged capillary refill time (CRT >2s centrally)
- Cool extremities
- Weak peripheral pulses
- Reduced urine output

Management:
- Fluid resuscitation: 10–20 ml/kg 0.9% NaCl. If concern for acute blood loss (e.g. feto-maternal haemorrhage, DIC), blood should be urgently administered in 10ml/kg aliquots as part of the fluid resuscitation.
- Inotropic support: persistent hypotension should be treated with inotrope infusion via a central line (consider dopamine, dobutamine, low-dose adrenaline or noradrenaline) +/- corticosteroids (hydrocortisone).
- Central arterial blood pressure monitoring recommended if requiring inotropic support (in-dwelling arterial line).
- Treatment of underlying cause.

Neonatal bleeding

Neonates are susceptible to bleeding for various reasons. The first step is to assess the infant and clinical history to determine if "sick" or "well" neonatal bleeding. Causes include:

Bleeding in a 'well' neonate:
- Immune thrombocytopenia
  - Alloimmune (NAIT) or Autoimmune (maternal ITP)
- Vitamin K deficiency
- Inherited coagulation factor deficiencies e.g. haemophilia
- Bleeding from anatomic lesions e.g. haemangioma, A-V malformation

Bleeding in a 'sick' neonate:
- Disseminated intravascular coagulation (DIC) - usually associated with sepsis, asphyxia, necrotising entero-colitis (NEC) or subgaleal haemorrhage
  - Consumption thrombocytopenia with coagulation factor depletion
- Liver failure

Clinical Pearl: DIC

Major bleeding from any primary cause may induce secondary DIC which can mask the original pathology.

Clinical presentation:
- Oozing from the umbilicus or stump
- Cephal- or Subgaleal haematoma
- Bruising more than anticipated after birth
- Bleeding: from venepuncture/procedure sites, mucous membranes, into scalp, post circumcision
- Petechiae
- Intracranial haemorrhage
- Unexplained anaemia and hypotension

Initial Investigations include:
- FBE with platelet count
- Coagulation studies: APTT, PT, fibrinogen, d-dimer
  - For interpretation of results: see chapter 23 Haematology.
- Specific factor assays (if suspected on history / presentation)

Management principles:
- Treatment of underlying cause
- DIC: Blood products (platelets and FFP) used on clinical grounds
  - FFP 10–15 ml/ kg to correct coagulopathy
  - Platelets 10–15ml/kg If platelets < 50 and actively bleeding
  - Cryoprecipitate (check local dosing) to correct a low fibrinogen in active bleeding
- Vitamin K Deficiency: vitamin K1 1 mg IV (effective within hours)
  - FFP 10–15 mL/kg immediately
- Inherited factor deficiency: FFP 10–15 mL/kg (after blood sent for factor assays)
  - Specific factor replacement once diagnosis known
- Paediatric Haematology input if bleeding is not responding to initial measures or underlying cause likely to require long-term management (e.g. haemophilia).

Subgaleal haemorrhage

Rare but potentially catastrophic complication of instrumental delivery, wherein fluid accumulates in the loose subgaleal space. Early recognition and appropriate management required for survival as exsanguination can occur rapidly.
- Differentiated from cephalhaematoma by palpation of a very fluctuant swelling that crosses suture lines.
- If moderate or severe, the affected infant will require full resuscitation including blood products & clotting factors to maintain heamodynamic stability.
- Urgent referral to a tertiary centre often required.

Respiratory Problems
Respiratory distress
Common neonatal presentation; most major causes will present within the first hours of life.
Clinical signs include:
- Increased work of breathing: intercostal and subcostal recession, sternal retraction, nasal flaring, tracheal tug
- Tachypnoea: > 60 breaths per minute
- Expiratory grunt
- Central cyanosis

Clinical Pearl: Respiratory distress
Babies should be considered for transfer to tertiary neonatal intensive care if they require >40% oxygen, with or without pressure support, to maintain saturations >88% (using pulse oximetry).

Management approach to neonatal respiratory distress
Antenatal considerations
- Anticipate high-risk babies and transfer to a tertiary hospital for delivery and neonatal care.
- Maternally administered steroids in threatened preterm labour reduces severity of hyaline membrane disease (HMD), halves mortality and incidence of brain haemorrhage, and improves long-term outcomes.

General care
- Routine resuscitation and stabilization (see section prior)
- Avoid enteral feeds initially as will worsen respiratory distress via splinting the diaphragm
- Give IV fluids
- Treat with benzylpenicillin and gentamicin until blood cultures are negative

Respiratory care
- A chest x-ray: supports diagnosis in most cases.
- Monitor cardiorespiratory & blood gas measurements, and escalate respiratory support aiming for:
  - Arterial pH 7.35–7.45
  - Arterial Pco_2 40–60 mmHg
  - Arterial Po_2 50–80mmHg
- Aim for oxygen saturations of 91–95%
- Babies with RDS, especially those <30 weeks' gestation need surfactant as early as possible (administer via ETT or minimally invasive technique according to centre preference)
- HFNC (2-4L/kg/min) or CPAP (5-8 cmH$_2$O) are effective treatments. Use early for a baby who is grunting or showing increased respiratory effort (start low and increased in stepwise fashion)
- *Caffeine citrate (loading dose; 20 mg/kg)*: give in the preterm infant, and the term infant presenting with apnoea (bronchiolitis/sepsis); consider maintenance therapy (5-10mg/kg/day) if preterm
- The decision to mechanically ventilate a baby is indicated in the setting of:
  - Apnoea unresponsive to other treatment
  - Unsatisfactory blood gases: pH <7.25 with PCO$_2$ >60 mmHg, or inspired oxygen >40% despite CPAP (up to 8 cm H$_2$O)

Respiratory distress syndrome (RDS)
Primarily caused by surfactant deficiency, immaturity of lung structure and delayed fluid clearance which results in insufficient lung expansion. It is the most common cause of respiratory symptoms in the premature newborn. Incidence decreases with increasing gestation. Diagnosis is made clinically and on chest X-ray features.

Clinical presentation:
- Respiratory distress typically increasing over 48-72 hours before clinical improvement.
- Rapid deterioration may occur leading to respiratory failure (hypoxia and rising arterial CO$_2$ level), particularly if newborn becomes cold, acidotic, or has an infection.
- Chest x-ray features: fine, generalised, reticulogranular (ground glass) appearance with air bronchograms.

Management:
- Respiratory support: oxygen, assisted ventilation (HFNC, CPAP, IPPV).
- Consideration of surfactant replacement therapy (200mg/kg) if Clinical RDS or at risk of developing RDS; *or* <30 weeks' gestation; *or* Intubated (any gestation) and requiring >40% oxygen.
  - Up to 2 repeat doses of 100mg/kg can be considered at 12-hour intervals.
  - Most children recover without consequence.
  - Some (particularly those born preterm) will develop chronic lung disease.

Transient tachypnoea of the newborn (TTN) or 'wet lung syndrome'

Caused by delayed clearance of fetal lung fluid. It is a diagnosis of exclusion commonly occurring in babies born near term by elective caesarean section.

Clinical presentation and management includes:
- Mild respiratory distress within the first 4 hours lasting 1 to 2 days.
- Chest x-ray demonstrates coarse streaking of lung fields with fluid in the fissures.
- Treatment: Respiratory support, usually 30–40% oxygen, rarely HFNC or CPAP required.

Pneumonia

Group B (β-haemolytic) streptococcus (GBS) is the most common and serious cause of pneumonia and septicaemia in the newborn. Usually acquired during perinatal period from a GBS colonised mother. Other organisms include *E. coli*.

Clinical presentation:
- Congenital pneumonia: early onset (<24 hours) with primary respiratory distress and progressive respiratory failure.
- Sepsis with secondary RDS.
- Later onset infection can present with lethargy, temperature instability, poor feeding, respiratory distress, apnoea or poor perfusion.
- If not treated early can lead to haemodynamic collapse and death from cardiovascular shock.
- Chest x-ray changes are similar to severe RDS and are not diagnostic. A non-homogenous (asymmetric) RDS pattern is concerning.

Treatment includes:
- Respiratory and cardiovascular support as required
- IV Antibiotic therapy:
  - Early onset: Benzylpenicillin and Gentamicin
  - Late onset: Flucloxacillin and Gentamicin

Bronchiolitis

Bronchiolitis is a viral lower respiratory tract infection diagnosed clinically based on characteristic history and examination findings (see Chapter 38, Respiratory medicine). Neonates, particularly preterm, ex-preterm or those with chronic lung disease are at particularly risk of severe bronchiolitis requiring respiratory support.

Meconium aspiration syndrome (MAS)

Hypoxia, causing fetal distress before delivery may cause an *in utero* gasp and inhalation of meconium. Occurs in 5% babies with meconium stained liquor at delivery.

Clinical presentation:
- Respiratory distress soon after birth from obstruction, pneumonitis and surfactant inhibition
- Chest x-ray shows hyperinflation and patchy consolidation
- Complications include:
  - Air leak syndrome (pneumothorax and pneumomediastinum)
  - Associated secondary pulmonary hypertension

Management:
- Oxygen as the mainstay of therapy
- Mechanical ventilation (and if severe ECMO) may be required
- Broad spectrum antibiotics to cover superimposed infection

Pneumothorax and tension pneumothorax

Pneumothorax occurs when air escapes from ruptured alveoli into the pleural cavity. This may occur spontaneously at birth, or secondary to other lung disease or positive pressure ventilation. Incidence has reduced since surfactant therapy and continuous positive airway pressure (CPAP) rather than mechanical ventilation have become routine care. However, 5–10% of babies with neonatal lung disease may develop an air leak. A small collection of air may not compromise the infant, however larger air volumes may result in collapse of the ipsilateral lung and shift of the mediastinum to the contralateral side. It is vital to recognise and treat early.

Clinical features and assessment:
- Acute deterioration with desaturation/increased oxygen requirement.
- Increase in respiratory distress and/or diminished chest movement.
- Circulatory compromise (indicates mediastinal shift/compression).
- On examination:
  - Decreased air entry and hyperresonance to percussion on affected side
  - Displaced apex beat
  - Hyperluminescence with transillumination using a cold light source
- Chest x-ray shows hyperlucency with absence of lung markings to the periphery on the affected side (this takes time to perform)

Management:
- Asymptomatic pneumothorax: usually no treatment required (will self resolve).
- Symptomatic pneumothorax: requires treatment.
  - Insertion of an intercostal catheter (see chapter 5 Procedures) with underwater drain at low negative pressure.
  - Needle aspiration may act as a temporising measure.

Tension pneumothorax is a medical emergency:
- Results if the accumulating air is under pressure.
- Consider in a rapidly deteriorating baby (despite full resuscitation) particularly with reduced air entry to one or both sides of the chest.
- Do not wait for a chest x-ray before initiating treatment.
- This is an acutely life threatening situation and immediate drainage will be required.
  - In the acute situation needle aspiration is performed
  - Definitive intercostal catheter (ICC) insertion once stabilised

Upper airway obstruction

All newborns with stridor require assessment of their airway. The neonatal airway is small and underdeveloped, making it vulnerable to the effects of external compression or internal obstruction. Causes are best considered according to their level in the airway:
- **Nasal:** URTI, choanal atresia/stenosis, deviated nasal septum (traumatic).
- **Oral:** macroglossia (BWS, T21, hypothyroidism), micrognathia, lingual thyroid, Pierre-Robin sequence (PRS; micrognathia, retrognathia, tongue base airway obstruction +/- cleft palate).
- **Glottic & subglottic**: laryngomalacia, laryngeal inflammation, laryngeal web, vocal cord palsy (VCP), subglottic stenosis, subglottic haemangiomata.
- **Intrathoracic:** tracheomalacia, tracheal stenosis, vascular ring/sling, mediastinal mass (e.g. teratoma).

Specific conditions:
- **Choanal atresia/stenosis:** Suspect when the breathing improves with opening the baby's mouth, and a 6F catheter cannot be passed through the nose to the nasopharynx.
- **PRS:** presentation at 2–4 weeks with airway obstruction & feeding difficulties common. Obstructive symptoms improve when prone. Severe cases require surgical correction.
- **Laryngomalacia:** presentation with inspiratory stridor, respiratory distress & feeding difficulties. Worse supine. Mild laryngomalacia usually needs no intervention (self resolves by 12–18m); severe cases require supraglottoplasty.
- **Management and prognosis** depends upon aetiology; seek specialty Ear Nose & Throat (ENT) advice.

Non pulmonary causes of respiratory distress
- Cardiac disease: Left-to-right shunts or left-sided obstructions can cause pulmonary oedema
- Pulmonary hypertension: secondary to cardiac, respiratory, other causes.
  - Presents with increased oxygen requirement but little respiratory difficulty
  - Chest x-ray often reveals clear lung fields

Gastrointestinal problems
Jaundice
Neonatal jaundice is common, but also clinically important because of (i) the potential for harm from high levels of bilirubin (SBR) and (ii) the need to identify rarer causes of jaundice which require more complex investigation and management. Skin colour change may not be detectible until the SBR exceeds 70–100 µmol/L in a Caucasian infant (and more difficult to detect with darker skin tones). Scleral jaundice may be detected with SBR of 25–40 µmol/L.

- **Neonatal unconjugated hyperbilirubinemia** is often transient and benign (up to 60% healthy term and 80% preterm infants develop 'physiological' jaundice). Less frequently, it can reach very high levels or be an early manifestation of an underlying disorder.
- Major risk factors for **severe hyperbilirubinemia** include:
  - Jaundice < 24 hours age
  - Blood group incompatibility (particularly Rhesus (Rh)) or other hemolytic disease
  - Cephalhaematoma / significant bruising
  - >10% weight loss from birth weight (+/-ineffective breastfeeding)
  - Family history RBC enzyme defects (e.g. *G6PD deficiency*) or RBC membrane defects (e.g. *hereditary spherocytosis*)
  - Prematurity
- **Bilirubin encephalopathy and kernicterus**
Severe unconjugated hyperbilirubinemia can lead to acute or chronic bilirubin encephalopathy. Infants present with behaviour changes and symptoms such as lethargy, hypotonia, and decreased suck even if the SBR is not high enough to require an exchange transfusion. The process can be transient with prompt treatment, however Kernicterus and long term sequelae may result if it progresses.
- Kernicterus presents with posturing and arching (opisthotonus), seizures, and risk of death.
- Sequelae of kernicterus include sensorineural hearing loss and irreversible brain damage with athetoid cerebral palsy.
- Well term infants with no haemolysis are at minimal risk of kernicterus.
- The risk of kernicterus increases with:
  - Increasing unconjugated hyperbilirubinemia (>340µmol/L in the term infant unsafe)
  - Comorbid illness (perinatal hypoxia, acidosis, hypothermia, meningitis, sepsis etc.)
  - Decreasing gestation; these infants should have active treatment started at lower SBR levels
- **Neonatal Conjugated hyperbilirubinemia** (neonatal cholestasis; conjugated SBR level > 20% of the total bilirubin level) occurring in the first 3 months of life *is always pathologic and requires thorough investigation.*

Physiological Jaundice
- Unconjugated jaundice.
- SBR rarely > 220 µmol/L.
- Develops day 2–7 of life, peaks day 4-5, & resolves within 2 weeks of birth.
- Newborn is well (alert, feeding well, afebrile) with normal coloured stool & urine.
- Aetiology is multifactorial: high RBC breakdown/turnover, immature liver conjugation, high intestinal reabsorption of bilirubin and hence reduced excretion.
- Consider pathological jaundice in the differential diagnosis particularly at higher SBR levels.

Pathological Jaundice:

Clinical Pearl: Pathological jaundice

A good rule of thumb in indentifying pathological jaundice is the catchphrase: ***"Too quick, too early, too high, and too long!"***. Features such as rapid progression, early onset, unexpectedly high SBR level, persistence beyond 2 weeks after birth, or association with other signs or symptoms suggest a pathologic process that requires investigation.

'Too quick' – Rapid progression
- SBR concentrations rising at greater than 8.5–10 μmol/L/hour are of concern and indicate a pathological process, usually haemolysis.
- Continued rise should be anticipated & monitored, with phototherapy treatment started promptly.

'Too early' – The first 24 hours
- Jaundice in the first 24 hours is always pathological.
- Unconjugated hyperbilirubinemia predominates.
- Newborns may be jaundiced at birth, SBR may rise rapidly over hours, or neonates may present with anaemia, hepatosplenomegaly and in severe cases foetal hydrops.
- Admit to a special care nursery, begin treatment immediately and investigate urgently.

Aetiology:
- Usually hemolysis secondary to immune-mediated blood group incompatibility between mother and foetus (haemolytic disease of the newborn):
  - ABO incompatibility; maternal anti-A or anti-B IgG antibodies target fetal ABO antigen(s)
  - Rhesus incompatibility; Rh-ve mother sensitised to Rh+ve fetal blood in previous pregnancy. (Incidence has significantly decreased with antenatal administration of anti-D immunoglobulin)
  - Other blood group antigen incompatibility
- Sepsis
- Less common causes: RBC enzyme or cell membrane defects eg. G6PD deficiency, pyruvate kinase deficiency, hereditary spherocytosis, hemoglobinopathies, rare genetic causes (eg. Crigler-Najjar syndrome), hepatitis.

'Too high' – 24 hours to 10 days old
If the SBR concentration exceeds 200-250 μmol/L during this time consider additional causes including:
- Breast *feeding* jaundice (mild dehydration with low milk supply)
- Breast *milk* jaundice (see below)
- Haemolysis
- Breakdown of extravasated blood (e.g. cephalhaematoma, bruising, CNS haemorrhage)
- Polycythemia
- Infection (eg. sepsis, UTI)

Breast milk Jaundice: unconjugated hyperbilirubinemia occurs in approximately 10% of breast fed infants.
- It is a diagnosis of exclusion, thought to be due to inhibition of UGT1A1 enzyme activity and increased enterohepatic circulation caused by compounds in breast milk.
- Typically develops after 7 days, is not associated with kernicterus and does not need treatment.
- *Breast milk jaundice does not need treatment; breastfeeding is important and should continue.*

'Too long' – Prolonged jaundice >10 days (especially if >2 weeks)
- Prolonged jaundice after 10 days of life can often be managed as an outpatient with caution, however, may require admission for investigation and/or management.
- Check SBR to determine whether hyperbilirubinemia is unconjugated (>85%) or conjugated (>15%).
- *Conjugated hyperbilirubinaemia is uncommon, always pathological and requires extensive investigation to determine the cause.*

Unconjugated hyperbilirubinaemia
- Continued poor milk intake
- Haemolysis: Sudden onset or reappearance of jaundice at this age suggests haemolysis caused by a red blood cell enzyme abnormality (G6PD most common; see Chapter 23, Haematology)
- Infection: especially UTI

- Hypothyroidism: jaundice may be the presenting sign
- Drugs e.g. cephalosporins
- Genetic e.g. Gilbert's syndrome

If the above are excluded in a well and breastfed baby, the likely diagnosis is breast milk jaundice.

Conjugated hyperbilirubinaemia – cholestasis

- Infection: causing neonatal hepatitis (TORCH).
- **Biliary atresia:** ascending inflammatory process of intra- and extrahepatic bile ducts (see Chapter 21, Gastroenterology). Early diagnosis important as prognosis is better with surgery (hepatoportoenterostomy or Kasai procedure) preferably before 8 weeks of age.
- Choledochal cyst: rare congenital anomaly with cystic dilatation of the intra- and extrahepatic biliary tree.
- Ischaemic liver injury: secondary to altered systemic circulation such as in perinatal asphyxia.
- Parenteral nutrition: especially in prolonged use (>2 weeks). Usually resolves 4-6 months after cessation of TPN but severe cases may progress to end stage liver disease.
- Gestational alloimmune liver disease (GALD): previously known as neonatal haemochromatosis. Rare, idiopathic, antenatal onset of liver disease with excess extrahepatic iron deposition.
- Inborn errors of metabolism / Genetic: galactosaemia, tyrosinaemia, mitochondrial disorders Alagille syndrome, α1-antitrypsin deficiency.

Jaundice Prevention, Investigation and Management

Prevention

- Primary prevention involves early and frequent breastfeeding (8–12 times per day initially)
- Secondary prevention involves the following;
  - Blood group, Rh (D) type and Coombs' test on the infant's (cord) blood if the mother is known to be Rh -ve or has not had antenatal blood grouping.
  - Monitor all newborns routinely for jaundice at least 12-hourly.
  - Assess the risk of developing hyperbilirubinaemia prior to discharge (eg. late preterm & early discharge <48 hours) and ensure follow up examination undertaken.

Investigation

Differentiating unconjugated from conjugated hyperbilirubinemia, and identifying haemolysis will direct further laboratory tests and imaging.

Clinical Pearl: SBR measurement

Jaundice is quantified by measuring transcutaneous and/or serum bilirubin levels. Transcutaneous bilirubi-nometers, most accurate at lower bilirubin levels, are helpful for initial screening and follow-up. *They should not be used if a baby is receiving or has received phototherapy.* Discrepancies are more likely in preterm babies and those with darker skin tones. Where there is doubt, confirm the result with a laboratory measured SBR (total SBR concentration, unconjugated and conjugated fractions).

First line bloods:

- SBR; total and conjugated
- Blood group and direct antiglobulin test (Coombs' / DAT)
  (compare with maternal blood group & Ab screen for risk of blood group incompatibility)
- FBE + film (haemolysis; fragmented red cells) +/- reticulocytes
- CRP (if infection is suspected)

Further investigations depend upon clinical suspicion and may include:

- Blood: LFT, coagulation screen serum bile acids, amino acids, culture, TORCH, toxin and/or drug screening
- Urine: culture, metabolic screen
- Imaging:
  - Abdominal ultrasound; biliary atresia, choledochal cyst, biliary sludge
  - MRI; abnormalities of the intra- and extrahepatobiliary system, GALD
- Disease-specific tests: e.g. α_1-antitrypsin phenotype, Gal-1-PUT (galactosaemia), urine succinylacetone, genetic testing
- Liver biopsy: especially when conventional investigations do not yield a diagnosis

Management Approach

- Ensure adequate enteral hydration;
  - Supplement with EBM/Formula if required (may reduce enterohepatic bilirubin circulation), or IVF (if enteral intake inadequate / contraindicated)
- Phototherapy including 'biliblankets' (see below)
- Exchange transfusion (ExT: if indicated – see below)
- IVIG (0.5–1.0 g/kg IV, repeated after 12 hours if needed) reduces need for exchange transfusion
- Treat the cause (e.g. infection, hypothyroidism)
- Ursodeoxycholic acid - for intrahepatic cholestasis

Phototherapy

Light therapy causes photo-isomerisation of the bilirubin molecule and transforms it into water soluble forms which can be excreted directly into the bile, and excreted in the baby's urine & faeces without being conjugated.

- Phototherapy effectiveness increases with blue light (460-490 nm), the intensity of the light (> 30 μW/cm-2/nm-1) and greater skin exposure (circumferential treatment maximises the exposed area and may require combined use of lights and a 'biliblanket').
- Good-quality lights should not need to be closer than 30 cm.
- Phototherapy treatment threshold levels differ for gestation, weight and degree of illness (Tables 27.13 and 27.14).

Phototherapy management principles include:

- **Measure SBR** 12–24 hourly whilst rising and then daily as it stabilises with phototherapy
- **Increase** to multiple (intense) phototherapy if:
  - Rate of rise >8.5μmol/L/hour prior to phototherapy
  - SBR rises by >50μmol/L in 24 hours during single unit phototherapy
  - SBR is within 50μmol/L of exchange level
- **Reduce phototherapy**: when SBR >50μmol/L below exchange level
- **Cease phototherapy**:
  - Consider when below treatment level based on risk
  - Stop when SBR 50μmol/L below treatment level

Table 27.13 Hyperbilirubinemia treatment thresholds for gestation (<27 weeks to 34+6 weeks) and birthweight.

Parameter: Use lowest	Total SBR concentration (μmol/L)							
	<27 weeks' gestation OR Birthweight <1000 g		27–30+6 weeks' gestation OR Birthweight 1000–1499 g		31–32+6 weeks' gestation OR Birthweight 1500–1999 g		33–34+6 weeks' gestation OR Birthweight >2000 g	
	Start single unit PTx	Intense PTx & consider ExT	Start single unit PTx	Intense PTx & consider ExT	Start single unit PTx	Intense PTx & consider ExT	Start single unit PTx	Intense PTx & consider ExT
	For DAT positive isoimmunisation start treatment at SBR 20μmoL/L below threshold							
Birth	70	150	80	170	90	190	100	210
12 hours	90	180	110	200	120	225	130	240
24 hours	110	205	140	230	155	255	165	260
36 hours	125	220	160	250	175	275	190	295
48 hours	140	235	175	270	195	295	210	315
60 hours	145	245	185	280	210	310	225	330
≥72 hours	150	250	190	290	220	320	240	340
>21 days	Prolonged hyperbilirubinaemia investigations							

Table 27.14 Hyperbilirubinemia treatment thresholds for gestation (>35 weeks), and birthweight, or risk factors for serious jaundice.

Parameter: Use lowest	Total SBR concentration (µmol/L)			
	35–37+6 weeks' gestation OR Birthweight <2500 g OR *With* risk factors for serious jaundice		>38 weeks' gestation OR Birthweight >2500 g *without* risk factors for serious jaundice	
	Start single unit PTx	Intense PTx & consider ExT	Start single unit PTx	Intense PTx & consider ExT
	For DAT positive isoimmunisation start treatment at SBR 20µmoL/L below threshold			
Birth	85	235	110	270
12 hours	130	260	160	295
24 hours	170	280	205	325
36 hours	200	300	235	350
48 hours	225	325	265	375
60 hours	240	340	290	390
72 hours	260	360	310	410
96 hours	290	385	340	430
>5 days	290	385	360	435
>14 days	Prolonged hyperbilirubinaemia investigations			

Note: PTx = Phototherapy; ExT = Exchange transfusion;
Risk factors for serious jaundice: jaundice <24 hours, DAT+, cephalhaematoma/significant bruising, >10% weight loss from birthweight, family Hx RBC enzyme/membrane defects.

- **Monitor for rebound**
  - ○ Check SBR 12–24 hours after cessation of phototherapy (~10% rebound is expected)
  - ○ If SBR is static or falling do further testing only if clinically indicated
  - ○ If SBR is rising repeat in 24 hours or restart phototherapy if above treatment threshold
- **Restart phototherapy:** if SBR above treatment threshold (e.g. rebound >10% or rate of rise is greater than expected for the day of life).

Exchange Transfusion (ExT)
- Rarely performed.
- Primarily corrects anaemia and removes antibodies in severe haemolytic disease of the newborn.
- Risks are uncommon but include; cardiorespiratory compromise, vasospasm, air embolism, infection, thrombosis, necrotising enterocolitis death (rarely).
- Any baby requiring an ExT should be discussed with and transferred to a tertiary centre.

Gastroesophageal reflux disease
Gastro-oesophageal reflux (GOR; see also Chapter 21, Gastroenterology) is the spontaneous and effortless passage of gastric contents into the oesophagus. It may result in vomiting and is self-limiting, usually resolving by 18 months whether treated or not.

GOR is common in healthy term babies (at least 40%) and is present in most preterm babies. It is physiological due to oesophageal sphincter relaxation (immature muscle), slower gastric motility and increased gastric acidity. Pathological GOR, or GOR disease (GORD) is more severe and associated with other symptoms.

Clinical Pearl: Gastroesophageal reflux
- Most preterm infants with recurrent apnoea and bradycardia do not have GORD.
- Non-pharmacological measures should be used first in the treatment of GOR; most infants do not require medication.
- Medication should only be used with proven GORD and if ineffective after a trial period (4 weeks) should be discontinued as they may cause harm.

Clinical presentation:
- Pronounced irritability with feeding
- Delayed acid clearance resulting in bleeding (haematemesis)
- Apnoea (*most apnoea is not due to GORD*)
- Cyanotic episodes
- Aspiration events
- Chronic cough, wheeze or exacerbation of chronic lung disease
- Failure to thrive with reduced intake and refusal to feed
- Apparent life-threatening events and SIDS (although controversial)

Investigation and treatment is reserved for babies with GORD. There is no gold standard for diagnosis ; this is predominantly clinical. Investigations are rarely necessary but may include:
- Contrast (barium) swallow: exclude structural abnormalities & may show reflux on dynamic assessment
- 24 hour pH probe; limited use if frequent or continuous feeds (including preterm) due to buffering of the gastric acid
- Oesophageal manometry - catheter size limits use in small babies
- Endoscopy and radio-nucleotide studies – not standardised / rarely indicated

Management approach:
Non-pharmacological treatment: GOR causes significant parental distress and requires education, reassurance, support and guidance. General measures may minimise symptoms.
- Positioning: holding infant upright with the head elevated for 20–30 minutes following a feed may help.
  - Elevating the sleeping surface has not been shown to reduce GOR and is not recommended.
  - Safe sleeping guidelines; prone sleeping or inclining the sleep surface is not recommended due to SIDS risk.
- Feeds: reduced volume with increased frequency may be possible in nursery environment.
  - Continuous gastric or jejunal feeds; in severe cases warranting admission.
  - Artificial thickening of milk; may reduce vomiting frequency although there is no current evidence to support this (and may contribute to constipation).
- Up to 40% of infants presenting with GORD have non-IgE mediated cow milk protein allergy; a 2–3 week trial of hydrolysed or elemental formula may be indicated with exclusion of the allergens (cow milk and soy protein) from the maternal diet.

Pharmacological treatment: aims to reduce the acidity of the regurgitated stomach contents rather than treat the GOR itself.
- Medication that lowers gastric acidity may alter GIT flora and increases the risk of NEC; avoid in the low birth weight and preterm infant.
- *There is no conclusive evidence that medications improve symptoms in those with reflux without demonstrated complications. Judicious use is recommended* (Table 27.15).

Table 27.15 Medications for GORD.

Medication class	Agent	Notes
Surface agents	Sodium or magnesium alginate	Long term use is not recommended
Proton pump inhibitors (PPI)	The mainstay of pharmacologic treatment *Omeprazole* • *<3kg: 0.7mg/kg up to 1.4mg/kg daily* • *>3kg: 5mg daily*	Studies indicate increased risk of lower respiratory tract infection, gastroenteritis, micronutrient deficiency and future fractures
H_2 blockers (histamine H_2 receptor antagonist)	*Ranitidine*	Oral use no longer recommended due to the ethanol content (7.5% w/v = 75 mg/mL).

Surgical Treatment: fundoplication is indicated for intractable or life-threatening GORD which has not responded to pharmacological therapies.

Cow's Milk Protein Enteropathy
See Chapter 13, Allergy

Renal Tract Diseases
See Chapter 37, Renal medicine
- Guidance on managing common finding of renal tract dilatation on antenatal ultrasound scans can also be found at https://www.bettersafercare.vic.gov.au/resources/clinical-guidance/maternity-and-newborn-clinical-network/hydronephrosis-in-neonates.

Neonatal Infection
This is one of the most common preventable causes of neonatal mortality and morbidity (see also Chapter 25, Infectious Diseases).
- **In utero infection**, which can occur any time before birth from transplacental transmission, results from overt or subclinical maternal infection. Consequences depend on the agent and timing of infection in gestation and include spontaneous abortion, intrauterine growth restriction, premature birth, stillbirth, congenital malformation (e.g. rubella), and symptomatic (e.g. cytomegalovirus [CMV], toxoplasmosis, syphilis) or asymptomatic (e.g. CMV) neonatal infection. HIV and hepatitis B are less commonly transmitted transplacentally.
- **Intrapartum (early-onset, <48hrs of life) neonatal infection** with herpes simplex viruses, HIV, hepatitis B, group B streptococci, enteric gram-negative organisms (primarily *escherichia coli*), *listeria monocytogenes*, gonococci, and chlamydiae usually occur from passage through an infected birth canal. Sometimes ascending infection can occur if delivery is delayed after rupture of membranes.
- **Postpartum (late-onset >48hrs of life) infections** are acquired from contact with an infected mother/visitor directly, via breastfeeding (e.g. HIV, CMV) or from the hospital or home environments (term infants: *Staphylococcus aureus*; preterm infants: coagulase-negative staphylococci (CONS), gram negative organisms [e.g. *E.coli*, Klebsiella, Enterobacter and Serratia spp.], fungi [Candida spp.] and viruses [e.g. Respiratory Syncytial Virus].

Risk factors include:
- **Early-onset sepsis:**
  - Prolonged ruptured membranes (PROM; > 18 hours)
  - Fetal distress
  - Maternal pyrexia (> 38 C) or overt infection such as a UTI/GIT/Diarrhoeal illness
  - Multiple obstetric procedures, including cervical sutures
  - Preterm delivery
  - GBS bacteriuria (current pregnancy) or GBS infection in previous infant
- **Late-onset sepsis:**
  - Prolonged hospitalisation
  - Presence of foreign bodies such as intravenous catheters, endotracheal tubes
  - Cross-infection (staff / visitors)
  - Congenital malformations (eg. urinary tract anomalies or neural tube defects)

Clinical presentation:
- Early symptoms and signs may be non-specific, however rapid progression to overwhelming sepsis may occur.
- Important warning signs of moderate-severe infection include:
  - Temperature instability
  - Respiratory distress
  - Poor feeding
  - Vomiting
  - Abdominal distension & tenderness
  - Drowsiness
  - Floppiness / Hypotonia
  - Pallor
  - Apnoea
  - Seizures

Investigations:
Have a low threshold to investigate and empirically treat if one or more of the warning signs are present.
- Blood culture (minimum 1ml)
- Urine MCS: after day 5 when primary UTI more likely (unless renal tract anomaly) via:
  - Suprapubic aspiration (SPA) under US imaging if possible
  - Catheter (size-5 French tube) if SPA unsuccessful
  - Bags should NOT be used to collect urine for MCS
- CSF for MCS, biochemistry and viral PCR (e.g. HSV 1/2, Enterovirus, Parechovirus) if meningitis suspected.
  - This should always be performed in the presence of fever in a newborn, or if blood culture is positive (except for CONS when LP may be avoided if responds appropriately to Vancomycin)
- Nasopharyngeal aspirate (NPA) for viral respiratory pathogens if symptoms present.
- CXR if focal respiratory signs, e.g. crepitations, are present.
- Throat and rectal swabs and swabs of any obviously infected lesion for MCS and/or PCR.

Latest Evidence: Early onset sepsis calculators
- Early-Onset Sepsis Calculators, many of which are freely available online, are now used as clinical risk stratification tools to guide the use of empirical antibiotics in newborns.
- Since their introduction within the last decade, they have contributed to a substantial reduction in the use of empirical antibiotics with no reported increase in adverse outcomes from EOS according to a recent systematic review and meta-analysis.
Source: JAMA Paediatrics 2019 [PMID 31479103].

Management
- Any unwell neonate must be considered at risk of sepsis and commenced on appropriate antibiotics as soon as possible (ideally) after cultures are taken.
- **Antibiotics should not be delayed if cultures cannot be obtained.**
- *Appropriate resuscitation is required if haemodynamic or respiratory instability present, and may include intubation and ventilation, fluid boluses and inotropic support.*

Tables 27.16 and 27.17 provide recommendations used in the Royal Children's Hospital (RCH) NICU on the choice of appropriate antimicrobial agents according to likely infectious agent or system affected.

Table 27.16 RCH neonatal antimicrobial recommendations – *Source undifferentiated.*

Type	Age	IV Empiric agent	Duration of treatment
Source Undifferentiated Meningitis excluded	<48 hrs	Benzylpenicillin[1] + Gentamicin **Add** Flucloxacillin if *S. aureus* suspected	Cease antibiotics after 48 hours if no growth on cultures and patient clinically improved
	>48 hrs	Flucloxacillin[1] + Gentamicin **Add** Benzylpenicillin if *Listeria* suspected[2] **Add** Fluconazole if *Candida* suspected[3]	If organisms isolated from samples, treat as per 'source differentiated'
Source Undifferentiated Meningitis NOT excluded	<48 hrs	Benzylpenicillin[1] + Cefotaxime **Add** Flucloxacillin if *S. aureus* suspected **Add** Aciclovir if HSV suspected	If CSF examination excludes meningitis, cease Cefotaxime and Aciclovir and treat as per *Source undifferentiated Meningitis Excluded*

Table 27.16 (*Continued*)

Type	Age	IV Empiric agent	Duration of treatment
	>48 hrs	Flucloxacillin[1] + Cefotaxime **Add** Benzylpenicillin if *Listeria* suspected[2] **Add** Aciclovir if HSV suspected **Add** Fluconazole if *Candida* suspected[3]	If CSF WCC is abnormal but no organism isolated from CSF, administer Cefotaxime for 14 days total duration.

Notes:
1. Use Vancomycin instead of Penicillin or Flucloxacillin for: septic shock, suspected MRSA (colonised, Indigenous, family history) or penicillin-resistant enterococcus
2. Consider Benzylpenicillin for Listeria if: >7 days old, maternal perinatal illness, preterm, chorioamnionitis, fetal distress, or green liquor present at time of birth
3. Consider Fluconazole for fungal infection if: fulminating course, <1500g and deteriorates whilst on antibiotics, ≥7 days antibiotics or on TPN and deteriorates

Table 27.17 RCH neonatal antimicrobial recommendations – *Source isolated*.

Source	Subtype	Antimicrobial agent (IV)	Duration of treatment	Notes
Blood	GBS *E.coli** CoNS	Benzylpenicillin Gentamicin (if susceptible) Vancomycin	7 days 10 days 5 days	*For *E.coli* – repeat blood culture until blood is sterile & continue gentamicin for 7 days from clear culture
CNS	Meningitis - GBS - *E.coli* / culture - HSV encephalitis EVD/Reservoir VP shunt	Benzylpenicillin Cefotaxime Aciclovir Vancomycin + Cefotaxime Vancomycin + Ceftazidime	14 days 21 days 21 days ID consult	ID advice for post-infection prophylaxis
Abdominal	NEC or other abdominal source	Amoxicillin + Gentamicin+ Metronidazole	7–10 days	If amoxicillin-resistant enterococci colonised consult ID
Urinary	UTI	Benzylpenicillin + Gentamicin	Mild: 3 days IV Gentamicin + 4 days oral antibiotics Mod/severe: 7–10 days IV Gentamicin	Difficult to differentiate between mild or mod/ severe in neonates. Consider Renal USS early to assess for pyelonephritis
Respiratory	Community acquired Pneumonia Hospital acquired Pneumonia Ventilator associated pneumonia Bronchiolitis	Benzylpenicillin + Gentamicin Flucloxacillin + Gentamicin Flucloxacillin + Gentamicin **NO** antibiotics	7 days 7 days ID consult	Consider IV-oral switch at 5 days if improved Diagnosed as HAP if occurs >48hrs after admission Recommend BAL if ventilated If antibiotics started, cease if clinically bronchiolitis
Skin and soft tissue	Post-op wound infection/cellulitis	Flucloxacillin	5 days	Swab + consider IV-oral switch at 3 days if improved

Endocrine conditions
Hypoglycaemia
Many newborns are at risk for hypoglycemia (Table 27.18).
- **Clinical presentation:**
  - Asymptomatic; OR
  - CNS excitation: jitteriness, high pitched cry, seizures; OR
  - CNS depression: lethargy, hypotonia, poor feeding, temperature instability, apnoea
- Bedside glucometers provide a blood glucose level (BGL) and are useful for *screening only* (reduced accuracy at low levels) – if hypoglycaemia suspected urgent true blood glucose (TBG) should be measured by a laboratory or a blood gas analyser.
- A definition of neonatal hypoglycaemia lacks consensus but is generally regarded as a **TBG <2.6mmol/L.**
- Treatment should not be delayed awaiting TBG in a symptomatic infant.
- Clinical intervention should be guided at the following thresholds:
  - BGL <2.0 mmol/L if asymptomatic newborn on postnatal ward (PNW)
  - BGL <2.6 mmol/L if symptomatic newborn on postnatal ward
  - TBG <2.6 for all newborns in SCN/NICU

Investigations:
- BGL screening < 1 hour of age for newborns with risk factors for neonatal hypoglycaemia
  - Screen Infants at low risk on PNW (to keep mother & baby together)
  - Preterm infants >34 weeks' gestation usually require screening before initial two feeds only

Management approach:
Prevention
- Advise maternal antenatal expression of breast milk for high risk newborns.
- Support early prolonged skin to skin contact and breastfeeding.
- Prevent hypothermia.
- Commence enteral feeds by 1–2 hours of age & feed frequently (2–3 hourly); EBM/formula at 60 mL/kg/d initially, increasing to 90 mL/kg by 24 hours if tolerated.
- IV 10% glucose at 60–90 mL/kg/day if unable to feed enterally (4–6 mg/kg/min of glucose; see glucose delivery / GUR calculation in Feeds and fluids section above).

Clinical Pearl: Normoglycemia
Infants provided with a steady glucose supply, who have normal hormonal pathways to regulate blood glucose should remain normoglycaemic on 4-8 mg/kg/min glucose.

Treatment
- Provide Buccal 40% glucose gel / Enteral feeds as directed (Figures 27.2 and 27.3).
- Treat the cause (e.g. commonly sepsis or hypothermia).
- Monitor response with frequent BGL's.
- If unable to obtain IV access & BGL is <1mmol/L give *glucagon 0.3units/kg IM.*

Table 27.18 Risk factors for neonatal hypoglycaemia.

Reduced glycogen stores / increased demand	Hyperinsulinaemic states	Other
• Prematurity	• Infant of diabetic mother	• Congenital adrenal hyperplasia (adrenaline and cortisol deficiency)
• IUGR (<10th percentile)	• Rhesus Isoimmunisation	
• Perinatal asphyxia	• Persistent hyperinsulinaemia	
• Hypothermia	• Islet cell hyperplasia / pancreatic tumour	
• RDS	• Beckwith-Weidemann syndrome	
• Sepsis / shock	• Macrosomia	
• Seizures		

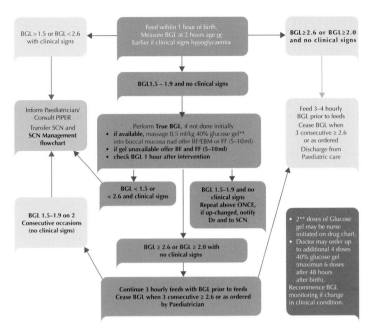

Figure 27.2 Postnatal ward management of infants at risk of hypoglycaemia. *Source:* Safer care Victoria – Hypoglycemia in Neonates. Reproduced with permission from authors.

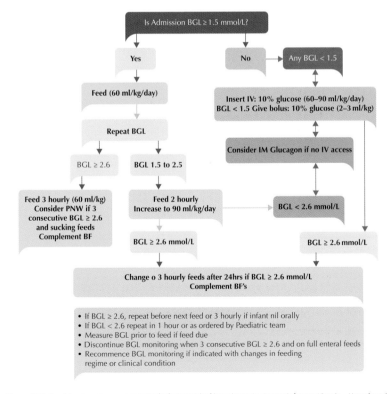

Figure 27.3 Special care nursery management of infants at risk of hypoglycaemia. *Source:* Safer care Victoria – Hypoglycemia in Neonates. Reproduced with permission from authors.

IV Glucose
- IV bolus 2–3 mL/kg 10% glucose (= 200–300 mg/kg glucose).
- Bolus should be followed by infusion to prevent rebound hypoglycaemia:
- 10% glucose infusion at 60-90 mL/kg/day (= 4–6mg/kg/min glucose).
- If fluid restriction required give a more concentrated glucose solution.
  Infusions >12.5% glucose should be given through a centrally placed line (such as a UVC) however inability to gain such access should not preclude their use. Be mindful of extravasation risk.
- Once BGL normalises, reintroduce enteral feeds & wean glucose infusion.

Glucagon
- IM glucagon 0.03–1.0 mg/kg (can repeat after 6–12 hours) if adequate glycogen stores & prolonged hypoglycemia despite glucose infusion (e.g. hyperinsulinaemic states).
- Infants of diabetic mothers may need up to 0.3 mg/kg (to maximum total dose of 1 mg).
- If hypoglycaemia continues despite 120 mL/kg/d of 12.5% glucose infusion (10.5 mg/kg/min glucose) then glucagon infusion should be considered (1–20 micrograms/kg/hr).

Corticosteroids
- Hydrocortisone 5–10 mg/kg/day IV/IM in divided doses can be used (rarely) to raise BGL.

Referral to tertiary NICU
- Infants with persistent hypoglycaemia despite treatment:
  - Infants receiving >100 mL/kg/d of >12.5% glucose (>8.75 mg/kg/min glucose)
  - Infants requiring glucagon infusion or corticosteroids

Hyperinsulinism
- Further investigation and treatment is necessary if the glucose requirement is 10 mg/kg/min or greater, as hyperinsulinism is suspected.
- The following tests ('critical hypoglycemia screen') should be performed when TBG <2.6 mmol/L:
  - Blood: BGL, ketones, insulin, growth hormone, cortisol, free fatty acids, lactate, UEC, LFT
- See Chapter 19, Endocrinology for more detailed information and management.

Congenital disorders of the thyroid gland
- Maternal thyroxine (T4) is transferred to the fetus where it is deiodinated to produce liothyronine (T3), which is essential for neurological development. Maternal T3 does not cross the placenta.
- The normal term newborn has a rapid thyroid stimulating hormone (TSH) surge within 30 minutes of birth that stimulates T4 secretion.
- fT4 and fT3 levels peak at 24-36 hours of life; TFTs conducted immediately after birth can be difficult to interpret and screening before 48 hours of age produces a high rate of false positive elevated TSH results.
- Investigation and treatment of neonatal thyroid disease depends upon maternal thyroid status and/or new-born screening test (NST) results (Figure 27.4).

Congenital Hypothyroidism
- Congenital Hypothyroidism (see Chapter 19, Endocrinology for detailed clinical investigation and management) is characterised by decreased thyroid hormone production, and in rare cases *no* thyroid hormones are produced.
- Most common presentation is a raised TSH on NST taken at 48–72 hours (except in secondary or tertiary disease).
- If raised TSH present, early treatment with thyroxine (either long or short term) is usually indicated to avoid neurodevelopmental morbidity.
- Transient disorders of thyroid function are more common than true congenital hypothyroidism, especially in preterm infants.
- Abnormal or difficult to interpret TFT's require specialty endocrinology input.

Congenital Hyperthyroidism
Trans-placental transfer passage of thyroid receptor antibodies (TRab), usually in maternal Graves' disease (and rarely from Hashimoto's thyroiditis) in the third trimester causes stimulation of the fetal thyroid gland.

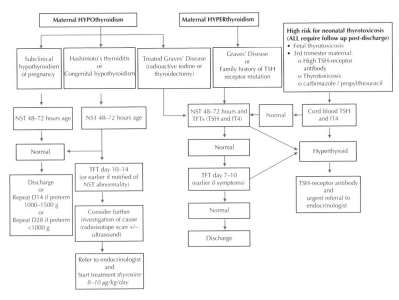

Figure 27.4 Neonatal thyroid disease investigation and management algorithm.

Neonatal thyrotoxicosis is rare, however can be life threatening.
Babies at high risk of neonatal thyrotoxicosis include those with:
- Maternal Graves' disease; AND
  o Elevated TRab in the third trimester
  o Carbimazole / propylthiouracil treatment during the third trimester
  o Antenatal evidence of foetal thyrotoxicosis (advanced bone age, craniosynostosis, hydrops associated with heart failure/tachycardia/arrhythmia, IUGR, preterm, hyperkinesis, goitre)
- Family history of TSH receptor mutation

Presentation
- Clinical features usually present by 10 days of age and include:
  o Irritability, restlessness, jitteriness
  o Exopthalmos
  o Tachycardia, arrhythmia, cardiac failure
  o Increased appetite, diarrhoea, vomiting, weight loss, failure to thrive
  o Advanced skeletal maturation: craniosynostosis, frontal bossing, microcephaly
  o Temperatirue instability, sweating
  o Hepatosplenomegaly, lymphadenopathy, thrombocytopenia
  o Goitre
- The TRab half-life is a few weeks; therefore resolution occurs in three to 12 weeks.

Management
- At risk babies require observation in hospital for at least four days.
- Known maternal Graves' disease:
  o TFTs with the NST 48–72 hours after birth (NST does not report low TSH or measure fT4).
  o Repeat TFT's on days 7–10 of life.
- **Suspected clinical neonatal thyrotoxicosis requires urgent referral to endocrinologist for advice on further investigations and therapy.**
- An approach to babies at high risk for neonatal thyrotoxicosis is illustrated in Figure 27.4.

Neonatal surgical conditions

Clinical Pearl: Red flags for neonatal surgical conditions

- Severe subgaleal haemorrhage is a life-threatening complication of instrumental delivery. Early recognition with appropriate resuscitation is required to prevent death.
- Excessive drooling of frothy secretions from the mouth may suggest oesophageal atresia.
- Bile-stained or green vomiting is always abnormal and requires prompt recognition (malrotation may be present and requires urgent treatment).
- Delayed passage of meconium (beyond 24 hours) is abnormal and may indicate Hirschsprung's disease.
- Inguinoscrotal hernias need urgent attention to avoid strangulation in the neonatal period.

Perioperative Care

Varies depending on the surgical problem but an ABC approach to the newborn infant requiring surgery is required (Table 27.19). Care of neonates with congenital cardiac disease is not outlined her (see Chapter 15, Cardiology).

Table 27.19 Neonatal perioperative care.

	Preoperative Care	Postoperative Care
Airway	• **CDH:** intubate early • **OA/TOF:** Avoid intubation if possible due to risk of gastric rupture with distal TOF, use CPAP with caution as upper pouch may overdistend • **UAO:** Airway adjuncts (NPA, Guedel, LMA) used if infant spontaneously ventilating	• If ETT in situ; CXR post operatively for tube position and lung inflation
Breathing	• Ventilation settings & saturation targets directed by gestation and pathology • **CDH:** low targeted tidal volume where possible (e.g. 4mls/kg)	• ETT often remains in-situ until analgesia and sedation weaned & respiratory drive adequate
Circulation	• Monitor HR, BP, CRT, UO, lactate • Ensure adequate access eg. UVC, PICC, UAC or PAL • Fluid resuscitation: 10ml/kg 0.9% NaCl boluses as required • Inotropes if MBP below targets for gestational age • A **pre-op echocardiogram** may be required if haemodynamically unstable or OA repair (to determine arch position)	• Ensure **normovolemic & normotensive** • Fluid bolus requirements (0.9% NaCl) can exceed 100mls/kg/day in first 48 hours post-op • Albumin, PRBC, platelet, FFP or cryoprecipiate may be indicated
Disability	• Ensure adequate analgesia (validated pain scores eg. mPAT may be used) • May require opiate analgesia +/-benzodiazepine sedation	• Analgesia & sedation weaned as quickly as possible to facilitate extubation • mPAT and NAS guide weaning
Examination	• Thorough examination to assess condition & for (associated) congenital anomalies	• Conclude anomaly screen (USS, x-rays, genetic tests) if required
Fluids	• Maintenance fluid administered (no PN during surgical procedures as line sites are often not visible) • NGT losses replaced ml for ml if > 20mls/kg/day# • **Gastroschisis:** high insensible losses from their exposed bowels requires high fluid replacement requirements. Losses into the silo or wrap added to NGT losses and replaced ml for ml with 0.9% or 0.45% NaCl + 10mmol/500ml KCL#	• Maintenance fluid usually restricted to 70–80 mls/kg/day for 48 hrs to avoid tissue oedema (fluids boluses are used) • Consider need for PN • Introduce feeds in liaison with the surgical team
General	• Pre-op bloods: gas, FBE, Coags, ASBT or Group&hold, UEC (if >24hrs old), LFTs	• Post –Op: gas FBE, Coags, UEC, LFTs. Results guide fluid and blood product requirements.

Head, neck and thorax

Post-haemorrhagic hydrocephalus

Obstruction to CSF flow from the lateral ventricles may occur following intraventricular haemorrhage. This is most common in preterm infants (see preterm infant section below).

- If lateral ventricular dilatation is seen on cranial ultrasound and/or head circumference increasing rapidly, referral to a paediatric neurosurgeon required.
- CSF may be drained via a Rickham's reservoir following insertion into one of the lateral ventricles; if unsuccessful at averting hydrocephalus, a ventriculo-peritoneal shunt will be required.

Oesophageal atresia

Oesophageal atresia (OA) denotes congenital interruption of the oesophagus, most often with an associated tracheo-oesophageal fistula (TOF). The two most common variants (Figure 27.5) are OA with a distal TOF (85%), and pure OA (8%).

- Suspected antenatally due to maternal polyhydramnios, a small/absent fetal stomach, and other anomalies associated with OA (e.g. cardiac lesions).
- Postnatally; excessive drooling, frothing at the mouth, feed intolerance, and/or respiratory distress (due to saliva (or milk) filling up the blind-ending upper oesophageal pouch & spilling into the trachea, and/or gastric contents refluxing through a distal TOF into airway).
- Diagnosis confirmed by failure to pass a 10-French OGT/NGT into stomach; tube arrests 9–11cm from the gums and often coils (normal distance to stomach is 20–25cm).
- A distal TOF is confirmed by x-ray of the chest and abdomen showing gas in the stomach (notably enlarged stomach may indicate preferential ventilation of the stomach through the TOF with risk of gastric perforation).
- Preoperative care: supporting neonate and identifying associated congenital anomalies or syndromes (e.g. trisomy 18, trisomy 13, trisomy 21, CHARGE, VACTERL).
- Echocardiography for major cardiac lesions, especially duct-dependent lesions requiring prostaglandin infusion.
- Intubation and positive pressure ventilation avoided if possible due to the gastric perforation risk.

Surgical management

- OA with a distal TOF (Figure 27.6): TOF ligation & oesophageal anastomosis to re-establish oesophageal continuity (early surgery within 12–24 h of admission).
- Premature infants, and OA cases with long anatomical gap between the upper and lower oesophageal ends ('long gap OA'), each require a staged & more complicated operative approach with prolonged NICU inpatient stay.

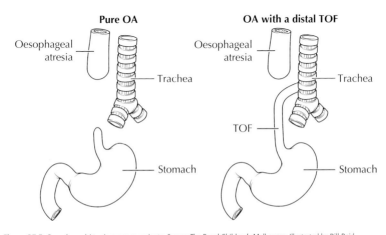

Figure 27.5 Oesophageal Atresia common variants. *Source:* The Royal Children's Melbourne. Illustrated by Bill Reid.

Repair of OA and TOF

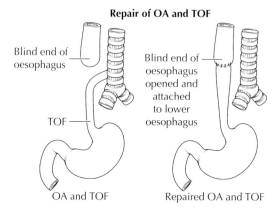

Figure 27.6 Oesophageal atresia with trachea-oesophageal fistula repair. *Source:* The Royal Children's Melbourne. Illustrated by Bill Reid.

- A trans-anastomotic tube (TAT) is passed at surgery to bridge the anastomosis and permit enteral feeding earlier than oral feeding might allow.
- Postoperative contrast study to assess the anastomosis common but not essential.
- Acute surgical complications include: oesophageal anastomotic leak.
- Longer term morbidity includes: oesophageal strictures (may require dilatations), recurrent TOF, gastro-oesophageal reflux, tracheomalacia & oesophageal dysmotility.

Congenital Diaphragmatic Hernia

Congenital diaphragmatic hernia (CDH) occurs in 1 in 5000 live births. The common diaphragmatic defect type is posterolateral (Bochdalek), of which 85% are left-sided, 13% right-sided and 2% bilateral. Anterior (retrosternal, Morgagni) hernial defects are usually asymptomatic but rarely present where strangulation occurs.

- Majority of CDH diagnosed on antenatal ultrasound (+/- MRI).
- Features associated with poorer outcome include earlier gestational age at diagnosis (worse pulmonary hypoplasia), liver in left chest, and reduced lung : head ratio (LHR).
- Further antenatal assessment for associated anomalies (present in 40%, cardiac 20–25%); may have significant implications for prognosis and treatment decision-making.
- Minority diagnosed postnatally, e.g. respiratory distress, scaphoid abdomen (bowel in thorax), heart sounds to the *right* of midline (if *left*-sided defect). Chest x-ray confirms diagnosis.
- Pre-operative CDH care includes:
  - Protecting the hypoplastic lung(s) from iatrogenic injury (intubate early, low pressure / oscillation / JET ventilation)
  - Management of pulmonary hypertension (may require inhaled nitric oxide and/or prostaglandin infusion)
  - Supporting adequate end-organ perfusion
  - NG tube decompression of chest cavity bowel

Surgical management

- CDH repair is not an emergency; undertaken once cardio-respiratory stabilization & optimization achieved (may be several days).
- Reduction of herniated contents & repair of CDH defect (may require synthetic patch if defect is large); operative approach typically open (laparotomy) however thoracoscopic repair possible for select cases.
- Post-operative complications: ipsilateral pneumothorax and later pleural effusion (avoid chest drains if at all possible as can precipitate rapid and dangerous mediastinal shifts).
- Post-operative outcomes: 80–90% survival rates post-surgery are now being achieved; however, poor outcomes persist for those with severe pulmonary hypoplasia and hypertension.

Clinical Controversy: Adjunctive CDH management approaches

The role of extracorporeal membrane oxygenation (ECMO) as an adjunct to medical and surgical management of CDH remains a matter of debate and some controversy. Even more controversial is the role of fetal intervention for CDH; Fetoscopic Endoluminal Tracheal Occlusion (FETO). International clinical trials of FETO are currently ongoing.

Congenital lung lesions

The majority of congenital lung lesions are diagnosed antenatally on ultrasound, and remain asymptomatic at birth. However, these conditions must also be considered as uncommon causes for respiratory distress in the newborn. Chest x-ray and other imaging can aid in diagnosis.

Congenital lobar emphysema (CLE)

CLE describes marked hyperinflation of a pulmonary lobe due to expiratory obstruction and air trapping in the affected lobe. The aetiology of CLE includes idiopathic (50%), intrinsic causes such as deficiency of bronchial cartilage, and extrinsic causes such as compression by thoracic vasculature or cysts. Half of CLE cases show neonatal respiratory distress, especially with feeding.

- Diagnosis is confirmed on:
  - Chest X-ray; increased radiolucency in the affected lobes (most frequently the left upper lobe or right middle lobe).
  - CT chest in selected cases (for aetiology).
  - Echocardiogram; 15–20% have associated cardiac lesions.
- The majority managed non-operatively; but when required operative management is lobectomy.

Pulmonary sequestration

Pulmonary sequestration describes a cystic lung lesion, in which there is non-functioning lung tissue without connection to the normal bronchial tree, and a blood supply which arises from an anomalous systemic artery, typically directly from the aorta. Sequestrations are more commonly left-sided and may be either intralobar or extralobar.

- Can also present postnatally with supra-infection or as incidental finding on chest x-ray.
- Treatment is surgical resection (thoracoscopic or open approach).

Congenital Pulmonary Airway Malformation (CPAM)

CPAM (previously termed 'congenital cystic adenomatous malformation, CCAM) include a range of congenital lesions and lung abnormalities characterised by abnormal bronchiolar tissue with communicating cysts and a relative paucity of cartilage. Many CPAMs are diagnosed antenatally, as a cystic or solid mass ± mediastinal shift and maternal polyhydramnios.

- Clinical presentation variable:
  - Antenatally diagnosed CPAMs may spontaneously regress before birth, but not always.
  - If present at birth; the majority are asymptomatic.
  - Less commonly CPAMs are symptomatic, and may present as neonatal respiratory distress, recurrent LRTI, pneumothorax, or as an incidental finding on chest x-ray.
- CT chest resolves diagnostic uncertainty and aids surgical planning, but is not a routine requirement.

Management

- Preferred management varies between centres.
  - Symptomatic or complicated CPAMs require surgical resection.
  - Asymptomatic, antenatally diagnosed CPAMs: there is disagreement between routine non-operative management with follow-up vs elective resection.

Clinical Controversy: CPAMs and risk of malignant transformation

A key argument for routine elective resection is the assertion that CPAMs have important malignant potential. This is controversial, with debate over whether the small number of documented malignancies reflect uncommon malignant transformation in a pre-existing CPAM (supporting routine elective resection) vs. whether primarily malignant lesions such as primary pulmonary blastoma (PPB) may uncommonly masquerade as a CPAM when initially identified (supporting routine non-operative management with follow-up). Currently, most antenatally-diagnosed asymptomatic CPAMs are managed at RCH with non-operative management and follow-up.

Abdomen and pelvis

Abdominal wall defects

Gastroschisis and exomphalos are abdominal wall defects that place the child at risk of heat and water loss from the exposed surface of the sac (exomphalos) or bowel (gastroschisis).

- The newborn should be kept warm (radiant warmer / incubator).
- The abdomen should be covered in Glad Wrap immediately (in delivery room).
- Care taken to ensure exposed bowel is not twisted and its blood supply is not compromised.
- Gastrointestinal decompression with a nasogastric tube, and IV fluid management commenced (Table 27.19) whilst transfer to a tertiary surgical centre is undertaken.

Midgut malrotation with volvulus

Normal midgut rotation and fixation achieves a stable and wide-based small bowel mesentery between the fixed points of the duodeno-jejunal (DJ) flexure (epigastrium to left of midline) and ileo-caecal junction (right iliac fossa). Midgut malrotation results in a small bowel mesentery which is is narrowed, with risk of midgut volvulus.

- Midgut volvulus occurs when the unfixed midgut twists around the narrow small bowel mesentery compromising the superior mesenteric vessels.
- A 360° twist may cause venous and lymphatic engorgement with bile-stained vomiting; emergency laparotomy at this point should have a good outcome.
- A 720° twist may result in arterial ischaemia of the entire midgut (duodenum to the mid transverse colon) which is potentially fatal.
- **The typical presentation** is of bile-stained vomiting (green) in a full-term baby that has been well prior.
- **Early presentation:** abdomen is typically soft and non-distended.
  Innocuous abdominal signs must not discourage urgency in proceeding to diagnostic upper GI contrast study.
  - Contrast study confirms an abnormal position of the DJ junction, and sometimes spiraling of contrast through the twisted bowel.
- **Later presentation:** may include abdominal distension, tenderness, and passage of blood per rectum. *These features indicate major gut ischaemia, which necessitates urgent laparotomy (without delay for radiology).*
- Preoperative care: NGT insertion, fluid resuscitation, intravenous antibiotics to cover intra-abdominal sepsis, and preparation for laparaotomy.

Surgical management

- Emergency laparotomy to avoid ischaemia leading to loss of the midgut.
- Surgical goals: confirm the diagnosis, devolve the midgut (usually untwisted anti-clockwise), and broaden the midgut mesentery to achieve a position which is no longer prone to twisting ('Ladd's procedure).
- If extensive midgut ischaemia and gangrene present, critical loss of bowel length may result.
- Post-operative complications: chylous ascites, abdominal sepsis.
- Longer term morbidity: short bowel syndrome with nutritional challenges (if extensive bowel loss; see Chapter 10, Nutrition), recurrent volvulus (rare), complications from adhesions.

Duodenal Atresia

Duodenal atresia (DA) occurs in 1 in 5000 live births. The aetiology of DA is unknown, and may be genetic. DA encompasses of spectrum of obstruction ranging from complete luminal discontinuity, incomplete luminal obstruction (allowing some passage of bowel contents), and rarely duodenal stenosis (rather than atresia).

- DA is diagnosed antenatally in 60%, antenatal ultrasound shows polyhydramnios and/or 'double bubble' (dilated stomach + dilated proximal duodenum), +/- supporting features of trisomy 21.
- Postnatally, abdominal x-ray showing a gas-filled 'double bubble' can be diagnostic.

- The neonate has feed intolerance with typically green (bile-stained) vomiting given the obstruction is distal to the ampulla of Vater in 80%.
- Phenotypic features of trisomy 21 are supportive of a DA diagnosis.
- Upper GI contrast study is recommended (if diagnostic uncertainty).
- Late-presenting DA is rare, but recognized (e.g. incomplete obstruction) in infants / young children.
- Pre-operative DA care: identification of clinically important associated conditions, e.g. trisomy 21 (20%) and congenital cardiac lesions (40%).

Surgical Management
- DA surgery is not an emergency; usually undertaken in the first week of life.
- Surgical goal: to restore continuity of the duodenum (open approach in majority); usually duodeno-duodenostomy, duodenoplasty or duodeno-jejunostomy; the anastomosis type varies with DA morphology and surgeon preference.
  - A secondary goal is to assess for associated abdominal anomalies (e.g. midgut malrotation) that can be corrected intra-operatively.
- Post-operative complications: rare; anastomotic complications are uncommon.
- Post-operative care is principally supportive (e.g. ventilatory support, analgesia, PN) whilst awaiting recovery from laparotomy, return of gut function and feed tolerance.
- Mortality approximately 10%; poor prognostic factors include serious associated anomalies and/or syndromes, low birth weight and prematurity.

Necrotising enterocolitis
Necrotising enterocolitis is the commonest gastrointestinal emergency in preterm infants with most cases (>85%) occurring in infants born before 28 weeks post-menstrual age, typically between days 14–21 of life. The pathophysiology is multifactorial and includes mucosal injury, poor perfusion and bacterial translocation.
- Medical management is bowel rest for 7–10 days, antibiotics cover for GIT and anaerobic organisms, intravenous nutrition and nasogastric tube drainage.
- Surgical management is required for failure of medical treatment and/or intestinal perforation.
- Laparotomy preferable; allows necrotic bowel to be resected and an anastomosis or stoma to be formed; however, insertion of a Penrose Drain as a temporary measure (to decompress the abdomen if compromised) may be required.
- NEC incidence & severity is reduced by feeding extremely preterm infants with exclusive breast milk and by administering a safe, multi-strain probiotic combination until at least 34 weeks PMA.

Inguinal Hernia
See Chapter 41, Surgery.

Ambiguous genitalia
Genitalia that are frankly ambiguous need urgent consultation with an experienced paediatric endocrinologist or surgeon on the first day of life (see Chapter 19, Endocrinology).
- An enlarged clitoris in an apparent female is also abnormal and needs immediate referral.
- Hypospadias may overlap with ambiguous genitalia. This needs a careful initial assessment; if the diagnosis of hypospadias has been made, someone has already assumed the gender is male.
- *If one or both testes are undescended, or the scrotum is bifid, or both, the baby should be treated as having ambiguous genitalia until proven otherwise with immediate referral for further investigation.*

Sacrococcygeal Teratoma
Any lump over the coccyx of a baby should be assumed to be a teratoma until proven otherwise (see newborn examination section above). This needs appropriate imaging (US or MRI) and immediate referral at birth to a tertiary centre for neurosurgical review.

The preterm infant

- Definitions:
Extremely preterm (EP): An infant born before 28 weeks of completed gestation.
Very preterm (VP): An infant born between 28 and 31+6 weeks of completed gestation.
Moderate preterm (MP): An infant born between 32 and 33+6 weeks of completed gestation.
Late preterm (LP): An infant born between 34 and 36+6 weeks of completed gestation.
- Preterm infant survival has improved dramatically over the past three decades in developed countries since the introduction of routine antenatal steroid and surfactant administration.
- Several countries are now offering active resuscitation for infants born from 22 weeks completed gestation.
- Despite improved survival, neurodevelopmental disability is an ongoing long-term consequence. It is worth noting however, that adults who were born EP rate their own quality of life highly.
- When counselling prospective parents in circumstances where EP birth is probable or imminent, it is essential to provide easy to understand, up-to-date information on local outcome data for preterm infants.

Strategies to optimise outcomes for preterm infants
- Obstetric factors include:
  - Delaying birth for as long as safely possible using tocolysis, vaginal progesterone and cervical cerclage.
  - Maternal corticosteroids (repeated doses if birth does not occur within seven days).
  - Maternal magnesium sulphate for foetal neuroprotection.
  - Maternal antibiotics in the setting of maternal chorioamnionitis.
- Ensure every effort is made for preterm infants to be delivered in tertiary centres with access to appropriately skilled staff, equipment for resuscitation, and capacity for ongoing neonatal intensive care.
- If infants are outborn, the local retrieval team should be contacted as soon as possible, even before birth if delivery is imminent.
- A clear, well-documented and practised team approach to newborn resuscitation and stabilisation to ensure appropriate systems-based management occurs in a timely and efficient manner.

Clinical Pearl: 'The Golden Hour'
The early stages following birth are often referred to as "The Golden Hour" to emphasise the need for rapid institution of therapies either in the delivery room or the NICU to optimise outcomes. These include but are not limited to:
- Maintaining normothermia.
- Commencing appropriate respiratory support.
- Obtaining IV access and commencing glucose infusion.
- Administering medications such as Vitamin K, antibiotics, caffeine or surfactant as indicated.
- Undertaking investigations, such as blood tests and CXR to guide further management.

Morbidity associated with preterm birth:
- All infants born before 37 weeks completed gestation have increased risk of both short-term (infection, poor feeding, hypoglycaemia) and long-term (neurodevelopmental impairment) complications when compared to term-born infants (Table 27.20).
- Complications of prematurity typically occur at a higher incidence and with greater severity in those born at lower gestational age ranges, particularly before 28 weeks completed gestation.
- Routine screening for complications should be undertaken; check you local guidelines for details.

Clinical Pearl: The late preterm infant
Acknowledgement of the risk of long term neurodevelopmental impairment in late preterm infants is essential to ensure ongoing developmental surveillance is undertaken in this group. Moderate to late preterm infants account for approximately 70% of all preterm births, and as such any small increase in neurodevelopmental morbidity within this cohort has the potential to place a significant burden on health resources. Increased vigilance and ongoing surveillance is recommended so these infants are not merely treated as 'small' term babies.

Table 27.20 Common morbidities associated with preterm birth.

System	Morbidities	Comments
Neurological	• Intraventricular haemorrhage • Post-haemorrhagic hydrocephalus • Cystic/Periventricular leukomalacia • White matter injury/loss • Cerebral palsy • Impaired cognitive & executive functions • Retinopathy of prematurity (ROP) • Sensorineural hearing loss	• Routine Cranial Ultrasound scans at regular intervals as per local guidelines • Neurodevelopmentally-appropriate care (e.g. clustering of handling episodes, limiting exposure to extreme sound or light) should be provided • ROP screening as per local guidelines to ensure laser therapy treatment and/or intravitreal monoclonal antibody injections administered to avoid blindness • Routine Audiology assessments in addition to the NBHS are recommended for all high-risk infants
Cardiovascular	• Anaemia of prematurity • Thrombocytopaenia • Patent Ductus Arteriosus (PDA) • Hypotension (1st week)	• Delayed cord clamping reduces requirement for blood transfusions • Iron supplementation for exclusively breastfed infants • Age, gestation (and respiratory support) based guidelines provide transfusion thresholds for PRBC and Plts; higher thresholds associate with reduced adverse effects • Echocardiography recommended for PDA surveillance for EP infants • PDA can be treated with indomethacin, ibuprofen, paracetamol or surgical ligation • Hypotension is typically treated with 10ml/kg 0.9% NaCl boluses x 2 before considering inotropes or blood.
Respiratory	• Apnoea of prematurity • Respiratory Distress Syndrome / Hyaline Membrane Disease • Pulmonary Interstitial Emphysema • Bronchopulmonary Dysplasia Chronic Lung Disease	• Caffeine for all infants born < 32 weeks to prophylactically treat apnoea of prematurity. Initial loading dose + daily maintenance dosing until cessation at 34 weeks. • Exogenous surfactant administered for RDS/HMD via ETT or under direct laryngoscopy. Given as soon as practical after birth but may be helpful up to 72 hours of age. • Targeted tidal volume ventilation strategies recommended to avoid barotrauma. (volutrauma and atelectotrauma also injurious to preterm lungs). • Antenatal steroids reduce the incidence and severity of preterm lung disease • Non-invasive respiratory support modes (nCPAP or HFNC) preferable to mechanical ventilation where possible • Postnatal steroid treatment after the 1st week of life reduces CLD. Adverse effects include hyperglycaemia, hypertension, hypertrophic cardiomyopathy (rare) & severe ROP. Long-term neurodevelopmental effects are not significantly increased by late treatment.
Gastrointestinal	• Intestinal perforation • Necrotising enterocolitis (NEC) • Feed intolerance • Growth impairment	• Human milk reduces the risk of gastrointestinal disease • Perforation risk increased by ibuprofen, indomethacin & corticosteroids (in 1st week of life) • Probiotics reduce NEC by approximately 50% if after feeds commenced until 34 weeks. • Grading feeds up by 30mls/kg/day is safe and does not increase the risk of NEC
Genitourinary	• Inguinal hernia	• Common; repair is usually deferred until term-corrected age. • If discharged prior, parents should present to hospital urgently if signs of strangulation

(continued)

Table 27.20 (*Continued*)

System	Morbidities	Comments
Infectious Diseases	Particular considerations for preterm infants: • CONS • Fungal infection • CMV • RSV (other respiratory tract viruses)	• Far greater risk of infection than term counterparts due to their immature immune system, prolonged hospitalisation and requirement for access lines • Prophylactic anti-fungal agents eg. nystatin as per local guidelines • Thrombocytopaenia may be a sign of CMV or fungal infection • More likely to require hospitalisation & respiratory support due to respiratory tract viral infections. Palivizumab (RSV-specific monoclonal antibody) for high-risk infants <12m as per local guidelines • Vaccinations: see Chapter 9, Immunisation for additional recommended vaccinations for preterm infants
Endocrine	• Hypo/hyperglycaemia • Bone disease of prematurity	• Monitor BGL to assess glucose requirements until PN or feeds established. • Hyperglycaemia with glycosuria common in 1st week of life for EP infants but often resolves spontaneously • Osteopaenia & fractures may occur if Ca, Vit D & PO4 intake insufficient. Supplement micronutrients until 36 weeks as per local guidelines
Metabolic	• Acidosis (1st week of life)	• Usually resolves over the first few days of life in response to routine fluid administration
Skin	• Fragile • Increased insensible fluids losses	• Transcutaneous probes (e.g. ECG leads or C02 estimation) should be closely monitored • Nurse in humidification and temperature-controlled isolettes until skin matures
Psychosocial	• Adverse effects on infant & parental mental health	• Parents of preterm infants are at increased risk of anxiety, depression and post-traumatic stress disorder • Programs facilitating parental engagement & attachment after birth (eg. delivery room cuddles, regular skin-to-skin/kangaroo care sessions, FiCare™) reduce adverse parental effects

USEFUL RESOURCES

• RCH Clinical practice guidelines: http://www.rch.org.au/clinicalguide/; multiple neonatal medicine focussed clinical practice guidelines.
• Neonatal e-handbook, c/o Safer Care Victoria website: https://www.bettersafercare.vic.gov.au/resources/clinical-guidance/maternity-and-newborn; clinical information & guidelines on specific common neonatal presentations.
• ANZCOR (Australian and New Zealand Committee on Resuscitation) Guidelines: https://resus.org.au/guidelines/anzcor-guidelines/; up to date neonatal (and paediatric) resuscitation guidelines and treatment algorithms.
• American academy of Paediatrics *Bilitool*: http://www.bilitool.org; online calculator for assessment & thresholds for jaundice treatment.
• Australian breastfeeding assessment website: http://www.breastfeeding.asn.au; patient breastfeeding information and resources.

CHAPTER 28

Neurodevelopment and disability

Daryl Efron
Gehan Roberts
Lynne Harrison
Gordon Baikie
Giuliana Antolovich
Deborah Marks
Catherine Marraffa

Key Points
- Persistent language delay not explained by another diagnosis or inadequate learning opportunities can be described as a Developmental Language Disorder.
- Learning difficulties are experienced by many children, may have a range of causes, and are usually responsive to educational interventions. Specific learning disabilities are lifelong conditions characterised by persistent, unexpected poor performance in an area of learning.
- The most effective treatment for children with ADHD is psychostimulant medication.
- Autism Spectrum Disorder (ASD) causes difficulties in social communication and repetitive and restricted behaviour and interests. Behavioural support, specialised educational strategies and manipulation of the environment provides the best chance for a child to achieve their full potential. Medication has a role in treating the associated (not core) symptoms of ASD.
- Cerebral palsy (CP) is a clinical descriptor only. An aetiological work-up is essential and should include an MRI brain, testing for genetic causes and consideration of metabolic conditions. A history of regression is a red flag for an alternative diagnosis.

Normal childhood development and developmental delay
Healthy early childhood development sets the stage for meeting future educational, social and economic goals. Positive developmental progress is a product of a complex interplay between genetic potential and environmental nurturing and stimulation.

Putting the Science into Practice: The first 1000 days
The earliest stages of development, from conception to the end of the 2nd year of life is also known as the First 1000 days. This period is so important for future health and development that it has been subject to a growing focus by scientists, early year educators and governments.

Developmental Monitoring and Surveillance is a flexible, continuous process of skills observation and periodic screening that is built into routine well-child care. It is designed to identify deviations from normal and expected developmental trajectories, across a range of developmental domains in early childhood (fine and gross motor, language, social/emotional and cognitive). Children who screen positive should be referred for

---

Paediatric Handbook, Tenth Edition. Edited by Kate Harding, Daniel S. Mason and Daryl Efron.
© 2021 John Wiley & Sons Ltd. Published 2021 by John Wiley & Sons Ltd.

further investigations, formal developmental assessment and early intervention. Monitoring and surveillance is usually carried out by primary care providers such as general practitioner/family doctor and maternal child health (MCH) nurses (or local area equivalent). Parental concern about development should always be respected and followed up; however a lack of parental concern is no guarantee that the child does not have a developmental problem.

Developmental Surveillance Example: MCH Nurses in Victoria, Australia

The MCH Nurses in Victoria provide a free, universal health and development surveillance system for children age 0 – 5, called the 'Key Ages and Stages'. During the 10 visits, the nurses carry out a two stage screening process. The parent or carer is asked to complete a screening questionnaire called the Parents' Evaluation of Developmental Status (PEDS). Children who score positive are then screened using the Brigance Inventory of Early Development. Children who screen positive for developmental concerns are referred for further assessment and intervention.

- **Developmental delay** is the term used when a child is slower than expected to develop skills in any developmental domain, and is seen in up to 20% of children. This can be quantified using a standardised developmental assessment tool such as the Bayley Scales of Infant Development.
  - The most common delay in early childhood is in language development.
- **Global developmental delay** (GDD) is defined as a significant delay in 2 or more developmental domains (for example language and social/emotional skills); this is much less common, affecting 2–3% of children. Many children with GDD are later diagnosed with an Intellectual Disability (see section below) or other more specific diagnosis.
- The role of the primary care doctor is to identify potential developmental delay, encourage activities and a lifestyle that promotes optimal development (e.g. socialisation, group childcare, appropriate stimulation, a language rich environment, good nutrition, optimisation of sleep and general health), and to have a low threshold to refer on for further assessment when indicated.
- The role of the paediatrician is to investigate for an underlying cause, organise formal assessment(s), monitor developmental progress and response to intervention, and advocate for family and educational supports.

Language delay and developmental language Disorder

- A child acquiring language milestones later than expected (Table 28.1), is described as having a language delay.
- A persistent language delay, not explained by another diagnosis and occurring despite adequate language-learning opportunities can be described as a Developmental Language Disorder (DLD. *Previously called Specific Language Impairment.*)
- DLD can include difficulties with language understanding/comprehension (receptive) and/or language production (expressive) and these difficulties impact on their everyday life.
- DLD can also include difficulties with pragmatic language skills (social use of language).
- Articulation/phonological problems may also occur, resulting in reduced speech intelligibility.
- DLD can occur in isolation, or as part of another disorder (eg autism spectrum disorder).

Prevalence

- 20% of 2-year olds (<50 words and few or no word combinations)
  - 30% of this group is still delayed at 4 years.
- DLD prevalence at school entry is between 5–20%, and this can have a profound impact on educational achievement.

Preschool children with persistent speech and language disorders tend to have:

- Learning and social difficulties at school.
- Increased risk for later literacy and numeracy problems.
- Increased rate of emotional and behavioural disorders which may persist into adolescence and adulthood and affect employment opportunities.

Factors raising concern about speech and language

- Parental concern regarding speech and language development.
- History or risk factors for hearing loss.

Table 28.1 Language delay red flags.

6 months	• No response to sound. • No cooing, laughing or vocalising.
12 months	• Not localising to sound or vocalising. • No babbling or babbling contains a low proportion of consonant vowel babble (e.g. baba). • Doesn't understand simple words (e.g. 'no', 'bye'), recognise names of common objects or respond to simple requests (e.g. clap hands) with an action. • Doesn't respond reliably to name by turning head.
18 months	• No meaningful words except 'mum/dad'. • Doesn't understand and hand over objects on request.
2 years	• Expressive vocabulary <50 words and no word combinations. • Cannot find 2–3 objects on request.
3 years	• Speech not understood by the family. • Not using simple grammatical structures (e.g. -ing ending on verbs). • Doesn't understand concepts such as colour and size.
4 years	• Speech not understood outside the family. • Not using complex sentences (4–6 words). • Unable to construct simple stories.
5 years	• Speech not intelligible. • Doesn't understand abstract words and ideas. • Can't reconstruct a story from a book.

- Delay in both receptive and expressive language skills.
- Delay in language *and* other developmental domains.
- Autistic features. (see autism spectrum disorder section below).
- Developmental plateau or regression.

Bilingualism
- The process of learning to speak a second language does not exacerbate a language disorder.
- Bilingual children with language delay need to be assessed across all spoken languages and should be encouraged to develop proficiency in their home language (this improves language outcomes in the medium to long term).

Clinical Pearl: Practical tips for language assessment in the consultation room
Language development is best assessed through play in addition to clinical history; try to utilise both parental report and direct observation of the child during the consultation. Toys such as tea-sets, picture books bubbles and animal figurines are helpful to make observations about how the child is expressing themselves and responding to the language interactions of others.

Management of language delay
- Assess other areas of the child's development (fine motor, gross motor, social) to determine isolated language delay vs global developmental delay.
- Audiology assessment to exclude hearing loss.
- Speech pathology referral as early as possible.
- Encourage a 'language rich environment' (engaging the child verbally, talking out loud, reading books etc).
- Where regression in language is suspected, or there are broader developmental concerns, refer to a paediatrician.

Speech disorder
- A Speech Disorder refers to difficulty with production of sound and sound units for speech.
- Usually a preschool child should be understood by people outside of the family ~ 75% of the time.

- Speech disorders can be caused by cognitive, linguistic, motor or structural issues and referral to a speech pathologist is important to determine the degree and nature of the problem and the most appropriate treatment approach.

Clinical Controversy: Tongue tie (Ankyloglossia)

With an increase in the number of professionals performing tongue tie surgery, the presence and impact of tongue tie (ankyloglossia) has become increasingly debated. There is no strong evidence to indicate that a tongue tie release improves a child's speech or prevents future speech problems, and the procedure is not without risk of complications. However, some parents and practitioners still support this intervention being undertaken. Providing clear and accurate information so that parents are fully informed about the evidence for the procedure, and the potential risk of procedure complications is essential.

Stuttering
- Stuttering is a disorder that affects the fluency of speech production.
- Stuttering behaviours can include repeated speech movements (repetitions), fixed postures, which include stretching out a sound in a word (prolongations), or not being able to produce any sound (blocks).
- 12% of children will stutter at some point up to 4 years of age.
  - ○ Majority of children will recover eventually.
  - ○ However, it is not possible to predict which children will recover.
- Strong genetic component; 50–75% have at least one relative with childhood stuttering.
- Cause unknown, but research suggests the onset is not associated with anxiety, stress or personality factors.
- Current best practice recommends waiting for up to 12 months before commencing treatment; however, if significant distress/impact, parental concern or the child becomes reluctant to communicate then referral to speech pathologist indicated.

Management
- Treatment of preschool children who stutter should be undertaken by speech pathologists trained in the Lidcombe Program (behavioural treatment programme for <6 year olds with stuttering), which has the best evidence for improved outcomes in this age group.
- Stuttering is more difficult to treat in older children so early referral for treatment is important.

Learning Difficulties & Learning Disabilities
About 20% of children will struggle to learn the foundation skills of literacy and numeracy in the early years of school. Without early identification and appropriate remediation, these difficulties are likely to persist over time and result in poor long-term outcomes such as school refusal, mood or behavioural difficulties and loss of confidence and self-esteem.

- Children experience **learning difficulties** due to a variety of underlying causes (e.g. chronic ill health, sensory difficulties, underlying mood or behavioural disorders, English as an additional language (EAL), or psycho-social stress).
- A **specific learning disability** is present in a minority of children (approximately 5%), and is best understood as persistent and unexpected underachievement in a specific area of learning, due to underlying neurodevelopmental differences, resulting from a complex interplay of genetic, cognitive and environmental factors.
- Children with **learning difficulties** are likely to close the gap with same-age peers if the underlying cause can be addressed and short-term remediation is provided.
- In contrast, for children with a **specific learning disability** the gap in educational achievement between the individual and their peers is likely to widen over time. These children are likely to make progress according to their own trajectory and, in the long-term should aim to fulfil their own personal academic/educational potential. To achieve this they will require:
  - ○ Consistent long-term classroom accommodations
  - ○ Ongoing remediation
  - ○ Measures to maintain their engagement and self-esteem

Table 28.2 DSM-5 criteria for specific learning disabilities.

Criterion	Description
A	Ongoing difficulty learning and using at least one academic skill (e.g. reading; spelling; writing; number facts). Difficulties persisted and failed to improve despite the provision of targeted, evidence-based intervention for at least six months.
B	The difficulties experienced by the individual are assessed using standardised achievement tests[a] and found to be at a level significantly lower than most individuals of the same age.
C	The difficulties experienced by the individual usually become apparent in the early years of schooling. The exception to this is where problems occur in upper-primary or secondary school once the demands on student performance increase significantly.
D	No other plausible explanation for the difficulties (e.g. intellectual disability(ID)[b]; sensory impairment; school absence/ inadequate teaching; ESL; psychosocial deprivation).

Source: Adapted from 'Understanding Learning Difficulties; a Guide for Parents. Revised Edition. AUSPELD. 2018.
[a] e.g. the Wechsler Individual Achievement Test (WIAT).
[b] A cognitive assessment (e.g. Wechsler Intelligence Scale for Children (WISC)) should be carried out together with the academic assessment in order to rule out an ID and identify the child's cognitive strengths and vulnerabilities.

- A **specific learning disability** can be diagnosed if all four of the criteria (Table 28.2) are met. The level of functional impairment caused by the learning disability relates to the degree to which the child struggles to perform compared with their peers and the amount of support required to enable the child to fully participate at school.
- The role of the primary care doctor and paediatrician is to assess the child for, and treat, underlying or co-morbid conditions (e.g. ADHD), carry out necessary medical investigations, monitor for emerging secondary issues such as a mood disorder, and advocate for school-based assessments and supports (such as an Individual Learning Plan and extra remediation).

Intellectual Disability

About 2% of children have an Intellectual Disability (ID). This is a statistical definition, based upon:

1. A Full Scale IQ score that is significantly below age expectations (<2 SD below the mean, or a score below 70, on a standardised test such as the Wechsler Intelligence Scale for Children (WISC), which has a population mean of 100, and a SD of 15), together with;
2. Significant impairment in functional or adaptive skills (<2 SD below the mean, or a score below 70, measured using a parent or teacher completed questionnaire such as the Vineland Adaptive Behaviour Scale (VABS)).

- Children with an ID usually have a history of globally delayed development during early childhood. Standardised testing should be carried out around the time of starting school, in order to better inform school supports and applications for support funding.
- ID can be described as mild, moderate, severe or profound, with each category defined by the number of SDs below the mean (i.e. mild ID= IQ score 55–70, between 2 and 3 SD below the mean of 100. This descriptor has some significance in predicting future functional capacity (eg. ability to live independently, and to work independently etc.)
- The more severe the ID, the more likely it is that investigations will reveal an underlying cause. Genetic tests (chromosome microarray and Fragile X testing) are the mainstay of investigations (approximately 15% yield), with metabolic and neurological testing depending on clinical indications.
- For non-syndromic ID, microarray has an approximately 10% likelihood of identifying a pathogenic copy number variant (deletion or duplication) that contributes to the risk. Whole exome sequencing will increase that yield to approximately 40–50%, and will likely be available to paediatricians in the near future.
- The role of the primary care doctor and paediatrician is to investigate for an underlying cause, assess the child for, and treat, underlying or co-morbid conditions (e.g. mood disorder), monitor for emerging or associated issues such as seizures, sensory deficit or pain syndromes, and advocate for school and community-based supports.

Tics/Tourette's disorder

Tics are sudden, rapid, involuntary, stereotypical movements (motor tic) or vocalisations (vocal tic) which occur repeatedly. They occur in up to 25% of children and affect boys approximately four times more frequently than girls. Onset is typically in the preschool or early primary school years. Most cases are transient, but some run a chronic course. Tics are substantially more common in children with neurodevelopment disorders such as attention deficit hyperactivity disorder (ADHD) and autism spectrum disorder.

DSM-5 criteria for **Tourette disorder (TD)** are two or more motor tics and at least one vocal tic occurring many times a day nearly every day for longer than a year, with onset <18 years of age. Prevalence estimates vary from 0.1% to 1%.

- Simple motor tics: these are the commonest type, where one muscle group twitches repeatedly, for example eye blinking, facial grimacing or limb jerking.
- Complex motor tics: involve sequences of coordinated stereotypic movement involving multiple muscle groups or limbs, sometimes recruiting the whole body, such as arm straightening, tapping, body gyrations, obscene gestures or bizarre gait.
- Tics occasionally become 'linked' such that one tic leads rapidly to another and then another, in a repertoire unique to the individual.
- Vocal tics are also common, including sniffing, throat clearing and various vocalisations. These are often misdiagnosed as medical problems such as allergies or upper respiratory infections.
- Complex vocal tics are less common. These may involve echolalia, coprolalia, or repeating certain phrases.
- Children with tics commonly have associated problems, including ADHD, anxiety disorders, OCD and learning disorders. These conditions are often more functionally impairing than the tics, and thus should be managed accordingly.

Clinical Pearl: Identifying tics

Tics are preceded by a premonitory urge, which is relieved transiently by the expression of the tic. Patients usually have some degree of voluntary control over the tics, such that they can suppress them for minutes to hours, at the cost of a build-up of tension. Typically, there are periods in which tics are hardly noticed (e.g. during school) followed by briefer periods of intense tic activity (e.g. after school). They tend to be less severe when the child is engaged in a task requiring concentration. Tics are often suggestible – talking about them can bring them on. Some children allocate great effort to camouflage tics, which can be distracting.

- The nature of the tics usually shifts over time, with one tic or repertoire of tics being replaced by another.
- The natural history of tics is to:
  - Wax and wane over years
  - Decrease in adolescence (some cases can persist into adulthood, usually at a milder severity)
  - Be more severe with stress, sleep deprivation and over-excitement. More severe periods may be associated with a clear environmental trigger e.g. new school year, though often no such trigger is able to be identified.

Management

- Most children with tics do not need any specific treatment; education about the condition and natural history is usually helpful.
- In severe cases tics can cause embarrassment and social exclusion, emotional disturbance and functional interference. These cases warrant intervention.
- Behavioural management: program called Comprehensive Behavioral Intervention for Tics (CBIT) has best evidence. Involves training the individual to recognise the premonitory urge, and to generate responses which are incompatible with the tic (habit reversal training), and/or increase their tolerance to the urge.
- Pharmacological management: medications can reduce the frequency of tics; however, effect sizes are generally small over and above the natural fluctuation in severity (Table 14.8 Psychotropic medications for children and adolescents, Chapter 14, Behaviour and mental health).
  - Alpha-2 adrenergic agonists clonidine or guanfacine first line (may cause sedation).
  - Antipsychotics, particularly haloperidol, risperidone and olanzapine are the most effective (significant side effect profile including acute dystonic reactions, sedation and weight gain).

○ Other medications with some anti-tic activity include clonazepam, topiramate and tetrabenazine.
○ Selective serotonin re-uptake inhibitors eg. fluoxetine or sertraline maybe helpful for comorbid OCD or anxiety, and may indirectly result in tic reduction.
○ Botulinum toxin injections can be effective for disabling focal motor tics.

Attention deficit hyperactivity disorder (ADHD)

ADHD is the most common neurodevelopmental disorder in childhood, with a prevalence of approximately 3–5%. It is highly heritable and approximately twice as common in boys than girls. The core features are impulsivity and inattention (Table 28.3). Younger children with ADHD often exhibit motor hyperactivity. Diagnosis is less reliable before school entry because of variation in normal development. Common associated problems include oppositional defiant disorder, anxiety disorders, learning disorders, autism spectrum disorder and tics. Risk factors include family history, prematurity, very low birth weight, in-utero exposure to neurotoxins such as alcohol, and environmental deprivation in infancy.

Assessment

- History: Early development, academic progress, social skills and the family context need to be explored. The timing and nature of initial concerns along with secondary effects such as depression, low self-esteem and social ostracism should be noted. It is important to identify the child's strengths as well as their weaknesses.
- Behaviour rating scales (e.g. Vanderbilt diagnostic scales or Child behavior checklists) completed by parents and teachers are an efficient way to gather information across settings.
- Exacerbating factors such as sleep deprivation or nutritional deficiencies should be identified and managed.
- Physical examination: A detailed examination should be performed to exclude medical conditions or genetic syndromes. Inviting the child to read some text and sampling handwriting may provide valuable information regarding literacy competence.

Table 28.3 DSM-5 diagnostic criteria for attention deficit hyperactivity disorder.

A persistent pattern of inattention and/or hyperactivity-impulsivity that is inconsistent with developmental level and that negatively impacts on social and academic functioning, as characterized by (1) and/or (2)
1. **Inattention:** At least six or more of the following symptoms have persisted for at least 6 months. • Often fails to give close attention to details or makes careless mistakes in schoolwork, at work or during other activities • Often has difficulty sustaining attention in tasks or play activities • Often does not seem to listen when spoken to directly • Often does not follow through on instructions and fails to finish schoolwork chores or duties in the workplace • Often has difficulty organising tasks and activities • Often avoids or dislikes tasks that require sustained mental effort • Often loses things necessary for tasks or activities • Is often easily distracted by extraneous stimuli • Is often forgetful in daily activities
2. **Hyperactivity/impulsivity:** Six of the following symptoms have persisted for at least 6 months • Often fidgets with or taps hands or feet and squirms in seat • Often leaves seat situations in which remaining seated is expected • Often runs about or climbs excessively in situations where it is inappropriate • Often has difficulty playing or engaging in leisure activities quietly • Is often 'on the go' and acts as if 'driven by a motor' • Often talks excessively • Often blurts out answers to questions before the questions have been completed • Often has difficulty awaiting his or her turn • Often interrupts or intrudes on others
Symptoms must have been noted prior to age 12 years, be present in two or more settings (e.g. home and school), and not be better accounted for by another mental disorder (e.g. mood disorder, anxiety disorder, personality disorder)

- Psychoeducational assessment: Children with significant learning difficulties should be referred to an educational psychologist for a formal assessment to identify their learning strengths and weaknesses. This can be arranged through the school or privately.
- Hearing should be tested with formal audiology. Other investigations are not helpful unless there are clinical indications.

Management

- A multimodal strategy is usually required. The child and family need sustained support over many years. This requires the doctor to work in collaboration with other health, educational and community professionals.
- Most children with ADHD have one or more comorbidities. These often need to be managed alongside the ADHD.
- Behaviour modifications include:
  - Behavioural modification methods (see chapter 14 Behaviour and Mental health) are generally helpful.
  - Parents and teachers need to apply structured behaviour modification strategies as calmly and consistently as possible. Good communication between home and school is important.
- Educational strategies include:
  - An individualised learning plan.
  - Classroom adaptations; including seating the child at the front of the classroom near a good role model, minimising distractions, and using written lists and other visual prompts.
  - Clear rules and predictable routines.
  - Positive reinforcement provided for acceptable behaviour.
  - As much 1:1 adult supervision as possible is helpful for children with ADHD to ensure they have understood instructions and to provide reminders to complete tasks.

Medication

- Psychostimulant medication is the single most effective intervention for children with ADHD:
  - Provides effective symptom reduction in about 80% of cases.
  - Secondary benefits including improved peer status, family functioning and self-esteem accrue over time.
  - Side effects include: appetite suppression (most common), increased anxiety and tics, irritability or subdued personality (less common). Side effects resolve when the medication is stopped.
  - Weight, height and blood pressure should be monitored.
  - Stimulant medications are not addictive in the doses used to treat ADHD. A number of different forms and preparations are available (Table 28.4).

Table 28.4 Medications to treat ADHD.

Trade name	Generic name	Formulation	Duration of action	Usual dosing times
Dexamphetamine	Dexamphetamine	5 mg tab	4–5 h	Morning and lunchtime
Vyvanse	Lisdexamfetamine	30, 50, 70mg caps	8-12 h	Morning
Ritalin 10	Methylphenidate	10 mg tab	2.5–4 h	Morning, lunchtime ± after school
Ritalin LA	Methylphenidate biphasic release	10, 20,30,40 mg caps	6–8 h	Morning
Concerta	Methylphenidate extended release	18, 27, 36, 54 mg tabs	8–10h	Morning
Strattera	Atomoxetine	10, 18, 25, 40, 60, 80, 100 mg caps	Steady state	Morning or evening

Note: All items are available in Australia on the PBS by authority prescription. In most states the prescribing of these medications is restricted to paediatricians, child psychiatrists and neurologists.

Other medications may be useful in some children with ADHD, these include:
- Atomoxetine, a selective noradrenaline reuptake inhibitor.
- The alpha-2 agonists clonidine or guanfacine, which can help with sleep onset, explosive behaviour and tics.
- Antidepressants (SSRI, SNRI, tricyclics) are beneficial to treat associated impairing anxiety.

Diet
Elimination of synthetic food colourings and preservatives is beneficial in some children with irritable mood. Fish oil supplementation may be helpful for some children.

Prognosis
Most children with ADHD will continue to have some difficulties through adolescence and into adulthood, although many develop compensating strategies and function well. A significant minority have adverse long-term outcomes including academic underachievement, vocational disadvantage, relationship difficulties, substance abuse, and mental health disorders.

Autism spectrum disorders
Autism Spectrum Disorder (ASD) is a complex neurodevelopmental condition that has a pervasive effect on social understanding, learning and flexibility. To meet the criteria for ASD, children need to have substantial difficulties in two areas:
1. Social communication and interaction
2. Restricted interests or repetitive behaviours

These difficulties must cause an impairment in functioning. Additionally, many children with ASD also have atypical sensory processing.

Terminology
In 2013, the DSM-5 defined autism as a spectrum of conditions (Table 28.5), replacing the previous diagnoses of Autistic Disorder, Asperger Syndrome and Pervasive Developmental Disorder Not otherwise specified. The term 'high-functioning autism' refers to children with intelligence in the normal range (previously called Asperger Syndrome).

Prevalence
The prevalence of ASD in Australia has been increasing rapidly over the past few decades. The increase is likely to be related to greater recognition of the condition in high-functioning children. The current prevalence is between 1.5 and 2.5%. The condition occurs more commonly in boys.

Aetiology
The precise aetiology of ASD is still unknown. It has a high degree of heritability (64–95%), with a wide variety of genes implicated. In 13% of children, ASD occurs as part of a known neurodevelopmental syndrome such as Tuberous Sclerosis and Fragile X Syndrome, with a causal genetic abnormality or in association with intrauterine damage, such in Foetal Alcohol Syndrome, Congenital Rubella or use of Valproate during pregnancy.

Table 28.5 Summary of DSM-5 criteria for autism spectrum disorder.

Persistent deficits in social communication and interaction (all of the following):
1. Deficits in social-emotional reciprocity (sharing of ideas and emotions in conversation or play)
2. Deficits in use of nonverbal communication (integration of eye contact, gesture and facial expressions to effectively communicate)
3. Deficits in maintaining relationships (ability to make and repair friendships and engage with others in play)
Restricted or repetitive patterns of behaviour, interests and activities (at least 2):
1. Repetitive motor movements or speech (eg. spinning, rocking, flapping, and using repetitive sounds or phrases)
2. Insistence of sameness and difficulties with change of routine (includes rigid thinking patterns)
3. Highly restricted interests of abnormal intensity and focus (eg. focus on parts of objects)
4. Hyper- or hypo-reactivity to sensory inputs or interest in sensory aspects of the environment

Diagnosis

The diagnosis is established by considering the following features in relation to the child's developmental level:

- The child's social behaviour and understanding of social situations
- A history of difficulties in early socialisation and communication with parents and siblings
- Observations and reports of repetitive behaviours, and need for sameness
- History of unusual sensory responses or sensory seeking behaviours

These features need to be considered in the light of the child's overall level of intellectual functioning and exposure to social opportunities. Deficits must occur in more than one context. The deficits become evident when social challenges exceed the capacity of the child, such as in middle childhood, and may be masked through parental 'scaffolding' in the home environment and learned strategies in later life.

- The severity of ASD is rated subjectively according to level specified in DSM-5, from level 1, 'requiring support' to level 3, "requiring very substantial support".
- In addition, children with ASD often experience difficulties with emotional regulation and are prone to rapid increases in distress linked to challenging behaviour commonly referred to as 'melt-downs'.

Autism presenting in infancy

In early life ASD presents with unusual interaction with primary caregivers, such as reduced eye contact, lack of response to name, lack of showing, pointing and attempts to interest others in their activities, and engagement in repetitive movements or non-functional play. Delays in language development may also be present. Some children develop single words and then regress in language use and social interest in the second year of life.

Autism presenting in adolescence

Children who have higher intelligence may present with challenging behaviour, social withdrawal, school refusal, or depressed or anxious mood. Features of ASD in earlier life should be sought. The presentation may be delayed where children are academically strong and families have a higher tolerance for 'quirky' behaviour.

Autism in girls

Girls more commonly present with difficulties in emotional control and anxiety. Girls often mask symptoms through copying others and joining in the periphery of social groups. Their interests are likely to be similar to typically developing girls but differ in intensity and level of creativity. Girls with intellectual impairment are more likely to present with classical features of ASD.

Diagnostic assessment process

There are two components to a comprehensive assessment:

1. Establishing the main diagnosis and presence of comorbidities
2. Assessing a child's functional learning and social capacities.

While it is possible for an individual clinician to make the diagnosis of ASD, the comprehensive assessment should include a multidisciplinary approach and may involve a combination of psychologists, speech pathologists or occupational therapists.

- A speech pathologist's evaluation of pragmatic language is valuable for understanding the extent of social communication difficulties.
- Audiology is needed to exclude hearing deficits in inattentive children.
- It is important to establish a child's cognitive abilities and receptive and expressive language level, especially in preparation for starting school.
- A medical examination should be performed to identify underlying causes.
- It is important for one clinician to oversee the process and to provide the child's family with coherent information about the diagnosis and help them to develop a management plan.

For some children, a multidisciplinary team is needed to establish a diagnosis in the first instance due to complexity of the child and family's situation, for example in situations of severe trauma, or complex medical comorbidity.

There is no one tool that can define all cases of ASD across the range of ages, genders and IQ levels. The Autism Diagnostic Observation Schedule-2 is widely used, particularly for research, as it is helpful in evaluating social skills through child interview. It is operator dependent. It has high specificity and moderate sensitivity. Sensitivity is lower in children with extremes of intellectual ability and in girls.

Comorbid conditions

Comorbid conditions occur frequently in ASD, with mental health problems occurring in 40–80%. It is important to monitor children with ASD for these conditions which can emerge at different life stages.

- **Intellectual disability**: Mild to moderate intellectual impairment occurs in approximately 30% of children with ASD and has a significant effect on long-term prognosis. It is important to perform cognitive testing before a child starts school, however the results may be affected by communication skills and compliance and the testing may need to be repeated. Severe intellectual disability can also be a differential diagnosis for ASD.
- **Attention-deficit hyperactivity disorder.** ADHD should be considered where a child with ASD is restless, overactive, impulsive and inattentive.
- **Anxiety disorders.** While anxiety is common in children with ASD in situations of change or social complexity, some children have severe symptoms that meet the criteria for Generalised Anxiety Disorders, Social Anxiety Disorder, Panic Attacks, Selective Mutism, Separation Anxiety Disorder or Specific Phobias.
- **Other comorbid conditions**. Specific Learning Difficulties, Language Disorders, Sleep Disorders, Eating Disorders, Hearing and Visual Impairments, Epilepsy, Depression, Psychosis, Gender Identity Disorder and Tourette's Disorder occur at a higher rate in individuals with ASD.

Management

- The role of the medical practitioner is to help parents deal with the challenges of receiving a diagnosis, provide evidence-based information, assist with referrals for intervention and monitor a child's progress with the aim of providing additional support at times of transition. There is no role for medication in the treatment of core symptoms of ASD. Comorbid conditions should be treated on their merits and may require medication.
- **Management of challenging behaviour or anxiety**. Challenging behaviours often arise as a result of the mismatch between social or academic expectations and a child's skills. Changing a child's environment to accommodate heightened sensory responses, differences in communication levels and social abilities can lead to greater engagement in school and the community and confidence-building for the child. This may involve such strategies as allowing planned breaks at school to reduce cognitive overload, avoiding noisy situations, modifying the school curriculum, or using visual strategies to support communication and planning. Specialist psychologists or mental health clinicians employ a number of techniques to help children develop their social-emotional awareness in different social contexts (eg. Social Stories™ or Tracking Better®).
- **Management in preschool**: The aim at this stage is to promote the development of joint attention and co-operative play, as well as developing communication skills. A multi-disciplinary early intervention program could include speech pathology, clinical psychology for behavioural modification, and occupational therapy support for sensory difficulties and play development, according to each individual's needs.
- **Management in primary school years**. Further development of communication skills and social skill development is the primary focus of this life stage. Ongoing speech therapy may include social skills and conversation training. Children often require a modified curriculum and some children will need a specific Education Support worker.
- **Management in adolescence**. Anxiety disorders and depression commonly begin in adolescence in response to increasing social complexity with peers and greater academic demands. Teenagers with ASD need different supports in developing their sexuality. Planning for transition to employment is important.
- **Medication.** A combination of medication and behavioural intervention is indicated for comorbid ADHD. Challenging behaviour resulting from emotional dysregulation may respond to risperidone. There is limited evidence to support the use of SSRIs such as fluoxetine for children with ASD to treat coexisting Anxiety or Depression.

Disorders of motor development
Cerebral palsy and complications

Cerebral palsy (CP) describes a group of permanent disorders of movement and posture causing activity limitation, following an insult to the developing foetal or infant brain. CP has a prevalence of 1.5–2.5 per 1000 live births.

The motor disorders of CP are often accompanied by disturbances of sensation, perception, cognition, communication and behaviour, by epilepsy and by secondary musculoskeletal problems. It is important to remember that 60% of people with CP are ambulant, and fewer than half have a learning disability.

Aetiology

There are many risk factors for CP (e.g. low birthweight and prematurity). The majority of CP is a result of antenatal insults. Perinatal asphyxia accounts for <10% of cases and post-neonatal illnesses or injuries for a further 10%. CP is a clinical descriptor, and there are many CP-like conditions. An aetiological diagnosis is an essential part of the assessment.

Classification

CP is classified according to the

- Type of motor disorder (e.g. spasticity, dyskinesia (includes dystonia and athetosis), ataxia, mixed).
- Distribution of the motor disorder (e.g. hemiplegia, diplegia, quadriplegia).
- Severity of the motor disorder on gross motor function and mobility, using the Gross Motor Function Classification System (GMFCS; Table 28.6, Figure 28.1).

Presentation

Children with CP may present with

- Delayed motor milestones
- Asymmetric movement patterns
- Abnormal muscle tone
- Associated problems (e.g. severe feeding difficulties and irritability)

Investigation

- A careful history and examination exploring potential aetiology, and making certain the neurological cause is central in origin. A history suggesting regression is a red flag requiring consultation and investigation.
- An MRI brain scan should be undertaken. This may provide information about underlying neuropathology and timing of the brain injury.
- Testing for genetic abnormalities, and consideration of metabolic conditions is often necessary.

Management

- A multidisciplinary team approach with family input to goal-setting is essential.
- Access to good paediatric care including immunisation, growth surveillance, emotional monitoring and good dental health are key to achieving best care.
- It is important to remember that fitness is a key goal for people with CP (see https://www.canchild.ca/en/research-in-practice/f-words-in-childhood-disability).

Associated impairments

- **Motor impairment** is the defining feature of CP, with an impact on mobility and reliance on aids to support mobility. Upper limb function may also be affected. Impacts include reduced independence, coordination and stamina.
- **Communication difficulties** vary and include receptive and expressive language problems and dysarthria. Take time to understand the best way each child communicates, *do not assume they can't* - ask the child and their carer. There are a range of assistive communication devices, including PODD (Pragmatic Organisation Dynamic Display) books and eye gaze.
- **Intellectual disability and specific learning problems** can occur and are present in < 50% of children with CP. A cognitive assessment characterises each child's strengths, vulnerabilities and learning styles. This particularly assists with planning of educational needs.

Table 28.6 General headings for each level of GMFCS.

GMFCS Level	Function
Level I	Walks without limitations
Level II	Walks with limitations
Level III	Walks using a hand held mobility device
Level IV	Self-Mobility with limitations; may use powered mobility device
Level V	Transported in manual wheelchair

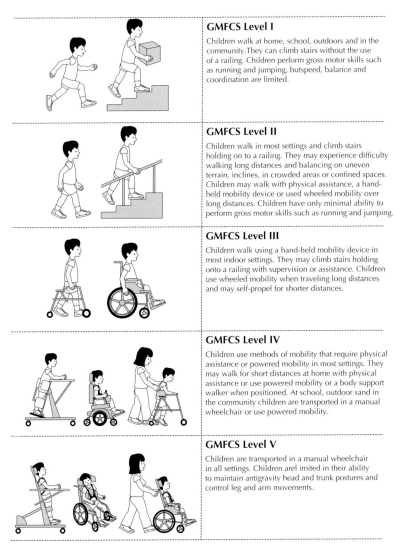

GMFCS Level I

Children walk at home, school, outdoors and in the community.They can climb stairs without the use of a railing. Children perform gross motor skills such as running and jumping, butspeed, balance and coordination are limited.

GMFCS Level II

Children walk in most settings and climb stairs holding on to a railing. They may experience difficulty walking long distances and balancing on uneven terrain, inclines, in crowded areas or confined spaces. Children may walk with physical assistance, a hand-held mobility device or used wheeled mobility over long distances. Children have only minimal ability to perform gross motor skills such as running and jumping.

GMFCS Level III

Children walk using a hand-held mobility device in most indoor settings. They may climb stairs holding onto a railing with supervision or assistance. Children use wheeled mobility when traveling long distances and may self-propel for shorter distances.

GMFCS Level IV

Children use methods of mobility that require physical assistance or powered mobility in most settings. They may walk for short distances at home with physical assistance or use powered mobility or a body support walker when positioned. At school, outdoor sand in the community children are transported in a manual wheelchair or use powered mobility.

GMFCS Level V

Children are transported in a manual wheelchair in all settings. Children arel imited in their ability to maintain antigravity head and trunk postures and control leg and arm movements.

Figure 28.1 Descriptors and illustrations of GMFCS levels for children aged 6th and 12th years. *Source*: The Royal Children's Melbourne. Illustrations by Bill Reid, Kate Willoughby, Adrienne Harvey and Kerr Graham. Reproduced with permission from the authors.

- **Visual problems** are found in about 45% of children with CP. All children require a visual assessment.
- **Hearing deficits** of at least moderate degree are found in about 7% of children with CP. All children require a hearing assessment.

Health problems

- **Growth and nutrition** as children with CP can be either underweight or overweight. Poor weight gain, from oromotor dysfunction, results in malnutrition and specific micronutrient deficiencies, with health, growth and neurodevelopmental consequences. Non-oral feeding by nasogastric, gastrostomy or jejunal routes may be indicated.
- **Aspiration** (that may lead to **chronic lung disease**) may be present; coughing or choking during meal-times or wheeze during or after meals may signal this. It can also occur without symptoms or signs. Careful feed assessment by a speech pathologist can assist with management and directing investigation.
- **Gastro-oesophageal reflux**, oesophagitis with associated pain, bleeding and resulting anaemia are common in CP.
- **Constipation** resulting from immobility, low-fibre diet, poor fluid intake and some medications is common.
- **Epilepsy** should be managed with optimal medication regimes.
- **Osteopenia** is frequent. Monitor vitamin D levels in all children. Insufficiency fractures are common in children functioning at GMFS IV-V level.
- **Undescended testes** are more frequent in this group.
- Actively monitor for emotional disorders such as **anxiety, depression** and **social difficulties**. These may impact more on the child's wellbeing than any physical issue.

Further consequences of the motor disorder

- **Poor saliva control** can be improved by speech pathology input, the use of medication and occasionally surgery.
- **Incontinence** is common and the causes are multifactorial. Centrally mediated bowel or bladder dysmotility, cognitive deficits, lack of opportunity and medication side-effects may all play a role.
- **Spasticity and dyskinesia** are common problems, which can impact on function and care, and can also cause pain and disturb sleep. A team approach is required:
  - A good history identifying potential drivers for dyskinesia, such as constipation, gastro-oesophageal reflux, or anxiety, is necessary as underlying problems such as these must be managed.
  - Assessment and prescription of aids and orthoses, including good seating, are critical for management.
  - Oral medications can be very helpful, and include baclofen, gabapentin, diazepam (see chapter 36 Rehabilitation medicine).
  - Targeted use of botulinum toxin can be extremely helpful
  - Neurosurgical interventions, such as intrathecal baclofen, selective dorsal rhizotomy and deep brain stimulation may be beneficial in a selected population of children with more severe symptoms.
- **Orthopaedic consequences**: Hip dysplasia and spinal deformity and other musculoskeletal complications are common, and surveillance for these problems should be part of routine care.
  - **Hips**: non-walkers (GMFCS IV, V) and those ambulant only with mobility devices (GMFCS III) are prone to hip subluxation and eventual dislocation. Dislocation causes severe pain and is extremely difficult to treat, but can usually be prevented by timely orthopaedic surgery. Early detection is vital. Hip X-rays should be performed according to hip surveillance guidelines.
  - **Spinal deformity:** Scoliosis and kyphosis are common in non-walkers. They can lead to postural deformity, restrictive lung disease and other health consequences. New surgical techniques allow for surgical correction when the spinal curve is small and flexible, and children are still growing. Early referral to spinal orthopaedics is essential for timely intervention.
  - **Knees**: Flexion contractures may require hamstring surgery.
  - **Ankles**: Equinus deformity is the most common orthopaedic problem in children with CP. It is treated conservatively in young children with orthoses +/- botulinum toxin. Older children may require surgery. A range of other problems around the foot and ankle may benefit from orthopaedic assessment.

Referrals

Liaising with the kindergarten, school and other members of the medical team is important. Referral to and ongoing liaison with allied health professionals is essential to enable children to achieve their optimal potential and independence. Access to the National Disability insurance Scheme (NDIS – see section later in chapter) is critical to adequate service provision.

- **Physiotherapists** aim to reduce impairments and optimise function. They also give advice regarding mobility aids, the use of orthoses and special seating.
- **Occupational therapists** provide parents with advice on developing their child's upper limb and self-care skills. They design and make arm and hand splints, can provide advice on specialised equipment (such as car seats and adapted cutlery) and recommend home modifications.
- **Speech pathologists** assist with severe eating and drinking difficulties, as well as communication and assistive communication systems for children with communication difficulties.
- **Orthotists** design, fabricate, fit and maintain various orthoses (braces). Orthoses are used to improve function, support, align, prevent or correct musculoskeletal deformities and improve function in different parts of the child's body, most commonly the lower limbs.
- **Continence Nurses** provide support advice and expertise to manage complex continence issues.
- Other professionals who may be helpful include **social workers, nurses, psychologists and special education teachers**.

Neural tube defects/myelomeningocele

The neural tube defects (NTDs) comprises a spectrum of disorders of abnormal folding and closure of the embryonic neural tube and are the most common severe congenital malformations of the nervous system. Of these, spina bifida with a myelomeningocele causes multi-system dysfunction. The degree of impairment from the spinal cord pathology varies and depends on the type and size of the defect. Most children have some lower limb motor weakness, sensory loss and a neurogenic bladder and bowel. Eighty per cent have an Arnold Chiari malformation leading to progressive hydrocephalus requiring surgery. Many children with NTDs have specific learning problems (even in the absence of hydrocephalus).

Prevention

Folic acid supplementation in the month before conception and in the first 3 months of pregnancy has been shown to reduce the risk of recurrence in any at-risk family (by ~75%). Recommended doses are

- 0.5 mg daily: low-risk women (no family history of NTDs).
- 5 mg daily: if there is a family history of NTD *or* if the woman is taking anticonvulsant medications.

Putting the Science into Practice: Antenatal surgery for NTDs

Some centres offer antenatal surgery for NTD's and there is some evidence that antenatal surgical closure of the defect improves motor function and hydrocephalus, but not urinary or bowel incontinence.

Management

Management requires collaboration between the child and family and an interdisciplinary team. Ideally, this includes a GP, paediatrician, neurosurgeon, urologist, orthopaedic surgeon, neuropsychologist, physiotherapist, orthotist, occupational therapist, social worker, continence and stomal therapists. Most children with NTDs attend regular schools.

Initial management

- Neurosurgical and paediatric assessment of the newborn infant to determine if early surgery is indicated to close the spinal defect.
- Clinical and ultrasound observation to detect and monitor hydrocephalus.
- Insertion of a ventriculoperitoneal shunt is often necessary.
- Urological consultation and investigation with an ultrasound of the bladder and kidneys in the neonatal period provides baseline information for subsequent management.
- Orthopaedic assessment includes clinical examination and an ultrasound of the hips. Infants with spina bifida have a higher than usual prevalence of developmental dysplasia of the hips and talipes.

Specific aspects of management
- **Mobility:**
  - Independent mobility is the primary goal. Upright experience in the early years and use of gait aides improves independence in adulthood, even if the person has progressed to using a wheelchair for ambulation.

- **Neurogenic bladder**
  - Neonates with myelomeningocoele are usually born with normal, functioning kidneys. The primary goal is the maintenance of satisfactory renal function and the secondary goal is the establishment of urinary continence.
  - Abnormal innervation causes bladder dysfunction in most children. At the extremes, the neuropathic bladder may be small and non-compliant, or compliant and floppy with poor emptying. The function of the sphincter and degree of reflux also influence the degree of leaking (incontinence) and intravesical pressures, which may render the kidneys at 'high risk' of long-term damage.
  - Urinary tract infection (UTI) is common. A midstream or catheter specimen of urine should be done and infection treated.
  - Renal function is monitored by checking creatinine.
  - Renal tract ultrasound (US) is regularly repeated to monitor for changes (e.g hydronephrosis & bladder trabeculation) and to assess normal renal structure and growth. Initially every 6–12 weeks, then 6 monthly in toddlers and children.
  - Urodynamic studies establish the filling and emptying pressures of the bladder to gauge 'risk' to kidneys and to inform treatment.
  - Clean intermittent catheterisation (CIC) is usually started in the neonatal period. Additional support may be necessary in the form of medication (e.g. oxybutynin 8–12 hourly).
  - Surgical interventions are aimed at protecting renal function and achieving continence (includes 'social dryness' – not wetting between CIC).
    - Vesicostomy – performed when high pressure bladder is causing hydronephrosis despite CIC, or where UTI is frequent, (usually in infancy).
    - Bladder augmentation. People with spina bifida who have undergone bladder augmentation, have an increased risk of malignant change and require lifelong urological supervision.
    - The Mitrofanoff procedure (fashioning a conduit from the bladder to the abdominal wall by using the appendix) is also used to facilitate independence in catheterization.
    - Insertion of artificial sphincter.
- **Neuropathic Bowel**
  - Difficulties in managing soiling, incontinence and chronic constipation affect the quality of life of patients and their carers.
  - Constipation is common, and dietary advice, laxatives, enemas and irrigation systems may be required.
  - The Malone procedure (fashioning of a non-refluxing appendicocaecostomy) can be performed so that an antegrade continence enema can be used to regularly evacuate the bowels and prevent soiling.
- **Neurological functioning**
  - Children with shunts should have neurosurgical assessment regularly (in infancy every 6–9 months; in childhood and adolescence at least every 1–2 years). Tethering of the spinal cord to surrounding structures occurs in most children. In a small number, traction on the cord causes deterioration in neurological functioning. Surgical de-tethering may be required.
  - Children often have specific cognitive difficulties and a neuropsychological assessment is usually carried out before school entry and repeated before transition to secondary school to ensure appropriate educational support is in place.
- **Co-morbid medical problems**
  - Scoliosis is a common management problem.
  - Pressure sores occur in all children with spina bifida at some time, most commonly on the feet or the buttocks.
  - Epilepsy occurs in 15% of people with myelomeningocoele.
  - Obesity is increasingly prevalent, especially as mobility changes, usually at puberty. Obesity can have significant implications for independence.

- **Adolescent issues**
  - Puberty may be delayed or precocious.
  - Specific adolescent issues including mental health sexuality, relationship difficulties, and contraception should be addressed.
  - Transition and transfer to adult services and vocational services is a major challenge and needs careful planning and support for the young person.

Irritability in children with profound intellectual and physical disability

Irritability in children with disabilities presents the clinician with diagnostic uncertainty, amplified in patients with difficulties in communication and/or complex medical illness. The following should be considered:

- Hunger
- Seizures
- Sleep deprivation
- Pain, secondary to:
  - Severe constipation
  - Infection e.g. ears, throat, respiratory tract, urine, skin
  - Gastro-oesophageal reflux
  - Dental abscess/caries
  - Muscle spasms
  - Surgical – appendicitis, intussusception, torsion of testes.
  - Corneal abrasion/foreign body in the eye
  - Renal colic
  - Subluxing or dislocated hips
  - Fractures – accidental or inflicted
  - Side-effects of medication, eg. anticonvulsants
  - Gynaecological
  - Pancreatitis
  - Raised intracranial pressure (eg. VP shunts which may become obstructed)
  - Anxiety and/or depression

The National disability insurance scheme

The National Disability Insurance Scheme (NDIS) has transformed how support is delivered to people with a disability in Australia. The Australian population contributes to the NDIS through taxation. The National Disability Insurance Agency (NDIA) is an independent body set up to develop and administer the NDIS. There is also an NDIS Quality and Safeguards Commission which is responsible for the quality of service delivery and to protect people with disabilities from neglect, abuse, restraint and seclusion.

The NDIS has largely replaced the fragmented and poorly funded services which were previously provided by State governments. Until a child is 7 years of age, they may receive funding for early intervention services through this scheme and it is open to all children with developmental problems. A formal diagnosis is not required for the provision of these services, which are provided by the NDIS Early Childhood Early Intervention (ECEI) partners. The aim is that reasonable and necessary supports are provided for people with disabilities in order to maintain and maximise function for independence and for participation in the social and economic life of their communities. The NDIS theoretically provides more flexibility and independence for the patient (or parent/guardian) to engage the services they feel are most necessary to help with social inclusion and participation.

Doctors are often asked to write a letter to confirm that a child has a developmental problem or disability. The application for funding is made by the family or individual and medical staff are discouraged from advocating specific therapies or supports. Further information is available at www.ndis.gov.au or via phone on 1800 800 110.

USEFUL RESOURCES

- Harvard centre on the developing child https://developingchild.harvard.edu/about/: links to summaries of the evidence behind early childhood development.
- Royal Children's Hospital; *Strong Foundations: Getting it Right in the First 1000 Days* https://www.rch.org.au/ccch/first-thousand-days/: research project and key finding regarding the significant first 1000 days of early childhood development.
- Developmental milestones https://www.healthdirect.gov.au/developmental-milestones: Department of Health (healthdirect) information on developmental milestones.
- The Raising Children Network https://raisingchildren.net.au/: Australian based essential early childhood and parenting information.
- Autism spectrum disorder parent and service information in Australia https://raisingchildren.net.au/autism/learning-about-asd/about-asd/asd-overview.
- NDIS Australia resources: Funding and general information https://www.ndis.gov.au/; General practitioner relevant information https://www.racgp.org.au/running-a-practice/practice-resources/general-practice-guides/ndis-information-for-general-practitioners; Paediatrician and Physician relevent information https://www.racp.edu.au/fellows/resources/ndis-guide-for-physicians.

CHAPTER 29

Neurology

Mark Mackay
Andrew Kornberg
Alison Wray

Key Points

- Benign focal epilepsy and absence epilepsy, which are the most common types of childhood epilepsy, typically do not require neuroimaging, respond well to medications and remit prior to adolescence.
- MRI is the investigation of choice in children with: (i) focal seizure in children aged less than three years, (ii) abnormal neurological examination, (iii) post-ictal Todd's paresis, or (iv) presence of a condition predisposing to seizures.
- In children with status epilepticus who have not responded to midazolam, phenytoin and levetiracetam have similar efficacy and safety.
- If symptoms of childhood stroke are present, urgent MRI brain and MRA should be performed in suspected arterial ischaemic stroke, and urgent non-contrast CT should be performed in suspected haemorrhagic stroke.
- Imaging the brain/skull using ionising radiation (particularly in young children) should be used judiciously and not as a routine screening assessment.

Febrile convulsions

- Febrile convulsions (FC) are usually brief, generalised seizures associated with a febrile illness, in the absence of any CNS infection or past history of afebrile seizures.
- Occur in 3–4% of children aged 6 months to 5 years.
- Recurrent in one-third (more likely if seizures occur in early infancy or if there is a family history).
- They can be divided into
  - *Simple* = brief, generalised and single convulsion.
  - *Complex* = either focal, >15 minutes, or multiple in a 24-hour period.
- In otherwise healthy children, FC are not accompanied by an increased risk of intellectual disability, cerebral palsy, other neurological disorders or death. However, there is a modest increase in the risk of epilepsy.

Management

- A careful search for the cause of fever is required; most will be due to viral respiratory infections.
- A lumbar puncture need not be done routinely following a simple FC, but meningitis should be considered in any unwell child, especially when there is a persistently depressed conscious state and in children with multiple or prolonged convulsions. The younger the child, the higher the index of suspicion of meningitis.
- General temperature lowering measures such as removing clothing and administering paracetamol 15 mg/kg may help reduce symptoms of fever. It will not, however, minimise the risk of recurrence.
- Stop a continuing convulsion (>5-minute duration) with buccal or intranasal midazolam 0.2–0.5 mg/kg (max. 10 mg).

Paediatric Handbook, Tenth Edition. Edited by Kate Harding, Daniel S. Mason and Daryl Efron.
© 2021 John Wiley & Sons Ltd. Published 2021 by John Wiley & Sons Ltd.

- *Anticonvulsants are not routinely recommended for children with recurrent FC.*
  FC are usually benign, anticonvulsant therapy may have significant side effects and do not alter long-term prognosis.
- In some circumstances (e.g. children with a history of prolonged FC) parents may be taught to administer buccal or intranasal midazolam.
- About 3% of children with FC subsequently develop afebrile seizures (epilepsy – as opposed to 0.5% of children in the general population).
  The risk is greater with:
  ○ Previous abnormal neurological development.
  ○ A history of epilepsy in first-degree relatives.
  ○ Prolonged (>10 minutes) FC.
  ○ Focal features present during, or after, the FC.
  ○ Multiple convulsions during a single febrile episode.
- Counsel parents; remember that many will have felt that their child nearly died.
  ○ It is important to emphasise the very low risk of neurological complications and excellent prognosis for eventual remission of FC, as well as the 1:3 risk of recurrence.
  ○ Advice on the management of future febrile illnesses and FC is required.
  ○ A follow-up visit is recommended to discuss what happened and help prevent the development of 'fever phobia' in parents.
  ○ An electroencephalogram (EEG) is of little value in single or recurrent, simple or complex FC.

Epilepsy

Epilepsy (defined as two or more unprovoked seizures) occurs in approximately 0.5–1% of children. Seizures may be focal and/or generalised and the aetiology may be due to structural (developmental malformation, tumour, or scar), genetic, infectious, metabolic or immune causes.

Self-limited focal epilepsies of childhood
- Onset is typically in mid-childhood (peak 7 years).
- Seizures are commonly nocturnal or early morning;
  ○ **Centrotemporal (Rolandic Epilepsy);** usually focal motor or sensory phenomena related to the face, mouth or jaw.
  ○ **Occipital (Panayiotopoulos and Gastaut)** varieties; may have visual manifestations.
  ○ Secondary generalised tonic–clonic seizures may occur.
- On EEG, spike discharges typically occur in the centrotemporal or occipital region.
- Imaging only necessary if clinical or EEG features are atypical or if seizure control is difficult.
- Prognosis is excellent as the seizures are usually infrequent and remit before the teenage years.
- Treatment only indicated if frequent or prolonged seizures;
  ○ Seizures are often controlled by a single night time dose of medication.
  ○ Low-dose carbamazepine or sodium valproate used for 1–2 years given the spontaneous remission of seizures.

Genetic generalised epilepsies
- Characterised by recurrent generalised tonic–clonic, absence or myoclonic seizures of presumed genetic cause.
- EEG shows generalised spike wave patterns.

Childhood absence epilepsy:
- Peak age of onset 6–7 years.
- EEG shows 3 Hz generalized spike wave epileptic discharges.
- Ethosuximide is first line treatment, followed by sodium valproate; the majority of children have a good response.
- Prognosis generally good for seizure control in later childhood or adulthood.

Juvenile myoclonic epilepsy:
- Initial presentation may be tonic–clonic seizures as the early morning myoclonus (characteristic of the condition) may go unrecognized by the patient/family.
- Sodium valproate is first line treatment.
- This condition has some overlap with the Juvenile Absence Epilepsy and Generalised Tonic Clonic Seizures Alone syndromes.

Focal epilepsies
- This term describes a heterogeneous group of seizure disorders in which children have focal seizures from particular brain regions.
- Usually caused by underlying developmental (congenital) or acquired structural lesions.
- Focal unaware seizures and focal motor seizures are the main seizure type.

Focal unaware seizures:
- Usually manifest by arrest of activity, staring, autonomic disturbances, semi-purposeful automatic movements (automatisms) and altered conscious state, sometimes preceded by an aura.
- Specific seizure manifestations depend on the brain region involved.
- Seizures may secondarily generalise.
- Seizures may be difficult to treat.
- Children may have associated learning and behavioural problems due to dysfunction in the affected brain region or the pervasive effect of uncontrolled seizures and medications.
- EEG may show localised epileptic activity.
- MRI may reveal structural pathology.

Developmental and epileptic encephalopathies
- Severe seizure disorders affecting infants and young children in which uncontrolled generalised seizures are associated with generalised epileptic disturbances on EEG and global developmental delay or regression.
- Examples include **Lennox–Gastaut syndrome** and **West syndrome**.
- Characteristic seizures in these syndromes are
  - Epileptic spasms (clusters of brief seizures that are usually generalised and in flexion or extension)
  - Tonic seizures
  - Myoclonic or atonic drop attacks
  - Tonic–clonic seizures
- Seizures are generally difficult to control with medication.
- **West syndrome** is also known as **Infantile spasms** and refers to the triad of:
  - Seizures (appearing usually in the third to fourth month of life)
  - Specific EEG pattern (hypsarrhythmia)
  - Developmental regression
- Infantile spasms are seen more frequently in association with other conditions, for example genetic disorders including Down syndrome, Tuberous sclerosis, and developmental or acquired structural CNS abnormalities.
- High dose corticosteroids are first line treatment (with the exception of Tuberous Sclerosis where vigabatrin is first line treatment).
- Early treatment (within two weeks) associated with better neurodevelopmental outcomes.

Investigation
The decision to investigate a child following a seizure depends on many factors.
- Children with FC do not generally need EEG or imaging investigation.
- EEG should generally be done in any child with a definite, non-febrile seizure, whether generalised or partial. EEG aids in the characterisation of seizures and epilepsies, *but should not be used to distinguish seizures from non-epileptic events.*
- Brain imaging is reserved for children with epilepsy in whom there is suspicion from history, examination or EEG that there may be an underlying cerebral lesion.
- Children with typical forms of uncomplicated and well-controlled self-limited rolandic or occipital focal or generalised epilepsies do not require imaging.

Clinical Pearl: Neuroimaging in epilepsy

- Clinical indicators for intracranial abnormalities requiring neuroimaging which are likely to change initial patient management include; (i) a focal seizure in children aged less than three years, (ii) abnormal neurological examination, (iii) Todd's post-ictal paresis, or (iv) presence of a condition predisposing to seizures.
- In children where an intracranial abnormality is considered likely, and neuroimaging is indicated, magnetic resonance imaging (MRI) is recommended over computed tomography (CT) because: (i) there is superior anatomic resolution and characterisation of pathologic processes from using MRI, and (ii) there is radiation exposure and escalated future cancer risk associated with CT.

Note: Adapted with permission from the Australia and New Zealand Child Neurology Society (ANZCNS) EVOLVE guidelines https://evolve.edu.au/recommendations/anzcns.

Management

- After the first afebrile seizure, only one-third of children experience further episodes; *Therefore treatment is not normally commenced unless there are features to suggest a significantly increased risk of recurrence.*
- It is important to characterise the epileptic syndrome from history, EEG and sometimes imaging. This guides prognosis and the need for treatment, including choice of anticonvulsant.
- Children with absence, myoclonic, complex partial seizures and epileptic spasms have usually had multiple seizures at presentation and require treatment.
- Prognosis:
  - Approximately 50% of childhood epilepsies have a favourable course.
  - 25% gradually improve with time.
  - 25% are refractory to treatment.

Principles of anticonvulsant therapy

- Antiepileptic medication (Table 29.1) is only indicated in children at risk of recurrent epileptic seizures.
- *Monotherapy:* most patients are well controlled with one anticonvulsant.
- *Titrate slowly:* most antiepileptic medications are commenced at a low dose and titrated up to the maintenance dose, to avoid side effects during their introduction (*'start low and go slow'*).
- *Changing medications:* introduce or change one anticonvulsant at a time, except in emergency situations.
- *Dosage variation:* individuals vary greatly in dosage requirements and tolerance. Young children and infants typically require relatively large doses per kg body weight.
- *Monitoring:* Routine monitoring of serum anticonvulsant levels is unnecessary as there is generally poor correlation between blood levels and clinical efficacy. Exceptions include:
  - Assessing compliance
  - Titrating AEDs in complex polypharmacy regimens
  - Adjusting for altered AED metabolism in disease states, puberty, young infants or intellectually disabled older children in whom side effects may not be identified as easily.
- Testing is reasonable for phenytoin, phenobarbitone and carbamazepine but other drugs are generally monitored with attention to usual prescribed doses and clinical markers.
- *Poor response to medication:* if seizure control is poor, the diagnosis and the choice of medication should be reviewed; *always consider non-compliance with therapy.*
- *Anticonvulsant cessation:* depending on the type of epilepsy, two years free of seizures are generally required before anticonvulsants are withdrawn; this is done gradually over several months.
- Parents need to be instructed in the first aid management of seizures, and be given a plan for what to do when seizures recur.
- Safety precautions such as supervision in water and avoidance of heights need to be discussed.
- Driving and other lifestyle and vocational restrictions apply to older teenagers and adults with epilepsy.

Status epilepticus

A convulsion involving the respiratory musculature and upper airways that does not cease within a few minutes may cause hypoventilation with hypoxaemia and hypercarbia.

- A recently proposed operational definition of status epilepticus (SE) is a seizure lasting more than 5 minutes, as this is the point at which emergency medications should be administered to terminate the seizure (Figure 29.1).

Table 29.1 Guidelines for the use of common anticonvulsants.

	Generalised tonic–clonic seizures	Focal or 2° generalized seizures	Absence (A) myoclonic(M) tonic (T)	Epileptic Spasms	Side effects (common or severe)
Carbazepine (Tegretol, Tegretol CR)	++	+++	Avoid	Avoid	Drowsiness, irritability, GIT, rash
Clobazam (Frisium)	+	+	A++, M++, T+	+	Drowsiness, irritability
Clonazepam (Rivotril)	+	+	A++, M++, T+	+	Irritability & behaviour disorder, increased secretions
Diazepam (Valium)	–	–	–	–	Drowsiness, respiratory depression
Ethosuximide (Zarontin)	–	–	A+++	–	GIT, thrombocytopenia
Gabapentin (Neurontin)	–	++	Avoid	Avoid	Drowsiness, dizziness, ataxia, fatigue
Lamotrigine (Lamictal)	++	++	++	+	Skin rash (3%) – may be severe. Increased risk if on sodium valproate
Lacosamide (Vimpat)	+	++	T++	–	Drowsiness, dizziness, GIT
Levetiracetam (Keppra)	+	++	M+, T+	–	Behaviour disturbance
Nitrazepam (Mogadon)	–	–	–	+	Drowsiness, increased bronchial secretions
Oxcarbazepine (Trileptal)	+	++	Avoid	Avoid	Drowsiness, hyponatraemia
Perampanel (Fycompa)	+	++	–	–	Drowsiness, dizziness, GIT, weight gain
Phenobarbitone	++	+	–	–	Cognitive, irritability, overactivity or drowsiness
Phenytoin sodium (Dilantin)	++	++	–	–	Gum hyperplasia, ataxia, nystagmus, serum sickness like illness, cognitive, rash
Prednisolone	–	–	–	+++	Weight gain, hypertension, irritability, immune suppression
Pregabalin (Lyrica)	–	+	–	–	Weight gain

(continued)

Table 29.1 (Continued)

	Generalised tonic–clonic seizures	Focal or 2° generalized seizures	Absence (A) myoclonic(M) tonic (T)	Epileptic Spasms	Side effects (common or severe)
Rufinamide (Inovelon)	+	−	T++ (Lennox Gastaut)		Drowsiness, dizziness, irritability, GIT, rash
Sodium valproate (Epilim)	+++	++	A++, M++, T+	+	Nausea, anorexia, vomiting, weight gain, severe hepatotoxicity (rare)
Tiagabine (Gabitril)	−	+	Avoid	Avoid	Headache, dizziness
Topiramate (Topamax)	+	++	−	+	Weight loss, sedation, cognitive nephrolithiasis, paraesthesia
Vigabatrin (Sabril)	−	+	Avoid	++	Excitation, agitation, drowsiness, dizziness, headache, weight gain, visual field constriction
Zonisamide (Zonegran)	++	++	M+	+	Weight loss, sedation, nephrolithiasis, paraesthesia

Notes:
* Table shows relative effectiveness of each drug against each of the major seizure types (does not represent a comparison of one drug against another).
* Table represents suggestions only; final decision of most appropriate anticonvulsant should take into consideration the patient's age, neurological status, co-morbidities, epilepsy syndromes, EEG, patient and parent attitudes and potential side effects.
* Anticonvulsants listed as to 'avoid' can potentially exacerbate seizures.
* Sodium valproate should be used with caution in children <3 years old, particularly if multiple anticonvulsants are used and there is developmental delay or regression.
* Cognitive side effects are seen with all anticonvulsants (particularly benzodiazepines and barbiturates).

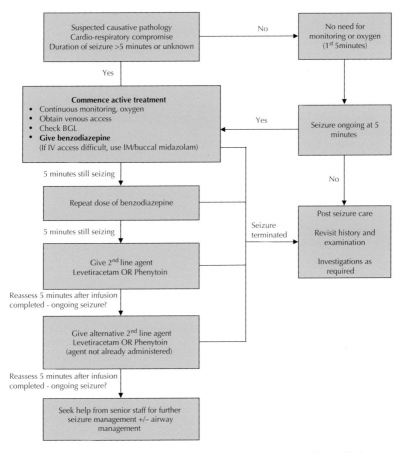

Figure 29.1 Acute seizure management. *Source*: Royal Children's Hospital Clinical Practice Guidelines – Afebrile seizures. Reproduced with permission from the Royal Children's Hospital.

Management

- Seek senior assistance early.
- Support airway and breathing, apply oxygen by mask, monitor.
- Be prepared to give mechanical ventilation, particularly if the child has meningitis.
- Secure IV access.
- Check BSL, UEC, CMP, blood gas. Consider blood culture if indicated.
- If hypoglycaemia present – correct low blood sugar (2ml/kg 10% dextrose; see Chapter 19 Endocrinology).
- **Anticonvulsant choices** include the following:
  - Initial treatment – Benzodiazepines
    - Midazolam: 0.15 mg/kg IV/IO/IM. Intranasal 0.2–0.5 mg/kg (max 10 mg) or buccal 0.3 mg/kg (max. 10 mg) can be given if no IV access.
    - Diazepam: 0.1–0.3 mg/kg (max 10–20 mg) IV/IO. May be given per rectum 0.3–0.5 mg/kg (max. 10 mg) if there is no IV access.

- o If the seizure does not terminate after two appropriate doses of benzodiazepines consider the following:
  - Phenytoin 20 mg/kg (max. 1.5 g) IV over 20 minutes in a monitored patient. Beware of negative inotropic effect – infuse under ECG monitoring.
  - Levetiracetam 20 mg/kg IV (maximum 1.0 g) as IV push
  - If no response after a further 5 minutes then give the alternative agent (Levetiracetam or Phenytoin).
- o For refractory status epilepticus
  - Involve senior ED / ICU / Anaesthetic staff for airway management
  - Midazolam infusion 1–5 mcg/kg/min IV/IO. This should only be given in a high-dependency setting with senior staff involvement and can serve as an alternative to rapid sequence induction (RSI) and ventilation.
  - Propofol 2.5 mg/kg stat followed by 1–3 mg/kg/h IV for no longer than 48 hours.
  - Thiopentone titrate dose slowly to effect (usually 2–5 mg/kg) slowly stat. Beware of hypotension and be ready to control the airway and breathing before administration. This should only be undertaken with ICU support.
- Consider IV ceftriaxone (100 mg/kg max. 2 g) and/or IV acyclovir (20 mg/kg 8H if age <3m, 500 mg/m^2 8H if age 3m – 12y, 10 mg/kg 8H if age >12y) if meningitis / encephalitis suspected.
- Prolonged convulsions may require large and repeated doses of anticonvulsant drugs or infusions and, consequently, mechanical ventilation.
- Suspect hyponatraemia as the cause of convulsions in meningitis and severe gastroenteritis-related dehydration.

Non-epileptic paroxysmal events
- Many children referred for assessment of epilepsy do not have epilepsy, but rather a non-epileptic paroxysmal disorder such as syncope, breath-holding spells, parasomnias or non-epileptic staring.
- In differentiating epileptic from non-epileptic events (Table 29.2), the description of the event is important, including the circumstances in which the event occurred and the details of what the child was doing immediately before the event.
- Most non-epileptic paroxysmal disorders can be diagnosed on history alone, or with the aid of a home video recording of a typical event. In some circumstances video-EEG monitoring may be required.
- The long Q–T syndrome should be considered in any episode of fainting or seizure that is not clearly due to typical breath-holding, vasovagal syncope or a definable epilepsy syndrome.

Weakness of acute onset
The acute onset of symmetrical limb weakness is usually of peripheral neuromuscular or spinal cord origin. Toxins (e.g. snake or tick bite), metabolic disturbance, systemic illness and psychogenic causes need to be considered under appropriate circumstances. Oral polio vaccine is a rare cause of acute flaccid paralysis.

Two key questions require urgent consideration:
- Is there a treatable cause?
- Is there respiratory or bulbar dysfunction of sufficient degree to warrant management in an intensive care unit?

Myasthenia gravis
- This diagnosis should be considered in any child with relatively acute-onset limb weakness, particularly if accompanied by ptosis, an eye movement disorder, pharyngeal or respiratory insufficiency.
- Parenteral anticholinesterase is rarely used for diagnostic testing. One may consider an ice-pack test (ice pack applied to upper eyelid transiently improves ptosis) instead if myasthenia gravis is a possibility.

Guillain–Barré syndrome
- Presents with weakness (ascending progression may be less clear in young children), pain and sensory loss.
  - o Weakness may be misinterpreted as ataxia.
  - o Back pain is common in childhood.
- The child should be transferred to a tertiary centre at the time of diagnosis, as respiratory weakness may occur rapidly.
- Intravenous gammaglobulin (IVIG) or plasma exchange need to be commenced early if they are to be effective.

Table 29.2 Non-epileptic paroxysmal events.

	Syncope	Breath-holding attacks	Shuddering	Benign paroxysmal vertigo	Self-stimulation	'Daydreams'	Confusional arousals[a]	Nightmares
Age	All ages	Infancy	Infancy	Preschool	Preschool	School age	Preschool/school age	All ages
Circumstance	Triggering factor or situational	Upset or a trigger is needed	Any time, anywhere	Any time, anywhere	Any time, anywhere	School, watching TV, times of inactivity	First one-third of sleep (non-REM)	Second half of sleep (REM)
Frequency	Occasional	Varies greatly	Sometimes many per day	1/month or less	Daily or less	Varies, small numbers per day	Nightly or less. Rarely >1/night	Nightly or less
Onset	Gradual or sudden	Sudden, with or without crying	Sudden	Sudden	Sudden	Vague	Sudden	Sudden
Recovery	Gradual	Slow if hypoxic Sz	Rapid	Rapid	Rapid	Vague. May 'snap out'	Returns to sleep	Remains asleep
Duration	Seconds to minutes	Seconds to minutes	Seconds	1–5 minutes	Minutes to hours	Seconds to minutes	Minutes	Minutes
Impairment of consciousness	Yes	Usually	No	No	No	Apparent but not real	Apparently awake but does not respond	Asleep
Observations	May have light headedness, dizziness or loss of vision. Tonic or tonic-clonic convulsion may occur at end	Cyanotic or pale, limp, may develop opisthotonos / convulsion	Rapid shivering movements maximal in head, trunk and arms	Frightened, pale, holds on to objects for balance or falls	Posturing with stiffening and while lying on side or supine, leaning against firm edge. Irregular breathing, flushing, sweating	Blank staring, no motor automations or blinking despite long episodes. Not precipitated by hyperventilation	Screaming, crying inconsolably, may get out of bed. Appears terrified	Nil
Post-event impairment	Minimal	Mild unless hypoxic Sz	No	No	No	No	No recollection of event	Good recall of event

[a] Including sleepwalking and night terrors.

Infant botulism

- Suspect in children 2–9 months of age with rapid onset of weakness and constipation, particularly with ophthalmoplegia and bulbar/respiratory weakness.
- A child with suspected infant botulism should be transferred urgently to a centre capable of undertaking long-term ventilation and providing specific therapies.

Spinal cord compression

- Persistent or severe back pain and stiffness are ominous symptoms requiring prompt attention.
- A myelopathy should always be considered when there is paraparesis or quadriparesis without neurological dysfunction at higher levels.
- Brisk deep tendon reflexes or extensor plantar responses may not be prominent early and a sensory level is often the most important clue to a myelopathy.
- The confirmation or exclusion of trauma, tumour, abscess, haematoma or skeletal pathology is an urgent priority.
- Spinal imaging with MRI is required urgently even when acute 'transverse' myelopathy is suspected.
- Steroid therapy is important in spinal cord compression, before surgical decompression.

Encephalopathies

- Encephalopathies are characterised predominantly (but not exclusively) by cerebral hemispheric dysfunction producing at least two of the following:
  - o Altered conscious state
  - o Altered cognitive state/personality
  - o Seizures
- Onset can be acute, subacute or chronic.
- Causes can be grouped into infective (or post-infective – see ADEM below), hypoxic, traumatic, epileptic, metabolic, migrainous, raised intracranial pressure and drug or toxin exposure. The primary cause may be systemic or originate in the CNS (see also chapter 25 Infectious diseases).

Clinical presentation

- Impaired conscious state or cognitive function (cardinal sign).
- There may be widespread upper motor neuron signs.
- Meningism may or may not be present.
  Investigations are guided by history and examination. Consider the following:
- Electrolytes
- Toxin and metabolic screen
- Lumbar Puncture (microscopy and culture; viral and mycoplasma PCR)
  (*Note*: for contra-indications to lumbar puncture see chapter 5 Procedures)
- EEG
- Neuroimaging: CT can exclude a mass lesion or acute bleed, but MRI is preferable in most circumstances.
  - o MRI brain & spinal cord may show multifocal demyelination in acute disseminated encephalomyelitis (ADEM).

Management

- Early specialist referral and neurosurgical involvement if raised intracranial pressure is suspected.
- Seizure control.
- Identify and treat the primary cause.
- Consider empiric antimicrobials, eg. cefotaxime and aciclovir.
- If ADEM suspected, consider high-dose IV corticosteroids.

Acute disseminated encephalomyelitis

ADEM is a monophasic inflammatory condition of the CNS that most commonly affects children and young adults. The usual presentation is with altered conscious state and multifocal neurological disturbance. It typically occurs following a viral prodrome and has been described following a variety of infections including measles, varicella, EBV, *Mycoplasma pneumoniae* as well as with non-specific febrile illnesses.

Clinical presentation & examination
- Prodrome of ataxia before onset is typical.
- Encephalopathy may vary in severity from irritability to coma.
- Multifocal neurological abnormalities such as ataxia, hemiparesis, optic neuritis, cranial nerve palsies and bladder dysfunction.
- A characteristic feature of ADEM is the evolution of symptoms and signs over time. New neurological symptoms and signs appear over the first few days (compared to other types of encephalitis where the onset is usually explosive without new manifestations after 24–48 hours).

Investigations
- MRI; usually demonstrates white matter changes (although grey matter involvement is not uncommon).

Management
- General principles as above.
- Steroids are used in the treatment of ADEM despite the lack of controlled studies to prove their efficacy.
  - Anecdotal evidence of their benefit is now strong.
  - Steroid therapy may improve the patient's condition
  - Withdrawal of treatment while the disease is still active may result in the return of original symptoms or the development of new symptoms.
- IVIG and plasma exchange can be used if response to steroids is suboptimal.
- Prognosis: Early studies indicate a mortality rate of up to 20% with a high incidence of neurological sequelae in those who survived.
  - Recent date suggests a more favourable prognosis, with most recovering fully.
  - Residual deficits in higher cognitive function may remain.

Chronic and recurrent headache
- Migraine is the most common identifiable cause of recurrent or chronic headache in childhood.
- In adolescence, muscle contraction (tension-type) headache is also common.
- Although rare, raised intracranial pressure and systemic illness must also be considered.

History
- Determine the location of headache and its quality, duration, frequency and time of onset.
- Identify trigger factors (food, sleep deprivation), associated symptoms (e.g. nausea or vomiting, visual disturbance and localising or focal symptoms) and the disruption to normal activities.
- Inquire as to whether the symptoms are progressive and if there is a history of recent head injury; development of visual, gait or coordination difficulties; or changes in personality or intellectual functioning; or a family history of migraine or cerebral tumours.
- Detailed social history and HEADDS screen in adolescent patients.
- Consider recording symptoms in a 'headache diary'.

Distinguishing / differentiating features
- *Tension headache (Chronic daily headaches):* tends to be persistent but usually does not interfere with sleep.
- *Migraine:* tends to have a fluctuating temporal pattern.
- *Migraine without aura:*
  - Usually frontotemporal, or bilateral in older children.
  - Frequently accompanied by nausea and vomiting initially, and followed by lethargy or sleep.
  - Marked pallor is common, and there is often a positive family history.
- *Migraine with aura or prolonged neurological symptoms:* uncommon in young children. Note that aura is not often reported by young children.
- *Intracranial pathology:* suggested by
  - Recurrent morning headaches
  - Headaches that are intense, prolonged and incapacitating or that show a progressive change in character over time.
  - Abnormal examination findings
  - Unusual migraine description and failure to respond to simple treatment measures.
  - *Such patients require urgent specialist referral.*

Examination
- Thorough neurological examination, including visual acuity and fields, eye movements, optic fundi, coordination and gait.
- Measure head circumference and blood pressure.
- Assess the child's growth and pubertal status.
- Inspect the skin for neurocutaneous stigmata.
- Palpate over the sinuses, cervical spine and teeth.
- Auscultate the skull for intracranial bruits.

Management of migraine
- Reassure the child and parents that migraine is not usually a serious condition.
- In an acute attack, all that is usually required is:
  - Trigger avoidance.
  - Stress management.
  - Early use of paracetamol 15 mg/kg per dose orally, 4 hourly (max. 90 mg/kg per 24 hours) and/or NSAIDs (e.g. ibuprofen 2.5–10 mg/kg per dose (max. 600 mg) oral 6–8 hourly).
  - If severe vomiting or unable to tolerate oral agents consider ondansetron, metoclopramide and chlorpromazine.
- Prophylactic therapy for those with severe or frequent attacks is best used in consultation with a specialist.
  - Propranolol or pizotifen are commonly used.
  - Sodium valproate, cyproheptadine, verapamil, clonidine and amitriptyline can also be effective in some children.
- Prognosis: Two-thirds of children cease having attacks but 50% of these will have recurrences in adult life.

Abnormal head shape and size
- Head shape and size are determined by intracranial components including brain tissue, cerebrospinal fluid and blood, and by the growth or lack thereof from the cranial sutures.
- The head grows rapidly in the first 12 months of life and serial measurements of occipital-frontal head circumference (OFC) are crucial to determine the need for and urgency of neuroimaging and other investigations.
- Measurement of both parental head circumferences is also important as benign familial macrocephaly is the most common cause of a large head in an otherwise normal child with no other indicators of hydrocephalus.
- Examination should include assessment of:
  - Head shape from above (for plagiocephaly, scaphocephaly, trigonocephaly or frontal bossing)
  - Head shape from the side (for brachycephaly)
  - Palpation of fontanelles, sutures size and auscultation for cranial bruits
- General inspection for dysmorphic features and a skin examination are important as they may provide clues to the underlying genetic causes.
- Fundoscopy to determine presence of papilloedema is essential, particularly when fontanelles are closed. *Note the absence of papilloedema does not exclude raised intracranial pressure.*

Abnormal head shape
Craniosynostosis is an uncommon disorder of childhood affecting 4/10,000 children. It is a condition of premature fusion of the cranial sutures resulting in an abnormal head shape. The resulting head shape depends on which suture fuses.
- The common shapes are:
  - Scaphocephaly (sagittal suture fusion)
  - Brachycephaly (coronal suture fusion)
  - Plagiocephaly (coronal or lambdoid suture fusion).
- Most cases are sporadic (non-syndromal) but rarely they occur in association with genetic conditions. Several of these syndromes are due to mutations in the fibroblast growth factor receptor (FGFR).
- Most children with posterior plagiocephaly have a postural deformation rather than craniosynostosis.
  - The incidence of postural (positional or deformational) plagiocephaly has increased with changes in sleeping position to prevent SIDS.
  - Children with developmental delay, abnormal bone quality or who spend longer times lying in a routine position are more likely to develop postural deformation.

Management depends upon aetiology:
- True sutural synostosis usually requires surgical correction.
- Posterior deformational plagiocephaly is not associated with fusion of sutures and does not require surgery.
  - It may partially correct spontaneously with changes in sleeping position and acquisition of motor skills allowing sitting.
  - The natural history of deformational plagiocephaly is for slow correction that continues until skeletal maturity.
  - In practice there is less concern about head shape with hair growth.

Microcephaly

Microcephaly is defined as an OFC more than 2 standard deviations below normal (i.e. below the 3rd percentile). Microcephaly can be divided into primary and secondary causes.
- In primary microcephaly the head is small at birth.
  - Causes include genetic disorders, disorders of early brain development (e.g. anencephaly, holoprosencephaly), neuronal migration and in-utero insults.
  - Dysmorphic features are clues to chromosomal disorders and microcephaly Vera.
- In secondary microcephaly, the OFC is typically normal at birth and slowed velocity of head growth becomes apparent in the first 3–6 months of life.
- Consideration should also be given to genetic craniosynostosis in which the head shape may not be abnormal if all sutures have fused.

Investigations
- MRI to assist with differentiating primary and secondary causes, identifying brain malformations, in utero or perinatal insults (including porencephaly, ischaemic or haemorrhagic stroke), and hypoxic ischaemic encephalopathy.
- Microarray should be performed in the absence of an identifiable peri- or post-natal insult.
- CMV testing on the Guthrie card should be requested

Clinical Pearl: Tips for assessment of head shape, fontanelles and cranial sutures
- Head shape should be assessed from above looking down onto the head, noting the general shape (normal is a mild tear drop shape), any asymmetry, and mobility (or fusion) of suture lines.
- The average age for closure of the anterior fontanelle is 12–18 months, but normal closure can range anywhere from 3–24 months.
- Absence of a 'soft spot' does not mean suture fusion. In a child with a normal head shape and normal growth along the centiles, the sutures may be aligned, open and growing.
- A large anterior fontanelle may be associated with vitamin D deficiency, metabolic bone disease, hypothyroidism, Down syndrome, rickets, syndromic craniosynostosis and raised intracranial pressure.
- In posterior (positional) plagiocephaly all structures on the deformed side are moved anteriorly (ear and potentially cheek) and the head assumes a parallelogram shape when viewed from above.
- In lamboid synostosis the affected side is constricted and there is contralateral compensatory growth giving a rhomboid shape with the ear in the normal position or posterior.

Macrocephaly

Macrocephaly is defined as an OFC more than 2 standard deviations above normal (i.e. above the 98th percentile).
- **Benign familial macrocephaly** is most common cause of a large head in otherwise normal infants. Serial OFC measurements typically show acceleration of head growth above the 98th percentile in the second six months of life followed by stabilisation in the second year of life.
- **Benign enlargement of the subarachnoid spaces (BESS)** is a relatively common cause of macrocephaly. Neuroimaging shows widening of the frontal subarachnoid spaces and normal ventricular size allows differentiation from cerebral atrophy.
- **Hydrocephalus** is the most important differential diagnosis, and can be divided into (i) Non-communicating hydrocephalus due to aqueductal stenosis or lesions obstructing CSF outflow, or

(ii) Communicating hydrocephalus due usually to failure of reabsorption at the level of the arachnoid granulations (which may occur following meningitis or subarachnoid haemorrhage) or very rarely to excessive CSF production (due to choroid plexus papilloma).
Urgent neuroimaging is essential in suspected hydrocephalus.
* **A large brain (megalencephaly)** may occur in the context of neurocutaneous syndromes such as neurofibromatosis or tuberous sclerosis, in genetic disorders such as Sotos syndrome or in rare metabolic disorders (including Alexander or Canavan disease).

Childhood stroke

Childhood stroke is more common than brain malignancy and is among the top ten causes of morbidity in childhood. More than half of survivors have long-term neurological impairment and 10–20% suffer recurrent strokes.
Subtypes include:
* Arterial ischaemic stroke (AIS)
* Cerebral sinovenous thrombosis (CSVT)
* Haemorrhagic stroke (HS)

Aetiology
* Arteriopathies
  ○ Transient; e.g. focal cerebral arteriopathy due to inflammation or infection (HSV and varicella), cervical or intracranial arterial dissection
  ○ Progressive; e.g. Moyamoya disease in AIS
* Congenital heart disease in AIS and CSVT
* Thrombophilias in AIS and CSVT
* Head and neck/ENT infections in CSVT
* Metabolic/mitochondrial disorders; e.g. homocystinuria
* Genetic conditions; e.g. Down Syndrome
* Haematological conditions; e.g. sickle cell disease

Clinical features
* Neonates: typically have non-specific presentation with seizures in the vast majority of cases, lethargy, apnoea. Focal neurological signs are rarely evident.
* Older infants and children: typically present with focal weakness, visual or speech disturbances, limb incoordination or ataxia (all more common in AIS), altered consciousness, acute headache with other neurological signs or symptoms or signs of raised intracranial pressure (all more common in HS).
* Patients with CSVT commonly present with seizures and signs of raised intracranial pressure.
* Older infants can also present with early hand preference due to clinically silent perinatal event (congenital hemiplegia).

Diagnosis
Urgent imaging is critical to confirm stroke diagnosis and guide management.
* In suspected haemorrhagic stroke, urgent non-contrast CT should be performed.
* In suspected arterial ischaemic stroke, urgent brain MRI and MRA should be performed.
  ○ Where urgent MRI is not possible within 30 minutes, CT (including CT angiography) should be performed.
* FBC, coagulation profile, UEC, glucose, LFTs, blood group and hold (to determine eligibility for reperfusion therapies (tPA and clot retrieval).
* ECG and transthoracic echocardiogram; to look for structural cardiac defects including patent foramen ovale (PFO) with paradoxical embolization.
* Prothrombotic workup – should be done *before* anticoagulation, and includes antithrombin, protein C, protein S, plasminogen, activated protein C resistance (APCR), prothrombin gene 20210 A, anticardiolipin antibody (ACLA), lupus anticoagulant, serum homocysteine.

Management

General measures shown to improve outcome in adults are likely to be beneficial in children and include:

- Maintain normothermia, normoglycaemia and normal blood pressure.
- Keep SaO$_2$ >93% in the first 24 hours.
- Close observations (hourly neurological observations initially).
- Maintain nil by mouth until assessment by speech pathologist.
- If seizures occurring; load with IV phenytoin or levetiracetam (or phenobarbitone in neonates).
- Early referral to a rehabilitation team should be made once child clinically stable.
- Discuss acute antiplatelet/anticoagulant treatment with the Neurologist and Haematologist on call.

Antithrombotic therapies
For neonates with AIS

- Cardioembolic AIS: Aspirin or anticoagulation is recommended for 6–12 weeks.
- Non-cardioembolic AIS: Do **not** use anticoagulation or aspirin unless there are recurrent events.

For children with AIS

- Reperfusion therapies may be appropriate in specific children but administration is time critical:
  - Alteplase within 4.5 hours of symptom onset.
  - Mechanical clot retrieval within 6 hours of symptom onset.
  - Acute treatment decisions should be coordinated by paediatric Neurology in consultation with paediatric Emergency department and Haematology.
- Initial secondary preventative measures: aspirin, 1–5 mg/kg per day, UFH or LMWH whilst being investigated for cardioembolic sources and vascular dissection.
- Continue LMWH or warfarin for another 3–6 months if dissection or cardioembolic source are confirmed.
- Conversion to aspirin, 1 to 5 mg/kg day is recommended for all other children for a minimum of 2 years.
- For children with sickle cell disease and arterial ischaemic stroke, initially treat with IV hydration and exchange transfusion to reduce the HbS levels to <30% total haemoglobin.

For children with CSVT

- Anticoagulation is usually recommended, except if associated with a significant haemorrhage, the patient is hypertensive or other risks for bleeding are present.
- For CSVT *without* significant intracranial haemorrhage, anticoagulation:
  - Initially with UFH or LMWH.
  - Subsequently with LMWH or warfarin for a minimum of 3 months (neonates 6 weeks to 3 months).
- For CSVT *with* significant intracranial haemorrhage:
  - Radiological monitoring at 5–7 days and anticoagulation if thrombus propagation occurs.

Head injuries
Assessment

- Determine the mechanism of the injury, its severity, the time of occurrence and the clinical course before the consultation.
- Always consider inflicted injury (abuse) in infants and young children with head injury (see Chapter 20, Forensic medicine).
- Assessment using the Glasgow coma scale is essential, once age appropriate (Table 29.3).
- General and neurological examination findings will provide a baseline for further assessment and must be carefully recorded. In the unconscious patient the presence of brain stem signs must be assessed.
- In all but minor cases of head injury, cervical spine injury must be assumed until excluded.

Radiological examination

- Skull radiograph: generally replaced by low dose CT scan.
- Cervical spine radiograph: necessary when there is a suggestion that the spine may have been injured and in all patients with moderate-to-severe head injuries.

Table 29.3 Level of consciousness – Glasgow coma scale.

Eye opening		Verbal response (modifications for small children in italics)		Motor response	
Spontaneous	4	Orientated *Appropriate words or social smile, fixes, follows*	5	Obeys commands	6
To speech	3	Confused *Cries but consolable*	4	Localises to stimuli Withdraws to stimuli	5 4
To pain	2	Inappropriate words *Persistently irritable*	3	Abnormal flexion	3
Nil	1	Incomprehensible words *Restless and agitated*	2	Extensor responses	2
		Nil	1	Nil	1

- Brain CT scan: indicated in patients with significant head injury, particularly if there is the possibility of an intracranial haematoma, as suggested by severe headache and vomiting, a depressed conscious state or focal neurological signs. Care is taken to avoid CT of the brain in the neonate due to the radiation exposure, as such MRI may be indicated.
- Brain MRI: indicated if there is suspicion of a brainstem injury, a spinal cord injury or a vascular injury or anomaly.

Blunt head injury

This form of injury is due to a non-penetrating impact that often produces an acceleration-deceleration type of injury. Spectrum of injury includes:

- **Scalp haematoma:** common in the infant or young child. They may be responsible for a significant reduction in the circulating blood volume.
- **Skull fracture:** significant injuries may not necessarily have a skull fracture, but the majority do. Conversely, a skull fracture may not be associated with significant brain injury. The fracture is usually linear and it may extend to the skull base. In the immature skull the bone often deforms at the point of impact and fractures at the margins running perpendicular to the cranial sutures. The involvement of the nasal, paranasal or middle ear spaces implies that the injury is compound, with a risk of infection. Check for CSF rhinorrhoea or otorrhoea. There is no evidence for prophylactic antibiotics for a fracture communicating with the paranasal or mastoid sinuses.
- **Concussion:** the most common type of traumatic brain injury, usually not requiring intervention. Involves transient loss of brain function, such as loss of awareness or memory of the event. The duration of unconsciousness is an indicator of the severity of the concussion.
- **Localised brain damage:** this is due to either local deformity at impact (which is not generally an important factor except for some injuries in infancy) or surface laceration of the brain due to brain movement within the skull.
- **Intracranial haemorrhage:** subarachnoid and subdural haemorrhages are usually due to a surface laceration of the brain. In extradural haemorrhage, a dural vessel is torn by distortion at or near the point of impact, especially if on the lateral aspect of the head.
- **Intracerebral haemorrhage:** may result from local damage or a shearing injury within the brain.

Clinical course

- **Scalp Haematoma:** spontaneously resolves but appear to enlarge as the collection liquefies. Delayed presentation at the point of the haematoma liquefying is not uncommon.
- **Fracture:** Undisplaced fractures of the skull will heal within 6-12 weeks without intervention. Caution should be taken regarding contact sports and high risk activities in the interim. In neonates and infants they can be complicated by growing skull fractures and as such a clinical review by Neurosurgery (no imaging) at least 6 weeks post injury is recommended.
- **Concussion:** Most patients rapidly recover from the effects of concussion in 12–24 hours. A delay or reversal of recovery suggests haemorrhage, brain swelling, infection or an extracranial complication – most commonly an impairment of ventilation, with hypercarbia leading to brain swelling.

Management
Mild
- A brief loss of consciousness (<5 minutes) without other neurological symptoms or signs suggests a mild head injury and these patients can be sent home after an initial 4-hour observation in emergency.
- Explanation and written information must be given to the parents regarding signs suggesting deterioration and indications for re-presentation (Table 29.4).
- The patient should be reviewed the following day, either by the local medical officer or in the emergency department.
- The Child SCAT5 is an online resource with concussion checklists for health practitioners, and handout sheets for families on how to best manage concussion.

Moderate – Severe
A more severe head injury is indicated by
- A longer period of unconsciousness.
- Increasingly severe headache with or without vomiting.
- A deterioration in conscious state, behaviour or vital signs.
- Neurological defects.
- Bleeding or CSF leak from the nose or ear.
- Severe bleeding from a scalp wound.
- A superficial haematoma on the side of the head. This may be associated with an extradural haematoma, even if no fracture is seen on the radiograph.

Children with these signs will require assessment and usually CT scanning. In the absence of scanning these patients should be observed carefully for at least 48 hours.

Delayed presentation
This can be grouped into four categories:
- Clinical features of potentially serious head injuries – admit.
- Patients with a wide linear fracture and a large scalp haematoma – Neurosurgical consultation for potential admission.
- Patients with a skull radiograph showing a narrow linear fracture, but who do not require admission on clinical grounds – discuss with a neurosurgeon and consider early involvement of a paediatrician.
- Apparently well patients – send home after appropriate advice, with instructions to return immediately if there is any deterioration.

Seizures and Head Injury
Seizures are a common response of the immature brain and are not predictive of subsequent epilepsy. Self limiting seizures at the time or within the first few hours following injury are not usually treated with anticonvulsants unless there is another risk factor such as a bleed or cortical laceration.

Penetrating head injury
In these injuries the damage is predominantly confined to a focal area of the head, however there may still have been an acceleration/deceleration component. These all require neurosurgical consultation, and there is a spectrum of presentations:
- Simple or compound depressed fractures are common.
- Infection may occur with compound injuries, but is delayed in its presentation.

Table 29.4 Mild head injuries: discharge instructions for parents.

For the next 24 hours keep a careful watch over the patient, who should be roused at least every 2 hours. The child must be reassessed immediately if you notice any of the following:
- The child becomes unconscious or more difficult to rouse.
- The child becomes confused, irrational or delirious.
- There are convulsions or spasms of the face and limbs.
- The child complains of persistent headache or has neck stiffness.
- Repeated vomiting.
- Bleeding from the ear or recurrent watery discharge from the ear or nose.

- Focal contusion or laceration of the brain may be present to a varying size or depth, and may produce neurological signs or seizures.
- Concussion may be absent.

Management
- Radiographs now replaced by low dose CT typically with 3D reconstruction as it allows assessment of associated injury such as bleeds/ intracranial air or parenchymal injury.
- Admission for neurosurgical assessment and monitoring is required in most cases.
- Prophylactic antibiotics are not routinely indicated.
- External compound head injuries: should receive antibiotics (flucloxacillin IV; also add gentamicin IV and metronidazole IV if there was contamination) and the wound covered by a head dressing. Consideration should also be given to the need for tetanus vaccination.
- Internal compound fractures (base of skull) with CSF leaks: should be initially observed and referred to Neurosurgery. At discharge it is important to educate about clinical signs of CSF leak and the need for medical attention with associated febrile illness.

Care of the unconscious patient
- Maintain the airway.
- Observe for vital and basal neurological signs.
- Protect the cervical spine.
- Ensure temperature regulation.
- Fluid and electrolyte balance.
- Nasogastric aspiration to avoid the inhalation of gastric contents (orogastric if the base of the skull is definitely or possibly fractured).

Anticipate complications
- Early evaluation essential to assess the development of complications such as compression and infection.
- Observing for complications associated with extracranial injury is also important.
- The patient who is not improving should be referred to a neurosurgeon.

Shunt Malfunction
Common causes include:
- *Obstruction:* the shunt may become blocked in either of the catheters (proximal or distal) or at the level of the valve. Obstruction may be from choroid plexus in the ventricular catheter, by blood or debris in the valve or by omentum in the peritoneum.
- *Fracture/dislocation:* with growth or movement the shunt may dislodge at insertion site or connections and with calcification around the components may fracture.
- *Infection:* usually occurs in proximity to shunt surgery or percutaneous tapping of a shunt. In atrial catheters infection can occur with a bacteremia and in peritoneal catheters may occur with peritonitis. Spontaneous infection of a shunt remote from surgery or other infection is very rare.

Symptoms
- Headache
- Drowsiness
- Vomiting
- The same symptoms as a previous episode(s)
- *Neck pain is an ominous sign and may indicate tonsillar herniation*
- Seizures are not are sign of shunt malfunction or raised pressure, but pressure waves may cause tonic posturing that can be mistaken for a seizure.

Pertinent clinical signs include:
- Increased fontanelle tension
- Focal neurological signs
- Change in vital signs
- Deterioration in conscious state

- Increasing head circumference in a child with open sutures
- Sunsetting eyes (upward gaze limitation)

Specific

- *Shunt Palpation:* many shunt systems now do not have a depressible reservoir. Palpation of the shunt cannot assess the patency of the system but may identify localized swelling or discontinuity of the catheter.
- *Cellulitis or infection:* the course of the shunt should be inspected for signs of overlying cellulitis or skin changes
- The type of shunt should be identified: VP (peritoneal) or VA (atrial) and any information on the shunt type and insertion/revision history if records are available.
- The presence of any intercurrent or other illness may be significant.

Clinical Pearl: Neuroimaging in suspected shunt malfunction

Historically possible shunt malfunction was investigated with a shunt series x-ray and a CT brain, which led to significant radiation exposure over the shunt lifetime. Such imaging is now not routinely ordered prior to full assessment. Consideration is given to using ultrasound in children with open fontanelles and even occasionally limited sequence MRI scans to reduce radiation exposure in young children. In particular, *shunt series X-rays are generally now only indicated when a decision has been made to take a shunt to theatre at the discretion of the treating surgeon.*

USEFUL RESOURCES

- Royal Children's Hospital epilepsy program http://www.rch.org.au/cep/; includes information about epilepsy, tests, treatments, proformas for seizure diary and management plans, and links to other resources.
- US National Headache Foundation https://headaches.org/resources/; information and links to headache resources.
- SCAT 5 proforma for health professionals https://bjsm.bmj.com/content/bjsports/early/2017/04/26/bjsports-2017-097492childscat5.full.pdf; free standardized tool for the evaluation of concussion in children aged 5–12y.

CHAPTER 30

Oncology

Diane Hanna
Rachel Conyers

Key Points

- Cancer in childhood is relatively rare but the expectation is cure for most cancers.
- Collaborative international clinical trials with optimized chemotherapeutic combinations and aggressive supportive care have improved clinical outcomes.
- Live virus vaccines must not be given to immunocompromised children.
- A neutrophil count of $<0.5 \times 10^6$/L (and particularly $<0.1 \times 10^9$/L) is associated with a significantly increased risk of bacteraemia; the longer the duration of neutropenia, the higher the risk of infection.
- Approximately 80% of children and adolescents who receive a diagnosis of cancer now become long-term survivors; who subsequently have a higher risk of chronic health conditions that require long term follow up and surveillance.

Presentation of childhood malignancies

Approximately 1 in 600 children will develop a malignancy before the age of 15 years. Malignancy should be considered in children presenting with any of the following:

- Fever, pallor, bruising or petechiae, bone pain.
- Lymphadenopathy – marked, progressive or persistent, localised or generalized.
- Hepatosplenomegaly.
- Recurring morning headache, particularly if associated with vomiting or visual disturbance.
- Ataxia, cranial nerve palsies, or other neurological signs; particularly when associated with headache or back pain.
- New onset of dry cough, or stridor, without other symptoms of respiratory infection, particularly if associated with orthopnoea.
- Any unusual mass or swelling.
- Persistent severe unexplained pain, especially involving bones or joints.
- Unexplained weight loss.

When suspicion of a malignancy arises, investigations should be undertaken in consultation with a paediatric oncologist.

Paediatric Handbook, Tenth Edition. Edited by Kate Harding, Daniel S. Mason and Daryl Efron.
© 2021 John Wiley & Sons Ltd. Published 2021 by John Wiley & Sons Ltd.

> **Putting the Science into Practice: Precision oncology**
> We are in the era of precision oncology, which includes molecular characterization for prognostication and novel and targeted therapy; host pharmacogenomics to predict and limit toxicity; and response based risk stratification.

Oncological emergencies

Emergency presentations (Table 30.1) include:

- Mass lesions: mediastinal masses (solid or liquid tumours), superior mediastinal syndrome, spinal cord compression, increased intracranial pressure (ICP)
- Haematologic/metabolic: hyperleukocytosis, tumour lysis syndrome (TLS), cerebrovascular accident (CVA)
- Immunosuppression: typhlitis

CNS tumours

- CNS tumours comprise approximately 20% of all childhood cancers (gliomas most common).
- Most CNS tumours (80–90%) originate in the supratentorial area (cerebral hemispheres or midline), but are infrequently located in the posterior fossa (3–12%) and spinal cord (5–10%).
- Causes of brain tumours largely unknown; certain autosomal genetic predisposition syndromes are associated with an increased risk including:
  - Neurofibromatosis type I (NF1 gene mutation)
  - Li-Fraumeni syndrome (TP53 gene mutation)
  - Turcot syndrome (APC gene mutation)
- Previous exposure to ionising radiation associated with malignant gliomas.

Clinical features

The presentation of brain tumours varies and depends largely on the age of the patient and tumour location. Compared with low-grade tumours, high-grade tumours tend to have a shorter interval of symptoms.

- Children with high-grade tumours frequently also present with symptoms related to raised ICP, including headache, nausea, and vomiting, which are classically worse in the morning.
- Infants present with non-specific symptoms, particularly developmental delay or regression of previously attained developmental milestones. If an infant's cranial sutures have not fused, they may present with an increasing head circumference and/or hydrocephalus.
- **Supratentorial tumours:** localised signs, such as hemiparesis or seizures; alterations in personality, mood changes, and declining school performance.
- **Posterior fossa tumours:** symptoms of raised increased ICP due to compression of the fourth ventricle, including headache, emesis, lethargy, behavioural changes and deterioration in school performance, and signs of obstructive hydrocephalus such as ataxia or torticollis.
- **Brainstem tumours:** cranial nerve palsies (VI and VII are the most commonly affected; infants with bulbar nerve involvement may present with failure to thrive); signs of long tract involvement; ataxia. Hydrocephalus is rare (<10%).
- **Cervicomedullary tumours:** signs of long tract involvement; no ataxia or cranial nerve involvement.

Table 30.1 Presentation, differential diagnosis and management of oncological emergencies.

Emergency	Presentation	Differential diagnosis	Management
Superior mediastinal syndrome (SVC)	Orthopnoea, cough, shortness of breath, respiratory arrest Venous engorgement: facial swelling, plethora, syncope	NHL – B or T Hodgkin lymphoma Acute lymphoblastic leukaemia(ALL); Acute myeloid leukaemia (AML) Germ cell tumour Thymoma Neuroblastoma Sarcoma	*Investigations:* CXR – wide mediastinum, tracheal deviation, narrowing CT chest Echocardiogram *Treatment:* Airway – use least invasive method with minimal sedation. VC heparinisation/thrombectomy, IV access (femoral) Tumour – steroids and chemotherapy (CTx).
Spinal cord compression	Back pain (80%) – especially if pain has radicular component or is not relieved in supine position Neurologic signs - weakness, sensory abnormalities, urinary and faecal incontinence or retention	Any tumour type. Most commonly: Neuroblastoma Sarcoma Leukaemia/lymphoma CNS tumour/ metastases	*Investigations:* MRI spine – contrast will show intra-spinal lesion. *Treatment:* Dexamethasone 0.25–0.5 mg/kg q.i.d. • If <80% compression: dexamethasone + radiotherapy (XRT) or CTx • If ≥80% compression: dexamethasone + XRT or surgery (laminectomy)
Hyperleukocytosis (WCC >100,000 cells/ mm³)	CNS leukostasis: headache, mental status change, seizures, coma, death *Note:* risk of intracranial haemorrhage if thrombocytopenic or coagulopathic. Pulmonary leukostasis: Triad of respiratory symptoms, hypoxia and infiltrates on CXR. *Note:* risk of pulmonary haemorrhage.	ALL – higher risk of tumour lysis syndrome AML – higher risk of hyperviscosity	*Treatment:* Hyperhydration (decrease hyperviscosity) Avoid diuretics initially Avoid PRBCs (increases hyperviscosity) Keep plts >20,000/mm³ and treat coagulopathy *Note:* FFP/cryoprecipitate do not increase overall viscosity Cytoreduction (lower WCC): CTx Leukapheresis: less commonly used as it produces a transient effect and does not reduce the risk of TLS
Tumour lysis syndrome (dying cell release their contents into blood stream spontaneously or in response to therapy	Hyperuricaemia → renal uric acid deposition, lethargy, nausea/vomiting, renal toxicity, CNS dysfunction Hyperkalaemia Hyperphosphataemia Hypocalcaemia Electrolyte abnormalities can cause renal insufficiency, cardiac arrhythmias, seizures and death due to multiorgan failure.	Tumours with a high rate of cell death: Burkitt lymphoma ALL ⊠AML	*Investigations:* Frequent blood monitoring *Treatment:* Hydration (with no potassium) at 1.5–2× maintenance or 125 ml/m2 /h ± NHCO3. Urine alkalinisation: aim for urine pH 7–8. CaPO4 Low risk: Allopurinol (xanthine oxidase) prevents hypoxanthine becoming xanthine and in turn, uric acid. High risk/established TLS: urate oxidase/rasburicase breaks down uric acid to allantoin which can be easily excreted.
Typhlitis (neutropenic enterocolitis)	Nausea, diarrhoea Fever	Most common in patients with leukaemia or lymphoma, especially after cytarabine.	*Investigations:* AXR/US Abdomen: pneumatosis, paucity of air, bowel wall oedema ±Abdominal CT *Treatment:* Nil orally IV antibiotics (enteric organism coverage)

Table 30.2 Leukemia and lymphoma.

	Acute lymphoblastic leukaemia (ALL) / Non-Hodgkin lymphoma (NHL)	Acute myeloid leukaemia (AML)
Background	ALL and NHL: family of genetically heterogeneous lymphoid neoplasms derived from B- (80%) & T-lymphoid progenitors (15%). Lymphoblastic leukaemia implies >25% bone marrow involvement; lymphoma is <25%. ALL is the most common cancer (30%) in children with a peak age of 2–5 years.	AML: group of relatively well-defined haematopoietic neoplasms involving precursor cells committed to the myeloid line of cellular development Childhood AML is a rare disease occurring in children < 15 years.
Aetiology	• Clonal proliferation of lymphoid progenitor cells, Accumulation of leukemic blasts or immature forms results in variable reduction in the production of normal red blood cells, platelets, and mature granulocytes. • Cause unknown. • Certain genetic syndromes have a higher incidence: including trisomy 21 (T21), neurofibromatosis type 1 (NF1), Bloom syndrome and ataxia-telangiectasia.	• Clonal proliferation of myeloid precursors with reduced capacity to differentiate. Accumulation of blasts as described in ALL. • Associated with genetic abnormalities including T21 and Fanconi anaemia.
Clinical features	*ALL:* Presenting symptoms and signs reflect bone marrow infiltration and extramedullary disease. History: • Bone pain, limp, refusal to weight bear • Fatigue, pallor • Easy bruising, bleeding, petechiae and fever/infection • If CNS involvement – headache, nausea, vomiting, irritability Examination • Lymphadenopathy >1cm, hepatosplenomegaly • Testicular involvement (painless, unilateral enlargement) *Note:* T-ALL often occurs in older boys with a large anterior mediastinal mass. *NHL:* mediastinal mass and/or matted lymphadenopathy	See ALL *Note:* Palpable lymphadenopathy and hepatosplenomegaly is uncommon (<20%)
Investigations	• FBE + film – anaemia, thrombocytopenia, neutropenia, peripheral blasts. • Bone marrow aspirate +/– trephine (BMAT). • CXR – for mediastinal mass. • If suspected NHL – excisional biopsy of the abnormal lymph node. • Consider LP	See ALL
Treatment	Current CTx protocols achieve an overall cure rate >80% in children *ALL:* Patients with ALL require prolonged Ctx (2–3 years) Pre-B ALL, T ALL/NHL: Tumour lysis syndrome or the presence of a mediastinal mass should be regarded as an oncological emergency (Table 30.1)	Improvements in supportive care have had a major impact on increased survival rates in childhood AML. Immunosuppression a/w significant morbidity and mortality from infection. Hyperleukocytosis and APML is a medical emergencies due to haemorrhage risk (Table 30.1).

Leukaemia and lymphoma
See Table 30.2.

Clinical Pearl: Transient leukemia in Trisomy 21

- A proportion of newborns (5%) with T21 have transient leukaemia (aka transient abnormal myelopoiesis (TAM) or transient myeloproliferative disorder).
- This condition usually resolves spontaneously, however can progress.
- Within the first 4 years of life 10–20% of these infants will develop myeloid leukaemia.

Bone tumours

See Table 30.3.

Table 30.3 Bone tumours.

	Osteosarcoma	Ewing's sarcoma
Background	Most common primary bone tumour. Predilection for age of pubertal growth spurt and sites of maximum growth. Cause: • Unknown in most • Exposure to radiation or alkylating agents • Increased risk with inherited disorders associated with alterations of tumour suppressor genes (eg. hereditary retinoblastoma, Li-Fraumeni syndrome)	Second most common primary bone tumour. Aggressive form of childhood cancer. 25% arise in soft tissues rather than bone. Cause: unknown
Clinical features	• Can occur in any bone – most commonly metaphyses of long bones (distal femur, proximal tibia, and proximal humerus). • 85% have localised disease and present with pain, swelling, limitation of joint movement, pathological fractures. • 15% present with radiographic metastases (lung, bone, rarely lymph nodes and soft tissue).	• Most common sites – bones of the pelvis, lower extremities, chest wall, axial skeleton. In long bones, they tend to arise from the diaphyseal–metaphyseal portion. • 75% localised disease. • 25% present with metastases (lung, bone, bone marrow most commonly). • Constitutional symptoms due to metastatic disease (malaise, fever, anorexia and weight loss).
Diagnosis	• X-ray – osteoblastic, osteolytic or mixed appearance of bone. Soft tissue patchy calcifications. A triangular area of periosteal calcification at the border of tumour and healthy tissue is known *as Codman triangle* – this is typical for osteosarcomas. • MRI – this should include the entire involved bone as well as the neighbouring joints, so as to not miss skip lesions. • Open or imaging guided biopsy.	• MRI – include the entire involved bone or compartment. • Imaging-guided core biopsy without fixation.

Treatment	• Local therapy alone is insufficient, as 80–90% of all patients with seemingly localised disease will develop metastases.
	• Current treatment regimens include
	  ○ Primary (preoperative; neoadjuvant) induction CTx
	  ○ Definite surgery – aim for complete tumour removal – postoperative (adjuvant) CTx leads to cure in approximately two-thirds of patients with seemingly localised disease
	• Approximately 30% of all patients with primary metastatic osteosarcoma and >40% of those who achieve a complete surgical remission can become long-term survivors.
		• Complete local control with surgery (preferred) and/or RTX is imperative for curative treatment + CTx.
		• The use of CTx has greatly improved survival rates for patients with localised ES from approximately 10 to 70–80%.

Table 30.4 Abdominal tumour differentiation.

	Neuroblastoma	Wilms tumour
Symptoms	Pain, Anemia	Abdominal mass
Mean age (months)	22	39
Predisposing syndromes	Rare	Frequent
Frequency metastasis	70%	10%
Site metastasis	Bones, bone marrow	Lung, liver
Prognostic factors	Age, biology, histology, stage	Stage, histology

Abdominal tumours

The two most common abdominal tumours in children are Neuroblastoma (NB: tumour of the sympathetic chain and adrenal gland) and Wilms tumour (WT: renal tumour). See Table 30.4.

Neuroblastoma

- NB are mainly localised in the abdomen but can occur anywhere along the sympathetic chain (neck, thorax, pelvis).
- It is the most common solid tumour outside the brain, and most frequent in infants.
- Some tumours in infants demonstrate spontaneous regression even if metastatic (Stage 4 S).
- The main prognostic factors are the age (better prognosis <18 months), the stage (localised or metastatic NB), the biology (amplification of MYCN, ploidy).

Clinical features

- If localized: abdominal mass, signs of spinal cord compression.
- In infants metastases are localised to the skin (blue tumours) and the liver (hepatomegaly).
- In older children, symptoms are related to metastases in bone marrow/bone (pain, fever, anaemia).

Investigations

- Urinary catecholamines (24 hours collection) positive in 90% of the cases.
- CT/MRI.
- A biopsy (or surgical resection) of the primary tumour is needed to obtain a definitive diagnosis and determine prognostic factors (histology, biology).

Treatment

- Surgical resection ± CTx.
- Prognosis is good in localised NB with favourable biology with a 5-year overall survival (OS) greater than 90%. In infants, with a small tumour detected by systematic ultrasound, NB may be safely observed as spontaneous regression can occur.

Wilms tumour

- WT is the second most common abdominal tumour and the most common renal tumour in children.
- 10% of children with WT have other abnormalities.
- Syndromes associated with WT include:
  - Overgrowth syndromes (Beckwith–Wiedemann syndrome, isolated hemihypertrophy, Sotos syndrome)
  - Non-overgrowth syndrome (WAGR syndrome – Wilms tumour, aniridia, genitourinary malformation and mental retardation).

Clinical features

- Well child with massive abdominal tumour.
- Severe hypertension.

Investigations
- On ultrasound, the tumour arises from the kidney
- Local and metastatic evaluation is done by a thoraco-abdominal CT scan. It confirms the renal tumour and assesses the contralateral kidney, patency of renal vein and inferior vena cava, lymph nodes, lungs and liver.
- Tumour markers (AFP, HCG, urinary catecholamines) are negative.

Treatment
- CTx + surgery at week 4.

Supportive care guidelines
Aggressive supportive care improves clinical outcomes.

Blood products
Blood products should be irradiated and leukodepleted.

Packed red blood cells (PRBC)
- Transfusion with PRBC indicated to correct Hb <70 g/L (aim for Hb 100–120), symptomatic anaemia or acute blood loss.
- Formula: amount required in mL = Desired rise in Hb (g/L) × Wt (kg) × 0.5
- Each unit PRBC is 200–250 mL.

Platelets (Plts)
- Transfusion with platelets is indicated to correct bleeding manifestations. Indications may include:
  - Plts <10,000/L without bleeding.
  - Plts <20,000/L if febrile or mucosal bleeding.
  - Plts <30,000/L prior to lumbar puncture or if brain tumour.
  - Plts <70,000/L prior to any other surgical procedure.
- Use apheresed platelets only if you anticipate the need for long-term support to minimise exposure to multiple donors.
- *Formula: one pedipack (approximately 50mL) per 10 kg up to 40 kg or 10–15 mL/kg.*

Infection
Risk factors for infection in immunocompromised patients are:
- Neutropenia: A neutrophil count of <0.5 × 10^6/L is associated with a significantly increased risk of bacteraemia. This risk is markedly increased with a neutrophil count <0.1 × 10^9/L. The longer the duration of neutropenia, the higher the risk of infection.
- Lymphopenia is associated with increased risk of opportunistic infection such as *Pneumocystis jirovecii* and reactivation of herpes simplex and herpes zoster viruses.
- Steroid therapy is a risk factor for invasive fungal infection.
- Central venous catheter: (CVC): Most children receiving chemotherapy have either a Hickman catheter (externalized CVC) or an infusaport (subcutaneous catheter).
- Breaches of the normal skin and mucosal barriers, particularly in heavily colonised sites around the perineum, in the mouth, nose and lower gastrointestinal tract, allow organisms' access to the bloodstream.

Febrile neutropenia
Fever and neutropenia (FN) are common complications in children who receive chemotherapy for cancer. It is associated with significant morbidity and mortality. Causes of an initial fever in a neutropenic child may be bacterial, viral, or fungal.
Definition:
- A temperature between 38.0–38.5°C twice in 1 hour, or ≥38.5 ° C on a single occasion and absolute neutrophil count (ANC) <500/µL or 1000/mm^3.

Assessment and management
- Initial management influenced by many factors, such as patient characteristics, clinical presentation, drug availability and cost, and local epidemiology, including resistance patterns.

- Careful clinical assessment and blood cultures essential.
- *Empiric antibiotics* are routinely indicated and should be administered down all lumens of the CVC without delay (see Appendix: Antimicrobial guidelines and RCH febrile neutropenia clinical practice guidelines http://www.rch.org.au/clinicalguide/guideline index/ Febrile Neutropenia/)
- Initial empiric antibiotics should be rationalised to include the clinically or microbiologically documented infection. It is reasonable to cease antimicrobials when the child is afebrile, there is platelet recovery and the absolute neutrophil count >100/uL and rising.
- Empiric antifungal therapy should be initiated for invasive fungal disease (IFD) in high-risk neutropenic patients after 96 hours of fever in the setting of broad-spectrum antibiotics. It should be continued until resolution of neutropenia (ANC >100–500/µL) in the absence of documented or suspected IFD.

Pneumocystis jirovecii pneumonia prophylaxis

- All patients should receive trimethoprim/sulfamethoxazole (TMP/SMX) at a dose of TMP 2.5 mg/kg/dose (maximum dose 160 mg/dose) orally twice daily on 2 or 3 sequential days per week.
- Consider *Pneumocystis jirovecii* pneumonia in an at-risk patient who presents with tachypnoea, lowered oxygen saturations and/or diffuse opacities on chest radiograph.

Infectious disease contacts in immunosuppressed patients

- Varicella and measles may lead to very severe illness in immunocompromised children.
- Measles: no effective antiviral agent is available and it may cause fatal pneumonitis. Although immunity may wane during chemotherapy, prior vaccination or infection is usually protective.
  - Give normal human immunoglobulin (NHIG) for measles contact within 72 hours
  - Dose: 0.25 mL/kg IM daily for 2 days.
- Varicella: if the patient's immune status is not known or negative, give zoster immunoglobulin (ZIG) for varicella contact at dose of:
  - Weight <20 kg or <5 years of age: 250 mg IM (1 × 2 mL/125 IU vial).
  - Weight, 20–40 kg or 5–10 years of age: 500 mg IM (2 × 2 mL/125 IU vial).
  - Weight >40 kg or age >10 years: 750 mg IM (3 × 2 mL/125 IU vials).

Long term line management

- Hickman catheters or port-a-caths are often required for administration of chemotherapeutic agents as well as supportive care
- In the setting of fever they require access and blood cultures to be taken to exclude a possible line infection
- If a line infection is identified, please obtain specialist infectious diseases advice regarding targeted antimicrobial treatment. In some cases the line needs to be removed.

Management of mucositis/perirectal cellulitis

- IV hydration and/or parenteral nutrition
- Effective analgesia (topical lignocaine gel and opioids such as oxycodone or morphine)
- Anti-infective therapy as indicated
- Salt baths
- Strong barrier cream (Calmoseptine cream)
- Mouthcare with Curasept

Antiemetic prophylaxis

- Chemotherapy-induced nausea and vomiting (CINV) are classified as acute, delayed or anticipatory.
- Actinomycin, cisplatin, carboplatin, cyclophosphamide/ifosfamide and doxorubicin/daunorubicin-based regimens are moderate/highly emetogenic agents.
- Anti-emetic options (Table 30.5):
  - Ondansetron: potent 5-HT3 receptor antagonist of 5-HT. Dosages up to 0.15 mg/kg QID orally or IV.
  - Aprepitant: potent, central nervous system-penetrant, selective NK-1 receptor antagonists of SP. Administered as a 3-day regimen: 125 mg orally 1 hour prior to chemotherapy administration (day 1) and 80 mg per day orally in the morning on days 2 and 3.
  - D2 receptor antagonists: include promethazine and metoclopramide.

Table 30.5 Antiemetic options.

Emesis risk	Antiemetics
High	Ondansetron, dexamethasone (small doses) and aprepitant +/- Olanzepine
Moderate	Ondansetron, dexamethasone (small doses) and aprepitant +/- Olanzepine
Low	Ondansetron alone
Minimal	Nil
Anticipatory	Addition of lorazepam or promethazine

Clinical Pearl: Anticipatory nausea and vomiting

Anticipatory nausea and vomiting is reported by 30% of patients and is a conditioned response that usually occurs prior to the actual administration of chemotherapy based on previous experiences of nausea and vomiting. It may be triggered by factors, such as tastes, odours, sights, thoughts or anxiety associated with the treatment, and is usually more difficult to control than acute or delayed CINV.

- Anti-histamines: include promethazine and cyclizine.
- The steroid dexamethasone, while not an anti-emetic, can potentiate the effect of Ondansetron.

Constipation
- Known side effect of vincristine therapy and can be particularly troublesome when the drug is used frequently.
- Commence prophylaxis with laxatives or stool softener at the beginning of therapy.
- If severe constipation persists despite prophylaxis ± addition of other agents, nasogastric colonic lavage solutions (e.g. Golytely) is usually successful.
- *Suppositories and enemas must not be used* because of the risk of causing small abrasions, which can predispose to secondary local infection and/or septicaemia.

Extravasation of chemotherapy
- Depending on the volume and type of drug extravasated, untreated damage can vary from mild irritation and erythema (irritant) to severe necrosis of the dermis and subcutaneous tissues (vesicant). These effects may be immediate or delayed.
- Vesicants include vincristine/vinblastine, anthracyclines, actinomycin-D.
- Treatment includes ceasing infusion, topical application of dimethyl sulphoxide (DMSO), and plastic surgery review if extensive.

Osteonecrosis or avascular necrosis
- May develop during or following steroid therapy in ALL.
- Often involves multiple joints over time, not limited to weight-bearing joints. Common sites include hip, knee, ankle, heel, shoulder and elbow.
- Symptoms and examination findings may include joint pain, joint stiffness, limited range of motion (e.g. pain with internal rotation of the hip), limited mobility or ambulation and/or gait abnormalities.
- MRI is superior in sensitivity and specificity to other modalities, especially with early bone changes.

Immunisation during and after chemotherapy
- Response to routine immunisations will not be optimal during therapy. Hence, routine immunisation programs should be interrupted while the child is on therapy.
- If required for treatment of a tetanus prone wound, tetanus toxoid can be safely given but concurrent use of tetanus immunoglobulin should also be considered.
- **Live virus vaccines must not be given to immunocompromised children.**

- **Siblings of patients should not receive oral polio vaccine (Sabin); give injectable polio vaccine inactivated instead.**
- It is strongly advised that unimmunised, non-immune siblings receive MMR and varicella vaccine.
- All family members including the immunocompromised child should be encouraged to have annual influenza vaccination.
- Approximately 6 months after completion of chemotherapy, interrupted immunisation programs should be completed. A booster dose of ADT or CDT, Sabin and MMR should be given to those who have previously been fully immunised. Hepatitis B immunisation should be commenced if not previously given.
- Consult with a specialist regarding immunisation after an allogeneic bone marrow transplant.

A new era of immuno- and cellular therapy

Targeted therapy is a treatment that has emerged as a potent therapy against the immune escape mechanism of relapsed and or refractory leukaemia, or is directed primarily at the genetic mutation/fusion causing the proliferative advantage in the cell type.

- **Molecular Inhibitors:** have a range of targets and include (but are not limited to) tyrosine kinase inhibitors, proteasomal inhibitors, VEGF inhibitors etc.
- **Immunotherapy:** recent expansion of the various immunotherapy approaches includes:
  - Monoclonal antibody drug conjugates (e.g. Inotuzumab) – binds to CD22 and injects a a cytotoxic drug directly into the leukaemia cell
  - Bi-specific T-cell engagers (BITE) – contains fragments that recognize CD19 (on ALL cell) and CD3 (on T cell) bringing the immune cell in direct contact with the leukaemia cell for killing
  - Chimeric antigen receptor –T cells (CAR-T) - use of autologous T cells that have been genetically reprogrammed identify and eliminate malignant cells through tumor-specific antigen recognition e.g. CD19.

Toxicity of immunotherapies

- **Cytokine release syndrome (CRS):** occurs commonly with Car T cell therapy. It is advantageous for efficacy of the therapy. It is an inflammatory process related to exponential T-cell proliferation with resultant marked elevations in cytokine levels (IFN gamma and soluble cd25).
  - Symptoms can range from mild flu-like symptoms to shock and multisystem organ failure and occasionally death.
  - IL6R inibitors (tocilizumab) improve the CRS without impacting the efficacy of the immunotherapy (CAR-T).
  - Steroids contraindicated
- **Neurological sequelae**
  - 'Immune effector cell-associated neurotoxicity syndrome' (ICANS). Disorder characterised by a pathologic process involving the central nervous system following any immune-effector cell (IEC) therapy that results in the activation or engagement of endogenous or infused T-cells and/or other immune-effector cells.
  - Symptoms include: tremor, dysgraphia, mild difficulty with expressive speech, impaired attention, apraxia and mild lethargy. Headache is non-specific)
  - Most neurological events will occur within 8 weeks of infusion, with a median time of onset of 7 days, and median time to resolution of 7 - 12 days.
- **B-cell aplasia**
  - B-cell aplasia and associated hypogammaglobulinaemia can occur after CAR-T cell therapy due to on-target/off-tumour effect (CAR-T cells target CD19, a biomarker that is expressed in malignant B-cells as well as in healthy B-cells in low levels)
  - Treatment: intravenous immunoglobulin replacement monthly for prevention of opportunistic infections.

Late effects of childhood cancer therapy

- Approximately 80% of children and adolescents who receive a diagnosis of cancer now become long-term survivors.
- Damage to the organ systems of children caused by CTX and RTX may not become clinically evident for many years.

- Survivors of childhood cancer have a higher risk of chronic health conditions that increases over time, and many die prematurely.
- Long-term follow-up of survivors of childhood cancer is necessary with an emphasis on surveillance for:
  - Second cancers (e.g. breast and colorectal, melanoma, and non-melanoma skin cancer).
  - Coronary artery disease.
  - Cardiomyopathy: late-onset anthracycline-related.
  - Pulmonary fibrosis.
  - Endocrinopathies (e.g. premature gonadal failure, thyroid disease, osteoporosis, and hypothalamic and pituitary dysfunction).
- More specific concerns include:
  - Bone-tumour survivors: most likely to have severe limitations in activity, which may further compound the risk of cardiovascular disease.
  - CNS tumour survivors: most likely to be functionally impaired.
  - Hodgkin's disease survivors: highest risk of second cancers and heart disease.

USEFUL RESOURCES
- The Children's Oncology group www.childrensoncologygroup.org; patient & family resources, as well as research & collaboration interests
- Cure4Kids online resource for health professionals https://www.cure4kids.org/; online education and collaboration tools.

CHAPTER 31
Ophthalmology

Anu Mathew

Key Points

- Always attempt to check monocular vision or objection to cover or each eye and red reflexes.
- Neonatal conjunctivitis requires urgent referral and treatment due to risk of corneal perforation especially if Neisseria infection, risk of systemic involvement.
- A child of any age with a constant large-angle squint or a child over 2 months with any squint (constant or intermittent) should be referred to an ophthalmologist.
- Orbital cellulitis should be differentiated from preseptal cellulitis and requires urgent admission and treatment due to potential for vision loss and intracranial complications.
- Consider infantile glaucoma if there is a hazy cornea, enlarged cornea, watery eyes and photophobia. Urgent referral is required.

Important principles
Eye examination

- Always test and record vision as the first part of any eye examination.
  - In infants, observe following and other visual behaviour and listen to the parents' impressions of their child's vision. Use colourful toys (preferably without sounds) to assess fixing and following. Also observe if they object to cover of one eye more than another.
  - In a toddler, pictures (e.g. Kay picture test) or single letter matching can be used to assess vision.
  - In an older child, a linear letter chart, similar to one used in adults can be used (e.g. Snellen chart).
- Check for misalignment/strabismus using corneal light reflections.
  - If equal: pseudosquint or an intermittent squint
  - If unequal and one light reflection is more nasal: exotropia
  - If unequal and one light reflection is more temporal: esotropia
- Check red reflex
- Examine the anterior structures of the eye with a torch or slit-lamp if possible.

Instilling eye drops

- Do not use local steroid drops unless corneal ulceration has been excluded by fluorescein staining and only when directed by an ophthalmologist.
- Instilling eye drops/ointment in a young child: carer sits on the floor with legs extended; lay child between carer's legs with child's arms under the carer's thighs and the child's feet near the carer's feet. This leaves the child's head secured and the carer with both hands free to hold open the child's eyelids and instill eye medication.

Padding eyes

- Never pad a discharging eye.
- Pad an eye or keep the child indoors if local anaesthetic has been instilled, until the effect of the local anaesthetic has worn off (10–20 minutes).

Paediatric Handbook, Tenth Edition. Edited by Kate Harding, Daniel S. Mason and Daryl Efron.
© 2021 John Wiley & Sons Ltd. Published 2021 by John Wiley & Sons Ltd.

Referral to an ophthalmologist
- Transient malalignment of the eyes is common up to 6 months of age. However, a child with a transient squint after 6 months or a constant squint at any age should be referred promptly to an ophthalmologist.
- True squints rarely improve spontaneously.
- All children with a white red reflex or white masses in the retina must be referred immediately to an ophthalmologist to exclude retinoblastoma.
- In cases of photophobia or watery eyes with no significant discharge in the first year of life, consider congenital glaucoma.

Trauma
Trauma to the eye can take many forms. Physical trauma to the eye and surrounding structures may be blunt or sharp. Trauma can also result from radiation (thermal and electromagnetic) and chemical agents.

Clinical Pearl: Australasian Triage Scale (ATS) Category for Ocular Trauma
- Potential penetrating eye injury: Category 3, recommended to start treatment within 30 min
- Blunt trauma: Category 3, recommended to start treatment within 30 min
- Chemical injury: Category 2, recommended to start treatment within 10 min
- Thermal burns: Category 4, recommended to start treatment within 60 min
- Corneal foreign body: Category 4, recommended to start treatment within 60 min
- Lid laceration: Category 4, recommended to start treatment within 60 min

---

Foreign bodies
Foreign bodies on the surface present with a painful, watery eye.
- If a foreign body or corneal ulcer is suspected, instill one drop of local anaesthetic to ease the pain and facilitate examination.
  - Suitable local anaesthetics are amethocaine (tetracaine) 0.5 or 1%, or benoxinate (oxybuprocaine) 0.4%.
  - **Do not use local anaesthetics for the continuing treatment of ocular pain under any circumstance.**
- Conjunctival foreign bodies are common and often found on the posterior surface of the upper lid. Therefore, eversion of the lid is essential.
  - To evert an eyelid: ask the child to look down, then with a cotton bud resting on the eyelid at the level of the top of the tarsal plate, gently push down on the cotton bud while grasping the eyelashes with the other hand and rotating the lid margin in an upward direction.
- Most foreign bodies are within 1–2 mm of the eyelid margin and are easily removed with a moist cotton wool swab.
- If they are embedded and/or difficult to remove, refer the child to an ophthalmologist.
- Beware of an iris naevus (small pigmented lesion on the iris that can be mistaken for a corneal foreign body) or iris prolapse through a perforating injury of the cornea mimicking a corneal foreign body.

Intraocular foreign bodies are generally the result of high-velocity fragments.
- Suspect them if the history involves an explosion, metal(s) striking on metal, or any other situation that involves high-speed objects (e.g. power tools or a lawn mower).
- If the history is at all suggestive, even in the absence of local signs, radiography of the orbit (AP and lateral) is necessary.
- If an intraocular foreign body is demonstrated or suspected, immediate referral to an ophthalmologist is mandatory.

Eyelid injuries
All eyelid lacerations except the most minor (that does not require stitches) should be repaired under general anaesthesia. Refer to an ophthalmologist if lacerations involve the lid margin or the medial aspect of the eyelids (canalicular injury is likely).

Hyphaema (blood in the anterior chamber)

This is the result of blunt trauma to the eye and all cases require referral to an ophthalmologist.

- The potential complications include other eye injuries, secondary haemorrhage and vision loss.
- Minor hyphaemas can be managed as an outpatient. More significant hyphaemas may require admission and bed rest.

Fracture of the orbital bones

A blowout fracture through the wall of the orbit is suspected if ≥1 of the following three cardinal signs are present:

- Restricted movement of the eye, particularly in a vertical plane, with double vision
- Infra-orbital nerve anaesthesia
- Enophthalmos, this may be difficult to assess initially because of eyelid haematoma

Diagnosis is usually clinical, but a CT scan is often obtained to assess the extent of the fracture and any associated injuries.

- A CT scan is used to demonstrate the fracture of the orbital wall and entrapped orbital tissue (the classic sign is a teardrop 'polyp' hanging from the roof of the maxillary antrum).

Penetrating injury (including intraocular foreign body)

This should always be considered in children with lacerations involving the eyelids, particularly after motor vehicle accidents.

- Clinical clues include distortion of the pupil, shallowed anterior chamber, prolapse of the iris through the cornea, or presence of pigmented tissue over the sclera.
- If suspected, protect the eye with a cone or shield that does not place pressure on the eyelids or eye and admit.
- Prevent vomiting with an antiemetic, as this may cause extrusion of eye contents.
- Refer to an ophthalmologist immediately.

Chemical burns

Irrigate the eye with saline or water copiously for at least 15 minutes using an IV giving set under local anaesthesia. Continue this until the fluid is neutral on pH testing or equal to the contralateral eye if a unilateral injury. The child may need to be sedated for adequate washout. Refer all chemical burns to an ophthalmologist.

Thermal burns

The ocular surface is rarely involved. Check for ulceration with fluorescein staining. Chloramphenicol ointment is suitable for use on superficial lid burns. Secondary lid swelling may result in corneal exposure and the exposed cornea should be protected with ocular lubricants until the swelling subsides.

Non-accidental injury

The presence of retinal haemorrhages in cases of unexplained head injury raises the possibility of non-accidental injury. An appropriate investigation of the circumstances of the injury should be initiated. The retinal haemorrhages must be assessed by an ophthalmologist (Chapter 20, Forensic medicine).

Acute red eye

See Table 31.1.

Conjunctivitis

Aetiology

- Bacterial: generally, pus is present
- Viral: generally, there is watery discharge
- Allergic: history of atopy and 'itchy eyes'

Neonatal conjunctivitis (ophthalmia neonatorum)

Neisseria gonorrhoea

- Clinical: Presents within a few days of birth with acute, severe, purulent discharge associated with marked conjunctival and lid oedema ('pus under pressure').

Table 31.1 The causes of red, watery and sticky eyes.

Condition	Pain	Itch	Epiphora	Discharge	Erythema	Photophobia	Reduced eye movements	Other
Neonatal conjunctivitis (ophthalmia neonatorum)	+++		++	+++	++-+++			
Congenital nasolacrimal duct obstruction			+-++	+-+++				
Infantile glaucoma			++		+	++		Enlarged and cloudy cornea
Viral conjunctivitis	++		++	+	+-++			
Bacterial conjunctivitis	++-+++		++	+++	++-+++			
Allergic conjunctivitis		++-+++	++-+++	Stringy	+			
Chemical conjunctivitis	+++		+++	+	++-+++			
Corneal abrasion	+++		++	Variable				
Foreign body	+++		++	Variable				Variable fluorescein staining
Preseptal cellulitis	++		+	Variable	+++ Swelling of eyelids			Conjunctiva not inflamed
Orbital cellulitis	+++		+	Variable	+++ Swelling of eyelids		+-+++	Eye is often inflamed and proptosed

- Diagnosis: Urgent Gram stain for Gram-negative intracellular diplococci and direct culture to appropriate culture media.
- Treatment: This is an ocular emergency because of the risk of corneal perforation. Admit and give IV ceftriaxone for 7 days. Penicillin (same duration) is an alternative if the organism is known to be susceptible. In all cases, local measures such as ocular lavage and topical antibiotics (chloramphenicol) may be helpful.
- Investigate and treat the mother and partner.

Chlamydia
- Clinical: Usually occurs at 10–14 days of age. Fails to respond to routine topical antibiotics. If left untreated, there is a risk of pneumonitis.
- Diagnosis: Giemsa stain of conjunctival scraping for intranuclear inclusions. Also antibodies in tears and immunofluorescent stains of conjunctival scrapes. Use a Chlamydia kit, ensuring conjunctival cells are collected.
- Treatment: Erythromycin 12.5 mg/kg oral q.i.d. for 14 days or azithromycin 20 mg/kg oral daily for 3 days. Eye toilet.
- Investigate and treat the mother and partner.

Other bacteria
- Other causes of conjunctivitis are Staphylococcus, Streptococcus or diphtheroids.
- Culture and treat with chloramphenicol eye drops/ointment. A rapid clinical response is anticipated.
- Occasionally, Neisseria meningitidis can cause conjunctivitis and should be treated as for invasive infection (see Chapter 25, Infectious diseases and immunisation).

Blocked nasolacrimal duct
- Presents with mucopurulent discharge with a watery eye. See Watering eyes below.

Conjunctivitis in older children
Viral
- This condition usually clears spontaneously.
- If it is unclear whether the infection is viral or bacterial, chloramphenicol eye drops may be given.

Bacterial
- Severe: chloramphenicol eye drops: 2 hourly by day and ointment at night.
- Less severe: chloramphenicol eye drops or ointment three times a day.

Herpes simplex conjunctivitis
- Suspect if the child has eyelid vesicles.
- Check for corneal ulceration and treat with 4 hourly aciclovir ointment if ulceration is present.
- Refer to an ophthalmologist.

Allergic
- In mild cases, use lubricants and oral antihistamines.
- In moderate cases, use a topical antihistamine and mast cell stabiliser (Ketotifen or Olopatadine).
- In severe cases, refer to an ophthalmologist. Topical steroid should only be given under the supervision of an ophthalmologist.

Corneal Ulceration
Ulceration causes pain, photophobia, lacrimation and blepharospasm. It is diagnosed by eye examination. For causes and management, see Table 31.2.

Table 31.2 Causes and management of corneal ulceration.

Cause	Appearance of ulcer (with fluorescein staining)	Management
Trauma (with or without a foreign body)	Scratch – linear Subtarsal foreign body – round or vertically linear	Chloramphenicol ointment (1%) or drops 3-4 times per day for 4 days. Review in 24 hours. If not healed in 48 hours, refer to an ophthalmologist.
Herpes simplex (dendritic ulcer)	Dendritic (occasionally 'geographic' if late presentation)	Aciclovir eye ointment (1 cm inside the lower conjunctival sac) five times a day for 14 days and refer to an ophthalmologist

Periorbital and orbital cellulitis

Both periorbital and orbital cellulitis present with erythematous, swollen lids in a febrile child.

Periorbital (preseptal) cellulitis

Periorbital cellulitis refers to infection in the soft tissues of the eyelids. This may arise from purulent conjunctivitis, dacryocystitis, or entry via local trauma or insect bite.

Distinguish this from a periorbital allergic reaction.

- A well child, who has eyelid swelling with minimal or no erythema, fever, tenderness nor local warmth, may simply have an allergic reaction to an allergen that has been blown or rubbed into the eye, or be secondary to an insect bite.
- In this case, no specific radiological imaging is required.
- An oral antihistamine may be used.
- The child should be reviewed if the swelling does not settle in the next 24 hours or if signs of inflammation develop.

For recommended antibiotic treatment for periorbital cellulitis see Appendix: Antimicrobial guidelines. Failure to respond in 24–48 hours may indicate orbital cellulitis or underlying sinus disease.

Orbital (septal) cellulitis

Orbital cellulitis occurs when infection is present around and behind the globe of the eye and is usually due to spread from sinus infection (especially the ethmoid sinuses). It usually occurs in children >2 years. Orbital cellulitis is a medical emergency and should be treated with the same level of urgency as meningitis or a brain abscess. The potential for loss of vision and suppurative intracranial complications is significant.

Orbital cellulitis is differentiated from periorbital cellulitis by the presence of:

- Chemosis
- Proptosis
- Ophthalmoplegia
- Reduced vision
- Systemic symptoms

If the features of orbital cellulitis are present, a CT scan of orbita, sinuses +/- brain is required to determine if the sinusitis is complicated by abscess formation. This is most commonly a subperiosteal abscess on the medial wall of the orbit adjacent to the ethmoid sinus (displacement of the medial rectus muscle is often an indication of abscess formation). An abscess will often require surgical drainage. If no abscess is present, treatment is by IV antibiotics alone; however, CT scanning may need to be repeated if there is clinical deterioration, or if there is lack of improvement with medical treatment.

For recommended antibiotic treatment of orbital cellulitis see Appendix: Antimicrobial guidelines. Urgent ENT and ophthalmology consultation are also required in suspected orbital cellulitis. Keep fasted until need for surgery is clarified.

Watering eyes

Watery eyes are common in children and are the result of either poor tear drainage or overproduction. The latter is usually the result of eye irritation and causes include foreign bodies (page 432), corneal ulcer (page 435), conjunctivitis (page 433) and infantile glaucoma (page 438).

Nasolacrimal duct obstruction is the most common cause of watery eyes and discharge that persists after the first 2 weeks of life. The discharge is worse on waking and the conjunctiva is not inflamed. It usually resolves spontaneously. Local eye cleaning is usually the only treatment indicated. If the eye is red and inflamed, topical chloramphenicol eye drops may be given (but avoid repeated courses of antibiotics). Secondary irritation of the skin can be minimised by protecting it with an application of soft white paraffin ointment after discharge is cleaned off. If the discharge and watering have not settled by 12 months of age, refer to an ophthalmologist for probing under general anaesthetic.

Strabismus or squint

Refer all children with squint or suspected squint to an ophthalmologist. This will allow early detection (and possibly prevention) of amblyopia and detection of any underlying pathology such as retinoblastoma or cataract. Urgent referral to an ophthalmologist is required if:

- The red reflex is abnormal (very dull or white).
- There is limitation of eye movement on one or both eyes.

A child does not 'grow out of' a squint. However, in the first few weeks of life, babies may have an intermittent squint, especially when feeding. A child of any age with a constant large-angle squint or a child over 2 months with any squint (constant or intermittent) should be referred to an ophthalmologist. All children with a first-degree relative with a squint should be seen by an ophthalmologist at about 3–3.5 years of age, even if there is no squint, as they may have a refractive error alone.

A pseudostrabismus (pseudosquint) is due to a broad nasal bridge or epicanthic folds, or both. This results in the appearance of a squint, but corneal light reflexes are central and there is no movement on cover testing (Figure 31.1). Only make the diagnosis of pseudostrabismus if absolutely certain. Refer doubtful cases to an ophthalmologist.

Putting Science into Practice: Strabismus

Both experimental and clinical data support the hypothesis that there is an early sensitive period during which strabismus and anisometropia (different refractive error between the two eyes) can lead to abnormal visual development. Conventionally this is considered to be the first 7 years of life. Thus, early detection and referral of any strabismus (intermittent or constant) is important.

Eyelid lumps and ptosis

Styes

Styes are acute bacterial infections of an eyelash follicle. They occur at the eyelid margin and are red and tender. Warm compresses and eyelid massage several times per day often hasten resolution. Local antibiotics are sometimes indicated. Systemic antibiotics are rarely needed.

Chalazion

A chalazion is an obstructed tarsal (or meibomian) gland. These glands are situated within the substance of the eyelid and help produce the lipid component of the tear film. Thus, a chalazion will present as a lump within the eyelid. There may be no associated symptoms. Redness associated with a chalazion is usually the result of sterile inflammation due to leakage of the contents, rather than a bacterial infection. Thus, local or systemic antibiotics

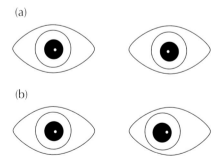

(a)

(b)

Figure 31.1 Corneal light reflex. Shine a light at the child's eyes and observe the reflection. (a) Eyes are straight and the corneal light reflex is symmetrical. (*Note*: It is displaced slightly to the nasal side of the centre in each eye.) (b) Left convergent strabismus or esotropia. The reflection from the deviated eye is displaced laterally.

seldom influence the natural history of these lesions. As with styes, warm compresses and eyelid massage often hasten resolution. If the chalazion is persistent (>6 months), large or causes discomfort and has not responded to conservative measures, incision and drainage under general anaesthesia may be indicated.

Ptosis

Ptosis is a droopy or lowered upper eyelid. In children, it is usually the result of a minor and isolated anomaly in the development of the levator muscle. It may be unilateral or bilateral, and is sometimes inherited in a dominant manner. If the lowered eyelid obstructs the pupil in a young child, visual loss will occur secondary to amblyopia. Semi-urgent referral to an ophthalmologist is appropriate in such cases. Referral is also indicated if there are associated pupil abnormalities. In more minor degrees of ptosis, surgical intervention is for cosmesis and is less urgent.

Rare but important eye conditions

Iritis

Acute iritis is very rare in children and presents with an acute red eye with symptoms of photophobia +/- reduced vision. The pupil is small and does not react well to light. Consider iritis in children with Juvenile Idiopathic Arthritis (JIA). This form of iritis (or uveitis) is chronic and painless. Refer to an ophthalmologist.

Infantile glaucoma

The presenting features are:
- A hazy cornea
- An enlarged cornea
- Watery eyes
- Photophobia

This is a rare condition, but early recognition is vital. Prompt surgery offers a chance of cure and preservation of vision. All infants with suspected glaucoma require urgent referral to an ophthalmologist for assessment and treatment.

Congenital cataracts

Congenital cataracts are rare, but early detection and removal with subsequent optical correction (contact lenses or spectacles) offers a good chance of visual preservation. All newborn infants should have their red reflexes examined before discharge from hospital. Check the red reflexes and fundi in any infant with poor visual performance (fixation and following). Nystagmus is a late sign of congenital cataracts. A unilateral cataract will often present as a squint. Any child suspected of having a congenital cataract must be referred urgently.

Retinoblastoma

This is a rare childhood cancer of the retina and presents with a white pupil (cat's eye reflex), squint, poor vision, or a family history of the tumour. Prompt recognition is vital to maximise the possibility of preserving vision. Untreated this is a fatal disorder. If suspected, refer urgently to an ophthalmologist.

CHAPTER 32

Orthopaedics

Michael B. Johnson
Leo Donnan

Key Points

- Infants with hip instability (Barlow or Ortolani positive developmental dysplasia of hip) require immediate referral for brace treatment, ideally before 3 months of age. Do not wait for ultrasound confirmation.
- The key to identifying pathological bowing (genu varum or genu valgum) is recognising asymmetry, inappropriate age, and beyond physiological normal range.
- In cases of torsional deformity (in-toeing, out-toeing) it is critical to examine with a rotational profile to determine the level of torsion: femur, tibia or foot. This determines the likely natural history and need for treatment, if any.
- Not all children's fractures are benign. Some have real risk of progressive angulation because of the intact periosteum. This needs to be counter-acted with a well applied, moulded cast.
- Bone and joint infection in children needs to be identified as early as possible. Use the Kocher's criteria to distinguish from other causes of limb pain and limp.

Developmental dysplasia of the hip

This condition was previously known as congenital dislocation of the hip; however, not all cases are present at birth and it describes a spectrum of disease ranging from under formation of the hip socket (dysplasia), hip instability, and in the severest cases hip dislocation.

- Risk factors: breech delivery, family history, congenital anomalies (especially foot abnormalities), being first-born and female, and swaddling legs in extension.
- Associations: oligohydramnios, caesarean section, packaging disorders e.g. torticollis and foot deformity.

Diagnosis

General screening

All neonates should have a clinical examination for hip joint instability, the Ortolani and Barlow tests.

- The baby should be relaxed. With the knee flexed, the thumb is placed over the lesser trochanter and the middle finger over the greater trochanter. The pelvis is steadied with the other hand and the flexed thigh is abducted and adducted.
- Any clunk or jerk where a dislocation reduces allowing the hip to abduct fully, is a positive Ortolani sign.
- The demonstration of dislocation by levering the femoral head in and out of the acetabulum is a positive Barlow sign (Figure 32.1).

Selective screening

Infants in high-risk groups and those with an abnormal routine clinical screening examination should have an ultrasound examination of their hips.

- As clinical diagnosis can be difficult and ultrasound has diagnostic limitations, the repeated examination of children with risk factors during the first year of life is important.

Paediatric Handbook, Tenth Edition. Edited by Kate Harding, Daniel S. Mason and Daryl Efron.
© 2021 John Wiley & Sons Ltd. Published 2021 by John Wiley & Sons Ltd.

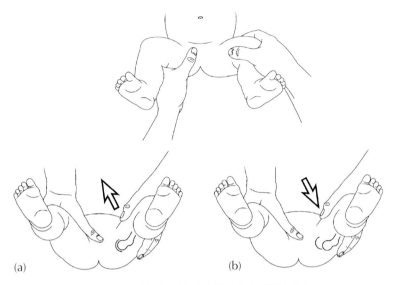

Figure 32.1 Screening for developmental dysplasia of the hip. (a) Ortolani's sign, (b) Barlow's sign.

- When the ossification nucleus of the femoral head develops, between 3 and 9 months, the preferred mode of imaging changes from ultrasound to plain radiograph. Generally, use ultrasound up to 9 months of age and radiography thereafter.

Management
The earlier the diagnosis, the easier the management.
- Most neonates can be successfully treated by abduction bracing with a Pavlik harness or Dennis-Browne bar.
- Operative treatments, including open reduction, may be required with later diagnosis.

Swaddling
Swaddling is a common technique used to settle infants. However, swaddling with the hips in an adducted and extended position is a risk factor for DDH.
- Parents and health professionals should be made aware of the risks associated with swaddling with the hips in extension. Safe swaddling involves the legs being wrapped loosely to allow for hip flexion and abduction.

Adolescence
Later presentation of acetabular dysplasia can occur with different patterns of involvement of the acetabulum.
- Presenting symptoms include Pain and activity limitation.
- Surgery in symptomatic individuals is aimed at preserving cartilage thickness, reduce shear forces, and removing impingements to movement in an effort to prevent or delay later arthritic changes.

Club foot (congenital talipes equinovarus)
"Talipes" is Latin for ankle-foot and needs to be followed by the description of the position of the foot.
- Common postural problems are usually mild and mobile; that is, they correct easily and fully with the pressure of one finger.
- Examples are: talipes calcaneovalgus (excessive dorsiflexion and eversion), talipes metatarsus varus (adduction of the forefoot) or postural talipes equinovarus (Figure 32.2).
- They resolve spontaneously with no treatment.
- The true club foot deformity (congenital talipes equinovarus: CTEV) is more severe and is often stiff. The foot is in equinus, with the hindfoot in varus and the forefoot supinated.

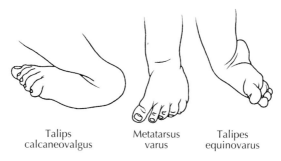

Talips
calcaneovalgus

Metatarsus
varus

Talipes
equinovarus

Figure 32.2 Congenital foot deformities.

Management

Stiff, non-resolving deformities require manipulation and casting.

- Soft tissue surgery is required for many.
- Bone surgery is required for a few.

Torsional and angular deformities in children

Many children are seen with normal angular or torsional variants of the lower limbs. It can be difficult to distinguish physiological variation from pathological conditions. The range of 'normality' is wide, but physiological variations can result in as much parental anxiety as pathological disorders.

In-toeing

In-toeing in childhood can be due to metatarsus varus, internal tibial torsion or medial femoral torsion (Table 32.1 and Figures 32.3–32.4).

Out-toeing

Infants and toddlers have restricted internal rotation at the hip because of an external rotation soft tissue contracture, not retroversion of the femur.

Infants

- Present with a 'Charlie Chaplin' posture between 3–12 months.
- The child weight-bears and walks normally.
- Resolution occurs with no treatment.

Table 32.1 In-toeing in childhood.

	Metatarsus varus (Figure 32.2)	Internal tibial torsion (Figure 32.3)	Internal femoral torsion (Figure 32.4)
Synonyms	Metatarsus adductus		Inset hips
Age at presentation	Birth	Toddler	Child
Site of problem	Foot	Tibia	Femur
Examination	Sole of foot bean shaped	Thigh–foot angle is inwards	Arc of hip rotation favours internal rotation
Management	Observe or cast	Observe and reassure	Observe, rarely surgery
When to refer if not resolved	3 months after presentation	6 months after presentation	8 years after presentation

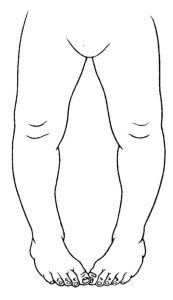

Figure 32.3 Internal tibial torsion.

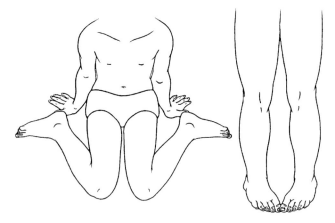

Figure 32.4 Internal femoral torsion.

Children
- May be due to neurologic disorder.
- Surgery may be necessary.

Bow legs (genu varum)
The vast majority are physiological. Rare causes include skeletal dysplasias, rickets and Blount disease (tibia vara).

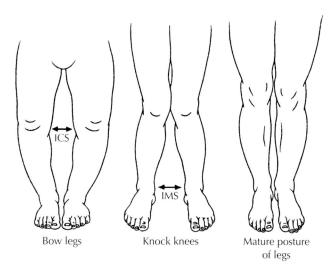

Figure 32.5 Postural variants in the lower limbs.

Presentation
- Toddlers are usually bowed until 3 years of age.
- Physiological bowing is symmetrical, not excessive and improves with time.

Management
- Monitor intercondylar separation (Figure 32.5)
- Refer when ICS is >6 cm, is not improving or is asymmetric.

Knock knees (genu valgum)
Most children with bow legs or knock knees are normal, with <1% having an underlying problem. Rare causes rickets and trauma.

Presentation
Children are usually knock-kneed from 3–8 years.
- Physiological knock knees are symmetrical, not excessive and improves with time.

Management
Monitor the intermalleolar separation (IMS) see Figure 32.5.
- Refer if IMS >8 cm.

Flat feet (pes plano valgus)
This condition is painless and asymptomatic. If pain or stiffness is present, referral is needed.

Causes
- Physiological (in the vast majority): all newborns have flat feet due to fat that fills the medial longitudinal arch; 80% of children develop a medial arch by their sixth birthday. Having the child stand on their toes may reveal the 'hidden' arch.
- Tarsal coalition (in older children and adolescents only), usually painful.

Management
No treatment is required unless symptomatic.
- The condition is unaffected by orthotics or exercises.
- Most cases resolve spontaneously.

Trauma

The management of fractures and dislocations is an integral part of the overall management of the trauma patient. Common fractures in children involve the wrist, elbow, clavicle, distal tibia, fibula and femur. Each has distinct management strategies but there are common themes.

Assessment

Fractures in children are more common than ligament rupture or strain.

- Fracture is most likely in cases of trauma with acute pain, swelling, and limb disuse.
- Children presenting with a suspected fracture or dislocation require a full evaluation of the fracture and exclusion of damage to other structures.
- An accurate history of the mechanism of injury will determine which structures may potentially be damaged.
- Consider Non-Accidental Injury in infants with fractures (see Chapter 20, Forensic medicine).

Examination

- Soft tissues: check for blistering, bruising, puckering of skin, or open fracture.
- Deformity or swelling.
- Neurological status distal to the injury.
- Peripheral pulses: if the blood flow to the limb is compromised, emergency orthopaedic consultation is necessary.
- Associated injuries.

Description of fractures

It is helpful to use specific, technical vocabulary to describe fractures for the purposes of documentation, and discussion with colleagues.

Important features include:

- The anatomical site of the fracture: bone, side, part of the bone (distal, middle or proximal), e.g. right midshaft humerus.
- The fracture type: open or closed. A closed fracture has an intact soft tissue envelope.
- Specific type of children's fracture. Bones are more elastic and are more likely to bend and buckle, rather than crack or break. This results in two common patterns of fracture that are seen in children and not in adults:
  - Buckle fractures (both cortices are intact on both AP and Lateral projections)
  - Greenstick fractures (one cortex broken, the other side intact.
- **Involvement of the growth plate** is described according to the Salter–Harris classification (Figure 32.6).
- **Displacement of the fracture** e.g. undisplaced, angulated or displaced.

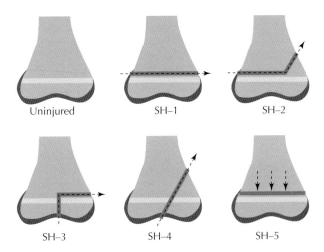

Figure 32.6 Salter–Harris (SH) classification of growth plate injuries.

Management

See Table 32.2 for specific fracture information.

General management

- The affected limb should be splinted by a board or plaster slab before radiography.
- Analgesia is required (e.g. fentanyl 0.15 μg/kg intranasally). See Chapter 6, Pain management.
- Anteroposterior and lateral views should be obtained of the suspected fracture site. Generally, the joint above and below should also be X-rayed.
- Some greenstick fractures with one cortex disrupted are at risk of late angulation (from intact periosteum) and need a molded cast to prevent angulation.
- A simple undisplaced buckle or torus fracture can be treated in a backslab.
- Open fractures usually require operative intervention.
- Generally, any displaced or angulated fracture should be discussed with orthopaedist and may require manipulation under either local anaesthesia block (e.g. Bier block, see Chapter 5, Procedures) or a general anaesthetic.
- Minor fractures of various types are discussed in the RCH Paediatric Fracture Guidelines (including their management and when to review etc.). Refer to www.rch.org.au/clinicalguide/fractures.
- For video on closed reduction and plastering, see www.rch.org.au/fracture-education/management_principles/Management_Principles/.

Home treatment after a full plaster

- Elevate the limb above the heart level for the next 24–48 hours.
- Forearm: a sling (after 48 hours) should keep the hand above the elbow.
- Lower limb: crutches should only be used by children over 6–7 years of age, who are coordinated enough to use them. A walking frame may be used by younger children.
- Written plaster instructions should be explained and given to parents.

Follow-up

For children who have had a manipulation of a fracture or a fracture involving both cortices of the bone, a repeat radiograph should be obtained in 1 week to ensure the correct position is maintained. Plaster should remain in place for 3–6 weeks, depending on the degree of injury and bone involved. Following the removal of the cast, the bone is still at risk of re-fracture for the next 8–12 weeks; therefore, contact sports are not recommended during this period.

Other common soft tissue and joint injuries

General management

Remember the RICE acronym:

- **Rest:** weight-bearing should occur as soon as able. If there is significant swelling and the child is unable to weight-bear, they may benefit from immobilisation but only for a few days.
- **Ice:** should be applied for 15 minutes every 2–3 hours during the first 48 hours, then heat can be applied.
- **Compression:** should be accomplished with a firm bandage or Tubigrip.
- **Elevation:** the limb should be elevated on a few pillows whenever possible to allow the swelling to subside.

Range of motion and balance exercises should start as soon as possible followed by strength exercises

Knee injuries: Acute patello-femoral dislocation

- There may be underlying predispositions to this injury: anatomical malalignment (valgus, internal femoral torsion, extensor mechanism) and generalized hypermobility.
- The dislocated patella presents as a fixed flexion deformity, pain and medial swelling.
- Reduction can be achieved by gentle traction and bringing the knee into extension with no force applied to the patella itself.
- The knee is then maintained in extension for a short period of time with early physio aimed at not losing quadriceps power.
- MRI investigation is warranted to identify chondral or osteo-chondral loose bodies which if present requires referral.

Table 32.2 Specific fractures.

Site of fracture	Type	Ortho consult	Treatment	Repeat x-ray	Follow-up	Return to sport	Potential complications
Clavicle	Greenstick	No	Sling	No	No	4–6 weeks	No
	Complete displaced, or distal	Yes	Sling (rarely operative)	Yes	1–2 weeks	8–12 weeks	Palpable lump
Humerus – surgical neck	Greenstick/undisplaced	No	Collar and cuff	No	2–3 weeks	6–8 weeks	No
Humeral shaft	Undisplaced	Yes	Collar and cuff ± backslab	Yes	1 week	6–8 weeks	Radial nerve
Supracondylar fracture	Undisplaced/minor posterior angulation	No	Backslab to wrist (90 deg angle at elbow)	Yes	1 week	6–8 weeks	Nerve or vessel injury check radial pulse, hand movement
Lateral condyle	Undisplaced	Yes	Backslab to wrist	Yes	1 week	6–8 weeks	Displacement of fragment
Proximal radius or ulna fracture	Undisplaced	Yes	Backslab to wrist	Yes	1 week	6–8 weeks	Intra-articular fracture may require pinning
Midshaft radius and ulna	Undisplaced	Yes	Above elbow plaster	Yes	1 week	6–8 weeks	
	Greenstick angulated only	Yes	Reduction LAMP or GA	Yes	1 week	8–12 weeks	Displacement
Distal radius	Buckle, torus	No	Backslab wrist only	No	No	2–4 weeks	
	Greenstick fracture (1 cortex disrupted), <20 deg angulation	No	Below elbow plaster	Yes	1 week	6–8 weeks	Late angulation
	Angulated >20 degrees or displaced	Yes	Reduction LAMP or GA	Yes	1 week	8–10 weeks	
Metacarpals	Undisplaced or angulated <30 degrees	No	Backslab involving fingers	No	2 weeks	4–6 weeks	Look for rotation of finger
Phalanx	Undisplaced	No	Buddy tape	Yes (if distal fracture)	1 week	2–6 weeks (buddy tape during play)	Rotation of fracture if distal
Tibia	Undisplaced, greenstick or torus	No	Nothing or backslab	No	2–3 weeks	8–12 weeks	Toddler fracture[a]
	Spiral undisplaced	Yes	Above knee plaster	Yes	1 week	12–16 weeks	
Fibula	Undisplaced shaft or distal	No	Backslab below knee	Yes	1 week	6–8 weeks	
Metatarsal	Undisplaced or mildly displaced	No	Backslab	Yes	1 week	4–6 weeks	

[a]Toddler fracture is usually following a fall, with the child limping or nonweight-bearing, tenderness over the tibia or fibula and a normal X-ray. Treatment outlined above.

Ankle injury

True sprains are common. Minor fractures of the growth plate or epiphysis should be treated like a sprain. These injuries are usually created by an inversion injury to the ankle.

Radiographs are required if:

- Deformity is present.
- Maximal tenderness occurs over the distal tibia or posterior aspect of the fibula.
- The child is unable to weight-bear at all.

Pulled elbow

The cause of this injury is either the child's arm being forcefully pulled or related to a fall. The radial head subluxates and jams in the annular ligament.

Clinical features

- Age: commonly 1–3 years.
- There may be a crack or popping sound at the time.
- On examination: the arm is pronated, slightly flexed, and limp by their side (pseudoparalysis), there is absence of tenderness or swelling along whole of arm, supination of the arm causes pain.

Management

- No investigations are necessary.
- Hold the child's hand as if to shake it and with your other hand, encircle the elbow with the thumb over the annular ligament of the radius.
- Gently apply traction and supinate the hand firmly and then flex the forearm at the elbow all the way to the shoulder. You may feel a pop as the radial head is relocated.
- The child should be moving the arm normally within 10–15 minutes. If there has been a delay in relocation, it may take longer for the child to resume using the arm.
- Note: If the history is not typical, there is swelling or attempts at reduction fail, a radiograph of the elbow should be obtained to exclude a fracture.

Orthopaedic infections

Infections involving bones and joint are common in children. Most often these originate from a haematogenous source, but children may also have a history of injury to the local region. Hallmark signs are fever, pain, swelling and disuse of the limb or joint. The infant hip can have both osteomyelitis and septic arthritis by virtue of the intra-articular portion of the metaphysis.

Investigations

- Blood tests: FBE, ESR, CRP and Blood culture
- Plain X-ray
- Ultrasound
- MRI (in non-resolving osteomyelitis or septic arthritis)

Clinical Pearl: Septic arthritis

Kocher signs

- Temp $>38.5°$
- Inability to bear weight
- White cell count $>12 \times 10^9/$ L
- ESR >40 mm

The presence of 4 signs indicates a 99.6% probability of septic arthritis, the presence of none of these signs indicates a <0.2% probability of septic arthritis.

Management

See Table 32.3

Antibiotic treatment

see Appendix: Antimicrobial guideline.

Table 32.3 Bone and joint infections and inflammation.

Condition	Clinical features	Treatment
Transient synovitis	Well, no fever, weightbearing but irritable joint Low or normal ESR / CRP Normal X-rays	NSAIDs No antibiotics until diagnosis made Review following day for improvement

Septic arthritis	Unwell child, febrile, not using limb, reduced
	    joint range of motion, swelling/effusion
	Elevated inflammatory markers
	X-ray may be normal or show large effusions
		Keep fasted
		Delay empiric antibiotics until synovial sample
		    taken **unless** signs of systemic sepsis (then
		    blood culture before antibiotics)
		General anaesthetic, aspirate, arthrotomy or
		    arthroscopic drainage and lavage

Osteomyelitis	Fever, pain, limited use of limb, tenderness and
	    swelling
	Elevated inflammatory markers
	X-ray (late changes): periosteal reaction,
	    cortical destruction
	Confirmed on advanced imaging
		IV antibiotics followed by 3 weeks of oral
		    antibiotics
		+/- aspiration/drainage if collection present **or**
		    failure to resolve

Table 32.4 Differential diagnosis of limp in childhood.

Acute	Subacute	Chronic
Fracture	Juvenile idiopathic arthritis	Cerebral palsy
Irritable hip	Tumour/leukaemia	Developmental dysplasia of the hips
Septic arthritis	Acute or chronic SCFE	Perthes disease
Osteomyelitis		Chronic SCFE

SCFE, slipped capital femoral epiphysis.

Limp in childhood

Limp is a common presenting complaint in childhood (Table 32.4).

Clinical assessment

Review musculoskeletal assessment (Chapter 39, Rheumatology).
Specifically:
- Acute, subacute or chronic limp
- Associated pain or fever
- Other constitutional symptoms
- Previous episodes of pain or limp
- What position is the leg held in (e.g. flexed and externally rotated)
- Pain on joint movement or bony pressure
- Limitation of movement

Investigations
- FBE with differential, ESR and CRP.
- Plain radiograph of the joint or affected limb.
- Ultrasound of hip (looking for fluid in the joint) if it is painful or tender with movement.
- MRI or bone scan (indicated rarely for further investigation of infection, tumour).

Management

This will depend on the underlying problem:
- Slipped capital femoral epiphysis (SCFE), tumours, Perthes disease or developmental dysplasia of the hip should be referred immediately to an orthopaedic surgeon.
- Toddlers' fractures may be occult and not seen on a radiograph. If the child is afebrile, then observation is appropriate.

Irritable hip (transient synovitis)

The usual presentation is a child who is constitutionally well with a partial limp and difficulty walking ± a painful hip.
- Common condition which needs to be distinguished from septic arthritis (Table 32.3).
- Although it is the most common reason for limp in the preschooler, irritable hip is a diagnosis of exclusion.

Usual clinical features and management

See Table 32.3.

Clinical Pearl: Hip examination

The easiest way to assess for significant hip irritability is to distract the child whilst gently rolling the hip with your hand.

Perthes disease

This is a specific hip disease of childhood. Affected children have a generalised disorder of growth with a tendency to low birthweight and delayed bone age. The pathology is necrosis of the capital femoral epiphysis followed by a sequence of resorption of necrotic bone, reossification and remodelling. This sequence of events is seen radiologically as increased density of the capital epiphysis, patchy osteolysis, new bone formation and remodelling with a variable degree of femoral head deformity.

Clinical features

- Age range: commonly 4 and 8 years, but can occur 2–12 years
- Sex ratio: five males to one female, 20% bilateral
- Symptoms: pain and limp, usually for at least 1 week
- Signs: restriction of hip motion

Investigations

- X-ray
- MRI or bone scan abnormality may precede Xray signs in early Perthes

Management principles

- Resting the hip in the early irritable phase
- Regaining motion if the hip is stiff
- Containing the hip by bracing or surgery in selected children

Slipped capital femoral epiphysis

Can occur acutely or chronically. High clinical suspicion is essential as early detection prevents later morbidity. Any adolescent with hip, thigh or knee pain should have this diagnosis considered.

Clinical features

- Age: late childhood to early adolescence. Maximum incidence in girls aged 10–12 years and boys 12–14 years.
- Weight is usually >90th percentile.
- Pain often described in the anterior thigh or knee, or groin.
- Limp.

- The hip appears externally rotated and shortened.
- Decreased hip movement, particularly internal rotation.
- May be bilateral (20% of cases).

Clinical Pearl: Slipped capital femoral epiphysis hip examination
As the hip is flexed the affected side will externally rotate and abduct even in the most minor slips.

Investigation
- X-ray of the pelvis and a frog-leg lateral x-ray of the affected hip.

Management
- The child should not weight-bear if this diagnosis is considered.
- Immediate transfer to hospital.
- Urgent orthopaedic referral and surgery to prevent further slipping is required. Most children can be managed with pinning.

Scoliosis
Scoliosis is a 3-dimensional deformity of the spine seen as a side-ways curvature when viewed from the frontal (coronal) plane, and rotation in the axial plane. **Non-structural or postural curves** may be secondary to a problem outside the spine, such as unequal leg lengths or muscular spasm.
Scoliosis causes, include:
- Congenital (embryological origin).
- Neuromuscular (Cerebral palsy, Spina bifida, Rett syndrome, Duchenne muscular dystrophy).
- Syndromic and other secondary causes (e.g. Marfan syndrome).
- Idiopathic: The most common type of scoliosis is adolescent idiopathic scoliosis (AIS), affecting girls in 90% of cases. 2% of female adolescents have curves of >10 degrees. There is evidence of genetic predisposition for AIS.

Detection
This is usually done by the forward bend test, in which the examiner observes the spine from behind as the subject bends forwards, demonstrating asymmetry of the ribs and chest wall. Detection of asymmetry warrants X-ray investigation. Low dose radiation scanogram images (EOS) films are preferable, when available, to show the whole spine.

Management
The risk of curve progression is related to the underlying pathological cause, age at presentation, and the size of the curve. Growth is a major cause of progression.
All children with scoliosis should be referred to a paediatric orthopaedic surgeon.
- If the curvature is <20 degrees: observe during growth.
- If the curvature is 20–40 degrees: a brace is often recommended.
- If the curvature is >40 degrees: surgery is indicated.

Clinical Pearl: Scoliosis
Growth is a key cause for progression of scoliosis; children do not grow straighter, so require early referral.

USEFUL RESOURCES
- Developmental dysplasia of the hip clinical resource *ddheducation.com*
- The RCH Paediatric fracture guidelines www.rch.org.au/clinicalguide/fractures

CHAPTER 33

Otolaryngology

Elizabeth Rose
Valerie Sung

Key Points

- For a possible airway foreign body or laryngeal trauma, the child should be kept fasted and the anaesthetic and otolaryngology teams should be involved in the management as early as possible.
- A child with acute otitis media will have pain, inflammation/redness of the tympanic membrane (TM) and bulging of the TM. This is manifest by the handle of the malleus being poorly seen. In otitis media with effusion the malleus is more prominent.
- The majority of children with acute otitis media do not benefit from antibiotic treatment. There are certain children who should be treated with antibiotics, and a 10-day course should be considered.
- For children with chronic rhinosinusitis, most can be managed with nasal saline irrigations. If snoring is a marked symptom, they may benefit from adenoidectomy.
- An ultrasound examination of the neck may not demonstrate a deep neck infection, including a possible peritonsillar abscess.

Emergencies

Possible aspirated foreign body

This may be above the larynx, within the larynx, or in the trachea or bronchus; a foreign body in the upper oesophagus may also cause noisy breathing but there will also be drooling.

Evaluate and manage the child in a resuscitation room

Partial obstruction (child has noisy breathing, is moving air, is able to cough, may have oxygen desaturations):

- Place child upright in the position that is most comfortable and contact an anaesthetist and ENT surgeon to arrange for urgent removal of the foreign body in the operating theatre.
- Do not instrument the airway if the child is coping.
- Give oxygen.

Complete obstruction:

- Contact an anaesthetist and ENT surgeon
- Under direct vision (preferably using a laryngoscope) check in the mouth and oropharynx for a foreign body, if present, remove it with Magill forceps.
- If no foreign body is seen:
  - Place child prone with the head down.
  - Apply five blows with the open hand to the interscapular area.
  - Turn child face up.
  - Apply five chest thrusts using the same technique as for chest compression during CPR.
  - Check in the mouth to see if the foreign body has appeared and remove it.

Paediatric Handbook, Tenth Edition. Edited by Kate Harding, Daniel S. Mason and Daryl Efron.
© 2021 John Wiley & Sons Ltd. Published 2021 by John Wiley & Sons Ltd.

- If no foreign body seen after this manoeuvre:
  - Apply five lateral chest thrusts.
  - If unsuccessful, repeat interscapular blows, central chest compressions and lateral chest thrusts.
  - It is possible the foreign body is lodged in the lower trachea or bronchi
  - Ventilation/oxygenation through an oral endotracheal tube should be attempted while organising endoscopic removal. Aid intermittent expiration by lateral chest compression.
  - If this is unsuccessful, perform cricothyrotomy or tracheostomy.

Surgical management of an obstructed upper airway

Emergency Departments will have a trolley for airway management, and staff should familiarise themselves with the equipment available.
- Insertion of an **IV cannula percutaneously** into the trachea through the cricothyroid membrane (between the thyroid and cricoid cartilages) allows oxygenation (but not ventilation).
- Use a 16 gauge BD Insyte IV cannula, angled towards the feet.
- Remove the needle and connect the cannula to a bagging circuit using a Rapid O_2 Insufflator.
- Oxygenate with 100% oxygen at an initial flow rate of 1 L/kg/min (higher flow rates may be required in the obstructed airway).
- Insufflate for up to 4 seconds looking for chest rise and improvement in oxygen saturations.
- Repeat insufflation once oxygen saturations begin to fall.
- Aid intermittent expiration by lateral chest compression.

or
Perform cricothyrotomy:
- Stabilise the cricoid cartilage with one hand.
- Incise the skin over the cricothyroid membrane.
  - In the midline bluntly dissect into the airway with forceps or incise vertically with a scalpel.
  - Insert an appropriately sized bougie into the trachea.
  - Railroad an appropriately sized endotracheal tube into the trachea.
  - Remove the bougie and oxygenate using a T-piece or self-inflating (Laerdal) bag.

or
Perform percutaneous mini-tracheostomy.

Laryngeal trauma

Laryngeal trauma may be internal or external, penetrating or blunt.
- Internal trauma is usually as a result of intubation injury or airway burns.
- Penetrating injuries (from a knife or falling on a sharp object) are less common than blunt trauma which usually results from motor vehicle accidents or sports injuries.
- Blunt trauma is less common in children compared with adults as the larynx is relatively higher in the neck and more protected by the mandible.

Diagnosis may be difficult as upper airway trauma is commonly associated with other injuries, especially head injuries, facial fractures, cervical spine injuries and chest trauma.

If there is suspected laryngeal trauma call the Anaesthetist and the Otolaryngologist to attend.

Major signs and symptoms

- Subcutaneous emphysema
- Dyspnoea
- Stridor
- Inability to tolerate the supine position: This indicates the possibility of cricotracheal separation and requires immediate airway management.

Other signs and symptoms include:
- Localised swelling and tenderness
- Hoarseness
- Dysphagia/pain on swallowing
- Haemoptysis

Investigations

- Lateral cervical spine: subcutaneous emphysema and cervical spine injury.
- Chest X-ray: pneumothorax and other injuries.
- CT scan if the child is stable or when the airway has been secured.
- Awake laryngoscopy with a nasendoscope may be performed if there are no immediate concerns with the airway, and will show integrity of the mucosa, vocal cord mobility and patency of the airway, especially above the level of the vocal cords.

Initial airway management

This depends on the individual case, especially the degree of obstruction and other possible injuries. The possibilities include:

- Observation for 24 hours if there is no concern about an unstable airway or obstruction.
- Surgical airway under local anaesthesia. This may be difficult in a child who is hypoxic and there is oedema and haematoma of the neck.
- Intubation in theatre under General anaesthesia. With rigid bronchoscopy an assessment is made about the severity and level of the injury, while securing the airway; a decision can be made whether to perform a tracheostomy.

Needle cricothyrotomy is not recommended as the cricoid cartilage is often the level of the injury.

Clinical Pearl: Laryngeal trauma

- The inability to lie supine with laryngeal trauma suggests there is cricotracheal separation and a plan must be made to secure the airway immediately.
- Needle cricothyrotomy is not recommended as there is often swelling and this is the area of the trauma.

Other trauma and foreign bodies

Aural trauma

Trauma to the external auditory canal is usually associated with bleeding, but usually heals well. The tympanic membrane can be perforated by direct trauma or a pressure wave (e.g. a slap across the ear or diving). Acute perforations usually heal within weeks and do not require acute intervention. Topical antibiotics are recommended for water-related injuries. Direct trauma may rarely cause ossicular disruption, facial paralysis or inner ear damage (with complete deafness and vertigo). Follow-up at 4 weeks after injury is required to ensure perforations have healed, usually with an audiogram.

Foreign bodies in the ear

These are often superficial and can be removed with the doctor wearing a head light and using a wax curette placed behind the foreign body to pull it out. Forceps may not grasp it and so push it in further, especially if the object is round and hard.

- Batteries should be removed as an emergency and with general anaesthesia if there is already swelling. This allows good aural cleaning and application of antibiotic/steroid ointment if necessary.
- Large foreign bodies wedged in the canal or deep in the ear canal may also need removal under general anaesthesia, to prevent trauma. The first attempt is often the best, so if there is doubt about the ability to remove it in the Emergency Department, it is best to consult with an ENT surgeon.

Nasal trauma

A nasal deformity due to a displaced nasal fracture should be reduced within 7–10 days of injury, and the child should be seen within a week of the injury, once the soft tissue swelling has resolved. The decision to reduce the nasal fracture is based on clinical grounds and radiology is unhelpful.

Nasal septal haematoma

- Pressure on cartilage causes necrosis and nasal collapse (saddle nose deformity).
- The child presents after trauma with nasal obstruction and pain associated with a bulge of the septum that can be confirmed by palpating with an instrument (e.g. wax curette) following application of a topical anaesthetic.

- The haematoma frequently forms an abscess and as this is the 'danger area of the face', there is also the possibility of cavernous sinus thrombosis.
- Treatment involves incision and drainage, nasal packing to prevent recurrence, and anti-staphylococcal antibiotics.

Epistaxis

This is usually due to bleeding from the vessels on the anterior nasal septum (Little's area), often in association with nasal crusting from infection or nose picking.

- Acute bleeding usually settles with local pressure to the lower nasal septum (on the soft part of the nose, not on the nasal bones).
- Recurrent bleeding can be treated by the application of an antibiotic ointment if significant nasal crusting is present, and by keeping the nasal mucosa moist with a water-based gel.
- Antibiotic treatment should continue for one month, and in dry weather the gel should be applied before going outside.
- For children with frequent bleeding, a prominent vessel can be cauterized with silver nitrate application after preparing the nose first with lignocaine and phenylephrine. This is rarely needed in pre-school age children, and the child needs to be co-operative for the procedure to be effective.
- Very rarely epistaxis in children can be from a nasal tumour (juvenile angiofibroma in adolescent males) or a previously undiagnosed coagulopathy.

Foreign bodies in the nose

Children with a foreign body in the nose may present at a later time with unilateral, offensive rhinorrhoea. It is often possible to see the foreign body. Older children may be able to blow it out.

For younger children 'Parent's kiss' technique can be used.

- The procedure should be fully explained to the parent (or other trusted adult) and the child told they will be given a 'big kiss'.
- The parent then:
  o places their mouth over the child's open mouth, forming a firm seal as if performing mouth-to-mouth resuscitation
  o occludes the unaffected nostril with a finger
  o blows until they feel resistance caused by the closure of the child's glottis
  o gives a sharp exhalation to deliver a short puff of air into the child's mouth (which passes through the nasopharynx and out through the unoccluded nostril)
- If necessary, the procedure can be repeated a number of times.
- There have been no reports of adverse events from this technique and it is successful in 60% of cases.

Removal in the Emergency Department

- Spray topical decongestant/anaesthetic into the nose and wait 10 minutes for this to be effective.
- Sit the child upright on a parent or assistant's lap.
- The doctor uses a headlight so that both hands are free.
- Use a wax curette or a hook to pass behind the foreign body to pull it out.
- Forceps may not grasp it and push it in further.
- Anticipate bleeding and warn the parents first.

If the foreign body has been there for more than a day there is often pus in the nose. This will clear once the foreign body is removed and there is no need to treat with antibiotics.

If there is a button battery it is best to remove this immediately without local anaesthesia as the additional moisture may cause more leakage from the battery.

- If it is not readily removed take the child to theatre for a general anaesthetic and removal as there is a risk of damage to the nasal septum.

Oral/oropharyngeal trauma

This may occur after a fall with a stick or similar object in the mouth and may sometimes be associated with a significant injury.

Evaluation of the child includes:

- Ability to feed/swallow.
- Upper airway obstruction.

- Significant laceration, requiring debridement, closure or both. Lacerations on the hard palate will usually heal within a few days but if there is a laceration on the free edge of the soft palate this may need suturing to avoid incompetence.
- Significant retropharyngeal injury may not be obvious on oral examination, and there is the potential for abscess formation with tracking inferiorly to the mediastinum.
- A lateral laceration of the oropharynx has the potential to cause trauma to the carotid artery with dissection. Investigations include:
- Lateral cervical spine radiograph to check for retropharyngeal air or swelling.
- Flexible nasopharyngoscopy for assessment of mucosal trauma to the retropharynx.
- Angiography if potential damage to the carotid artery.

Consider involvement of the teeth in cases of oral trauma, and referral to a Dentist (see Chapter 17, Dentistry).

Foreign bodies in the throat
Fish bones
Most fish bones lodge in the tonsil and can be seen and readily removed in the Emergency Department.
- Use a headlight and spray the tonsil with lignocaine or co-phenylcaine spray first.
- Remove the bone using Magill forceps.
- If the bone is not visible, nasendoscopy is performed. If a bone is seen in the back of the tongue it may be removed using a tongue depressor and Magill forceps, but if lower in the pharynx a general anaesthetic may be required.
- If no foreign body is seen the child should be reviewed within 48 hours and if there are still symptoms, a CT scan may be useful to show the bone or swelling.

Upper respiratory tract infections (URTIs)
Young children, especially pre-school age, may have up to 12 URTIs a year.
- The aetiology is from a number of viruses, and improvement is usually by 10 days.
- There is usually nasal obstruction, rhinorrhoea, sore throat, earaches and cough.
- There may be fever, and infants and young children may be quite lethargic and have reduced feeding; it is important to exclude serious bacterial infections.
- Often there is purulent rhinorrhoea. This does not mean that there is a superimposed bacterial sinusitis.

Management
- Symptomatic, ensuring adequate fluid intake and administering paracetamol for pain.
- Saline drops and sprays may help clear the rhinorrhoea to assist nasal obstruction and difficulty with feeding and sleeping.

Otitis media
The peak age for middle ear problems is 9 months, and it is common in pre-school age children, but can occur at any age. An acute infection is often followed by middle ear fluid for a variable time.

Predisposing factors
- Family history of otitis media, and especially in older siblings
- Attendance in day care
- Exposure to tobacco smoke
- Use of a dummy/pacifier
- Exposure to chlorine swimming pools
- Season – winter and spring
- Known immunological deficiencies

Acute otitis media
- History of *acute* onset of symptoms and signs of pain and fever, often in the setting of an URTI
- A middle ear effusion or perforation of the tympanic membrane (TM) with otorrhoea
  - The TM is opaque due to the fluid in the middle ear.
  - Reduced TM mobility, as assessed by pneumatic otoscopy and/or tympanometry, if available.

- Signs and symptoms of middle ear inflammation, characterised by redness of the TM. There are prominent vessels and erythema due to the inflammation.

Note: Be wary of accepting AOM as the sole diagnosis in an unwell infant with a fever. There may be a coexistent serious bacterial infection. Consider a septic work-up or careful observation.

Clinical Pearl: Tympanic Membrane (TM)

The presence or absence of the light reflex on the TM is not a useful sign to determine if the middle ear is healthy.

- If there is acute otitis media the handle of the malleus is not seen well due to bulging of the TM.
- If there is a middle ear effusion the handle of the malleus is more prominent and more horizontal.

ATM may be red from fever or crying.

Management

All children should have analgesia with paracetamol or ibuprofen.

Most cases of AOM in children resolve spontaneously. The routine use of antibiotic treatment should be avoided.

Antibiotic treatment is recommended if the child:

- Is sick with severe pain, high fever, possible complication
  - Mastoiditis
  - Facial nerve palsy
  - Possible intracranial complication with abscess or venous sinus thrombosis
- Has bilateral disease
- Has a perforated TM (implies more virulent organism)
- Has a known immune deficiency
- Is Aboriginal or Torres Strait or Pacific Islander
- Has a cochlear implant
- Has an infection in an only hearing ear
- Has unresolved pain after 48 hours of symptomatic otitis media
- Is 23 months or younger

The usual antibiotic treatment, if required, is amoxicillin 15 mg/kg (max. 500 mg) orally 8 hourly for 10 days.

- If there has been treatment with amoxicillin in the last 30 days or no improvement in acute symptoms after 48 hours of amoxycillin then consider treatment with amoxycillin+clavulanate 22.5 + 3.2 mg/kg up to 875 + 125 mg orally, 12 hourly for 10 days.
- If there is an allergy to penicillin, treatment with cefuroxime is recommended (children 3 months and older) 15 mg/kg up to 500 mg orally, 12-hourly or trimethoprim+sulfamethoxazole (child 1 month or older) 4 + 20 mg/kg up to 160 + 800 mg orally, 12-hourly.
- As an adjunct, short-term use of topical 2% lignocaine, 1-2 drops applied to an INTACT TM may be effective for severe acute ear pain.
- Decongestants, antihistamines and corticosteroids are NOT effective in AOM or in the resolution of otitis media with effusion.

Follow up

- Review the child in 1–2 days if there is unresolved pain or fever.
- A middle ear effusion is present for a variable period following AOM and may be associated with noticeable hearing loss, particularly if bilateral. Most resolve by 3 months after the infection, so a review at this time with possible audiogram can be arranged.

Putting Evidence into Practice: Acute otitis media

Among children 6 to 23 months of age with acute otitis media, 5 days of antimicrobial treatment resulted in less favorable outcomes than 10 days of treatment; in addition, neither the rate of adverse events nor the rate of emergence of antimicrobial resistance was lower with the shorter regimen.

Source: Hoberman A., et al. (2016) *N Engl J Med 375(25):2446–2456.*

Mastoiditis

This is a severe complication of AOM. Children are unwell, presenting with features of AOM associated with more severe systemic symptoms and post-auricular inflammation (ranging from cellulitis to subperiosteal abscess). Management involves referral to otolaryngologist and IV antibiotics. Unless mild, children will require insertion of middle ear ventilation tubes and drainage of the subperiosteal abscess. Mastoidectomy is performed where cholesteatoma is suspected or in the presence of an additional suppurative complication.

Recurrent acute otitis media

Defined as three or more episodes in six months or four or more episodes in twelve months.
To prevent this:
- Reduce contact with people with upper respiratory infections.
- Avoid pacifiers/dummy (5.4 episodes of OM vs 3.6 if no dummy).
- Breast feed for at least six months, and preferably twelve months. If the baby is bottle fed, do not prop the bottle up with the baby lying flat as the milk may pass into the eustachian tubes.
- Avoid tobacco smoke as there is a 38% higher rate of AOM, and middle ear effusions (MEE) of longer duration especially if the child attends day care.
- Vaccinate with PCV-13. There is a reduction in OM episodes by 8%, and a reduction in the number of children requiring operative treatment with ventilation tubes by 20%.
- Avoid chlorine pools.

Otitis Media with Effusion (OME)

OME (also called serous otitis or glue ear) is fluid in the middle ear without signs and symptoms of infection, although there is variable hearing impairment.
- Antibiotics and ENT referral are not routinely required for OME, as the majority of cases occur after an episode of AOM and resolve spontaneously with no long term effects on language, literacy or cognitive development.
- Persistent effusion beyond 3 months should trigger a hearing assessment and ENT involvement/referral.

Management

Medical
- For most children the effusions resolve with time and with the end of winter.
- Balloon insufflation: this needs the ability to co-ordinate blowing the balloon and then swallowing, and so is not usually possible in young children. It does have short term benefits but not long term.

Surgery with insertion of middle ear ventilation tubes:
- Middle ear ventilation tubes provide good short-term benefit, without altering the underlying Eustachian tube dysfunction responsible for OME.
- There is relief of symptoms by providing an alternative means for middle ear ventilation.
- In the months that the tubes remain in place there is normalisation of the middle ear mucosa, a change in season, and maturation of the child's immune system.
- Depending on the growth of the child and the design of the tube, these remain in place for months to years before extruding.
- The long-term impact of tube insertion on language, literacy and cognitive function is the subject of ongoing research, and the most important factor for language enhancement for young children is interaction with their carers and a rich language environment.

Insertion of middle ear ventilation tubes is considered if:
- The middle ear effusions are present for at least three months and appear likely to persist long term, especially if this is bilateral, and
- There are significant symptoms: either recurrent AOM or functionally significant hearing loss (e.g. speech delay, behavioural disturbance or poor school performance).
- Other children with only a mild hearing impairment who may benefit include:
  ○ Suspected or diagnosed speech and language delay or disorder.
  ○ Autism-spectrum disorder and other pervasive developmental disorders.
  ○ Children with blindness or uncorrectable visual impairment.

Other reasons for recommending insertion of middle ear ventilation tubes include:
- Unresolved acute otitis media (especially young children in winter)
- Complications of acute otitis media such as facial palsy, mastoiditis
- Recurrent acute otitis media
  - 3 or more well-documented and separate AOM episodes in the past 6 months.
  - 4 or more well-documented and separate AOM episodes in the past 12 months.
  - Atelectasis or retraction pocket in the TM.

Management of discharging ears in children with tubes or perforated TMs
- Ear toilet using tissue spears
- Topical antibiotics, for example ciprofloxacin (avoid aminoglycosides)
- For refractory discharge:
  - Sample for microscopy, culture and sensitivity
  - 1.5% hydrogen peroxide ear washes
  - Refer to an ENT Surgeon
  - Consider the possibility of an underlying immunodeficiency or cholesteatoma

Otitis externa
Commonly occurs due to water contamination following swimming, or in children with dermatitis of the external auditory canal. It is characterised by:
- Pain (often severe).
- Inflammation of the ear canal, which may include the TM (mobility of the TM on pneumatic otoscopy excludes otitis media).
- Pre-auricular or post-auricular tenderness.

Management
- Ear toilet.
- Topical antibiotics combined with steroids (e.g. ciprofloxacin HC).
- An ear wick should be inserted when the ear canal is very oedematous (to maintain patency of the ear canal and allow topical antibiotics to enter the ear canal) and moistened frequently with topical antibiotics.
- Swab for microscopy, culture and sensitivity if the infection is slow to resolve.
- Hospital admission for administration of (anti-pseudomonal) intravenous antibiotics when ear pain is severe and not relieved by regular analgesics, or where cellulitis has extended beyond the ear canal.
- Children with fungal otitis externa need treatment with anti-fungal drops or cream, and review for ear toileting until there is no further accumulation of debris.

Acute sinusitis
The child is unwell and has nasal obstruction or purulent rhinorrhoea. There may also be frontal headache or cough.
- Anterior rhinoscopy can be performed using an otoscope and will show swollen, red mucosa; it may be possible to see pus from the middle meatus under the middle turbinate.
- Imaging, including plain films and CT, are not recommended unless there is a possible complication.
- Symptoms for fewer than 10 days are likely to be a viral infection and can be treated with symptomatic relief including analgesia, saline irrigations and topical nasal decongestants if there is significant nasal obstruction.
- If symptoms continue for longer than 10 days, consider treatment with topical nasal steroids as well.
- Immediate referral should be made if there is:
  - Periorbital swelling or erythema or concerns with displaced globe or double vision.
  - Reduced visual acuity.
  - Severe frontal headache or swelling.
  - Concerns with meningitis or any neurological signs.
- If CT imaging is requested, this should be with contrast to demonstrate any intracranial complications, and the views requested should include complete views of the paranasal sinuses in case surgery is needed.
- The management includes intravenous antibiotics, nasal saline irrigations; topical decongestants; topical nasal steroids; systemic steroids; imaging with a CT scan with contrast; and surgery if needed.

- Antibiotic treatment is considered if there is:
  - Clinically severe sinusitis with purulent rhinorrhoea, fever, localised pain
  - Possible complication of sinusitis
- Hospital admission should be considered if there are severe symptoms and/or possible complications.

Chronic rhinosinusitis

There is chronic inflammation of both the nasal mucosa and the paranasal sinuses.

- The main symptoms are nasal obstruction and rhinorrhoea although there may be a cough.
- The aetiology is multifactorial and usually improves by 8 years, largely due to maturity of the immune system.
- Predisposing factors include attendance in day care, exposure to tobacco smoke and chlorinated pools.
- Medical imaging is not helpful in deciding if there is significant sinusitis as many children who no longer have symptoms, have changes in the sinuses on scans for weeks after recovering from an URTI.
- Most children do not need investigation but if there is irritability, failure to thrive and other infections including chest problems, consider testing for allergy, immunological competence and cilial function.
- The mainstays of treatment for happy children are reassurance, saline sprays, learning to blow the nose, and topical nasal steroids.
- If there is significant nasal obstruction, an adenoidectomy may be helpful.

Note: Antihistamines are not indicated in URTIs unless coexistent allergic rhinitis is suspected. Refer to Chapter 13, Allergy. Antihistamines, especially sedating varieties, should be avoided in children younger than 24 months old; they can make the obstructive symptoms worse and tend to make secretions thicker.

Acute pharyngitis/tonsillitis

The combination of fever and sore throat is a common presenting problem in children.
Acute tonsillitis is a clinical diagnosis:

- Sore throat
- Fever
- Red tonsils sometimes with exudate
- Tender cervical lymphadenopathy
- Absence of cough

Commonly associated symptoms:

- Headache
- Dysphagia
- Snoring
- There may also be abdominal pain, vomiting, earache

Most sore throats are due to a viral infection (almost all sore throats in children 4 years old or younger).

- The only clinically important bacterial pathogen is group A β-haemolytic streptococcus (GABHS), *Streptococcus pyogenes*.
  - GABHS is less likely if the child has associated coryza, cough, generalised lymphadenopathy or splenomegaly.
  - Treatment with penicillin reduces the incidence of acute rheumatic fever but not of acute glomerulonephritis. Although penicillin reduces the duration of symptoms this is by only a few hours and is not of clinical significance. See Chapter 25, Infectious diseases.
- Infectious mononucleosis is a relatively common cause of acute pharyngitis in older children.
  - The diagnosis often becomes apparent when other characteristic features develop (e.g. generalised lymphadenopathy, splenomegaly, mild jaundice and rashes), there is no response to penicillin and the illness follows a more prolonged course.
  - A rash commonly occurs if amoxicillin is prescribed.

Alerts for possible complications of tonsillitis

- Stertor
- Drooling/difficulty swallowing

> **Clinical Pearl: Tonsilitis**
> The presence of exudate on the tonsils does not distinguish between a viral cause and Group A β-haemolytic streptococcus (GABHS).

Investigations

Throat cultures are not helpful in the diagnosis as:

- There is a high asymptomatic carrier rate.
- Superficial throat swabs are a poor guide to the microflora in the tonsil crypts.

Streptococcal serology is also not helpful in diagnosis.

Management

- Children who probably **do not** need antibiotics are those aged 4 years or younger, and/or those with associated cough or coryza.
- Children who benefit from antibiotic treatment for acute sore throat include:
  - Children 2 to 25 years with sore throat in communities with a high incidence of acute rheumatic fever, (e.g. some Indigenous communities in central and northern Australia, and some other communities such as Pacific islanders)
  - Children of any age with existing rheumatic heart disease
  - Children with scarlet fever (with a distinctive rash)
- Antibiotic treatment is oral phenoxymethylpenicillin 250 mg (500 mg if >10 years) BD for 10 days
- For children with true penicillin allergy, Azithromycin 500 mg (child: 12 mg/kg up to 500 mg) orally, daily for 5 days, may be used.

> **Clinical Pearl: Duration of antibiotic treatment in tonsillitis**
> Symptoms of streptococcal pharyngitis and tonsillitis usually last 7 days. However, a 10-day treatment duration is recommended for phenoxymethylpenicillin and cefalexin to eradicate *S. pyogenes* from the pharynx and prevent nonsuppurative complications. Azithromycin has a long intracellular half-life, so 5 days of treatment is sufficient.

Quinsy (peritonsillar abscess)

Infection can extend beyond the tonsil as cellulitis (peritonsillar cellulitis) or as a peritonsillar abscess (quinsy). In addition to features of severe tonsillitis, quinsy presents with drooling, a 'hot potato' voice, and trismus. There is inflammation of the palate adjacent to the tonsil with the uvula pushed to the other side. In the earlier cellulitic stage, the condition will settle with IV antibiotics, but where an abscess is present, drainage is necessary.

Recurrent acute pharyngitis/tonsillitis

Recurrent sore throats are a normal part of growing up for many children, and when starting to have contact with other young children, 6 infections in a year is common. Some have a year of recurrent infections and then have fewer the subsequent years, but there are children who continue to have recurrent infections with considerable pain, dysphagia, and time at home.

Tonsillectomy (with or without adenoidectomy) should be considered if the pattern of infection (i.e. frequency, severity and duration of infections) is such that significant morbidity is expected to continue for a prolonged and unacceptable period of time. The presence of associated airway obstruction may influence the decision about the benefits of tonsillectomy and adenoidectomy.

Neck masses

Diagnosis

A differential diagnosis can usually be made based on history and examination findings including clinical history (congenital or acquired, presence or absence of fever and tenderness), location (midline or lateral) and imaging characteristics (cystic versus solid).

Infectious/inflammatory (reactive) lymphadenopathy
- Most common.
- Usually results from a URTI.
- Most resolve in 6 weeks.

Congenital
- Thyroglossal duct cysts are in the midline, usually near the hyoid bone and thyroid cartilage.
- Branchial cysts are in the lateral neck. These may become apparent after a cold with increase in size and pain from an abscess.
- Branchial cleft cyst (usually second) presents as a painless enlarging neck mass anterior to the sternomastoid muscle, or with infection after a URTI.

Neoplastic
- Rare.
- Majority are lymphomas but may be from sarcomas, or thyroid gland tumours.

Management
If it is likely to be an inflamed lymph node, either observe for 6 weeks or treat with a course of antibiotics. At 6 weeks if it is unchanged or enlarged, consider investigation:
- FBE and film, LFT including LDH and serology for CMV, EBV, toxoplasmosis, Bartonella and Quantiferon Gold.
- Ultrasound if concerns about possible abscess, typical or atypical mycobacterium, rapidly enlarging painless mass larger than 2 cm, or if the mass has not resolved by 2 months.
- If the mass is deep in the neck imaging with MRI will give more information than an ultrasound.

Consider referral to Infectious Diseases physician if concern about infection, and to an ENT surgeon if an abscess, possible malignancy or likely congenital neck mass.

Hearing loss

Children with hearing loss are at risk of speech and language delay, which may contribute to learning, behavioural and social problems. The more severe and prolonged the hearing loss, the greater the chance of developmental impairment. Some children may be affected by even mild levels of impairment (e.g. difficulty learning in a noisy classroom). Associated disabilities may magnify the adverse effects of hearing loss.

Hearing threshold (loudness) is measured in decibels (dB) and represent the softest sounds that the child can hear (Table 33.1). Frequency (or pitch) is measured in Hertz (Hz).

Screening
Almost all infants born in Australia are offered Universal Newborn Hearing Screening (UNHS). Infants who have a 'refer' from either or both ears will have confirmatory testing at an audiology centre. Approximately half of the babies who are referred for full testing have hearing loss in one or both ears.

Formal audiological testing
There are two main types of audiological testing: objective and behavioural. Objective testing, e.g. auditory brainstem response (ABR) and auditory steady state responses (ASSR), is most commonly used for infants and

Table 33.1 Degrees of hearing loss.

Hearing loss	Hearing thresholds in decibels (dB)	Possible impacts on speech
Normal hearing	≤20 dB	Normal speech
Mild	21 – 40 dB	Difficulty hearing soft speech and in background noise.
Moderate	41 – 60 dB	Miss most of the conversation. Reduced vocabulary. Poor pronunciation.
Severe	61 – 80 dB	Speech and language very limited without amplification.
Severe to profound	81 – 90 dB	Very limited speech without a cochlear implant. Will need to learn sign language if no implant.
Profound	≥ 91 dB	

children who have developmental delay, and relies on the child's electrophysiological responses to noise. Behavioural testing, e.g. visual reinforcement audiometry (VRA) and pure tone audiometry (PTA), relies on the child physically responding to a noise, and depending on the child's development, can be used from age six months or older.

Medical assessment of hearing-impaired children

Around 40% of children with hearing loss have medical and developmental co-morbidities including visual, language and learning problems. Assessment is aimed at identifying important causes and associations of hearing loss to guide management. Most parents of hearing-impaired children have normal hearing, because most genetic causes of hearing loss are of autosomal recessive inheritance.

Hearing loss may be conductive, sensorineural or mixed, and may be unilateral or bilateral.

- The most common cause of hearing loss in children is transient conductive loss from middle ear fluid, usually as a result of otitis media.
- More than 50% of children with sensorineural hearing loss have an underlying genetic aetiology.
  - Most children with genetic hearing loss are non-syndromic (no other physical features apart from hearing loss), while around 25% have an identifiable syndrome.
  - At least 100 different genetic mutations have been identified to cause hearing loss, with the majority of autosomal recessive inheritance. Of these, the most common is the connexin 26/30 gene GJB2/6.

History

- Antenatal history: spontaneous/recurrent miscarriages, maternal immunisation status and serological results, infections or febrile/flu-like illnesses (particularly cytomegalovirus (CMV), toxoplasmosis, herpes simplex virus (HSV), varicella, rubella, syphilis, human immunodeficiency virus (HIV)), medication use (e.g. ototoxic medications), drug/alcohol use.
- Birth history: gestation, delivery type, condition at birth (e.g. Apgar scores), birth growth parameters, complications/interventions at delivery, abnormalities noted/suspected/diagnosed at birth.
- Postnatal/medical history: jaundice requiring phototherapy/exchange transfusion, peak serum bilirubin, bacterial meningitis, head injuries, proven/suspected congenital infections, exposure to ototoxic medications (e.g. aminoglycosides, loop diuretics, cisplatin), cranial irradiation, motor delay/balance issues (consider vestibular dysfunction), haematuria (Alport syndrome).
- Family history: three-generation family tree, audiograms from first-degree relatives, family history of:
  - Hearing loss
  - Goitre (Pendred syndrome)
  - Pigment abnormalities (Waardenburg syndrome, neurofibromatosis type 2),
  - Congenital renal anomalies or renal failure (Alport syndrome, branchio-oto-renal syndrome BOR)
  - Short stature (Stickler syndrome, 22q deletion)
  - Cardiac malformations (22q deletion, CHARGE)
  - Arrhythmias/sudden death (Jervell Lange Nielson)
  - Vision issues (Usher syndrome)

Examination

See Table 33.2.

Investigations and further assessments to consider for hearing loss

- **Ophthalmology / vision assessment:** Ophthalmic abnormalities affect 30–60% of children with hearing loss. Multisensory deficits can have compounding effects on the child's development.
- **Family audiograms for first-degree family members:** To help complete the family pedigree and may detect subclinical hearing loss in family members, especially siblings.
- **CMV saliva or dried blood spot PCR:** Congenital cytomegalovirus (cCMV) infection is the most common infectious cause of childhood hearing loss. It can cause fluctuating or progressive hearing loss. If diagnosed early (by saliva PCR within 21 days of birth), there may be treatment options available. After 21 days of age, testing for cCMV should be completed by checking CMV PCR on the newborn screening dried blood spot (Guthrie) card.
- **Other perinatal infection testing:** Should be considered for 'at risk' babies i.e. known maternal infection (serological or clinical evidence), ophthalmology findings

Table 33.2 Key characteristics on physical examination.

Examination systems	Physical features	Examples of diagnoses to consider
Growth	Microcephaly Low birth weight	Congenital infections

Development	Developmental delay/regression
	Gross motor delay*
		Congenital infections / metabolic disorders
		Neurological causes (e.g. prematurity, hypoxic
		   ischaemia encephalopathy)
		*Gross motor delay may be an early manifestation of
		   vestibular dysfunction (consider Pendred, Usher)

General	Dysmorphology Pigmentation: skin / hair /eyes Coarse features Blood pressure	Syndromic causes Waardenburg syndrome Metabolic / storage disorders Renal causes

Head and neck	Facial asymmetry
	Abnormal external ears
	Abnormal ear canals
	Preauricular sinuses / pits / tags
	Bifid uvula
	Cleft palate / submucous cleft
	Tympanic membrane status
	Goitre
		Developmental causes (especially with unilateral
		   hearing loss e.g. branchio-oto-renal syndrome)
		
		Middle ear fluid
		Pendred Syndrome (goitre onset usually in mid-late
		   childhood)

Eyes	Cataracts
	Retinal scarring (fundoscopy)
	Microphthalmia
	Hypertelorism
	Heterochromia iridium
	Retinitis pigmentosa
	   (fundoscopy)
		Congenital infections
		
		Syndromic causes
		Waardenburg Syndrome
		Usher Syndrome (retinitis pigmentosa onset usually in
		   mid-late childhood; electroretinography best
		   screening tool)

Neurologic	Hypotonia Ataxia Focal neurological signs	Neurological causes (e.g. prematurity, hypoxic ischaemia encephalopathy, space occupying lesions)
Cardiac	Murmur	Related cardiac conditions
Skeletal	Spine Digits Nails Hyperextendable joints	Bony dysplasias Connective tissue disorders
Abdominal	Organomegaly	Storage disorders
Urine dipstick / microscopy	Haematuria	Alport (onset usually late childhood)

- **Thyroid function:** Should be considered where there is clinical indication of thyroid dysfunction (developmental delay, abnormal growth), a history of early newborn bloodspot screen (before 48 hours of age), or presence of goiter. In Pendred syndrome, children develop hearing loss early, with goitre and/or thyroid dysfunction occurring later.
- **Genetic testing:** The option of genetic testing should be offered to children with bilateral sensorineural hearing loss, as more than half will have a genetic aetiology. Testing for connexin 26/30 (GJB2/6) mutation is first-line. Other genetic testing options, such as genomic sequencing, depend on funding and availability. Genetic testing is not indicated for unilateral loss.

- **Metabolic testing:** Genetic testing for mitochondrial DNA variants (MT-RNR1) should be considered if there is suspicion of or a family history of aminoglycoside-induced hearing loss. Urine metabolic testing to be considered where there is progressive hearing loss or other clinical indications (e.g. developmental regression).
- **Urinalysis for haematuria / proteinuria:** Should be considered for delayed onset or progressive hearing loss, or family history of renal diseases associated with hearing loss
- **Resting ECG:** Should be considered for children with bilateral severe to profound hearing loss to exclude Jervell and Lange–Nielsen syndrome. It is characterised by prolonged QT interval on ECG and is associated with tachyarrhythmias and risk of sudden death.
- **MRI brain and parasagittal sections of internal acoustic canal:** MRI is important for diagnosis of large endolymphatic ducts and sacs (LEDS), associated with enlarged vestibular aqueducts (EVA), also known as large vestibular aqueduct syndrome (LVAS). LEDS/EVA/LVAS is associated with progressive hearing loss and deterioration can occur with mild head trauma. In unilateral hearing loss, MRI abnormalities are identified in more than 50% of cases. MRI is essential before cochlear implantation.
- **CT scan:** Should be considered for permanent conductive hearing loss, or if further information required beyond MRI
- **Renal Ultrasound:** Should be considered if there are multi-system abnormalities, family history of renal malformations associated with hearing loss, maternal history of hearing loss and diabetes or the following physical features: isolated pre-auricular pits, cup ears or other ear anomaly accompanied by one or more of the following: cochlear/vestibular malformations (seen on imaging), other branchial abnormalities (e.g. branchial cleft fistulae or cysts).

Management of children with hearing loss

Management options will be considered by the otolaryngologist, audiologist and family. Some causes will be amenable to surgical interventions (e.g. grommet insertion for middle ear fluid) but most permanent causes of hearing loss require optimisation of communication potential by other means, including sign language, amplification (with hearing aids) or cochlear implant.

CHAPTER 34
Palliative care

Bronwyn Sacks
Molly Williams
Sidharth Vemuri
Jenny Hynson

Key Points
- Palliative care can start at any time, even when a child is receiving curative or disease-directed treatment and continues for as long as needed.
- Do not be afraid of sadness or silence, important things are often said after a long pause in the conversation. Try to find a quiet place and allow sufficient time to speak with families.
- Wherever possible, it is useful to discuss goals of care and key decisions before a crisis occurs and when the child is well. Advanced Care Planning (ACP) is a process of discussions between families and health care providers about preferences for care, treatments and goals in the context of the child's current and anticipated future health.
- Families and children can simultaneously hold realistic insight and maintain hope. The clinician's task is to understand the full breadth of hopes (from the mundane to the miraculous), and offer realistic hope in terms of ongoing support, attention to symptoms and help to maximise the child's quality of life.
- Treatment of symptoms by exploring and addressing all contributing factors is likely to be far more effective than medications alone.

Paediatric palliative care is an active and holistic approach to care that aims to improve the well-being of infants, children, and young people with life-limiting conditions and their families. It includes, but is not restricted to, end of life care; and is much more about living well than dying.

This approach to care involves:
- Provision of developmentally appropriate assessment and management.
- Discussions regarding a child's diagnosis, prognosis and goals of treatment, including advance care planning (ACP).
- Provision of, or referral to, psychosocial and practical support services.
- Assessment and management of troublesome symptoms.
- End-of-life care.

Who can provide palliative care?
All paediatric health care providers who care for children living with life-limiting conditions and their families can provide elements of palliative care. Parents prefer their child's trusted clinician to provide key elements of palliative care, such as ACP at times when their child is medically well. However, there are times when the assistance of specialist paediatric palliative care (SPPC) services is needed.

Specialists in palliative care are available in all states in Australia and can help in the provision of direct care to children with complex palliative care needs, such as difficult symptoms and complex decision-making, and practical supports to live well with their illness. They can also help children achieve personal goals (e.g. returning to school). SPPC teams provide care in a variety of locations, including hospital, home, respite centres or hospices.

Paediatric Handbook, Tenth Edition. Edited by Kate Harding, Daniel S. Mason and Daryl Efron.
© 2021 John Wiley & Sons Ltd. Published 2021 by John Wiley & Sons Ltd.

SPPC services often work in a consultative role, to support and educate others who are partnering in palliative care. This is because parents prefer an approach that integrates palliative care with their primary treating team.

When should palliative care start?

Palliative care should start when it is needed. This can be at diagnosis, when the prognosis is uncertain and treatment is still being given in the hope of a cure, when a disease has become unresponsive to treatment, or when the child is deteriorating. Often it is helpful to ask, "would I be surprised if this child died within a year?" If the answer is no, elements of palliative care should be incorporated into the child's care, and referral to SPPC considered.

Is it too early to involve a SPPC team?

Clinicians may worry about introducing palliative care 'too early'. However, evidence shows that children and their families are receptive to early integration of palliative care, and parallel disease-directed treatment alongside palliative care is widely recommended. Early involvement of a palliative care team has been shown to:

- Improve symptom management
- Improve quality of life
- Improve overall child and caregiver satisfaction with care
- Reduce caregiver burden and improve caregiver wellbeing.
- Improve communication

In contrast to adult medicine, most children requiring SPPC have non-malignant conditions. Children can be involved with SPPC for months or even years. Some children will have fluctuating palliative care needs and may dip in and out of SPPC services.

Helpful ways to introduce the SPPC team include:

'I'd like to get some help from the palliative care team because they can provide an extra layer of support and advice for us to give Mohammad the best possible care'

'I'm not sure what the future holds for Jane but I am worried that things might not work out as we hope. We routinely ask the palliative care team to help at times like these, so we can face this uncertainty together'

'Palliative care can help us hope for the best and have plans in case things work out differently'

Decision-making for children with life-limiting conditions

Talking with families about their child's prognosis and making decisions about care can be extremely difficult. Staff should be aware of the impact of their own feelings of anxiety, sadness and impotence. Most families appreciate honest information given in an empathic way, tempered with a sense of hope.

Wherever possible, it is useful to discuss goals of care and key decisions before a crisis occurs and when the child is well. Advanced Care Planning (ACP) is 'a process of discussions between families and health care providers about preferences for care, treatments and goals in the context of the child's current and anticipated future health.' The Thinking Ahead Framework provides a stepwise approach in which the clinical team shares knowledge about the child's condition, prognosis and the potential efficacy, benefits and burdens of various interventions, and the child and family share their values, goals and hopes, and what they believe the child might experience as a benefit or burden. It is not imperative to make clear decisions in advance. The value of ACP is in laying the groundwork so that better decisions can be made in times of crisis. The Thinking Ahead Framework is available from The Victorian department of health and human services, www2.health.vic.gov.au/about/publications/policiesandguidelines/thinking-ahead-resources.

It is important to establish child and parents' preferred roles in discussions and decision-making. Some will find shared decision-making empowering, whilst others may find it burdensome. Medical leadership is very important. Parents should not feel that they are solely responsible for decisions. The team should talk before meeting with the family, in order to minimise the risk of confusion or delivery of mixed messages. A trusted clinician known to the family should lead the discussion and provide guidance and direction about what they believe to be the best way forward.

This conversation is often best started by talking in very general terms and asking some fundamental questions. It may be helpful to outline a plan of what you'd like to cover in the meeting. Ensure that the child and family have ample opportunity to express their expectations for the meeting, and to articulate their values, hopes, concerns and fears. Remember to acknowledge and empathise with emotions; it is difficult to do any cognitive processing when feeling emotionally overwhelmed. Do not be afraid of sadness or silence, important things are often said after a long pause in the conversation. Try to find a quiet place and allow sufficient time to speak with the family. Ensure those who need to be present are but be mindful of having too many people in the room. Suggested questions and phrasing might include:

- *Tell me about your child: what does she enjoy? What things frighten her? What is it like for her to be in hospital?*
- *What do you understand about her condition right now?*
- *What is most important to you?*
- *What are the most frightening things for you?*

Where there is disagreement, resolution is usually achieved with time and good communication. Try to avoid 'convincing' parents of the reality of their child's situation. They usually know but strong emotions are at play. Helping them acknowledge, express and explore these emotions can be a helpful intervention. Where disagreement cannot be resolved, a second opinion, consultation with a clinical ethics service and/or legal advice may be helpful. It is always important to tell parents that you can see how much they love their child and that they are trying to do the best they can.

Clinical Pearl: Advanced care planning
- ACP is an iterative process, not an event.
- There is value in discussing and reviewing goals, values, hopes and fears in the context of a life limiting condition, even when no agreed ACP can be achieved.
- ACP should begin when the child is well wherever possible.
- Goals may change over time, and it is okay for a child to die without an ACP.
- A resuscitation order is a communication tool regarding medical treatment. It is not a legally binding document, and does not require parents' signatures.
- Hope is an important therapeutic tool which can enhance communication with respect to ACP. Hope does not necessarily reflect lack of insight or denial on the part of the child and family.
- The Thinking Ahead Framework provides a useful guide to having conversations about ACP.

Approach to symptom management

Distressing symptoms are extremely common in children with life-limiting conditions. Recognising, assessing and holistically treating these symptoms in order to maximise functioning and preserve quality of life is the core business of paediatric palliative care. A child's experience of symptoms is influenced by individual physical, psychological, social and spiritual factors. Treatment of symptoms by exploring and addressing these factors is likely to be far more effective than medications alone (Table 34.1). A comprehensive approach to symptom management in the child with palliative care needs is summarised in Figure 34.1.

Pain

Pain is present in more than 80% of children with cancer who are receiving palliative care and more than 70% of children with severe neurological impairment (SNI). Pain is frequently under-recognised and under-treated, particularly in non-verbal children. The investigation for the cause of pain should not preclude or delay appropriate analgesia.

Pain can be categorised as neuropathic, visceral or nociceptive. Most pain, regardless of cause, will respond to opioids; the addition of adjuvant pain medications may optimise comfort and function in children with neuropathic pain. Many parents fear that opioids will cause respiratory depression or hasten death. This is incorrect. Appropriate analgesia has been found to extend life in the palliative phase, and the risk of respiratory depression is extremely low when opioids are titrated appropriately.

For pain in the palliative phase, analgesia should be given regularly rather than PRN, starting with simple agents and adding opioids and adjuvants if pain is more severe, and by a route and in a formulation that is most acceptable to the individual. Enteral routes are generally preferred, with subcutaneous routes reserved for those with impairment in swallow or gut absorption (doses are equivalent to IV route). Children can receive subcutaneous analgesia at home with the support of community palliative care teams.

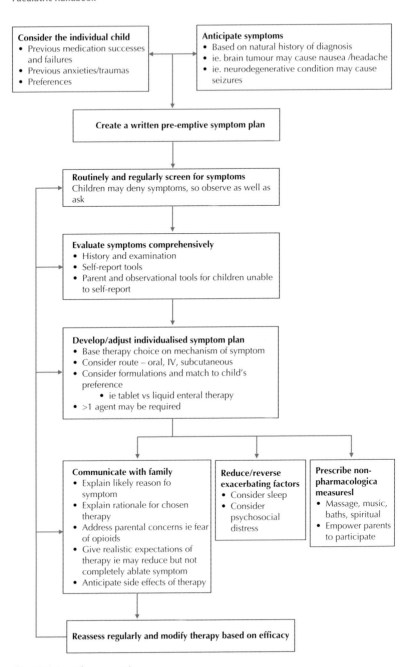

Figure 34.1 Approach to symptomatic management.

Table 34.1 Common symptom control medications.

Symptom	Common medication	Starting dose	Second line therapies
Pain	Morphine	**ORAL** **1-12m**: 0.1mg/kg q4h PRN **>12m**: 0.2mg/kg q4h PRN (max dose 5mg) **IV/SC** **0-1m**: 0.025mg/kg q6h PRN **1-6m**: 0.1mg/kg q6h PRN **>6m**: 0.1mg/kg q4h PRN (max dose 2.5mg)	Oxycodone Hydromorphone Fentanyl Methadone
	Gabapentin	10mg/kg PO TDS	Pregabalin Amitriptyline Ketamine
Dyspnoea	Morphine	50% of pain dose, see above	
	Clonazepam	0.01-0.02mg/kg buccal Q6h PRN	Midazolam
Agitation	Midazolam	0.1-0.2mg/kg IV/SC q4h PRN	Levomepromazine
	Clonazepam	0.01-0.02mg/kg buccal Q6h PRN	
Nausea	Ondansetron	0.15mg/kg PO/IV TDS PRN (max 8mg/dose)	Levomepromazine
	Metoclopramide	0.15mg/kg PO/IV/SC TDS PRN (max 10mg/dose)	
	Cyclizine	0.5-1mg/kg PO/IV/SC TDS PRN (max 50mg/dose)	
Constipation	Macrogol	½-1 sachet PO daily	Bisacodyl Glycerol supps Microlax enema
	Sodium picosulfate	5-10 drops PO nocte	
Fatigue	Methylphenidate	6-12y: 5mg daily >12y: 10mg daily	

Dyspnoea

Dyspnoea is the unpleasant sensation of breathlessness. It may be present with or without tachypnoea (rapid breathing). Laboured breathing/gasping may be present in an unconscious child at end-of-life and is not necessarily uncomfortable. A hand-held fan directed at the face is effective in reducing dyspnoea. Low dose opioids may also treat dyspnoea through modulation of the reflexive drive to breathe and reduction in awareness of breathlessness, as well as improved breathing efficiency. Benzodiazepines may also reduce associated anxiety.

Terminal agitation

Restlessness and agitation in the terminal phase appear to be less common in children than in adults; it is an extremely distressing symptom to staff and parents as well as to children. Creating calm and familiar surroundings with the child's family and belongings may reduce this symptom. Agitation may be associated with reversible factors including urinary retention, infection, pain and medication side effects, and these should be actively considered and reversed if possible.

Sedation with benzodiazepines is the mainstay of pharmacological treatment, with other sedating therapies, including levomepromazine or phenobarbitone, available for refractory symptoms. There is some controversy around the use of antipsychotic agents in adult palliative populations, with recent trials showing no benefit of these agents over placebo in agitation.

Constipation

Constipation is an unpleasant and avoidable symptom, often associated with opioid use. Combined softeners and stimulants via the oral and rectal routes may be required to relieve this symptom. Aperients should always be prescribed when offering opioid medications. The choice of aperient depends on the preferences of the child. Macrogol is very effective but requires a relatively large volume to be ingested for efficacy; while sodium picosulfate comes in small volume drops but may cause cramping.

Nausea and vomiting

There are multiple causes of nausea. The choice of antiemetic depends on the likely cause: chemotherapy-associated nausea should be treated with serotonin receptor antagonists (i.e. ondansetron), while vomiting from gut stasis may respond better to prokinetics or dopamine receptor antagonists (i.e. domperidone). If good control of nausea is not achieved with the first agent, it is rational to trial a second treatment with alternate receptor activity. Reducing feeds, giving smaller bland meals, avoiding strong odours and attending to anxiety and distress that nausea may cause, are all invaluable in improving the child's experience.

Loss of appetite and feed intolerance

Children who are dying commonly reduce their oral intake. This is an emotionally charged symptom for parents; when food is unable to be tolerated, parents often describe a feeling of failure and loss of parental identity. Reduced feeding should be sensitively discussed pre-emptively as a natural part of the 'body winding down' and the dying process. Parents may fear their child is 'starving'. It can be useful to explain how artificial feeds can increase discomfort (i.e. by increasing nausea, worsening oedema and increasing respiratory secretions).

Feed intolerance is increasingly recognised as a pre-terminal phenomenon in children with SNI. Visceral hyperalgesia, presenting as pain behaviours associated with feeds, may be treated with neuropathic adjuvants. Recurrent episodes of abdominal pain, vomiting and reduced absorption of enteral medication are a worrying sign in this population, as the gut is a vital organ and its failure is not compatible with life.

It should be noted that the cessation of feeds in a dying child may not rapidly precipitate death. Children can live for some weeks without any intake at all. It is important to counsel families and staff about the physical changes of cachexia in the child unable to feed, and to reassure all parties that any discomfort or distress will be actively managed.

Fatigue

Fatigue is a common distressing symptom in children with malignancy, but often goes untreated. Managing pain and psychological distress, and reducing physical factors such as anaemia or infection, are important initial steps in managing fatigue. Gentle exercise, sleep hygiene and energy conservation are also helpful measures. Stimulants such as methylphenidate may be useful in more severe cases.

Psychological symptoms

Children who are dying are can experience sadness and anxiety. Allowing opportunities to communicate their emotions lightens the burden of these symptoms. While we may not be able to reassure them that they will survive their illness, we can assure them that they and their families will be cared for, will never be alone, and are loved. Music, art, play and physical therapies as well input from mental health professionals may be valuable in allowing children to explore and express their emotions.

Clinical Pearl: Symptomatic management

- The treatment of symptoms requires a holistic approach, engaging with physical, psychological, social and spiritual factors as well as pharmacology.
- Opioids are safe and effective medications for pain and dyspnoea. The risk of respiratory depression with appropriate dose titration is extremely low.
- Children with severe neurological impairment report more pain but receive less treatment than children who are verbal.
- Children may survive weeks without oral intake, if feeds are ceased in the palliative setting. Family and staff should be counselled to anticipate this.

End-of-life care & bereavement

'Life is meaningful because it is a story. . . and in stories, endings matter.' - Atul Gawande.

How a child dies significantly affects not only the child, but has a lasting impact on parents and siblings. For this reason, it is crucial that the health-care team provides skilled and sensitive care to minimise the child's suffering.

Communicating with children about death and dying

Children often know a great deal about their disease and prognosis even when they have not been 'told'. Attempts to protect the child from information may leave them feeling anxious and isolated as they sense others' distress and generate incorrect explanations for this, such as *'Mummy and Daddy are angry with me'*. Additionally, bereaved parents are likely to regret not having spoken with their terminally ill children. In general, it is best to encourage parents to be honest with children, using cognitively and developmentally appropriate information. This applies to both the child who is unwell, and their siblings.

It is important to listen to what the child is asking, and approach conversations with curiosity and sensitivity. The child who asks *'Am I going to die?'* may be most concerned about who will look after their parents, what their friends will think, or whether they will be in pain. Asking, *'What makes you ask me that?'* will provide further information upon which to base an answer. Stories, artwork, music and play allow alternative avenues for expression, build trust and facilitate communication. Just as adults do, children may wish to 'put their affairs in order'. They may want to do and say certain things to those they love and may even wish to give possessions away.

Planning for end-of-life care

Often the death of a child can be anticipated, with time to consider preferred location of care, religious and spiritual needs, and memory-making opportunities. What constitutes a 'good death' varies according to the values of children and their families. It is crucial that staff do not impose their ideas of what a good death is on the families they care for.

Most (but not all) children and families wish to spend as much time as possible at home. Most symptoms can be controlled effectively at home, with planning and the support of community-based palliative care services and the GP in consultation with SPPC staff. Although home-care offers many advantages, it may result in physical, emotional and financial stress. Re-admission to hospital or hospice should be readily available. A letter detailing the child's condition, plans in case of deterioration and people to contact, should be held by the family and forwarded to the ambulance service to facilitate appropriate care.

In most cases, reassurance that dying is generally peaceful is possible. It is often helpful to talk with parents about what to expect (e.g. reduced consciousness, reduced desire for food and fluids, reduced urine output, changes in breathing with prolonged apnoeas before their final breath).

Death needs to be clinically verified, and a medical cause of death certificate completed. Some child deaths require further investigation and are reportable to the Coroner. If in doubt, it is best to contact the Coroner's office directly for advice. Families should be prepared that care after death (including timing of funeral proceedings) may be influenced by the coronial process. The Coroner decides the extent of investigation required, including the need for autopsy.

Clinical Pearl: End of life care
- Prognostication is difficult
- The dying process may be prolonged
- Preferences for end of life care may change over time
- Truth telling is a process, not an event. It involves providing a space for children to ask questions and express themselves, and to control what information they receive.
- Truth telling does not mean burdening children with information they don't want or need.

Care after death

After a child has died, families should feel able to spend as long (or as little time) as they need with their child and offered the opportunity to wash and dress their child as a last act of love and care. Families who wish to take their child home after death should consult with a funeral director, as some preparation of the body may be necessary. Parents can usually transport their child's body from hospital to home, with the medical team providing an explanatory document. In the case of an infant death, the breastfeeding mother should be advised regarding lactation suppression.

The health-care team should be available to the family after death, and follow-up arranged. Notify other health professionals who have been and who will continue to be involved with the family, including the referring doctor, GP and maternal and child health nurse. Families should be given information regarding bereavement supports and counselling.

The death of a child often affects the parents of other children in the hospital ward or local community. Acknowledgement of a child's death with these families is important, whilst respecting confidentiality.

Bereavement

The course of parental grief following the death of a child varies greatly. When assessing bereavement risk, consider the preparedness of the family for their child's death, their view of pre-death care, their perception of available supports, their own physical and mental health, and life stressors.

Children react in their own way to a sibling's death. They may blame themselves and may fear their own death or that of others close to them. Distress may be expressed through developmental regression, school failure and physical symptoms. Staff can help siblings prepare and grieve for their sibling's death by dedicating special time to share information and answer questions. Reassurance that the illness is not their fault may be needed, especially for siblings who have donated organs. A return to family routines can help children to feel more secure.

Over time (usually years, not months) most families develop ways of living with their loss such that they are able to regain some sense of purpose and happiness. Functional grief is supported by ongoing parental and sibling bonds to the child who has died.

Clinical Controversy: Medical Assistance in Dying (MAID) in Paediatrics

- MAID broadly refers to prescription and/or administration of a lethal drug to a competent patient requesting assistance to die. MAID for adults with life-limiting conditions has recently been legalised in the state of Victoria.
- The ethical considerations in support of MAID include respect for autonomy, avoidance of suffering, harm minimisation, and a view of MAID as being on the continuum of end-of-life care. In opposition to MAID, are the value of life and community interest in not taking life, elusiveness of true autonomy, risk to the doctor-patient relationship, and risk to vulnerable groups.
- Palliative Care and MAID provide clinically and philosophically distinct health care. The Royal Australasian College of Physicians has taken a position of 'critical neutrality' with respect to MAID for adults. This approach avoids imposing one's own values on another person in favour of helping them find their way to a conclusion consistent with their own set of values.
- At present, the Netherlands and Belgium are the only two jurisdictions where legislation extends the practice of MAID to infants and/or children.

USEFUL RESOURCES

- **Thinking ahead framework** https://www2.health.vic.gov.au/about/publications/policiesandguidelines/thinking-ahead-resources Paediatric ACP framework and discussion guide
- **Paediatric Palliative Care** https://palliativecare.org.au/children Information for families and health professionals on navigating the palliative journey. CALD supported
- **Together for short lives** www.togetherforshortlives.org.uk/resource/basic-symptom-control-paediatric-palliative-care/ Multimodal approach to symptomatic management
- **Association for paediatric palliative medicine** www.appm.org.uk/guidelines-resources/appm-master-formulary/ Paediatric medication information
- **The Conversation project paediatric starter kit** https://theconversationproject.org/wp-content/uploads/2017/02/ConversationProject-StarterKit-Pediatric-English.pdf Guide to discussing serious illness with child, primarily for parents, but excellent insights for health professionals

CHAPTER 35

Refugee health

Georgia Paxton

Key Points

- All refugees and asylum seekers should have a comprehensive health assessment is after arrival in Australia. Assessment includes review of migration history, physical and mental health, development, education, immunisation status, and screening medical investigations.
- Refugee-background populations have experienced forced migration, with trauma and disruption of community, education, and health systems. These factors need to be considered in health consultations in Australia.
- Cohorts that warrant specific paediatric assessment include all unaccompanied minors or children on orphan relative visas; any children/young people with complex medical issues; malnutrition; rickets; developmental concerns; disability; mental health concerns; where age is queried; and all children who have experienced immigration detention.

Definitions

A refugee is someone who 'owing to a well-founded fear of being persecuted for reasons of race, religion, nationality, membership of a particular social group or political opinion, is outside the country of his/her nationality, and is unable to, or owing to such fear, is unwilling to avail himself/herself of the protection of that country'.

An asylum seeker is someone who has applied for refugee status and who is awaiting a decision on this application.

In this chapter, **refugee background** is used to describe both refugees and asylum seekers, and children born in Australia to refugee families.

Introduction

Australia accepts 18750 refugees each year under the Humanitarian Program. Around 40% of refugee arrivals are children and adolescents (age <18 years), and there are small numbers of unaccompanied/separated children each year. Demographics change annually, current arrivals are mainly from the Middle East, Asia, and Africa. Refugees arriving under this offshore resettlement program are Australian permanent residents from the time of arrival, with full access to Australia's health and welfare system.

Additionally, there are approximately 20,000 people arriving as asylum seekers annually. People who arrived by boat (prior to 2014) will have spent time in immigration detention (onshore, offshore, or community detention). Many asylum seekers do not have pathways for settlement in Australia, and migration uncertainty affects health. Asylum seekers may have limited access to Australian health and welfare resources.

The ongoing annual refugee intake, children born in Australia to refugee parents, and asylum seeker arrivals mean there are large numbers of refugee background children in Australia, and refugee health is an increasing consideration in paediatric practice.

Paediatric Handbook, Tenth Edition. Edited by Kate Harding, Daniel S. Mason and Daryl Efron.

Background

People of a refugee background:

- Are usually resourceful and resilient.
- Will have experienced conflict and transitions with migration and resettlement, including disruption to family, schooling and community.
- May be separated from immediate family members.
- May have witnessed or experienced physical or sexual violence, including torture and severe human rights violations.
- May have spent long periods in refugee camps or immigration detention.
- Usually arrive from countries where health facilities and programs are minimal or have been disrupted and are more likely to have been exposed to communicable and vaccine-preventable diseases.
- Have often had interrupted education.
- May have an incorrect date of birth recorded on their migration paperwork.
- Almost always require catch-up immunisations.
- Are at increased risk of mental health problems, especially unaccompanied minors and those who have been held in immigration detention.
- May be less familiar with preventive health care.
- May be worried about medical consultations.
- Will nearly always require the assistance of an interpreter in the initial (and often later) stages of settlement.
- Face challenges with resettlement, including educational transitions and accessing services.

Pre-departure screening

Pre-departure screening (Figure 35.1) and treatment is limited for children and young adolescents, and varies with country of departure, means of arrival and services available. All permanent migrants to Australia (humanitarian, skilled and family visa entrants) have to complete a compulsory immigration medical examination (IME) 3-12 months before travel. Humanitarian entrants may also complete a voluntary departure health check (DHC) in the week prior to travel. Health assessment information is stored in an electronic medical record system held by the Department of Home Affairs (DHA) and can be accessed by providers in Australia.

People seeking asylum do not have health assessments prior to travel, and their post arrival health assessments are variable. Adults in immigration detention usually have an equivalent check to the IME, however the assessment of children and early adolescents in detention varied widely, and both health screening and vaccinations are usually incomplete.

Post arrival settlement support and service access

Australia provides settlement support for refugees arriving under the offshore Humanitarian program. This includes on-arrival reception and accommodation, case work, orientation to life in Australia, English language classes and support to access healthcare, welfare (Centrelink and Medicare), education, and employment services. More intensive case work is usually available for a 6-month period, although many families have significant support needs over a much longer period. Unaccompanied/separated children receive intensive case work support until they reach 18 years. Support and healthcare for asylum seekers varies widely, and some asylum seekers may not be eligible for Medicare.

In some states of Australia (including Victoria), there are no routine post-arrival health checks. Barriers to accessing healthcare include patients not being familiar with the Australian healthcare system, providers not being familiar with refugee health issues, low English proficiency and difficulty accessing language services, financial constraints, and transport stressors. Patients often move houses in the early months after arrival and clinical follow-up can be challenging.

Working with interpreters

An interpreter will be needed with a majority of newly arrived families. It is never appropriate to utilise a family member as an interpreter. Establishing trust is essential - recently arrived communities may be small, and interpreters may be known to the family. Specific techniques can help when working with interpreters (Table 35.1).

Post-arrival health screening

All refugee and asylum seeker arrivals should be offered a comprehensive health assessment after arrival, ideally within one month. The assessment can be offered at any time after arrival if access to healthcare is delayed.

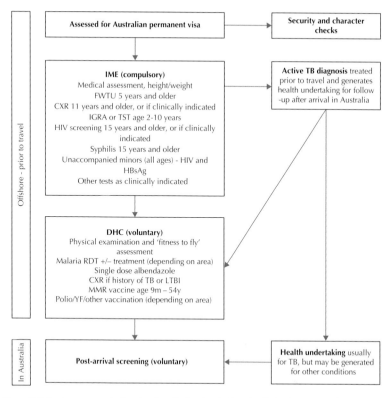

Figure 35.1 Pre-departure screening flowchart *Note*: this flow chart has been simplified to show screening for Humanitarian entrants, which includes routine tuberculosis (TB) screening in children 2–10 years and syphilis testing. FWTU = full ward test urine, CXR = chest x-ray, IGRA = interferon-gamma release assay, TST = tuberculin skin test, HIV = Human Immunodeficiency virus, HBsAg = hepatitis B surface antigen, RDT = rapid diagnostic test, LTBI - latent tuberculosis infection, MMR = measles, mumps, rubella, YF = yellow fever.

It is important to explain the concepts of health assessment, screening and disease prevention; families need to understand the implications of health screening and give informed consent. Individual counselling and an explanation of the bounds of confidentiality, including interpreter confidentiality, will be required in adolescents.

History
Assessment of newly arrived children and adolescents should consider:
- Migration background, including countries or origin and transit and language transitions
- Parent (or self-identified) concerns
- Excluding acute illness
- Immunisation status and catch-up plan
- Communicable diseases screening (including tuberculosis (TB), hepatitis, parasites and malaria)
- Nutrition and growth (including consideration of anaemia, iron deficiency, and vitamin D)
- Oral health
- Vision and hearing
- Concerns about development, education history
- Mental health and trauma exposure

- Previous childhood illness or physical trauma, female circumcision where relevant
- Confirming the child's reported birthdate
- Issues arising with resettlement in Australia.

Clinical Pearl: Post arrival history taking

Family and migration history can be complex and may reveal significant trauma. Useful questions that are respectful and helpful:

- Who is in your family in Australia, and who is in your family overseas? This allows the child/family to define relationships, and can reveal people who are lost/separated without asking directly
- Have you had access to school? Is more respectful than asking about education level directly
- What work did you do before Australia? People are not defined by their refugee status, and understanding their education and occupation is always helpful and usually appreciated
- Have there been times when your family was separated?

Other tips

- TB contact history is almost never disclosed initially – ask again if the screening test comes back positive
- Asking if the child was admitted to hospital overseas is useful
- Trauma history may not be disclosed for years after arrival
- When relevant, ask about female circumcision/cutting (with a female interpreter) – not female genital mutilation (FGM)
- Dual permission is a useful concept, especially with adolescents – e.g. you don't have to tell me information if you do not want to (you have control) but you can tell me if you would like to (I have heard stories like this before and I will not be surprised, we can make a plan together).

Table 35.1 Tips for working effectively with interpreters.

Bookings and set up
- Allow extra time - consultations take twice as long
- Clarify the preferred language, and gender if relevant
- Ensure interpreters wait in staff areas, not patient areas - this maintains boundaries and recognises their role as professional colleagues
- Arrange seating and aim for a triangle - across patient-interpreter-clinician
- Brief the interpreter prior to the consultation - background, what you are hoping to achieve.

During the consultation
- Face the patient, maintain eye contact and direct conversation to the patient (not interpreter)
- Introduce yourself and the interpreter and define confidentiality
- Use clear, simple language, short sentences, and avoid jargon.
- It is OK to ask for clarification - e.g. if a brief summary has shifted to a longer conversation, or where you need to define terms.
- Allow time for questions - they are an excellent gauge of patient understanding.

After the consultation
- Debrief and check in with the interpreter, especially for complex/trauma histories. In refugee background communities, the interpreters may have been through similar migration pathways, and hearing patients' stories may be a source of significant stress.
- Work with the same interpreter for repeat consultations where possible.

Working with interpreters is a skill like any other clinical skill – it takes time and practise to become confident and fluent, but it will enrich your clinical care.

Examination

Children and adolescents need a thorough physical examination. Particular features include:
- Growth parameters and nutritional status
- Anaemia
- Rickets
- Oral health and ear, nose, throat (ENT) disease
- Presence of a Bacillus Calmette Guerin (BCG) scar (location varies) and respiratory examination

Table 35.2 Recommended initial screening investigations.

	Initial screening investigations
i. All children and adolescents	• Full blood examination • Ferritin • **Hepatitis B serology** - surface antigen (HBsAg), surface antibody (HBsAb) and core antibody (HBcAb) • Strongyloides serology • **TB screening** - either tuberculin skin test (TST) or interferon gamma release assay (IGRA). TST should not be completed within 1 month of live viral vaccines (including pre-departure MMR vaccine). • **Faecal specimen** for cysts, ova, parasites (COP, ideally fixed specimen).
ii. Risk-based	• **Vitamin D, calcium, phosphate and alkaline phosphatase (ALP)** - if risk factors (lack of skin exposure to sun, dark skin, conditions affecting vitamin D metabolism, and exclusively breastfed infants with at least one other risk factor) • **Serum active B12** - if arrival <6 months and any of food insecurity, vegan, from Bhutan, Afghanistan, Iran or Horn of Africa • **Varicella serology** age 14 years and older if no history of clinical varicella infection and no documented vaccination • **Rubella serology** in females of childbearing age - not needed if catch-up vaccination in place • **Sexually transmitted infection (STI)** screening - *N. gonorrhoea* and *C. trachomatis* urine nucleic acid detection, syphilis serology (*note: also HIV, hepatitis B*) in sexually active adolescents, or if there is a history of sexual violence/abuse • **Syphilis screening** in all unaccompanied/separated children. Children should also be screened if their mother has positive serology • **HIV testing** – 15 years and older, <15 years if unaccompanied/separated minor, or clinical risk factors (sexually active, history of sexual violence/abuse, where parents are deceased/missing/known to be HIV positive, other STIs, TB, HBV, HCV, history of blood transfusions, or where there are clinical symptoms/signs) • *Helicobacter pylori* **screening** (faecal antigen test on fresh specimen) in children with family history gastric cancer, or symptoms/signs of dyspepsia/ulcer disease.
iii. Country-based	• **Malaria** - rapid diagnostic test (RDT) and thick/thin film, if arrival less than 3 months from *endemic area** or later if symptoms. Endemic - Africa (except Egypt), Burma, Bhutan, India, Pakistan, Sri Lanka- *not Middle East* • **Hepatitis C serology** - Hepatitis C virus (HCV) antibodies, if from *endemic area* or if clinical risk factors. Endemic - Congo, Egypt, Iraq, Pakistan, consider in Syrians - *not other African/Middle Eastern or Asian countries* • **Schistosoma serology** – if travel from/through *endemic area*. Africa, Burma, Iraq and Syria - *not other Middle Eastern or Asian countries.*

• Lymphadenopathy, hepatosplenomegaly
• Skin (scars, infections)
• There may be particular cultural practices noted, such as scarification or excision of the uvula.

Suggested initial screening investigations

Recommended first line investigations (Table 35.2) are grouped into:
  i.   Baseline tests
 ii.   Screening based on risk factors
iii.   Screening based on countries of origin/transit

Additional investigations may be needed depending on the clinical scenario; eg. recently arrived children who are febrile and unwell may require further investigation and consultation with an infectious diseases specialist.

Physical health issues

Refugee background children and adolescents have typical paediatric health problems and may also have health issues specific to their background or forced migration experience (Table 35.3).

Table 35.3 Common and specific health considerations in refugee background children and adolescents.

Presentation	Common causes	Additional considerations in refugee children *More likely shortly after arrival
Fever	Common viral infections Common bacterial infections (check for localising features)	Malaria (endemic areas)* Hepatitis TB any site, especially if prolonged Dengue and other arboviral infections* Typhoid* Dysentery*
Respiratory symptoms	Consider usual causes of respiratory symptoms for age, e.g. viral respiratory tract infection, bronchiolitis, croup, asthma, pneumonia	Whooping cough (pertussis): lack of vaccination TB – consider if contact, or cough >2 weeks Sickle cell disease acute chest syndrome Parasite infections may (very rarely) cause wheeze/ respiratory symptoms
Abdominal pain	Acute infection Constipation Surgical causes Gynaecological causes	Parasite infection *Helicobacter pylori* gastritis – epigastric pain, early satiety, anorexia, nausea/vomiting, family history Hepatitis
Diarrhoea	Viral gastroenteritis Bacterial gastroenteritis Malabsorption	Parasitic infections common Lactose intolerance may be more common Bacillary* and amoebic dysentery
Rashes	Infective Eczema Dermatophyte (tinea) infections	*Strongyloides* infection may cause an intermittent urticarial rash lasting a few days (larva currens): most typically on the buttocks/perianal region
Continence issues	Nocturnal or diurnal enuresis UTI Irritable bladder	Chronic UTI may not have been detected/treated Mental health issues can cause secondary enuresis Consider female circumcision in girls
Musculoskeletal pain	Injury Growing pains Joint pathology/inflammation	Low vitamin D is an extremely common cause: look for rickets (bossing, swelling of wrists and ankles, bony deformity).
Fussy eating	Behavioural issues Excess milk intake Enlarged tonsils	Food insecurity Iron deficiency is common *Helicobacter pylori* gastritis Other gastrointestinal infections Dental disease – pain can restrict food intake
Poor growth (failure to thrive, malnutrition)	Poor intake Increased losses (gut, urine) Increased requirements	Review food access overseas and in Australia Rickets may restrict linear growth Severe malnutrition may require admission
Seizures	Febrile convulsions Epilepsy Central nervous system (CNS) infection	Consider malaria if new arrival/endemic area/ febrile Consider TB meningitis as a differential Neurocystocercosis is a (rare) cause of seizures
Developmental or learning concerns, disability	Genetic Environmental Trauma: injury	Often multifactorial: combination of antenatal, peri- and post-natal contributors. Be wary of attributing delay to English as an additional language. Check age in older children. Consider interrupted schooling. Consider mental health and trauma.
Mental health/parent concern	Behaviour concerns Sleep issues Anxiety/separation issues	Clarify family background, separations and migration history, parental mental health & detention experience for asylum seekers. A paediatric assessment can be a useful first step to provide comprehensive assessment and facilitate mental health referral

Immunisation

Immunisation records are not a pre-departure requirement and most refugees/asylum seekers do not have written records. Check for a BCG scar and a past history of varicella infection, and clarify vaccinations given as part of pre-departure medical assessment.

Principles of catch-up vaccination (see also Chapter 9, Immunisation) include:

- People of refugee background should be vaccinated so they are up to date by the Australian immunisation schedule, equivalent to an Australian-born person of the same age.
- Catch-up vaccination is required unless written documentation of immunisation is available.
- Serology for immunity to vaccine preventable diseases (VPD) is not routinely recommended (post arrival screening includes hepatitis B and varicella serology as above).
- Vaccination information, including offshore records and pre-departure vaccinations, should be entered into the Australian Immunisation Register (AIR). Children need to have commenced catch-up, and vaccinations need to be on AIR to enable full Centrelink payments for families.
- In general, vaccination can be completed in three visits over four months in children 10 years and older, and four visits over 10 months in younger children using minimum dosing intervals.
- For most vaccines there are no adverse events associated with additional doses in immune individuals, and the benefits of immunisation are substantial.
- Provide a written record and clear plan for ongoing immunisations.
- For specific information on catch-up vaccination information see: *The Australian Immunisation Handbook* https://immunisationhandbook.health.gov.au/; and https://www.rch.org.au/immigranthealth/clinical/Catchup_immunisation_in_refugees/.

Nutrition and growth

- Nutritional issues are common; fussy eating and concerns about weight gain (too little or too much) may be a family priority (see Chapter 10 Nutrition, and Chapter 11 Growth).
- Specific issues include malnutrition, iron deficiency, anaemia, vitamin D deficiency, vitamin A deficiency, and vitamin B12/folate deficiency.
- Severe malnutrition has become more frequent, especially with complex disability.
- An early severe/prolonged nutritional insult or chronic disease during infancy will affect long-term growth and may affect final height ('stunting').
- Monitor growth parameters and clarify the correct age; linear growth is similar in children aged <5 years worldwide.
- Consider gastrointestinal and other infections (including TB), vitamin D deficiency, rickets, dental caries and thyroid dysfunction.
- Once an initial screen has been completed (with treatment as needed), a period of monitoring is often appropriate.
- Fussy eating is often due to high caloric intake in the form of excessive milk/juice consumption at the expense of solids/mealtimes. Consider organic disease early in children of a refugee background, including gastrointestinal (*Giardia*, other parasites, *Helicobacter pylori*) and other infections.
- The principles of healthy eating are universal and should be discussed with families.

Anaemia

Anaemia is usually multifactorial: consider low maternal iron stores, poor food access, iron deficiency, low B12/folate, malaria and other parasites.

- Iron deficiency is usually nutritional but may be due to gastrointestinal loss.
- Vitamin B12 deficiency is more common in refugee background populations.
- Consider folate deficiency in children with malnutrition or limited access to fresh foods.
- Consider haemoglobinopathies (particularly African and Asian populations).
- Consider lead toxicity if pica, unexplained microcytosis, developmental issues, or exposure risks (including through traditional medicine).

Vitamin D

Vitamin D is essential for bone and muscle health, and low vitamin D is common in refugee background populations in Australia (33–100%). Most vitamin D is made in the skin through the action of ultraviolet B (UVB) in sunlight, and diet is a poor source of vitamin D. Rickets remains a disease of dark-skinned migrant children, predominantly infants with prolonged exclusive breastfeeding.

25-hydroxy vitamin D levels (25(OH)D) are used to measure vitamin D status; levels ≥50 nmol/L at all ages are recommended.

Definitions of vitamin D deficiency
- Severe deficiency <12.5 nmol/L
- Moderate deficiency 12.5–29 nmol/L
- Mild deficiency 30–49 nmol/L

In the absence of sun exposure, recommended dietary intakes of vitamin D are:
- Age <12 months: 400 IU daily
- 1–18 years: 400 IU - 600 IU daily

  Note: 1 mcg of vitamin D = 40 International Units (IU).

Risk factors for low vitamin D
- Lack of sun exposure (time indoors, chronic illness, covering clothing, southerly latitude).
- Dark skin.
- Medical conditions (obesity, liver failure, renal failure, malabsorption) or medications affecting vitamin D metabolism.
- Infants: maternal vitamin D deficiency and exclusive breastfeeding with other risk factor.

Assessment
- Bone or muscle pain, especially with exercise.
- Irritability, delayed motor milestones (young children).
- Dairy intake, symptoms of hypocalcemia (muscle cramps, seizures rare >6m age).
- Previous vitamin D levels and/or treatment.
- Rickets – deformity in growing bones: peak incidence in infancy; look for long bone deformity, splaying (wrists, ankles), bossing, delayed fontanelle closure, and rachitic rosary.
- Delayed dental eruption (no incisors by 10 months, no molars by 18 months).

Screening
- Screen all children with ≥ 1 risk factor.
- Measure 25(OH)D, calcium, phosphate and ALP.
- Measure parathyroid hormone (PTH) in children with low calcium intake, symptoms/signs of low vitamin D or multiple risk factors.
- In exclusively breastfed infants with ≥ 1 risk factor, start supplements without screening.
- Children with rickets require additional investigations to exclude renal pathology and rarer causes of rickets (25(OH)D, calcium, phosphate, ALP, PTH, urea, electrolytes, creatinine, urine calcium, phosphate and creatinine, wrist x-ray, leg x-rays and clinical photos if deformity).

Management
- Children with symptomatic rickets or hypocalcaemia require urgent hospital assessment; *do not* give high dose vitamin D in the outpatient setting to this group.
- Children with low vitamin D should be treated to restore levels to the normal range with either daily dosing or high (stoss) dose therapy.
- Treatment is usually with 1000–2000 IU daily for 3-6m, or 150 000 IU stoss dosing (lower doses if <12m). There is inadequate evidence to support the use of high dose therapy in children <3 months.
- Ensure adequate calcium intake. Consider supplements if dietary intake poor
- Sun exposure: encourage outside activity; children with dark skin can tolerate intermittent sun exposure without sunscreen.
- Repeat 25(OH)D at 3 months (earlier in infants with moderate to severe deficiency).
- Encourage self-management – aim for behavioural change where possible and supplementation (e.g. 400-600 IU daily over the cooler months – May-September).

- Breastfed babies with ≥ 1 risk factor should have 400 IU vitamin D daily for at least the first 12 months of life. Exclusive formula feeding should provide adequate vitamin D. Consider checking levels or supplementing if mixed feeds and after weaning.
- Vitamin D deficient rickets requires supplementing vitamin D, calcium, +/- phosphate in consultation with endocrinology.

Tuberculosis
See Chapter 25, Infectious diseases.

Hepatitis B infection
See Chapter 25, Infectious diseases.

Intestinal and other parasites
Refugee children tend to have a higher prevalence of parasitic infections than adults. These infections may be chronic and have sequelae for nutrition, growth and wellbeing. Symptoms may be non-specific:
- Abdominal pain, constipation, diarrhoea, bloody diarrhoea and slow growth.
- Bladder symptoms and haematuria (*Schistosoma haematobium*).
  - *Strongyloides* infection (positive serology) may persist lifelong if not treated.
  - Strongyloides hyperinfection syndrome can develop with immunosuppression and has a high mortality, even with treatment.
  - Consider, screen (and treat) if commencing immunosuppressive therapy.

Management
- Parasite screening should be part of the initial assessment (see section above).
- Treatment is usually short course (often single dose) and well tolerated; see http://www.rch. org.au/immigranthealth/clinical/Intestinal Parasites/.

Human immunodeficiency virus
See Chapter 25, Infectious diseases.

Oral health
Oral health assessment is important, as refugee background children may have had poor diet, dental injuries and limited access to dental care/oral health promotion.

Female circumcision/cutting
Girls and women from refugee background communities may have had female circumcision/cutting (female genital mutilation, FGM). This is rarely disclosed initially, even with direct questioning. Assessment requires sensitive discussion, often over more than one visit, and specialised clinics are available. It is illegal to practice or to obtain FGM in Australia, or to take a child from Australia for this purpose. Any impending threat of FGM should be reported to child protection immediately (mandatory reporting applies). Questions about FGM should be considered in pre-travel assessment, as there may be pressure from family overseas for this procedure.

Trauma, developmental and mental health issues
Development
Development may be affected by any combination of biological, environmental, social and emotional factors (see chapter 28 Neurodevelopment and Disability). Migration and trauma experiences overlay these domains. Considerations in children and adolescents of a refugee background include:
- **Biological:** pre-, peri- and post-natal complications, malnutrition, chronic disease, severe infections (including meningitis and malaria), injury/accidents, hearing impairment, visual impairment, family history, genetic conditions, consanguinity.
- **Environmental:** living conditions, food security, safety, access to schooling/education, healthcare access, exposure to communicable diseases, toxins, environmental hazards, injuries.
- **Social:** migration and language transitions (and timing in relation to developmental milestones) parenting roles, family disruption/separation, parent/family education, occupation and circumstances, roles and responsibilities, detention experience, trauma, settlement experience.
- **Emotional:** temperament, stress, response to trauma experiences, loss, displacement, uncertainty around future, mental health issues, parent/family mental health.

Adolescence is also a critical developmental stage (see chapter 12 Adolescent medicine). Refugee background adolescents face expected adolescent transitions alongside the challenges of settlement – negotiating a new culture, new language, new schooling, and new technology while balancing the expectations of their parents/cultural background with those of their new peers. They may make new meaning from past trauma, and present with mental health concerns in relation to trauma during childhood.

Language acquisition and educational transitions

Immigrants learning a new language generally achieve conversational proficiency after 2–3 years, however it takes longer (at least 5–7 years) to achieve academic language proficiency. The amount of first language schooling is the most important predictor of success in the new language, and late primary/early secondary age students achieve academic language proficiency most quickly. It is important to encourage the first language (mother tongue) in order to achieve success in the new language.

Students from refugee backgrounds are likely to have multiple risk factors for educational disadvantage, however available evidence suggests they have similar school outcomes to their local born peers. Resilience factors include high academic ambition, parent involvement in education, a supportive home environment, accurate grade placement, teacher understanding of background, culturally appropriate school transition, supportive peers and successful acculturation – many of these are modifiable with long-term support.

Assessment of development and learning issues

Specific areas for review are:
- Confirming reported birthdate – age assessment may be required.
- Languages spoken, preferred language, timing of language acquisition.
- School history (including access, type, language of teaching).
- Sleep, screen, attention, behaviour and mental health history.
- Family developmental and education history.
- Home and family environment, settlement stressors, racism or bullying experiences.

Management

- Early audiology and formal visual assessment.
- Early screening for treatable medical contributors (iron deficiency, vitamin B12 deficiency, hypothyroidism, and consider blood lead levels).
- Encourage a healthy diet, adequate sleep, and appropriately limited screen use/content.
- Encourage first language, and provide education on additional language acquisition.
- Ensure opportunities for play, relaxation, exercise, and success – sporting activities are often important for connections and success.
- Financial supports where eligible, e.g. Carer allowance.
- Mental health supports and trauma counselling where needed.
- Consider grade placement carefully – consider placement with same age children in the younger grade level, and kindergarten in children aged 5 years.
- If clear history of developmental delay/disability, seek formal cognitive/language assessments early even though there are significant issues with standardised testing. Repeat testing will be needed over time.
- Enlist additional supports early, e.g. maternal and child health nursing, childcare/playgroups, early childhood education, and early intervention for younger children; and school-based/homework support and mentoring for older children/adolescents.
- Be prepared to advocate – accessing the National Disability Insurance Scheme (NDIS), Centrelink payments, and service system is challenging for new arrivals and those with low English proficiency.

Mental health

Children and adolescents from refugee backgrounds are likely to have experienced trauma and adversity before and after arrival in Australia. They will have experienced forced migration, and may have witnessed or experienced physical or sexual violence. Concern for remaining family overseas, or ongoing migration uncertainty for people seeking asylum may be overwhelming, with significant effects on settlement and wellbeing. While it is important to understand the influence of trauma, it is often not appropriate to ask about trauma directly – frequently children/families will disclose their trauma history after the initial health assessment, once trust and rapport are established.

- Clinical manifestations of trauma exposure reflect a child's age and developmental stage.
- Presentations include behavioural problems, sleep concerns (including nightmares and enuresis), developmental or learning concerns, attention difficulties, low self-esteem, friendship difficulties or psychosomatic symptoms, as well as more typical symptoms of depression, anxiety or post-traumatic stress disorder.
- Unaccompanied/separated children have specific vulnerabilities and are at increased risk of violence (including sexual violence).
- Many asylum seeker children who have experienced Australian immigration detention have had severe mental health issues, and infants held in detention may have had severe attachment issues.

Consider mental health in the broad family and settlement context. Parents with mental health issues and settlement related stressors will have reduced coping and parenting skills and parent mental health influences child/adolescent mental health.

Management

- Address mental health issues in the whole family – link parents with mental health or trauma counselling services where relevant.
- Support primary attachment relationships.
- Ensure predictability and support routine, including school attendance.
- Address sleep and screen use issues.
- Encourage play, enjoyable activities, exercise, and peer connections.
- Encourage expression of emotions.
- Set practical and realistic goals for behavior: reinforce positive behaviour, implement consistent consequences for negative behavior, and avoid over-reactions to difficult behaviour during transitions.
- Promote engagement with early childhood education services, school and community.
- Facilitate long-term care and a safe space to explore mental health concerns.

Although people from refugee backgrounds may have experienced significant trauma, there is good evidence that they often have great resilience and positive social adjustment. Trauma exposure does not always predict poor mental health outcomes and functional impairment. Most refugee-background children and adolescents grow to become well-adjusted adults and make significant contributions to their countries of settlement.

USEFUL RESOURCES
- RCH immigrant health service website http://www.rch.org.au/immigranthealth; wide variety of clinical and non-clinical resources relating to refugee and asylum seeker health.
- RACP Refugee and Immigrant Health curated collection.

CHAPTER 36

Rehabilitation medicine

Adam Scheinberg
Neil Wimalasundera

Key Points
- Rehabilitation focuses on function and independence rather than impairment.
- Goal setting is vital for engagement and motivation of children and families.
- Acquired brain injury (ABI) has life-long effects on psychosocial function. Young children have worse long-term outcomes than older children with equivalent severity ABI.
- Paediatric spinal cord injury (SCI) is rare; affected children should be seen within a specialist SCI service.
- Bladder and Bowel dysfunction has the greatest impact on reduced quality of life.

Introduction

Paediatric rehabilitation medicine involves the provision of comprehensive rehabilitation services to children and young people with disability due to injury or disease, with the aim of enabling the highest-level possible of physical, cognitive, psychological and social functioning (AFRM Standards 2015). Rehabilitation is focused on helping the child to develop as much independence as possible.

Children and adolescents with complex conditions where function is significantly impacted benefit from a rehabilitation approach to care. Children with acquired brain injury, spinal cord injury/disease, limb deficiency, neuromuscular disease and movement disorders form the largest populations likely to benefit, though children with other conditions such as chronic fatigue syndrome and those who are deconditioned (e.g post cardiac surgery) can also benefit.

Due to the complexity of these conditions and their impact on both the child's development and family function, a large team of health professionals are involved in delivering optimal care. The success of multidisciplinary teams depends on effective communication between and among the family and health professionals, collaborative leadership, and family centered goal setting. Communication strategies include regular care planning and family meetings, the provision of written information or online tools to assist with self-management, and linking with community organisations to provide peer support and mentoring.

Paediatric rehabilitation is focused on both regaining function *and* providing scaffolding from which they can develop previously unlearned skills in order to effectively engage with their family, school and social lives.

The rehabilitation assessment

The International Classification of Functioning, Disability and Health (ICF; Figure 36.1) is a framework for describing and organising information on functioning and disability. It provides a standard language and a conceptual basis for the definition and measurement of health and disability.

The ICF framework (see Figure 36.2) was further adapted by Rosenbaum et al. into the 6Fs. This model encourages rehabilitation teams to holistically assess and intervene in attempting to build functional capacity in the patients they see.

Paediatric Handbook, Tenth Edition. Edited by Kate Harding, Daniel S. Mason and Daryl Efron.
© 2021 John Wiley & Sons Ltd. Published 2021 by John Wiley & Sons Ltd.

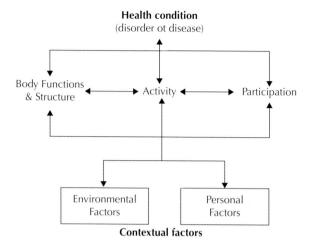

Health condition
(disorder ot disease)

Figure 36.1 ICF Conceptual framework. *Source*: World Health Organisation; https://www.who.int/classifications/icf/icfbeginnersguide.pdf?ua=1; p9 (Geneva, 2002). Reproduced with permission from the authors.

These two frameworks provide a basis for history taking, physical examination and specialised assessment of children referred for rehabilitation. The assessment is further tailored to the child's goals, for example focused on return to a sporting activity. As rehabilitation is primarily focused on building functional capacity (irrespective of the diagnosis), functional assessment is a core component of the overall assessment.

Functional assessment tools such as the WeeFIM II™ as in Table 36.1 cover a range of daily tasks, and have normed references for when the child is expected to be functionally independent.

Goal setting is another core component of the rehabilitation assessment. Goal setting can help engage and motivate the child in rehabilitation, as long as the goals are meaningful to the child and family. Various goal setting tools are used to help set and describe goals, and score them on completion of the program to monitor outcomes (e.g Canadian Occupational Performance Measure, Goal Attainment Scaling).

Acquired brain injury (ABI)

Acquired brain injuries are categorised into two groups, based on their aetiology:
- **Traumatic brain injuries (TBI):** including motor vehicle accidents, falls, assaults, and sport injuries.
- **Non-traumatic brain injuries (nTBI):** stroke (ischaemic and haemorrhagic), hypoxia, tumours, and encephalomyelitis.

TBI is the most common cause of interrupted normal child development and the leading cause of death in those under the age of 19. TBI is most likely to occur in in the 0–4y and 15–19y age groups.

Children and adolescents with ABI often have long term changes in both physical and cognitive/behavioural function. Many (25–75%) children with an ABI experience school failure or require special education services in the first five years post injury.

Severity

Classification of the severity of brain injury is undertaken by using a combination of the Glasgow Coma Scale (GCS), duration of loss of consciousness (LOC) and length of post-traumatic amnesia (PTA). See Table 36.2.

Common physical symptoms
- Headaches
- Fatigue
- Post traumatic seizures (12–18%, may contribute to secondary injury following an ABI)
- Poor balance and coordination

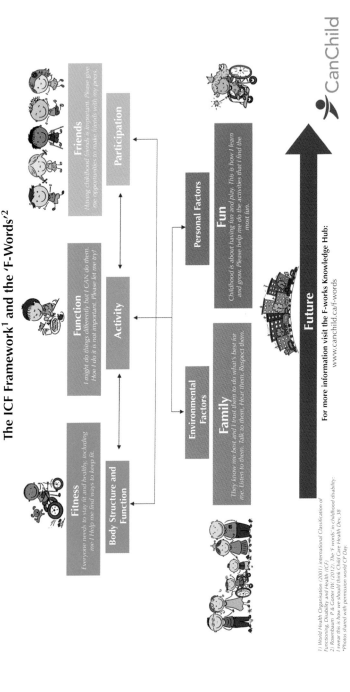

The ICF Framework[1] and the 'F-Words'[2]

Fitness
Everyone needs to stay fit and healthy, including me. Help me find ways to keep fit.

Function
I might do things differently but I CAN do them. How I do it is not important. Please let me try!

Friends
Having childhood friends is important. Please give me opportunities to make friends with my peers.

Body Structure and Function

Activity

Participation

Environmental Factors

Personal Factors

Family
They know me best and I trust them to do what's best for me. Listen to them. Talk to them. Hear them. Respect them.

Fun
Childhood is about having fun and play. This is how I learn and grow. Please help me do the activities that I find the most fun.

Future

For more information visit the F-works Knowledge Hub:
www.canchild.ca/f-words

CanChild

1) World Health Organisation (2001) International Classification of Functioning, Disability and Health (ICF)
2) Rosenbaum, P & Gorter JW. (2012). The 'F-words' in childhood disability: I swear this is how we should think! Child Care Health Dev, 38
*Photos shared with permission world CP Day

Figure 36.2 ICF conceptual framework representation as the '6Fs'; Fitness, Function, Friends, Family, Fun, Future. *Source:* World Health Organization. (2001) International Classification of Functioning, Disability and Health (ICF); Rosenbaum P, Gorter JW. Child Care Health Dev, 2012 Jul;38(4):457–63. *The 'F-words' in childhood disability: I swear this is how we should think!* Reproduced with permission from the authors.

Table 36.1 The Functional domains of the WeeFIM II™.

Functional Task	Age independent (years)
Self-cares	
Eating (using utensils to feed self once food is prepared)	6
Grooming (washing hands, brushing teeth, washing face)	7
Bathing (washing and drying self once bath is prepared)	7
Dressing (upper and lower body once clothes are set out)	7
Toileting (perineal hygiene)	6.5
Bladder management (continence)	6
Bowel management (continence)	4.5
Mobility	
Transfers (moving onto a chair, toilet, transferring into shower/bathtub)	5
Walking (at least 50m independently)	4
Stairs (going up and down a flight of stairs)	5
Cognition	
Comprehension (understanding everyday conversations and follow unrelated 3 step command)	5.5
Expression (expresses basic needs and ideas clearly and fluently)	3
Social interaction (safely and appropriately interacts with peers)	7
Problem solving (safely recognises if there is a problem, makes appropriate decisions, carries a sequence of steps to solve everyday problems)	5
Memory (recognises people frequently encountered, remembers daily routines, executes request without being reminded)	6

Table 36.2 Assessing severity of acquired brain injury.

	Mild	Moderate	Severe	Profound
GCS	13–15	9–12	3–8	
PTA	<1 hr	1–24 hr	>24 hr	> 7 days
Duration LOC	<15–30 min	15m–24 hr	1–90 days	>90 days

- Chronic pain
- Anosmia
- Hearing and vision impairment & disturbance
- Tremor, spasticity and dystonia
- Epilepsy (7–12%)

Common cognitive and behavioural problems
- Poor memory and concentration
- Difficulty with planning and organisation
- Difficulty with problem solving
- Difficulty with attention and arousal
- Personality and behavioural changes

Assessments
- Psychometric evaluation: generally, a test battery administer by an experienced neuropsychologist to give directions to the child, family and school about where to provide therapy intervention and environmental supports. For most, full scale IQ score relatively unchanged despite changes in attention, emotional control and working memory.

- Speech and language: formal receptive, expressive, and speech production to delineate deficits.
- Family function (e.g. family needs questionnaire): psychosocial function shown to be a key determinant of long-term outcome. Check for post-traumatic stress disorder in both the child and extended family.

Investigations
- Cerebral imaging is rarely required after the acute phase of an ABI (consider if suspicion of hydrocephalus or growing skull fracture). Generally, not helpful in prognosis.
- Bloods rarely indicated (nutritional bloods yearly if enteral nutrition, vitamin D if immobile).
- EEG generally not indicated in diagnosis or monitoring of post trauma epilepsy.

Management
There are few evidenced based interventions to remediate the behavioural and cognitive effects of an ABI. Children benefit from access to a specialised ABI rehabilitation program.
- Treatment approaches include:
  - Memory aides and timetables.
  - Minimising classroom distraction (provide ABI education to school/teacher).
  - Breaking down information into smaller chunks.
  - Instructions: repeated, verbal and written form.
  - Graded return to school.
  - Regular rest periods to avoid cognitive fatigue.
- More specific therapy approaches include;
  - Cognitive behavioural therapy for anxiety, depression, and internalising behaviours.
  - Programs to support family function and behaviour (e.g. Stepping Stones, Triple P, Acceptance and Commitment Therapy).
  - Face to face family problem solving therapy may improve internalising behavioural problems.
- Pharmacologic therapy
  - No medications proven to be effective in modifying outcomes for the child with ABI.
  - Methylphenidate may be of benefit to improve attention.
  - Amantadine may be of benefit to improve level of consciousness, and reduce aggression and agitation.
  - Anti-psychotic medication is rarely indicated in extreme aggression and should be used in liaison with psychiatry teams only.
- Return to sport
  - Return to sport guidelines for children with more severe ABI are not clear; risk of further brain injury must be balanced against benefits of fitness and social participation.
  - High risk sports such as skiing, motocross riding and horse riding may be contraindicated.
  - Children with post traumatic epilepsy should be supervised for swimming/watersports.

Clinical Pearl: ABI
- ABI at a younger age (<4y) results in poorer outcomes.
- Long term outcomes are better for focal rather than diffuse injury.
- Rehabilitation must be across multiple environments such as home, school and recreation activities.
- Consider hydrocephalus in the child with late onset headaches, vomiting and worsening ataxia.
- Long term anticonvulsant therapy is not effective in reducing the incidence of late seizures.
- Children post ABI perform better in evaluation settings than during their daily activities & social situations.
- The most important predictors of long term outcome following ABI are ongoing education, family function and behaviour.

Spinal cord injury and disease (SCD)
SCD in children and adolescents is relatively rare, however the impact of SCD on the child's growing body and the accompanying psychological effects are significant.

Very young children (<2y) are at increased risk of cervical spine injury due to poorly developed neck muscles, ligamentous laxity, incomplete ossification of vertebral bodies, and relatively large head size in relation to torso. As there is greater mobility and elasticity in the infant spine, infants with spinal cord injury may present with SCIWORA (spinal cord injury without radiological abnormality). Spine MRI is indicated in suspected paediatric SCD.

- Paediatric SCD includes both traumatic (60%) and non-traumatic (40%) causes.
- Causes of paediatric SCD include:
  - Motor vehicle accidents
  - Infections, e.g. transverse myelitis
  - Falls
  - Sports injuries
  - Atlanto-axial injury (Trisomy 21, juvenile rheumatoid arthritis)
  - Spinal tumours
  - Spinal vascular malformations

Classification of paediatric SCD

The most common method of classifying impairment from SCD is with the American Spinal Cord Injury Association (ASIA) scale:

- Uses a combination of muscle strength and sensation to determine a score, and motor and sensory levels.
- Helps to determine complete from incomplete injuries.
- Used after 72 hours can inform prognosis.
- *The assessment is unreliable in children under 5 years.*

Function

- SCD below C6: expectation of independence in self-cares & chair mobility.
- SCD at higher levels: upper limb orthoses, power chairs and communication technology is needed to assist independence.
- Bladder and bowel incontinence common after SCD; neurogenic bladder & bowel (alongside pain) are the most important factors impacting on quality of life for adults with paediatric onset SCD.
- Rehabilitation programs should aim for social continence and preservation of renal function.

Neurogenic bladder

- Clean intermittent catheterisation (CIC) is the standard of care for bladder management.
  Typical CIC routines aim for catheters 4–5 x daily, with expected bladder volumes calculated ((age+2) x 30 mls) and residuals less than 10% expected bladder volume.
- Children can be taught self CIC from 5–6y age.
- Long-term suprapubic catheters rarely used in children (risk of infection and bladder damage).
- Anticholinergic medication may be required to increase bladder compliance (typically Ditropan).
- Consider intravesical Botulinum toxin or bladder augmentation for the hypertrophic non-storing bladder.
- If hand function is impaired, an appendicovesicostomy/Mitrofanoff procedure may be recommended.

Neurogenic bowel

- Aim to replicate premorbid bowel habit (where possible).
- Time bowel movements to utilise gastro-colic reflex.
- Ensure supported sitting with hips in flexion and feet on floor.
- Diet should include adequate fluids and fibre.
- Digital stimulation may be all that is needed to initiate defecation.
- Medications include stool softeners and glycerin suppositories.
- Peristeen® washout (https://www.coloplast.com.au/peristeen-anal-irrigation-system-en-au.aspx) is a newer effective water-based enema.

Autonomic dysreflexia

- Dysfunction of the autonomic nervous system after SCD ≥ T6.
- Hypertension may be an emergency presentation.
- Older children typically present with throbbing headache, blurred vision, sweating and red skin discolouration on face, chest and arms.
- Younger children < 5y presentations are unreliable – may just be irritable.

- Management: sit up, evaluate & treat triggers such as urinary retention. Occasionally antihypertensive medication necessary.
- Children with autonomic dysreflexia should have an emergency information card easily available (e.g. on the back of the wheelchair).

Medical complications of SCD

- **Hypercalcaemia:** 10–20%, adolescent males most commonly, within 3m of injury. Monitor serum calcium regularly during this time.
- **Latex allergy:** up to 20% of SCD patients.
- **Scoliosis:** nearly all children injured pre-puberty develop scoliosis. Regular physical assessment and early referral to orthopaedics recommended.
- **Hip subluxation:** all children injured <5y, up to 80% <10y. Surgery to relocate the hip joint may be indicated if pelvic asymmetry impacting on sitting posture.
- **Osteopaenia/osteoporosis:** adults with pediatric-onset SCD have decreased bone mineral density (BMD) and increased fracture risk. Pathologic fractures can occur in up to 15% of children and adolescents with SCD.
- **Temperature regulation:** children with cervical level injury may have difficulty controlling their body temperature. Consider climate control and appropriate clothing to avoid overheating.
- **Puberty:** menarche expected at the normal age, consider referral to gynecology to assist with menses management.
- **Sexuality** is often overlooked. Should be addressed in a developmentally appropriate manner.

Hypertonia, spasticity, dystonia and other movement disorders

Cerebral palsy is the most common cause of paediatric neurological movement disorders; but not every child with a movement disorder has cerebral palsy. Accurate diagnosis of the aetiology of the movement disorder is essential in helping to predict prognosis and to identify appropriate treatment pathways.

Cerebral Palsy (see also Chapter 28, Neurodevelopment and disability)

If there is any diagnostic uncertainty regarding a prenatal, perinatal or postanatal cause of cerebral palsy then referral to neurology and futher more detailed neurogenetic investigation is warranted (Table 36.3).

The movement disorder in cerebral palsy can be broadly thought of in two categories:

- **Positive signs:** include spasticity and dyskensia which encompasses dystonia, chorea and athetosis.
- **Negative signs:** include weakness, reduced selective motor control and sensory deficits.

Negative symptoms can have just as much of an impact on function as the positve signs, but are often underestimated and overlooked. Motor function is also dependent on cogntive function and this is an important factor to consider when discussing motor prognosis with families.

Classifications of tone and movement abnormalities

Spasticity

- Velocity dependent increased tone with hyperreflexia and upper motor neurone signs.

Table 36.3 Features which may suggest an alternative diagnosis to cerebral palsy.

1. Lack of aetiological history.
2. Pure signs i.e. pure dystonia or pure spasticity – Cerebral palsy often has a dominant motor type but usually there is a mix of motor signs and often subtle arm involvement in leg dominant patterns. This is due to the 'crude' cause of the original brain injury.
3. Deteriorating or fluctuant course.
4. Diurnal variation in motor symptoms.
5. Strong family history.
6. Dysmorphic features.
7. Functional level not in keeping with motor classification and distribution.
8. Neuroimaging not consistent with clinical history or examination.

Dyskinesia

- Recurring, uncontrolled and involuntary movements that may be stereotyped.
- Tone abnormality varies and dyskinetic movements diminish in sleep.
  Dyskinesia encompasses:
  - **Dystonia**: characterized by hypokinesia (reduced activity) and hypertonia (increased tone) resulting in stiff movements – often stereotyped and twisting in nature.
  - **Choreoathetoid movement**: characterised by hyperkinesia (increased activity) and hypotonia (reduced tone) resulting in uncoordinated writhing and jerky movements (chorea are fast jerky movements whereas athetosis are slow writhing movements).

Ataxia

- Generalised hypotonia with loss of muscle coordination; characterised by abnormal force, rhythm, and control or accuracy of movement.

Mixed

- No single tone abnormality and movement disorder predominates. A combination of spasticity with dyskinesia is the commonest mixed type.

Management of movement disorders

There is no single therapeutic approach for managing paediatric movement disorders and any intervention should be guided by the child's overall mobility capacity using systems such as the gross motor function classification system (GMFCS; see Chapter 28, Child development and disability), and should also be related to participation goals.

- Physical therapy: all interventions should be task focused, repetitive and high in intensity to be effective. Overall intensive blocks of therapy are more successful than non-task focused, infrequent interventions.
- Hypertonia management (Table 36.4).

Table 36.4 Hypertonia management in childhood.

Treatment	Comments	Spasticity	Dystonia
Oral Medication			
Baclofen		Y	Y
Diazepam		Y	Y
Tizanidine		Y	N
Dantrolene	Rarely used in paediatrics due to liver toxicity	Y	N
Levodopa	Limited effectiveness in paediatric secondary dystonias	N	Y
Trihexyphenidyl	Often first line in treating secondary dystonias	N	Y
Gabapentin	Increasing utility in difficult to control dystonias	N	Y
Tetrabenezine	Rarely used in paediatrics due to effect on mood	N	Y
Clonidine	Sedative and hypotensive side effects	Y	Y
Injectables			
Botulinum toxin A	IM in all muscle groups	Y	Y
Ethanol	IM in larger muscle groups	Y	Y
Phenol	Nerve block in larger muscle groups	Y	Y
Surgical			
Orthopaedic	Muscle and tendon lengthening, transfers, disconnection	Y	Y
Intrathecal baclofen	Higher doses needed for dystonia	Y	Y
Selective dorsal rhizotomy	Lower limb spasticity	Y	N
Deep brain stimulation	Useful for primary dystonia, limited effectiveness for secondary dystonia	N	Y

USEFUL RESOURCES

- WHO website https://www.who.int/classifications/icf/en/; information and details regarding the ICF framework.
- CanChild Centre for Childhood Disability Research http://www.canchild.ca; information on ICF, 6Fs, goal setting, knowledge translation and Family Centred Care.
- Royal Children's Hospital ABI resources https://www.rch.org.au/rehab/abi_resources/; RCH fact sheets on rehabilitation for paediatric brain injury.
- Evidence based review of ABI https://erabi.ca; has a separate paediatric section with up to date evidence on best treatment approaches for ABI.
- SCI Australia https://scia.org.au; mostly related to adults but good library and links for support groups.
- Australasian Academy of Cerebral Palsy and Developmental Medicine https://www.ausacpdm.org.au/resources. Information on CP including hip surveillance guidelines, links to excellent CP Alliance newsletter, dyskinesia toolkit, CP registers and more.
- The Cerebral Palsy Foundation https://www.yourcpf.org; a wide selection of information, factsheets and resources available for patients/families.

CHAPTER 37

Renal medicine

Joshua Kausman
Susan Gibb

Key Points

- UTIs are very common in children. There is a high chance of underlying abnormality on imaging, but in most cases, this does not merit additional intervention. Correct microbiological diagnosis and prompt treatment are the initial priorities, with consideration of further investigation directed to younger children and those with recurrent infections.
- Haematuria and proteinuria are common findings in children. Many will be transient or orthostatic in origin and do not require specialist assessment. Correct collection and timing of urine samples is important. Persistent abnormalities or high grade blood and protein excretion should prompt referral to a specialist.
- Nephrotic syndrome is an uncommon condition, but due to a high risk of relapse, it imposes a major burden of care on children and families. During an episode there are significant risks of complications due to hypoperfusion, thrombosis and infection, but with good education and surveillance, many relapses can be detected and treated early prior to clinical deterioration.
- AKI is commonly associated with dehydration in children. This is generally associated with a bland urine and reduced intravascular state and responds well to fluid repletion. Assessment should include investigation for active urine sediment, fluid overload and progressive renal impairment, in which case specialist involvement is required.
- Hypertension is a common finding in children. Elevated BP or stage 1 hypertension should be confirmed with correct cuff and technique on 3 occasions before proceeding to further investigation or intervention. For stage 2 hypertension, prompt specialist referral should be made.

Continence

Nocturnal enuresis

Enuresis is defined as intermittent incontinence of urine during periods of sleep, in children aged 5 years or older, in the absence of congenital or acquired defects of the central nervous system or urinary tract.

- The threshold is >1 episode per month continuing over three months.
- It is a common condition in childhood with the prevalence being 15%–20% of 5 year olds, 9.7% of 7 year olds, 5.5% of 10 year olds, 2–3% of 12–14 year olds, and 1–2% of people aged 15 years and over.
- Bedwetting in the absence of daytime urinary symptoms is called 'monosymptomatic' nocturnal enuresis (MNE) whereas if day symptoms occur it is 'non-monosymptomatic' nocturnal enuresis (NMNE).
- Primary NE refers to a child who has never been dry for at least 6 months.
- Secondary NE refers to children who start to wet again.
- Although secondary NE may suggest an organic or psychological cause, in practice most secondary NE is simply primary NE that never fully resolved.

Paediatric Handbook, Tenth Edition. Edited by Kate Harding, Daniel S. Mason and Daryl Efron.
© 2021 John Wiley & Sons Ltd. Published 2021 by John Wiley & Sons Ltd.

Aetiology and pathophysiology

Enuresis is usually inherited as an autosomal dominant trait with variable penetrance.

The pathophysiology involves a combination of:

- Poor arousal to stimulus of full bladder.
- Nocturnal polyuria – relative deficiency of vasopressin at night.
- Overactive bladder with reduced nocturnal functional bladder capacity.

Enuresis is associated with low self-esteem, depression, reduced social participation and other behavioural co-morbidities particularly in children over 9 years of age. Treatment has been shown to improve self-esteem, even if is only partially successful.

Children with NMNE have symptoms indicating bladder dysfunction: wetting, frequency, jiggling or urgency.

- Urgency with associated posturing can occur with voiding postponement, 'waiting until the last minute' but commonly it is due to an overactive bladder with a small functional bladder capacity and small urgently voided volumes.
- These children often have NE that is refractory to initial treatment and persists beyond 10 years of age.

Following physical examination and urinalysis, treatment can be offered. Further investigation is not usually necessary. Red flags indicating rare physical causes are included in Table 37.1. Other associated conditions are obstructive sleep apnoea and sexual abuse.

Management

The spontaneous remission rate is approximately 15% per year. Those least likely to resolve spontaneously are those with NMNE. Treatment should be offered to children ≥6 years for whom wetting has become a problem. See Figure 37.1 for management algorithm.

Monosymptomatic NE

Alarms: First line treatment is with a pad and bell alarm or personal (body-worn) alarm, used nightly for 8–12 weeks. Relapses may be minimised by 'overlearning' – using a fluid load before bed for the last 1–2 weeks of treatment. A wetting diary may help in motivation and monitoring. When symptoms are refractory to treatment, unsuspected nocturnal bladder dysfunction with detrusor overactivity is often the cause.

Desmopressin (DDAVP): A synthetic analogue of vasopressin. In Australia it is available for those who have not responded to or are unsuitable for an alarm. It is useful in the short-term (school camps and sleepovers) and medium-term (adolescents who are fed up). Side effects are uncommon. Hyponatremia with convulsions has been reported and it is important to ensure that appropriate advice regarding fluid intake is given to minimise this risk. The child should **not** drink for 1 hour before and 8 hours after the administration of DDAVP. The oral dose of DDAVP is 120–240 mcg (1–2 melts) placed under the tongue 1 hour before sleep.

Other treatments: There is no evidence to suggest that fluid restriction or liberalisation influences outcome. There is insufficient evidence to recommend lifting or waking the child, psychotherapy, hypnosis, acupuncture, rewards, chiropractic or bladder training.

Non-monosymptomatic NE

Treatment plan

- Treat constipation/faecal incontinence first and exclude UTI.
- Use anticholinergics to treat detrusor instability if significant
- Then use alarm if needed as above.
- Frequent, regular voiding may help.

Table 37.1 Red flags in enuresis.

Red flags in enuresis	
Acute onset	Poor growth
Recurrent UTI	Poor urinary stream
Polyuria	Distended bladder
Polydipsia	Physical signs suggestive of occult spinal dysraphism or tethered cord

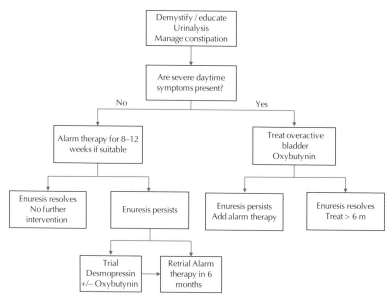

Figure 37.1 Management of nocturnal enuresis.

Table 37.2 Red flags in Day wetting without NE.

Red flags in day wetting	
Continuous wetting or dribbling	Tiredness
Weight loss	Abnormal urinary stream
Polyuria/Polydipsia	Distended bladder
Hypertension	Renal mass

Anticholinergics
- First line is Oxybutynin (Ditropan). Dose: 2.5–5 mg bd. Dry mouth is common. Less common side effects include rash, mood changes, constipation, headache, epistaxis, blurred vision. Treatment is often needed for many months to years.
- If poorly tolerated or ineffective other medication may be tried: more bladder specific anticholinergics, transdermal oxybutynin, mirabegron.

Daytime wetting without NE
Urinary incontinence is defined as wetting in Children ≥5 years occurring at least once a month for ≥3months. It is important to distinguish continuous wetting which likely has a structural cause from intermittent wetting. Further evaluation needs to distinguish neurological from functional disorders. Table 37.2 lists red flag features for underlying conditions. Initial treatment of day wetting involves education and a regular fluid intake and toileting program, sometimes called urotherapy.

Investigation
Children with day-wetting should have a urine microscopy, culture and glucose and a renal and bladder ultrasound including an assessment of residual urine volume. A 2-day voiding frequency/volume diary, and uroflowmetry with post-void bladder scanning can provide diagnostic information and further guide management.

Diagnostic subgroups

1. Overactive Bladder
   - The condition is caused by overactivity during bladder filling.
   - Symptoms include urgency, frequency, posturing (squatting) and wetting.
   - Management includes treating any coexistent UTI and constipation, regular voiding, and anticholinergic medication to reduce bladder spasms (see NMNE above). Second line therapies include neuromodulation.
2. Dysfunctional voiding
   - There is poor coordination between detrusor and bladder neck with poor relaxation of the external sphincter during voiding.
   - The condition is associated with increased intravesical pressure, high residual urine volumes and, at times, upper tract dilatation.
   - Management relies on teaching sphincter relaxation (i.e. pelvic floor relaxation) and ensuring optimal voiding techniques.
3. Other conditions
   - Wetting can also occur in giggle incontinence, stress incontinence or underactive bladder.
   - Bladder neck and urethral obstruction and neurogenic bladder may have large or expressible bladders.

Clinical Pearl: Vesicovaginal reflux

An important and easily treatable cause of day wetting in girls
- Dribbling post void, small leaks 5 to 10 mins after voiding during the day
- A trial of voiding whilst straddling the toilet facing the cistern should eliminate reflux of urine into the vagina and dribbling post voiding and can be a useful diagnostic test.
- Management is to change voiding posture:
  - Sit on the toilet with legs supported and well apart.
  - Lean forward making the urinary stream more vertical.
  - At end of voiding, use toilet paper to press and lift the perineum forward/upward to empty urine from the vagina.

Urinary tract infections

Symptomatic lower urinary tract infections (UTIs) during childhood are common and generally carry little long-term risk. Important but uncommon associations of febrile UTIs during childhood include pyelonephritis, renal impairment and hypertension (HTN). The primary aim of investigation of childhood UTIs is to reduce the risk of sepsis and identify children at risk of chronic kidney disease (CKD).

Clinical features

- UTIs may present with nonspecific clinical features. Fever may be the sole symptom. This is more common in younger children.
- Cystitis refers to urinary infections limited to the bladder and urethra. It may present with dysuria, frequency, wetting, urgency, cloudy or malodorous urine and lower abdominal pain. Fever is often absent although irritability and other minor constitutional symptoms are common in young children.
- Pyelonephritis usually presents with additional symptoms of fever, lethargy, vomiting, loin or generalised abdominal pain. Pyelonephritis in neonates and infants may present as an undifferentiated fever.
- Offensive urine is neither sensitive nor specific for UTIs in children.

Remember that finding a UTI in a sick child does not exclude another site of serious infection (e.g. meningitis).

Pathogens

- *Escherichia coli* (80%)
- *Enterococcus faecalis* (10%)
- Other gram-negatives: *Klebsiella* spp., *Proteus* spp., *Enterobacter* spp., *Citrobacter* spp.
- Other gram-positives: *Staphylococcus saprophyticus*

Diagnosis

The most reliable collection technique appropriate to the clinical setting should be used. This may be suprapubic bladder aspiration (SPA), in/out catheter specimen urine, clean catch or midstream urine sample. Urine bag samples should be used only in specific settings as contamination risk is high.

Urine 'ward test' strips

These are useful as a screening test in a child with low suspicion of a UTI (>6 months, without known renal tract abnormality and with an alternative focus for fever). Ward test should not be used in a child with a high chance of a UTI. If leukocyte esterase and nitrites are both positive, then a UTI is likely. The ward test strips for leucocytes or nitrites are negative in up to 50% of UTIs in children. This is because the production of nitrites by bacteria is time-dependent and infant bladder capacity necessitates frequent voiding.

Bag urine specimen collection

- Do not send for culture.
- Use for chemical strip screening only.
- In sick infants or those where the suspicion of UTI is high (e.g. renal tract anomaly or previous UTI), a bag specimen should not be taken, as it only delays the diagnosis. An SPA (preferred) or CSU sample should be obtained as part of the septic workup.

Midstream urine specimen collection

This can be obtained from children who are able to void on request (usually by 3–4 years of age). The child's genitalia are first washed with warm water. In girls the labia should be separated. The child is asked to void. After passing the first few millilitres, a specimen is collected.

- A pure growth of 10^8 c.f.u./L in an MSU is proof of a UTI.
- A pure growth of $>10^5$–10^8 c.f.u./L in an MSU is suggestive of a UTI (correlate with clinical setting).

Catheter specimen collection

See Chapter 5, Procedures.

- These are useful in infants after a failed SPA or in older children who are unable to void on request.
- A pure growth of $>10^5$ c.f.u./L indicates infection.

Suprapubic aspirate collection

See Chapter 5, Procedures.

- This is the preferred method of urine collection in infants.
- Aspirated urine should be sterile; hence any pure growth of bacteria indicates infection.

Additional investigations

It is important to identify bacteraemia, meningitis and sepsis in neonates and young infants with UTI, consider:

- Blood culture and electrolytes.
- Lumbar puncture. Do not omit a lumbar puncture in a sick child just because a UTI has been diagnosed. Collection of CSF should be undertaken in infants <3 months with UTI and considered in children <2 years.

Treatment

Treatment is directed by clinical severity, ability to tolerate oral medications and previous antibiotic sensitivities.

- Most infants <12 months of age with a UTI require benzylpenicillin 60 mg/kg IV (max. 2 g) 6 hourly and gentamicin 7.5 mg/kg IV (<10 years) or 6 mg/kg IV max. 240 mg (>10 years) daily.
- In children who are well and not vomiting (even those with clinical pyelonephritis), a course of oral antibiotics has been shown to be as effective as IV antibiotics (see Appendix: Antimicrobial guidelines). Antibiotic sensitivity should be checked when available (usually at 48 hours).

Recurrent UTIs

Ten to thirty per cent of children with a UTI will have a recurrence, usually within 12 months.

- A greater risk of recurrence is associated with the first UTI occurring <6 months of age, dysfunctional voiding, constipation, the presence of dilating VUR or evidence of renal parenchymal loss on initial scanning.

- Factors contributing to kidney vulnerability and risk of CKD
  - Family history of kidney disease
  - Structural renal disorders, chronic systemic illnesses

Further investigations

Screened population: antenatal ultrasound known to be normal:

- First infection
  - Lower tract, afebrile UTI in girl <3 years old. Consider renal ultrasound.
  - Lower tract, afebrile UTI in toddler or boy. Arrange renal ultrasound.
  - UTI at any age with unusual microbiology or clinical features. Arrange renal ultrasound.
  - Upper tract, febrile UTI
    - Renal ultrasound. If <3 years old perform dimercaptosuccinic acid (DMSA) scan at least 3–6 months after the UTI. This nuclear medicine scan looks for renal parenchymal defects (primarily renal scarring).
    - Consider micturating cystourethrogram (MCU) if presenting during infancy. Radiographic contrast is instilled in the bladder via a urethral catheter and subsequent radiographs taken to image the bladder and urethra to evaluate bladder emptying, exclude PUV and vesicoureteric reflux.
- Recurrent UTIs
  - Lower tract: bladder function evaluation by 2-day voiding volume diary and renal ultrasound.
  - Upper tract: as per lower tract, then DMSA at 3–6 months, consider referral to nephrologist or urologist.

Unscreened population: antenatal scans not performed

- Earlier renal ultrasound.

Management of recurrent UTIs

- Manage wetting and voiding dysfunction
- Manage constipation
- If >3 UTI's in 12 months then review history and management adherence, consider referral and prophylactic antibiotics.

Clinical Controversy: UTI

For many years there has been controversy over the role of VUR and UTIs in the progression of CKD. This has had implications for the use of MCU in the investigation of UTIs and surgical intervention in children, as there is a significant likelihood of detecting VUR in young children with UTI. However, data has failed to demonstrate a benefit of intervention with either reflux surgery or antibiotics for mitigating the progression of CKD, but they can reduce the recurrence rate of UTIs. Progression of CKD appears to be a result of underlying associated dysplasia in the majority of cases. MCU is therefore selectively used for cases with recurrent pyelonephritis and abnormal urinary tracts (particularly to diagnose posterior urethral valves), where surgical intervention may have a benefit.

Abnormalities of urinary sediment
Isolated microscopic haematuria

Isolated microscopic haematuria may be observed transiently in febrile children with a normal renal tract or following vigorous exercise. It is important to differentiate these from the children whose haematuria represents more significant renal pathology. Concerning features that should prompt further investigation:

- Persisting microhaematuria or recurrent macrohaematuria
- Proteinuria confirmed by morning urinary protein: creatinine (UPr:Cr) ratio
- High-level microhaematuria (>50 RBC/mL) particularly if associated with casts
- HTN, oliguria or oedema: would suggest acute glomerulonephritis
- Features suggesting systemic or chronic illness
- Painful haematuria: suggests bladder pathology (e.g. UTI), renal calculi or other urologic disorders.

The initial steps are to confirm isolated haematuria on three separate occasions when the child is well. Children with heavy isolated microhaematuria (>50 dysmorphic (glomerular) RBC/μL) should be referred. If low-level haematuria only is present, then these children may potentially be followed clinically. Blood pressure, general

pubertal and genital examination should be performed, and abnormalities managed. If these are normal, then the following management plan may be followed:
- If proteinuria (UPr:Cr >60 mg/mmol) is present, then consider acute nephritis and refer to paediatrician/ paediatric nephrologist.
- If proteinuria is absent, then the following should be performed:
  - Urinary Ca:Cr ratio. If ≥0.7 mmol/mmol on more than one morning sample then hypercalciuria likely, arrange renal ultrasound and refer.
  - Urinalysis or urine M&C on immediate family members. If isolated microhaematuria identified, then consider familial haematuria and refer.
  - Renal ultrasound. If abnormalities identified, then refer.
- If screening investigations are normal then annual review with general heath check, BP, urine M&C and UPr:Cr ratio is appropriate until haematuria has been absent for 2 years.
  - Children should be referred if they demonstrate persistence of haematuria after 4 years or into adolescence or if heavy microhaematuria (>50 dysmorphic (glomerular) RBC/μL) is consistently noted.

Macroscopic haematuria without proteinuria
Bleeding from any site within the renal tract may present with macroscopic haematuria. Generally glomerular inflammation (glomerulonephritis) presents with both haematuria and proteinuria, although IgA nephropathy may commonly present with recurrent episodes of painless macroscopic haematuria without proteinuria.

Pain associated with macro/microhaematuria may be helpful in directing investigations (Table 37.3).

Haematuria with proteinuria
The presence of both haematuria and proteinuria suggests pathological changes within the glomerulus (glomerulonephritis), endothelium (haemolytic uraemic syndrome) or renal interstitium.
- The most common cause is glomerulonephritis.
- Associated features may include tea coloured urine, oliguria, fluid retention with oedema and HTN (nephritic syndrome).
- Renal function may be impaired and electrolyte abnormalities are common.

Table 37.3 Causes of haematuria.

Symptoms	Causes	Clinical examples
Painless	Glomerular inflammation Tumour cell infiltration Genetic defects of the glomerulus	Glomerulonephritis Wilms tumour Alport's syndrome
Loin pain	Renal pelvis obstruction Renal engorgement with stretch of renal capsule	Obstructing calculi Blood • Renal vein thrombosis • Nutcracker syndrome • Cortical necrosis • Renal trauma • Haematoma Inflammatory infiltrate • Glomerulonephritis • Interstitial nephritis Infection • Complicated pyelonephritis Tumour • Wilms (may be painless)
Renal colic	Ureteric obstruction/peristalsis	• Obstructing calculi • Upper tract bleeding → clot colic
Suprapubic pain	Bladder mucosa	Infection • Haemorrhagic cystitis (bacterial/viral) Cytotoxic agents: • Cyclophosphamide cystitis

Evaluation should include careful history for antecedent infections, systemic illnesses and medication exposure. Examination should evaluate aetiology and consequences of acute kidney injury (AKI). Management should be discussed with a nephrologist.

Considerations should include:
- Assessment of AKI: see 'Acute kidney injury' section, p. 502.
- Aetiology of acute glomerulonephritis: C3, C4, ASOT, ANA, ± ANCA, ± AntiGBM Ab
  - Post infectious GN: nephritic syndrome typically follows throat or skin infection.
  - HSP nephritis: palpable purpura, arthralgia.
  - IgA nephritis: microhaematuria with episodic macrohaematuria coincident with mucosal infection.
  - SLE nephritis: nephritic or mixed nephrotic/nephritic picture, multisystem disorder.
  - ANCA associated and anti-GBM diseases: often associated with respiratory tract involvement. ANCA or Anti-GBM Ab positive.
- Other pathologies presenting with microhaematuria and some proteinuria
  - HUS: Coombs negative haemolytic anaemia with red cell fragmentation, thrombocytopaenia, increased LDH, low haptoglobin, AKI, HTN common. May or may not be associated with bloody diarrhoea.
  - Acute interstitial nephritis: haematuria, low-grade proteinuria, WBC casts ± eosinophiluria, eosinophilia, AKI. Commonly due to medications or infection.
  - Alport syndrome – a genetic defect of collagen in the glomerular basement membrane associated with sensorineural hearing loss and visual defects.

Isolated low-level proteinuria

Isolated proteinuria (+ or >0.3 g/L) is commonly detected on routine health checks, following exercise, during unrelated febrile illnesses or with UTIs. It is important to differentiate this transient physiologic proteinuria from persistent pathological causes.
- When low grade (+) proteinuria without haematuria is detected, a thorough history and physical examination including measurement of BP should be performed.
  - An early morning urine M&C and UPr:Cr ratio should be checked when systemically well.
  - If examination and urine investigations are normal, transient physiological proteinuria is the likely diagnosis. No further investigation is required in this setting.
- If high-grade proteinuria (+++ or >1.0 g/L) without haematuria is identified, then careful examination for evidence of generalised oedema suggestive of nephrotic syndrome should be performed (see Heavy isolated proteinuria and Nephrotic syndrome section below).
- If proteinuria with haematuria is noted, then the child should be investigated further as outlined above.
- If isolated proteinuria is persistent then orthostatic proteinuria or pathological proteinuria needs to be considered:
  - Orthostatic proteinuria is indicated by a normal early morning UPr:Cr ratio (after recumbent overnight) and elevated UPr:Cr ratio in afternoon after being upright during the day. This diagnosis carries a good long-term renal prognosis and reflects alteration in glomerular haemodynamics with changes in body position.
  - Pathologic proteinuria demonstrates a similar diurnal pattern. It may be differentiated from orthostatic proteinuria by the presence of elevated UPr:Cr ratio in an early morning sample. Daily protein excretion measured by 24-hour urine collection will be elevated in pathological proteinuria. Long-term renal prognosis will be determined by underlying renal pathology; persisting proteinuria requires further investigation and management.

Preliminary evaluation should include careful history of renal symptoms, medication exposure and family history. Thorough physical examination including growth, BP and general examination followed by repeat urine M&C, UPr:Cr, serum U&E, Cr, FBE, LFT and renal ultrasound. Children with screening test abnormalities or persisting proteinuria should be referred for specialist management.

Clinical Pearl: Proteinuria and Haematuria
- Where there is concern about proteinuria or CKD, perform a quantified urine protein (UPr:Cr) on an early morning urine.
- For a child with a history of haematuria, perform a spot urine, ideally in the early morning, for Pr:Cr, Ca:Cr and microscopy with phase contrast (red cell morphology).

Nephrotic syndrome

Nephrotic syndrome is characterised by heavy isolated proteinuria (≥+++ or UPr:Cr ≥200 mg/mmol), hypoalbuminaemia (≤25 g/L) and generalised oedema. Renal function is usually preserved. It is usually idiopathic and steroid sensitive. Initial evaluation and management should be directed towards confirming the diagnosis, optimising fluid status, management of complications, followed by specific treatment and family education.

Confirming the diagnosis of idiopathic nephrotic syndrome (INS)

Generalised oedema

- Usually dependent oedema. Scrotal/labial oedema is common and secondary cellulitis can occur in the setting of skin breakdown.
- Ascites and pleural effusions indicate significant oedema.
- Clinical monitoring of oedema and daily weights are required.

Hypoalbuminaemia

- Although less common, consider nutritional or gastrointestinal protein loss on history and examination.

Proteinuria without significant haematuria

- Confirm on formal measurement: UPr:Cr ratio ≥200 mg/mmol. Timed urinary excretion is not usually required in most cases of childhood INS.
- Haematuria should be mild (+/++) or absent.
- Hyaline casts may be present but granular or RBC casts should alert to the diagnosis being acute glomerulonephritis (GN) rather than INS.
- Macroscopic haematuria should alert to possible renal vein thrombosis or acute GN.

Preserved renal function

Optimisation of fluid status

Extravascular fluid/oedema

- Monitor oedema, body weight (daily or bd), BP, fluid balance, urine output.
- No added salt diet whilst oedematous.
- Fluids may be restricted to 1.0 L/m^2 per day.
- IV 20% albumin (1 g/kg = 5 mL/kg) over 4–6 hours with frusemide 1 mg/kg at midway and end of infusion, may be considered if gross oedema, evidence of imminent skin breakdown, symptomatic pleural effusions.

Intravascular volume depletion

- Likely if cool extremities, postural hypotension, oliguria, abdominal cramps (may represent bowel wall oedema or peritonitis).
- If evidence of severe hypoalbuminaemia and proteinuria, may consider IV albumin supplementation (IV 20% albumin 1 mg/kg over 6 hours ± frusemide 1 mg/kg).

Recognition and management of complications

Primary peritonitis or sepsis:

- Multifactorial including loss of complement factors, immunoglobulins and impaired T cell function in addition to bowel wall oedema, venous stasis and bacterial translocation into ascitic fluid.
- Most common organisms: *Streptococcus pneumoniae* or Gram negative organisms.
- Initial treatment should cover resistant pneumococci and bowel organisms, (e.g. cefotaxime, amoxicillin and metronidazole). Advice should be sought from a nephrologist and infectious disease physician.

Thromboembolism:

- Contributing factors include intravascular depletion, haemoconcentration, urinary loss of antithrombin III and increased hepatic synthesis of clotting factors.
- May occur as lower limb or pelvic deep venous thrombosis (80%), venous sinus thrombosis (seizures or altered conscious state), renal vein thrombosis (macrohaematuria) or arterial thrombosis.
- Evaluation and management should be in consultation with haematologist and nephrologist.

Skin breakdown and cellulitis.

Induction of remission and adjunct treatment

- Prednisolone is first-line treatment for INS. Commence at 60 mg/m^2 per day (max 80 mg) orally. Remission would be expected within 14 days. If failure to remit, discussion with a nephrologist is appropriate.

- Phenoxymethylpenicillin 12.5 mg/kg (max. 1 g) orally bd until gross oedema clears.
- Management once into remission
  - Prednisolone: Weaning schedules vary across nephrology services. Recent data has shown that prednisolone courses of 2–3 months are equally effective to those of 6 months duration. See The RCH clinical practice guideline: Nephrotic Syndrome for details.
  - Until oedema has resolved and high-dose prednisolone reduced: Low salt diet, penicillin and fluid restriction (if used).
- Immunisation: The child should receive the 13-valent conjugate pneumococcal vaccine (13vPCV) once in remission if no previous booster given after 12 months age. A follow-up dose should be given if the child did not complete primary vaccination.

Interim treatment and follow-up
- Children should be monitored regularly for steroid side effects including HTN, obesity, poor growth and mood disturbance whilst receiving steroids.
- 23-valent polysaccharide pneumococcal vaccination should be given at 4–5 years of age and ≥ 2 months after 13vPCV. Ideally this should be given after cessation of steroids. Influenza vaccine should be administered annually.
- Home monitoring for relapse by daily urinalysis. Recommendations regarding frequency of subsequent monitoring varies across different centres but often continues beyond 6–12 months after cessation of steroids.

Management of relapse
- Relapse is defined as recurrence of proteinuria (UPr:Cr >200 mg/mmol or >++ protein or urinary protein >40 mg/m^2/h) on three consecutive days.
- Relapse may be precipitated by infectious or immunologic factors or may occur without a clear trigger.
- There is no consensus regarding use of prophylactic penicillin; however, we recommend it when children have significant ascites. It is continued until ascites or gross oedema has resolved.
- Low-dose aspirin (2–5 mg/kg per day) is no longer routine in management.
- Prednisolone course is shorter, when treating relapse. Again, there is some variation across centres but a suitable weaning program is outlined in The RCH clinical practice guideline: Nephrotic Syndrome.

Indications for referral
- Uncertain diagnosis
  - Acute nephritis features
  - Other multi-systemic features
- Complications of nephrotic syndrome
- Failure to respond by 2 weeks
- Frequent relapses or steroid dependence

Clinical Pearl: Idiopathic nephrotic syndrome

Idiopathic nephrotic syndrome has high risk of relapse (>70%). To prevent redevelopment of symptomatic oedema, requiring admission to hospital, it is critical families are educated about the need to monitor the urine for early detection of proteinuria. Every family should know how to perform and record the urine dipstick for protein, have a relapse plan for prednisolone dosing and a sick day plan for prednisolone to prevent relapses with intercurrent infections.

Abnormalities of renal function
Estimation of GFR
Schwartz formula allows for estimation of renal function: $eGFR\ (mL/min/1.73\ m^2) \approx (36.5 \times Ht\ (cm))/sCr\ (umol/L)$.

Acute kidney injury
An acute decline in renal function may be evidenced by inability to maintain normal chemical homeostasis and fluid balance. Classification is based on changes in serum creatinine (sCr) and urine output. Evaluation of fluid status, nephrotoxins etc. should be undertaken even with small changes. Table 37.4 describes the aetiologies of AKI.

Table 37.4 Aetiology of AKI (GFR = nephron number × single nephron GFR).

Nephron number	
Reduced renal mass	Underlying structural renal disease Solitary kidney Ex IUGR Previous renal injury Chronic systemic disorders CKD
Single nephron GFR	
Reduced glomerular blood flow	Dehydration, hypotension Renal arterial embolism or obstruction Capillary endothelial damage; for example, HUS, acute severe HTN Renal vein obstruction
Reduced glomerular permeability and surface area	Capillary endothelial cell damage; for example, HUS, acute severe HTN. Glomerular pathologies; for example, glomerulonephritis
Reduced glomerular–tubular pressure difference or tubular damage	Tubular obstruction; for example, calculi, tumour lysis, rhabdomyolysis Tubular swelling and damage; for example, ATN, nephrotoxins, interstitial nephritis, pyelonephritis Tubular ischemia; for example, hypoxic injury
Distal tubule obstruction (tubular–glomerular feedback)	Obstruction at pelviureteric, ureter, vesicoureteric junction, bladder wall, bladder outlet

Evaluation of AKI
- Assess kidney function: U&E, sCr, calcium, magnesium, phosphate, acid-base, FBE, LFT and urine output
- Acute or chronic kidney disease (CKD)?
  - Clinical indicators of CKD (growth, Hb, baseline sCr, PTH)
  - Anuric non-catabolic acute renal failure
  - Serum urea (sUrea) usually rises 3–5 mmol/L per day
  - sCr usually rises 50–100 μmol/L per day
  - Does the sUrea and sCr match with known duration of current kidney injury
- Nephron number
  - Renal ultrasound: kidney number, size, cortical thickness, echotexture, cortico-medullary differentiation
- Glomerular blood flow
  - Hypoperfusion: often sUrea (μmol/L) >100 × sCr (μmol/L)
  - Renal Doppler ultrasound
- Glomerular permeability and surface area: markers of specific disease entities
  - HUS: haemolytic anaemia, thrombocytopaenia, LDH, haptoglobin, complement (if atypical)
  - Glomerulonephritis: haematuria, proteinuria, urinary casts, complement, GN serology
- Loss of glomerular–tubular pressure differences or tubular damage
  - Nephrotoxic drug levels, contrast exposure, rhabdomyolysis, interstitial nephritis
  - Urine M&C including eosinophils
- Distal tubular obstruction
  - Renal ultrasound: hydronephrosis, hydroureter, bladder wall thickness

Management of AKI
- Minimisation of primary insult
- Minimisation of secondary insult
  - Careful fluid management, avoid fluid overload or dehydration.
  - Avoid hypoxia.
  - Maintain normotension.

- ○ Remove nephrotoxin exposure, minimise diuretic exposure.
- ○ Treat infection.
- Maintain metabolic homeostasis: careful fluid, electrolyte and glucose balance
  - ○ Limit fluids to insensible losses (300–400 mL/m^2/d) plus urine output.
  - ○ Sodium: if anuric, for minimal intake. If polyuric, measure Urinary Na and volume of urine, often 75 mmol/L required.
  - ○ Potassium: monitor for ECG changes of hyperkalaemia (decreased P waves, prolonged PR interval, widened QRS, decreased Q wave, depressed ST segment, peaked T waves, prolonged QT interval).
  - ○ Hypocalcaemia: usually due to hyperphosphataemia. Correct before correcting acidosis.
  - ○ Acidosis: correct with sodium bicarbonate (mmol = base deficit × weight (kg) × 0.3). Take care with correction if the child is fluid overloaded (excess sodium) or hypocalcaemic (will be lowered further with correction of acidosis).
  - ○ Hyperphosphataemia: low phosphate diet, phosphate binders (calcium carbonate).
  - ○ Uraemia: acute rise to >30 mmol/L may cause CNS symptoms. Protein restrict if able. Consider dialysis if nutrition affected by fluid restriction or biochemical abnormalities unable to be corrected.
- Enhance recovery
  - ○ Provide adequate nutrition for recovery.

> **Clinical Pearl: Acute kidney injury**
> Most AKI in children is due to pre-renal insult (dehydration). Always consider the role of ibuprofen (NSAIDs), which exacerbates this injury by reducing renal perfusion and can also cause an interstitial nephritis. This is also a reason it should be avoided in individuals with CKD.

Hypertension
Measurement of BP in childhood
- Children >3 years of age should have BP measured.
- Children <3 years should have BP measured if risk factors have been identified. They include:
  - ○ Prematurity, VLBW or NICU graduate
  - ○ Congenital heart disease
  - ○ Recurrent UTIs, haematuria, proteinuria
  - ○ Known personal or family history of congenital kidney or urologic disease

Definitions and measurement of blood pressure in children
- HTN in childhood is defined as the 95th percentile for gender, age and height (Table 37.5). This is a statistical definition. It differs from the definition used in adulthood which is based on the risk of adverse cardiovascular outcomes. Nevertheless, significant sustained elevation of blood pressure in childhood is associated with end organ damage and should be treated.
- Blood pressure should be measured when the child is quiet and cooperative. The widest BP cuff that can fit around the arm should be used. The cuff bladder should cover at least 80% of arm circumference.
- Oscillometric BP measurements may overestimate BP and few are validated for use in young children.

Table 37.5 Interpretation of BP measurement.

Classification	Definition	Management
Normal BP	Systolic BP (SBP) and diastolic BP (DBP) <90th percentile	Check 1 year
Elevated BP (previously 'pre-HTN')	SBP or DBP ≥90th but <95th percentile; or BP >120/80	Recheck 6 months; begin weight management if appropriate
Stage 1 hypertension (HTN)	SBP and/or DBP 95th – 95th percentile plus 12 mmHg; or age >13yr: >130/80-139/89	Recheck 1–2 weeks, if remains high then begin evaluation and treatment including weight management if appropriate
Stage 2 HTN	SBP and/or DBP >95th percentile plus 12 mmHg; or age >13yr: ≥140/90	Begin evaluation and treatment within 1 week, more rapidly if symptomatic

- For all high results, especially if oscillometric measurements used, confirm in ideal setting with correct cuff size. A smaller cuff size is associated with higher readings.
- For children 8 years and older ambulatory blood pressure monitoring provides important information in:
  - Discriminating white coat HTN from true HTN
  - Assessment of diurnal variation and severity of HTN
  - Monitoring of adequacy of response to treatment

BP reference values
Available at:
- www.rch.org.au/uploadedFiles/Main/Content/clinicalguide/bp_charts_boys.pdf
- www.rch.org.au/uploadedFiles/Main/Content/clinicalguide/bp_charts_girls.pdf
- Flynn et al. Clinical Practice Guideline for Screening and Management of High Blood Pressure in Children and Adolescents. *Pediatrics*. 2017;140(3)

Rough rule of thumb
- BP systolic 99% ≈ 100 +2 × age in years
- BP diastolic 99% ≈ 60 +2 × age in years (<10 years) or 70 + 2 × age in years (>10 years)

Aetiology and assessment of HTN in children
HTN in young children and infants warrants thorough investigation for secondary causes and complications. HTN in adolescents, however, is not uncommon and may be primary in nature, related to obesity or may be due to secondary causes (Table 37.6). The extent of investigations will be determined by severity, likely aetiology and clinical findings.

- Stage 1 and 2 HTN should be investigated. Aetiologic evaluation should include:
  - Careful history including sleep (OSA), drugs, FHx, risk factors
  - Thorough examination including evaluation of obesity, 4-limb BP and pulses
  - Renal function, electrolytes, Ca, FBE, TFT
  - Urine M&C, UPr:Cr
  - Renal ultrasound with Doppler
  - Lipids, fasting glucose if overweight or family history
  - Drug screen/sleep study as appropriate
- Additional investigations for young children with Stage 1 and all children stage with 2 HTN
  - Plasma renin and aldosterone: low renin suggests mineralocorticoid-mediated HTN
  - Plasma and urinary steroid profile
  - Plasma and urinary catecholamines

Table 37.6 Causes of secondary HTN.

Obesity

Renal
• Acute glomerulonephritis
• Cystic kidney disease – ADPKD, ARPKD, syndromic
• Haemolytic uremic syndrome

Renal artery stenosis
• Idiopathic, fibromuscular dysplasia, NF1

CVS
• Coarctation of aorta
• Mid-aortic syndrome

Endocrine
• Aldosterone mediated – CAH, primary aldosteronism
• Glucocorticoid mediated – exogenous steroids and Cushing syndrome
• Catecholamine mediated – phaeochromocytoma, neuroblastoma, medications
• Thyroid mediated – hyperthyroidism

CNS
• Raised intracranial pressure

Medications

- End organ evaluation in Stage 1 and 2 HTN should include
  - Echocardiogram: LVH and exclude coarctation of aorta
  - Retinal examination: acute and chronic HTN changes

Management of HTN in children
- Prehypertension
  - Recommend physical activity, salt restriction and weight reduction if overweight
  - Pharmacological treatment only if significant additional CVS risk factors
- Stage 1 HTN
  - General management as per Pre-HTN
  - Pharmacological treatment if symptomatic, secondary cause or additional risk factor (diabetes mellitus, chronic kidney disease, LV hypertrophy, heart failure, or persists despite general measures)
- Stage 2 HTN
  - General management as per Stage 1 HTN
  - Commence antihypertensive treatment

Pharmacological treatment of HTN
- Commence a low-dose single agent to avoid rapid fall in BP, then increase over several weeks to maximum weight-based or adult dose, whichever is lower.
- Short-acting agents allow more rapid changes in dosing. Once HTN is controlled then change to long-acting daily medication.
- Choice of agents may be guided by aetiology in cases of secondary HTN, however, generally HTN in children responds well to agents that block the renin system (ACE inhibitors, angiotensin II receptor blockers (ARB)) and β blockers. Ensure renin and aldosterone levels are collected prior to commencement. If there is a delay in this, then consider a calcium channel blocker.
  Note: ACE inhibitors and ARBs are teratogenic and children with CKD require counselling about the risks and monitoring of creatinine and potassium.
- If a second agent is required add a calcium channel blocker then, after this, diuretics may be considered.
- Nephrology referral should be considered for HTN requiring more than one agent.

Symptomatic HTN / HTN urgencies
HTN emergency: severe HTN with acute target organ dysfunction (CNS, CVS, renal)
- Management should be discussed with an appropriate specialist with the aim to reduce BP by ≤25% over first 6–8 hours followed by a further reduction over the next 1–2 days.
- Management should be in ICU usually with titratable infusions (e.g. labetalol, nitroprusside).
HTN urgency: severe HTN without acute target organ dysfunction
- Management should be in conjunction with nephrologist and usually involves oral and bolus IV agents.
- This may include: Short-acting nifedipine, Frusemide, Captopril, Hydralazine, Propranolol, Prazosin (oral), Clonidine, Labetalol.

Clinical Pearl: Hypertension
- Stage 1 HTN without end-organ damage in adolescents who are overweight should initially be managed with lifestyle modification (exercise, salt restriction and weight loss) for 6 months before considering medications.
- Ambulatory blood pressure is very helpful in assessing and monitoring response to interventions for HTN, but for children <8 years is more often not tolerated and may require brief admission for monitored serial BPs if pharmacological treatment is being considered.

USEFUL RESOURCES
- Pocket guide to blood pressure measurement in children: National Institute of Health www.nhlbi.nih.gov/files/docs/bp_child_pocket.pdf
- The RCH clinical practice guideline: Nephrotic Syndrome www.rch.org.au/clinicalguide/guideline_index/Nephrotic_syndrome/

CHAPTER 38

Respiratory medicine

Danielle Wurzel
Sarath Ranganathan
John Massie

Key Points

- Cough alone, in the absence of wheeze, is rarely due to asthma.
- Antibiotics are rarely indicated for acute and subacute cough (i.e. cough lasting <4 weeks) in children.
- Sudden onset wheeze with a history of choking suggests foreign body inhalation and requires urgent specialist evaluation.
- Persistent fever (>48 hours) in the setting of pneumonia may indicate empyema and chest x-ray is indicated.
- Wheeze occurs commonly in preschoolers in the absence of asthma.

Respiratory Illness

Respiratory illness is one of the most common reasons for acute paediatric presentations. Infants and young children tire quickly and can rapidly present in acute respiratory failure. This can be due to:

- Airway compromise (e.g. asthma, bronchiectasis, croup). This results in noisy breathing (stertor above the larynx, stridor if extrathoracic or wheeze if intrathoracic).
- Parenchymal compromise (e.g. pneumonia). This may cause ventilation-perfusion mismatch and result in hypoxaemia.
- Poor respiratory mechanics, common in infants and young children < 2 years old because of a compliant chest wall.

Asthma

See also Chapter 13, Allergy.

Pathology

The two main components include:

- Airway inflammation, oedema and mucous production (chronic)
- Smooth muscle bronchoconstriction and airway hyper-responsiveness (acute)

Risk factors

- Individuals with allergic disease (i.e. allergic rhinitis, hay fever, eczema)
- First-degree relatives with asthma and/or atopic disease

Common triggers

- Upper respiratory tract infections (URTIs)
- Exercise

Paediatric Handbook, Tenth Edition. Edited by Kate Harding, Daniel S. Mason and Daryl Efron.
© 2021 John Wiley & Sons Ltd. Published 2021 by John Wiley & Sons Ltd.

- Exposure to cold air
- Allergen exposure
- Laughing (in preschool children)

Clinical features

- Wheeze
- Shortness of breath
- Chest tightness
- Cough
- Symptomatic improvement with short-acting bronchodilators.
- Interval symptoms: may be present; that is symptoms at night (waking the patient), early in the morning, at rest during the day or during physical activity.
- Some children have symptoms with exercise only.

Clinical Pearl: Cough in the setting of Asthma
Cough alone, in the absence of wheeze, is rarely due to asthma.

There may be few physical signs found between acute attacks, however undertreated or chronic asthma may be associated with:
- Hyperinflation
- Chest wall abnormalities, eg. pectus carinatum or flaring of the lower ribs (Harrison sulcus)
- Expiratory wheeze (generalised)
- Slowed growth parameters
- Medication side effects (e.g. oral candidiasis or reduced growth velocity in those taking inhaled steroids)

Other causes of wheeze to consider

- Small airway calibre (usually improves by 6 years)
- Suppurative lung disease (history of persistent wet cough, may have clubbing)
- Mediastinal mass (may have tracheal shift)
- Inhaled foreign body (localised monophonic wheeze)
- Cardiac failure (may have other cardiac signs or history of heart disease)

Diagnosis

- In pre-school children, the diagnosis of asthma is usually a clinical one; a therapeutic trial of bronchodilator often aids in the diagnosis.
- *Peak flow measurements are unreliable in children and are not routinely used.*

Spirometry assists in the diagnosis and management of older children with asthma. Children over the age of 5 years can learn to do spirometry accurately.

- **Airway obstruction** is defined as:
  - FEV_1 <80% predicted
  - FEV_1/FVC <80% (but this figure varies with age)
  - MMEF 25–75 <67% predicted
- If there is evidence of airway obstruction, bronchodilator reversibility should be assessed (an improvement in FEV_1 of ≥12% in absolute values).
- In most cases, spirometry is unhelpful during an acute presentation unless there is a difference between the perceived symptoms and objective clinical measures.

Exercise broncho-provocation challenge

- Most children with asthma have exercise-induced bronchoconstriction.
- Exercise challenge can be useful to confirm a diagnosis of asthma in children with normal baseline spirometry and a clinical history of asthma.
- 12-15% reduction in FEV_1 following exercise is considered significant.
- Graded dose inhalation of dry powder mannitol is an alternative to the exercise challenge in adolescents.

Table 38.1 Rapid primary assessment of the severity of acute asthma.

Mild/Moderate	Severe	Life-threatening
• Can walk, speak whole sentences in one breath (For young children: can move around, speak in phrases) • Oxygen saturation >94%	**Any** of these findings: • Use of accessory muscles of neck or intercostal muscles or 'tracheal tug' during inspiration or subcostal recession ('abdominal breathing') • Unable to complete sentences in one breath due to dyspnea • Obvious respiratory distress • Oxygen saturation 90–94%	**Any** of these findings: • Reduced consciousness or collapse • Exhaustion • Cyanosis • Oxygen saturation <90% • Poor respiratory effort, soft/absent breath sounds

Source: Adapted from Australian Asthma Handbook at publication of Version 2.0 (March 2019). © National Asthma Council Australia Ltd, 2019. Reproduced with permission from the authors.

Notes:
- If features of more than one severity category are present, record the higher (worse) category as overall severity level. The severity category may change over time.
- Pulsus paradoxus (systolic paradox) is not a reliable indicator of the severity of acute asthma.

Chest radiograph (CXR)
- CXR is not routinely required in either the acute or interval management of asthma.
- CXR may be required if there is evidence of an acute complication (e.g. mucous plugging) or patients with difficult-to-control, persistent asthma (particularly if they have not had a previous CXR).
- CXR is helpful if symptoms and signs are not wholly explained by asthma and may be caused by another disease (e.g. mediastinal mass, suppurative lung disease or foreign body).

Assessment of the severity of an attack
Acute asthma can be classified as mild-moderate, severe or life-threatening. The most reliable indicators are mental state and work of breathing (comprising accessory muscle use and recession).
- Initial arterial O_2 saturation (SaO_2) in air and ability to talk are additional features in assessing the severity of acute asthma (see Table 38.1).
- Arterial blood gases, chest x-ray and spirometry should not be routinely used in assessing the severity of acute asthma.

Management of acute asthma
The management of acute asthma is dependent upon its severity (Table 38.2).

Medication Doses
- **Salbutamol:**
  - < 6 years old: 6 puffs MDI
  - 6 years or older: 12 puffs MDI
- **Ipratropium bromide (21 mcg/puff) dose:**
  - < 6 years old: 4 puffs MDI
  - 6 years or older: 8 puffs MDI
- **Oral prednisolone**
- Give prednisolone 1 mg/kg (maximum 50 mg) orally each morning for 3 days

Treatment at home (discharge from hospital or ED)
- Patients are usually safe to be treated at home when they
  - Require salbutamol 3–4 hourly or less frequently;
  - Have adequate oxygenation AND
  - Their carer is well educated in asthma management and demonstrates the ability to administer salbutamol via a spacer.
- All children should have an *asthma action plan* provided to them, which should be reviewed and updated every 6–12 months or after any changes to their asthma medications.

Table 38.2 Management of acute asthma.

Severity	Signs of Severity	Management
Mild	Normal mental state Subtle / no increased work of breathing. Able to talk normally.	**Salbutamol** by MDI/spacer (see dosing below) and review after 20 mins. Ensure device / technique appropriate. Good response • Discharge on short acting B2-agonist as needed & **consider oral prednisolone** (see below) • Provide written advice on what to do if symptoms worsen. Consider overall control and family's knowledge. Arrange early follow-up. Poor response: treat as Moderate.
Moderate	Normal mental state Some increased work of breathing Tachycardia. Reduced ability to talk.	**Salbutamol** by MDI/spacer - 1 dose every 20 minutes for 1 hour; review 10-20 min after 3rd dose to decide on timing of next dose. See doses below. **Oxygen** if O2 saturation is < 90%. DO NOT give oxygen for wheeze or increased work of breathing. **Oral prednisolone** (see below)
Severe	Agitated/distressed Moderate-marked increased work of breathing accessory muscle use/recession. Tachycardia Marked limitation of ability to talk. **Note: wheeze is a poor predictor of severity.**	**Involve senior staff.** **Oxygen** if O2 saturation is < 90%. **Salbutamol** by MDI/spacer -1 dose (see below) every 20 minutes for 1 hour; review ongoing requirements 10-20 min after 3rd dose. If improving, reduce frequency. If no change, continue 20 minutely. If deteriorating at any stage, treat as critical. **Ipratropium** by MDI/spacer - 1 dose every 20 minutes for 1 hour only **Oral prednisolone** (see dosing below). If vomiting give **IV Methylprednisolone** (1 mg/kg; max. 60mg) 6 hourly If poor response to above treatment give: **Aminophylline** Loading dose: 10 mg/kg IV (maximum dose 500 mg) over 60 min. Unless markedly improved following loading dose, give continuous infusion (usually in ICU), or 6 hourly dosing (usually in ward). **Magnesium sulfate 50% (500 mg/mL = 2 mmol/mL)** Dilute to 0.8 mmol/mL (by adding 1.5mLs of sodium chloride 0.9% to each 1mL of Magnesium Sulfate) for intravenous administration • 0.2 mmol/kg over 20 mins (maximum 8 mmol) • If going to ICU, this may be continued with 0.12 mmol/kg/hour by infusion Arrange admission after initial assessment.
Critical	Confused/drowsy Maximal work of breathing accessory muscle use/recession Exhaustion Marked tachycardia Unable to talk. **SILENT CHEST, wheeze may be absent if there is poor air entry.**	**Involve senior staff and consider transfer to PICU** **Oxygen** **Continuous nebulised salbutamol:** use 2 x 5mg nebules undiluted. Monitor for hypokalaemia and toxicity (see below table) **Nebulised ipratropium** 250 mcg, added to salbutamol, every 20 minutes for 3 doses only. **Methylprednisolone** 1 mg/kg (maximum 60mg) IV 6-hourly. **Aminophylline** as above **Magnesium sulfate** as above. In ICU, children on magnesium sulfate infusion, aim to keep serum magnesium between 1.5 and 2.5mmol/L. Consider **IV salbutamol** (limited evidence for benefit) Aminophylline, magnesium and salbutamol must be given via separate IV lines. Intensive care admission for respiratory support (facemask CPAP, BiPAP, or intubation/IPPV) may be needed.

Source: The Royal Children's Hospital Clinical practice guidelines – Asthma acute. © 2018. Reproduced with permission from the Royal Children's Hospital.
Notes:
• Consider **Adrenaline. 10 microg/kg or 0.01mL/kg of 1:1000 (maximum 0.5mL) intramuscular**, if other signs of Anaphylaxis present.
• Beware salbutamol toxicity: tachycardia, tachypnoea, metabolic acidosis. Can occur with both IV and inhaled treatment. Lactate commonly high.
• Beware severe Hypokalaemia with frequent Salbutamol use. Consider monitoring Potassium levels.

- The key elements in the plan are:
  - Daily treatment detailed (including preventer therapy if appropriate and delivery system)
  - Reliever treatment before exercise (if it is a known trigger)
  - Treatment of minor symptoms
  - Treatment of acute exacerbation and appropriate emergency plan
- Parents of children of school-age or older, who are familiar with their child's asthma may be directed to initiate prednisolone at home at the start of an exacerbation.
- Early medical follow-up (within 2 weeks) after an acute exacerbation should be arranged, to ensure the patient and carer are well-educated on asthma management, to review preventer effectiveness and address any possible adherence issues.

Clinical Pearl: Prednisolone in preschool wheeze/asthma
There is no evidence for the effectiveness of prednisolone in preschool aged children with recurrent wheeze. It should thus be reserved for those with severe acute wheezing who require hospitalisation.

Drug delivery
- All MDI doses should be given through a spacer, regardless of age. In young children (usually 4 years and below), a mask is also used.
  - Shake the MDI prior to use.
  - Load spacer with one actuation at a time.
  - If the child uses tidal breathing, allow four breaths between each actuation.
  - Spacers should be washed in household detergent weekly and air-dried (spacers should not be rinsed or towel dried).
- All patients using inhaled corticosteroids should rinse their mouths afterwards to reduce risk of oral thrush.

Follow-up and outpatient management
Consultation with a Paediatrician is recommended if:
- The attack is moderate or severe.
- There is poor response to bronchodilators.
- Attacks occur frequently.
- Determine the pattern of asthma to prescribe the appropriate treatment (Table 38.3).
- Review medication regimen and asthma action plan.
- Check adherence to and administration of medication (eg. effective spacer technique).
- Educate regarding avoidance of cigarette smoking (active and environmental).
- Promote annual influenza vaccine
- Monitor growth and development.
- After an acute exacerbation, early medical follow-up (within 2 weeks) should be arranged to ensure the patient and carer are well-educated on asthma management, review preventer effectiveness and address adherence issues.

Prognosis
- Most children with episodic (infrequent or frequent) asthma will improve over time.
- Those with atopy or a strong family history in first-degree relatives are more likely to have asthma throughout their life.

Preschool wheeze
- Wheeze is common in preschool children; it is heard as a high-pitched whistling sound on expiration.
- It is usually triggered by viral infections.
- The majority of children with wheeze will not develop asthma.
- Some children will wheeze in response to multiple triggers e.g. allergen exposure, exercise, laughing etc and have wheeze between viral infections.
  - These children are more likely to develop asthma.
  - Other risk factors for asthma include: onset of wheeze over the age of 18 months; history of atopy e.g. eczema, hay fever, food allergy and family history of asthma.

Table 38.3 Classification of asthma and indications for initiating preventer treatment in children 6–11 years.

Severity of flare-ups	Average frequency of flare-ups and symptoms between flare-ups		
	Infrequent intermittent: Flare-ups every 6 weeks or less and no symptoms between flare-ups	**Frequent intermittent:** Flare-ups more than once every 6 weeks and no symptoms between flare-ups	**Persistent** Between flare-ups (any of): Daytime symptoms > once per week Night-time symptoms > twice per month Symptoms restrict activity or sleep
Mild flare-ups (Usually salbutamol Rx in community)	Not indicated	Consider	Indicated
Moderate–severe flare-ups (>2 requiring ED or oral corticosteroids in 12m)	Consider	Indicated	Indicated
Life-threatening flare-ups (require hospitalisation or PICU)	Indicated	Indicated	Indicated

Source: Australian Asthma Handbook at publication of Version 2.0 (March 2019). © National Asthma Council Australia Ltd, 2019. Reproduced with permission from the authors.

Notes:

- Preventer should be started as a treatment trial; assess response after 4–6 weeks and review before prescribing long term.
- Consider prescribing preventer according to overall risk for severe flare-ups; a flare-up is defined as a period of worsening asthma symptoms, from mild to severe.
- In children 1–5 years of age:
  - If occasional (e.g. 2–4 monthly or less) mild flare-ups – SABA alone is considered appropriate therapy.
  - If more frequent flare-ups or moderate-severe exacerbations, preventer therapy is indicated.

Diagnosis

- Parental accuracy in reporting wheeze is often poor; it is important to confirm presence of wheeze by clinician assessment.
- There are many causes of wheeze e.g. viral associated, aspiration, foreign body, cardiac failure and large airway abnormality.
- The onset, frequency and triggers for wheeze are important in determining the cause.

Investigations

- CXR is not routinely indicated in the evaluation of wheeze.
- CXR should however be considered in any child with atypical symptoms or whose wheeze does not respond to initial therapy.

Management

- Salbutamol (bronchodilator) should be trialed in all children presenting with wheeze; refer to asthma guideline for acute management.
- Steroids are not recommended in pre-school children with first presentation of mild to moderate wheeze. They should however be given to any child presenting with frequent, severe or life-threatening symptoms and/or ongoing frequent bronchodilator use.
- Preventer therapy should be considered in any child with recurrent or severe episodes of wheeze.
  - 3-month trial of inhaled corticosteroids (e.g. fluticasone diproprionate) is usually first-line.
  - Leukotriene receptor antagonists (e.g. Montelukast) can be considered in children with mild disease or in whom the inhaled route of administration is very difficult. (Parents should be counselled on the risk of mood and behavioural side-effects and headaches in children taking Montelukast).

Acute viral bronchiolitis

Aetiology
- Bronchiolitis is a generalised lower respiratory tract infection.
- Respiratory viruses are the most common cause of bronchiolitis in young infants; the most common is respiratory syncytial virus (RSV).

Clinical features
- Cough, wheeze, tachypnoea, fever and poor feeding in an infant (Table 38.4).
- There may be signs of respiratory distress including:
  - Tracheal tug
  - Intercostal & subcostal recession
  - Accessory muscle use
  - Grunting
  - Generalised crackles & wheeze on auscultation
  - Apnoea in young infants (<3 months)

Risk factors for severe bronchiolitis
- Younger age, especially infants <12 weeks of age
- Ex-premature infants (regardless of presence/absence of chronic lung disease)
- Chronic respiratory disease e.g. bronchopulmonary dysplasia, cystic fibrosis
- Congenital heart disease
- Neurological conditions (neuromuscular weakness or aspiration risk)
- Pulmonary hypertension
- Aboriginal or Torres Strait Islander

Management
- Treatment is supportive with oxygen, fluid support (NGT or IV) and minimal handling as the mainstays of management (Table 38.5).
- High flow nasal prong oxygen or CPAP may prevent intubation in severe cases.
- CXR and nasopharyngeal aspirates are not routine investigations for bronchiolitis.
- Bronchodilators do not work and may exacerbate hypoxia by worsening V/Q mismatch.

Table 38.4 Bronchiolitis: Assessment of severity.

	Assessment of severity		
	Mild	**Moderate**	**Severe**
Behaviour	Normal	Some / intermittent irritability	Increasing irritability and / or lethargy. Fatigue
Respiratory rate	Normal – mild tachypnoea	Increased respiratory rate	Marked increase or decrease in respiratory rate
Use of accessory muscles	Nil to mild chest wall retraction	Moderate chest wall retractions Suprasternal retraction Nasal flaring	Marked chest wall retractions Marked suprasternal retraction Marked nasal flaring
Oxygen saturation	O2 saturations > than 92% (in room air)	O2 saturations 90 –92% (in room air)	O2 saturations < 90% (in room air)
Apnoeic episodes	None	May have brief apnoea	May have frequent or prolonged apnoea
Feeding	Normal	May have difficulty with feeding or reduced feeding	Reluctant or unable to feed

Source: The Royal Children's Hospital Clinical practice guidelines – Bronchiolitis. © 2017. Reproduced with permission from the Royal Children's Hospital.

Table 38.5 Management of bronchiolitis.

	Mild	Moderate	Severe
Need for admission	Suitable for discharge (Consider risk factors)	Likely admission, may discharge after period of observation	Requires admission & consider need for PICU Refer early if signs severe disease
Observations Vital signs	Adequate assessment in ED prior to discharge (minimum of two recorded measurements or every four hours)	One to two hourly (not continuous) Cease SaO2 monitoring once improving and off oxygen for 2 hours	Hourly with continuous cardiorespiratory (including SaO2) monitoring and close nursing observation
Hydration/nutrition	Small frequent feeds	If not feeding adequately (< 50% over 12 hours), administer NG hydration	If not feeding adequately (< 50% over 12 hours), or unable to feed, administer NG hydration
Oxygen requirement	Nil requirement	O2 to maintain SaO2 ≥ 90% Cease SaO2 monitoring once improving and off oxygen for 2 hours	O2 to maintain SaO2 ≥ 90%
Respiratory support		Begin with NPO2 HFNC only if NPO2 has failed	Consider HFNC or CPAP
Disposition / Escalation	Consider further medical review if early in illness, risk factors present, or if child deteriorates post discharge	Decision to admit should be supported by clinical assessment (inc. risk factors), social and geographical factors, and phase of illness	Escalate therapy if severity does not improve Consider ICU review/ admission, or transfer to tertiary centre if: • Severity does not improve • Persistent desaturations • Significant / recurrent apnoea with desaturation • Risk factors present
Parental Education	Advice on the expected course of illness & when to return (worsening symptoms & inability to feed adequately) Provide parental information sheet	Advice on the expected course of illness & when to return (worsening symptoms & inability to feed adequately) Provide parental information sheet	Provide advice on the expected course of illness Provide parental information sheet

Source: The Royal Children's Hospital Clinical practice guidelines – Bronchiolitis. © 2017. Reproduced with permission from the Royal Children's Hospital.

- Use the respiratory rate, accessory muscle use and recessions to judge the work of breathing.
- Very young infants and infants with risk factors for severe bronchiolitis may need admission for observation even if they have mild bronchiolitis at presentation.
- Infants <3 months and those with severe bronchiolitis are more likely to become hyponatraemic (due to the syndrome of 'inappropriate' ADH secretion [SIADH]) and warrant close attention to fluid balance.

Community-acquired pneumonia
Aetiology
- *Respiratory viruses* (especially RSV) are the most common cause of community-acquired pneumonia (CAP) in children. There is usually only mild to moderate constitutional disturbance. Cough is usually present often with nasal discharge or congestion. There may be scattered inspiratory crackles and/or wheeze on auscultation.

- *Streptococcus pneumoniae* is the most common bacterial pathogen in all age groups, followed by non-typeable *Haemophilus influenzae* and *Staphylococcus aureus*.
- *Staphylococcus aureus* is an important cause of severe CAP and may be complicated by lung abscess and empyema.
- Group A β-haemolytic streptococcus is less common but may cause severe pneumonia (toxin mediated effects may exacerbate signs of sepsis and cause a rash).
- *Mycoplasma pneumoniae* is a common pathogen in children, including toddlers. Typically, symptoms (high fever and headache are typical) develop over several days before the cough. Cough is prominent and crackles may be focal or widespread.
- *Bordetella pertussis* (whooping cough) is an important, but uncommon, cause of CAP. Children often present with paroxysms of cough with cyanosis or apnoea. Pertussis pneumonia can be life-threatening in infants, particularly infants under 6 months of age.

Clinical features
- Cough, tachypnoea, increased work of breathing.
- Persistent fever is usually present.
- Focal signs in the chest may be difficult to detect in young infants.
- Clinical features are often similar between viral and bacterial pneumonia.

Investigations
- A diagnosis of pneumonia can be made clinically and a chest X-ray (CXR) is not routinely recommended in children with mild disease.
- CXR changes do not reliably distinguish viral from bacterial pneumonia with the exception of lobar changes, which, when present, are more likely to be associated with bacterial (than viral) pneumonia.
- In more severe disease i.e. requiring hospital admission, or when complicated pneumonia is suspected, a CXR is recommended.
  Respiratory viral nucleic acid testing (e.g. PCR) may assist in the management of children requiring hospitalization for CAP e.g. to evaluate for influenza infection, treatable with neuraminidase inhibitors.

Management
- Antibiotic therapy (Figure 38.1)
- Supportive care (oxygen and fluid management)
- Airway clearance (chest physiotherapy) is not required
- Young infants and those with severe disease are at risk of SIADH. Monitor sodium and consider limiting parenteral fluids to ½ or 2/3rds maintenance (see Chapter 7, Fluid and electrolytes).

Pleural effusion / empyema
- The most common cause of pleural effusion in children is a parapneumonic effusion occurring secondary to pneumonia. Other causes of pleural effusion e.g. inflammatory, traumatic, chylothorax are not discussed.
- Any child with CAP complicated by large parapneumonic effusion or empyema requires admission to hospital for intravenous antibiotics +/- drainage. Early consultation with a respiratory physician and paediatric surgeon is recommended.
- In children, Streptococcus pneumoniae, followed by Staphylococcus aureus are the most common pathogens, hence empirical antibiotic therapy are initiated to target these pathogens.

Clinical features
- Presentation as per pneumonia (see pneumonia).
- If persistent fever despite 48 hours of appropriate antibiotics, chest x-ray should be performed to evaluate for empyema.
- Examination findings include:
  - Localised decreased air entry
  - Dullness to percussion
  - Antalgic scoliosis (appearance of spinal scoliosis due to underlying pleuritic inflammation and muscle spasm).

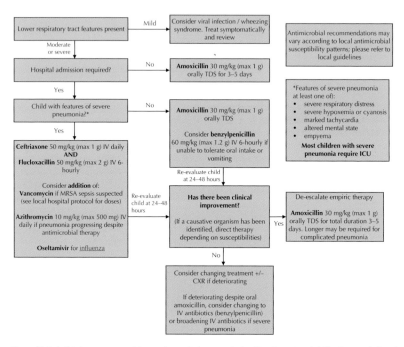

Figure 38.1 Antibiotic management of Community acquired pneumonia algorithm. *Source*: Royal Children's Hospital Clinical Practice Guidelines – Community acquired pneumonia. Reproduced with permission from the Royal Children's Hospital.

Investigations

- CXR – blunting of costophrenic angle initially evolving to dense opacification at periphery of lung +/- "meniscus sign" (rim of fluid on lateral chest wall). Scoliosis may be present with raised hemidiaphragn and mediastinal shift away from the effusion.
- Ultrasound – confirms presence of effusion and differentiates between simple (parapneumonic effusion) or complicated (empyema).
- Bloods: FBE & film (leukocytosis, neutrophilia and thrombocytosis), Blood culture, UECs (SIADH)
- Pleural fluid for:
  - ○ Gram stain, MCS
  - ○ Pneumococcal PCR
  - ○ AFB and mycobacterial culture/PCR if risk factors

Management

- Antibiotic cover for Streptococcus pneumoniae and Staphylococcus aureus. Consider additional cover for methicillin-resistant *S aureus*.
- Consider surgical management if large effusion, persistent fevers, clinical deterioration (Figure 38.2).

Pharyngitis/tonsillitis, acute otitis media and URTI

See Chapter 33, Otolaryngology.

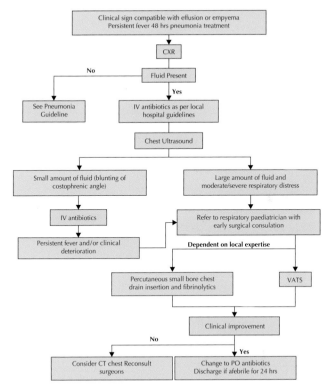

Figure 38.2 Pleural Effusion / Empyema management algorithm. *Source*: Royal Children's Hospital Clinical Practice Guidelines – Pleural effusion and empyema. Reproduced with permission from the Royal Children's Hospital.

Laryngotracheobronchitis (Croup)
- Croup (acute laryngotracheobronchitis) is usually due by a viral infection which causes inflammation and oedema of the upper airway.
- Croup most commonly occurs in children aged 6 months to 6 years and lasts for up to 5 days.
- Parainfluenza viruses are the most common causes of croup.

Clinical Features
- Characterised by hoarse voice, stridor and barking cough with variable degrees of airway obstruction.
- A coryzal prodrome with or without fever usually occurs.
- Symptoms typically worst at night.
- There should be no systemic signs of toxicity to indicate bacterial infection.
  If present, an alternative diagnosis e.g. epiglottitis, retropharyngeal abscess or bacterial tracheitis must be considered.

Investigation
- Blood tests, nasal/throat swabs or X-rays are rarely indicated and should be avoided when possible as they may exacerbate airway obstruction.

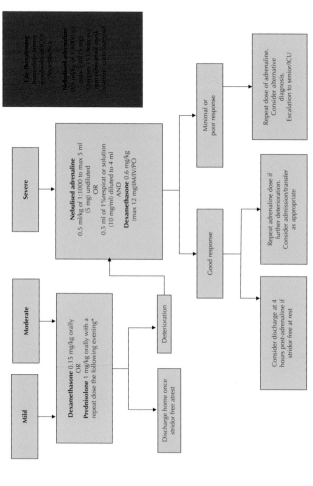

Figure 38.3 Croup (laryngotracheobronchitis) management algorithm. *Source:* Royal Children's Hospital Clinical Practice Guidelines – Croup. Reproduced with permission from the Royal Children's Hospital.

The following are the contents within the figure:

Mild

Moderate → Dexamethasone 0.15 mg/kg orally OR Prednisolone 1 mg/kg orally with a repeat dose the following evening* → Discharge home once stridor free atrest / Deterioration

Severe → Nebulised adrenaline 0.5 ml/kg of 1:1000 to max 5 ml (5 mg) undiluted OR 0.5 ml of 1%respirat or solution (10 mg/ml) diluted to 4 ml AND Dexamethasone 0.6 mg/kg (max 12 mg)IM/IV/PO

Good response → Consider discharge at 4 hours post-adrenaline if stridor free at rest / Repeat adrenaline dose if further deterioration. Consider admission/transfer as appropriate

Minimal or poor response → Repeat dose of adrenaline. Consider alternative diagnosis. Escalation to senior/ICU

Life-threatening: Immediate senior involvement/ICU/ Anaesthetics / Nebulised adrenaline 0.5 ml/kg of 1:1000 to max 5 ml (5 mg) Oxygen 15 L/min via non-rebreather mask Severe: continue/repeat

*Consider nebulized Budesonide 2mg if oral corticosteroids not tolerated

Management

- Avoid handling and limit examination to minimise distress.
- Keep children with carers for comfort and allow them to adopt a position of comfort to minimise airway obstruction.
- Mild–moderate croup (no stridor at rest) is treated with steroids (Figure 38.3).
- Nebulised adrenaline should be used if symptoms are persisting or worsening or if signs of severe airway obstruction.
- In a child with mild croup, consider discharge when there is no stridor at rest and it is at least 30 minutes post oral steroids or four hours post nebulised adrenaline (if this has been required).

Bacterial tracheitis: is an important differential diagnosis of any child presenting with fever and acute airway obstruction. It is due to invasive bacterial infection of the soft tissues of the trachea.

- The trachea is often markedly tender and symptoms are usually preceded by a viral respiratory tract infection.
- Staphyloccocus aureus is the most common pathogen.
- Treatment includes antibiotic therapy and airway management.
- Discuss all children with severe or worsening upper airway obstruction with a consultant urgently.

Epiglottitis

Acute epiglottitis is a life-threatening bacterial infection of the supraglottis. Since the introduction of *Haemophilus influenzae* type b (Hib) immunisation, incidence has fallen markedly. However, it continues to occur (e.g. child not immunised, immunisation failure, other bacteria i.e. *Streptococcus pneumoniae*) and if the diagnosis is not made promptly, the mortality rate is high.

Clinical features

Epiglottitis differs from croup in the following ways:

- The onset is with fever and lethargy.
- Cough is not a prominent feature.
- Most children appear toxic due to the associated sepsis.
- The stridor is soft, and the expiratory element is often dominant with a snoring or gurgling quality.
- Symptoms of respiratory obstruction develop rapidly.
- Difficulty in swallowing with drooling of saliva is common.

Management

- Complete obstruction may occur in just a few hours; therefore, patients require urgent, escorted transfer to hospital.
- Keep the child as calm as possible in a seated position and administer oxygen by mask.
- Antibiotic therapy should be initiated within 1 hour of presentation.
  - Ceftriaxone 100 mg/kg (max 2 g) IV followed by 50 mg/kg (max. 2 g) 24 hours later, for a 5-day course.
- Consider addition of dexamethasone (0.15mg/kg up to 10mg) intravenously, repeat after 24 hours if required.
- In general, tracheal intubation under anaesthesia is required.
- If complete obstruction is imminent, summon immediate help from an intensivist or anaesthetist. If inexperienced, do not attempt intubation unless the child becomes comatosed. Intubate orally initially with a small endotracheal tube.
- If intubation is not possible, attempt to ventilate with bag–valve–mask; a good technique may achieve adequate oxygenation and ventilation. If ventilation is impossible, perform cricothyrotomy or tracheostomy.
- Treat contacts prophylactically with rifampicin 20 mg/kg (max 600 mg) PO daily for 4 days.

Whooping cough (pertussis)

Whooping cough is caused by Bordetella pertussis and despite immunisation, continues to occur due to subop-timal uptake of childhood immunisation and/or waning immunity in adolescents and adults without booster (current vaccines give protection for only 5 to 10 years).

Clinical features
- Starts with a coryzal illness that resembles an URTI (infectious period).
- Persistent cough (>2 weeks) that may continue for weeks to months:
  - The cough is paroxysmal and may be associated with facial suffusion and post-tussive vomiting.
  - The paroxysm may be terminated by an inspiratory whoop.
  - The cough is often only recognised as pertussis at this stage (paroxysmal phase).
  - The child often appears well between coughing paroxysms.
- Older children may present with a persistent cough in isolation.
- *In young infants <12 weeks of age, pertussis can present with apnoea alone.*

Diagnosis
- Diagnosis can be made on clinical grounds, however nucleic acid testing (e.g. polymerase chain reaction) from nasopharyngeal swab is recommended to confirm the diagnosis in the acute phase (e.g. usually the first 3 weeks of illness).
- Lymphocyte count may be markedly elevated (>20×10^9/L).

Management
Pharmacological treatment
- There is no clear evidence that pharmacological agents improve the clinical course of whooping cough.
- However, treatment may reduce the likelihood of transmission by eradicating B. pertussis from an infected individual if they are within 3 weeks of onset of cough and symptoms.
- The current recommendation for antimicrobial management is:
  - Clarithromycin 7.5 mg/kg (max 500 mg) twice daily for 7 days.
  - Azithromycin (10 mg/kg daily for 5 days) is an alternative and preferred treatment for neonates.
- Contact prophylaxis is recommended, particularly if a contact is in the late phase of pregnancy or there is an incompletely immunised child in the family. Use clarithromycin (same dosage) for 7 days.
- Catch up pertussis containing vaccine of contacts due for vaccine.
- Infants with proven pertussis should continue with routine vaccinations (which will include DTPa).

Inpatient hospital treatment
- Admit those who are
  - Infants <6 months
  - Apnoeic
  - Cyanotic
  - Not coping with the cough
  - Feeding poorly
  - Systemically unwell
- Careful observation, including the use of an apnoea monitor is recommended.
- Supportive care (fluids and supplementary oxygen) which may delay time to cough induced desaturation.

Cough
Cough is a common symptom in children. The degree to which a family becomes concerned about the frequency and severity of a child's cough is extremely variable. There is often a poor correlation between a parental report of cough and objective measures.

Acute cough
The cause of an acute onset cough is generally easy to recognise, most commonly with a respiratory infection (commonly with coryza), asthma (associated with known triggers and wheeze) or occasionally an inhaled foreign body (in typical aged child, 12–36 months and characterized by sudden onset).

Persistent or recurrent cough
The history and characteristics of the cough usually inform diagnosis. Whilst asthma, gastro-oesophageal reflux and post-nasal drip are the three favoured diagnoses in adults, these occur less commonly in children. In children think of:
- Onset in infancy (and barking): Tracheomalacia.
- Dry (worse at night): post-viral cough, chronic non-specific cough of childhood (cough-receptor hypersensitivity), asthma.

- Dry (paroxysmal): pertussis (may be a modified illness in an immunised child).
- Wet (productive): Suppurative lung disease (protracted bacterial bronchitis, bronchiectasis, cystic fibrosis (CF), immunodeficiency, primary ciliary dyskinesia, inhaled foreign body).
- Onset in older childhood (bizarre, honking): 'habit cough', now called somatic cough syndrome (previously psychogenic cough). The cough is often intrusive, intensifies before sleep and is characteristically absent during sleep.

Cough due to asthma
Although cough can be a troublesome symptom of asthma, it rarely occurs without some evidence of airways obstruction (e.g. wheeze or shortness of breath with exertion).

Clinical Controversy: 'Cough variant Asthma'
There is considerable doubt as to whether the entity of 'cough variant asthma', in which cough is the only symptom of asthma, exists in children. *Be very reluctant to diagnose asthma in the absence of evidence of airways obstruction.* The management of asthma is based on the severity and duration of the airway obstruction, not on the cough.

Physical examination
This is usually normal, but to gauge the quality of the cough ask the child to cough or ask to hear a recording from the parents.
- Red flags include:
  - Poor growth and nutrition.
  - Digital clubbing (suppurative lung disease).
  - Chest wall deformity (pectus carinatum suggesting chronic airway obstruction).
  - Localised wheeze (inhaled foreign body).

Investigations
- Specific investigations for persistent cough depend on the clinical suspicion after history and examination.
- In some circumstances, it can be reassuring to the family to have a normal CXR and lung function.

Cough management
- Diagnosing the cause of cough may not always be possible on a first consultation, a treatment trial is often appropriate and provides clues as to the underlying cause.
- The effects of passive smoking should be discussed when relevant.
- Cough suppressants are not recommended and may be harmful.
- If a foreign body is suspected, urgent referral to a paediatric respiratory physician or ENT surgeon for bronchoscopic removal is necessary.

Airway foreign body
- Toddlers 12–36 months are most at risk of inhaled foreign bodies, but they can occur at any age.
- Nuts and small plastic toys are also common.
- What is retrieved from the airway is not always what was initially suspected to have been inhaled.

Symptoms
- Coughing, choking or spluttering episodes while eating solid foods or while sucking a small plastic toy or similar object. *This history should never be dismissed.*
- Sudden onset of persistent coughing and wheezing (in most other causes the cough and wheeze build up).
- 50% of inhaled foreign bodies are not witnessed.

Signs
- There may be no physical signs or alternatively reduced breath sounds over the whole or part of one lung.
- Localised wheeze.

Investigations
- Children >3 years old can often have a CXR taken in full inspiration and full expiration to enhance the appearance of obstructive hyperinflation. The radiograph should include the nasopharynx to the chest.

- Children <3 years of age should have an AP film and both a left and right lateral decubitus film. If the bronchus is obstructed, the affected side will not deflate.
- Normal radiographs do not exclude a foreign body.

Management
Bronchoscopy is indicated for all patients with a suspected inhaled foreign body. There needs to be a high index of suspicion as aspirated foreign body is frequently missed.

- Bronchoscopy in children is difficult and requires an expert paediatric endoscopist teamed with an experienced paediatric anaesthetist. It should only be done in a tertiary children's hospital. Rigid bronchoscopy is the procedure of choice.
- In most cases, the removal of the foreign body improves symptoms and there is rarely an indication for corticosteroids or antibiotics.

Cystic fibrosis
- Cystic Fibrosis (CF) is the most common life-shortening inherited disease of childhood.
- It is autosomal recessive, the incidence is 1:2500 and carrier frequency in people of European origin is 1:25.
- CF is caused by mutations in the cystic fibrosis transmembrane conductance regulator (CFTR) gene.
- Most babies with CF are born to families with no history of CF.

Screening
- Newborn screening (NBS) for CF detects 90% of affected babies.
- All babies have a heel prick on day 2 to 4 of life and the blood is placed on a filter paper card. Serum trypsinogen is measured by immunoreactive assay (IRT).
- Babies with an IRT >99th percentile have gene mutation testing for common CFTR gene mutations (mutation panels vary between centres).
- Babies with two CFTR gene mutations have CF and are referred to the CF clinic.
- Babies with one CFTR gene mutation are referred for a sweat test at an approved laboratory (Figure 38.4).
- Most babies with an elevated IRT and no CFTR gene mutations do not have CF.
- This screening test can miss babies who have a falsely low IRT or an uncommon CFTR gene mutation (there are >2000 CFTR gene mutations, although a panel of 12 mutations will detect 90% of people with CF).
- Screening only began in Australia in the 1980s and many other countries do not have the same screening program. So, if there is clinical suspicion, refer for a sweat test (this will avoid the possibility of missing a child who may not have a common mutation in a screening or diagnostic CFTR mutation panel).

Diagnosis
The diagnosis of CF is based on clinical findings (or a positive newborn screening test) associated with abnormalities of CFTR by gene test or sweat test.
- *A family history of CF should raise concern*
- Classic clinical features of CF include
  - Suppurative lung disease.
  - Pancreatic exocrine insufficiency (85% of patients), which manifests as steatorrhoea and failure to thrive.
  - Meconium ileus (15–20% babies with CF in Australia).
  - Multifocal biliary cirrhosis (may rarely present as prolong neonatal jaundice).
  - Elevated sweat electrolytes (occasionally presenting as hyponatraemic, hypochloraemic metabolic alkalosis).

Genetic counselling after NBS
- Genetic counselling for the family of patients with CF is offered routinely. Many elect to use IVF with pre-implantation genetic diagnosis or pre-natal testing for subsequent pregnancies.
- Siblings of an affected child should be offered a sweat test to exclude CF (and preserve their rights to have carrier testing at a later stage).
- Preconception and prenatal carrier testing of all prospective parents, regardless of family history, is available.
- The diagnosis and management of CF is best achieved in a specialist CF centre (with physiotherapy, dietetics, social work and CF nurse support).

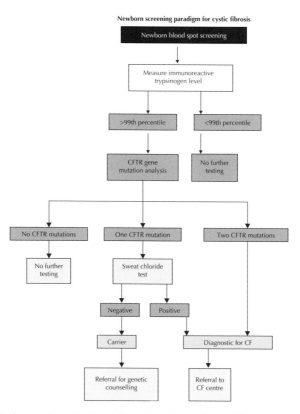

Newborn screening paradigm for cystic fibrosis

Newborn blood spot screening

Measure immunoreactive trypsinogen level

>99th percentile | <99th percentile

CFTR gene mutation analysis | No further testing

No CFTR mutations | One CFTR mutation | Two CFTR mutations

No further testing | Sweat chloride test

Negative | Positive

Carrier | Diagnostic for CF

Referral for genetic counselling | Referral to CF centre

Figure 38.4 Newborn screening paradigm for cystic fibrosis. *Source*: Pham and Massie (2019). Paediatric cystic fibrosis. Part 1: diagnosis. *Respiratory Medicine Today* 4(1): 31–33. Reproduced with permission from the authors.

CF management
Medications that activate CFTR
In the last few years there are new medications that activate CFTR, improving electrolyte transport at the epithelial surfaces and reducing morbidity.

Putting the Science into Practice: CFTR activating medications

Ivacaftor (CFTR potentiator) is used for patients with gating or conductance mutations. Ivacaftor and lumacaftor or tezocaftor (CFTR correctors) are used for patients with the common CFTR gene mutation p.F508del. The field is advancing rapidly and soon 90% of patients will be on one of the combinations under development. These drugs are very expensive, and traditional CF treatments are still required.

Traditional principles of CF treatment
- Nutrition:
  - High-fat, high-calorie diet
  - Pancreatic enzyme replacement
  - Vitamin supplementation (A, D, E and K)

- Salt supplementation
- Pulmonary care:
  - Airway clearance (chest physiotherapy), at least once daily (twice daily with an exacerbation). Mucolytic agents (anti-DNaseB or hypertonic saline) are usually added.
  - Antibiotic regimens are largely dependent on which organism infects the lungs (Table 38.6). Patients should be on antibiotics whenever they have a productive cough. Common CF pathogens include *S.aureus*, *H. influenzae, S. maltophilia and P. aeruginosa*. Non-tuberculous mycobacteria are increasingly being identified in CF sputum.

Table 38.6 Management of bacterial infection in CF.

	S. aureus	H. influenzae	P. aeruginosa
Prophylaxis	Antibiotic prophylaxis is given soon after diagnosis for 2 years	Antibiotic prophylaxis is given soon after diagnosis for 1 year, or until cultures in early infancy are clear	Not used
Acute infection	2 weeks oral antibiotics	2 weeks (Augmentin) if isolated in sputum. Continue for a further 2 weeks if symptoms persist	If child well & treatment adherence good, inhaled therapy alone is used (with the exception of very young children in whom IV therapy is often given as first-line).For symptomatic or younger children, initial 2 weeks of dual-agent IV anti-pseudomonal therapy is given followed by inhaled therapy.
		If symptoms persist after a total of 4 weeks, consider IV antibiotics	First-line IV therapy is ceftazidine & tobramycin pending sensitivities
		A bronchoalveolar lavage is indicated in patients not responding to treatment	
Chronic infection	Prophylactic anti-staphylococcal antibiotics if (1) *S. aureus* regularly cultured in sputum, (2) annual bronchoalveolar lavage is positive on 2 consecutive occasions, or (3) symptoms return when anti-staphylococcal antibiotics stopped If patients develop an intercurrent respiratory tract infection, change to another anti-staphylococcal agent for 2 weeks If this is unsuccessful, IV piperacillin/tazobactam (Tazocin) for 2 weeks may be necessary. Consider BAL in patients not responding to rule out *Pseudomonas* infection After treatment, oral antibiotics recommended	Consider long-term prophylaxis (Augmentin) if repeatedly sputum culture+ Augmentin also antibiotic of choice for acute exacerbations in those with chronic *H. influenzae* infection	Long-term nebulised tobramycin commenced if 3 consecutive positive cultures obtained at least 1 month apart If ongoing deterioration then switch to either nebulised colistin, nebulised preservative-free tobramycin (TOBI), or oral ciprofloxacin alternating with nebulised tobramycin on a monthly basis An exacerbation is characterised by an increase in cough, sputum production, change in sputum colour, loss of weight, decreased activity & deterioration in lung function. Fever may occur but is not typical

o Surveillance for airway pathogens: cough-suction specimens (infants) or sputum specimens (older children) are taken at each clinic visit. Bronchoalveolar lavage is used by some centres as needed with exacerbations in children too young to expectorate or annually for surveillance.

o The acquisition of *P. aeruginosa* infection is commonly associated with deterioration in lung function. P. aeruginosa can often be eradicated (~90% success using 2 months nebulized tobramycin) after initial acquisition, delaying the time to chronic lower airway infection and improving outcomes.

o Viral infections are a common cause of pulmonary exacerbations, but still require antibiotic cover. Thorough treatment of pulmonary symptoms is required to return the patient to baseline.

Non-pulmonary complications of CF
Distal intestinal obstruction syndrome

• Distal intestinal obstruction syndrome (DIOS) presents with signs of abdominal obstruction or more commonly, sub-acutely with colicky abdominal pain and constipation.

• Due to the accumulation of tenacious, muco-faeculent masses in the distal ileum or caecum. The cause is unclear but appears to be associated with dehydration, fever, missing pancreatic enzymes, liver disease and the use of anticholinergic and opiate drugs.

• The management varies according to severity (Table 38.7).

• Other conditions which should be considered in the differential diagnosis include

  o Constipation
  o Intussusception
  o Adhesions (previous surgery)
  o Acute appendicitis

Table 38.7 Management of distal intestinal obstruction syndrome.

Acute–mild severity (incomplete/ impending DIOS) Intermittent abdominal pain, no vomiting	Outpatient treatment	Single-agent laxative, polyethylene glycol*, given at the dose of 2 g/kg/day and titrated as per response (maximum 80–100 g/day). Simple analgesia (paracetamol) 'as needed'. If not responding within 5–7 days, escalate treatment. Ensure adequate hydration.
Acute–moderate severity (incomplete/ impending DIOS) Continuous pain with nausea ± anorexia but no (or minimal, non-bilious) vomiting	Outpatient / inpatient treatment	Per oral (older children >12 years) or nasogastric *polyethylene glycol solution, at a dose of 20–40 mL/kg/h up to a maximum of 1L/h (maximum of 2-4 L/day). Ensure adequate hydration.
Acute–severe (complete DIOS) Continuous pain, bilious vomiting, abdominal distension	Inpatient treatment	Insert wide-bore NGT for free drainage. IV fluids: Maintenance and correction. If not responding, or unable to tolerate oral/NGT agents due to complete obstruction, consider contrast enema. Gastrograffin can be used for enema (100 mL diluted four times with water).

Source: Bolia et al. (2018). Practical approach to the gastrointestinal manifestations of cystic fibrosis. *J Paediatr Child Health* 54: 609–619. Reproduced with permission from John Wiley & Sons.
Notes:
• Lactulose causes flatulence and abdominal cramps and is not preferred.
• Larger doses of polyethylene glycol solution have been recommended but we urge caution.
• Per oral or nasogastric gastrograffin has been recommended but is largely empirical and we urge caution with its use due to the risk of large fluid shifts.
• DIOS = distal intestinal obstruction syndrome; NGT = nasogastric tube.
*e.g. Movicol™ or Osmolax.™ Movicol (Full strength) sachet =13 g; Osmolax (Large Scoop) =17 g;

CF associated liver disease

- Most patients with CF will eventually have some biochemical or ultrasound evidence of liver disease that progresses from fatty infiltration to focal biliary cirrhosis to extensive cirrhosis with portal hypertension and complications such as variceal bleeding and hypersplenism.
- Approximately 5% of children have severe liver disease.
- Liver function tests are monitored annually and ultrasound performed every 2–3 years.
- Ursodeoxycholic acid may help delay progression.

CF related diabetes (CFRD)

- This is a combination of paucity of insulin production and insulin resistance.
- It develops through teenage years; about 40–50% of adults with CF will eventually develop CFRD.
- Development of CFRD is usually associated with slow weight loss and decline in lung function. Most centers now screen with an oral glucose tolerance test from early teenage years.
- Treatment is with insulin.

Spontaneous pneumothorax

This is an air leak into the pleural cavity that occurs in patients without underlying lung disease) and when there is no provoking factor (eg trauma, surgery, or diagnostic intervention).

Incidence

- 8 to 16 per 100 000 in the general population.

Clinical features

- Acute onset of chest pain that is severe and/or stabbing pain, radiating to ipsilateral shoulder and increasing with inspiration (pleuritic).
- Sudden shortness of breath.
- Asymmetric lung expansion – mediastinal and tracheal shift to the contralateral side with a large pneumothorax.
- Decreased or absent breath sounds and hyper-resonance on percussion.

Tension pneumothorax

- Tracheal deviation (to opposite side of pneumothorax), tachycardia, hypotension, cyanosis.
- This is considered a medical emergency and requires urgent needle thoracocentesis.

Investigations

- CXR

Management

- As per algorithm (Figure 38.5).
- Humidified 100% oxygen may accelerate the resorption of air in the pleural cavity (not recommended for premature neonates or any child at risk of hypoxic respiratory drive due to risk of oxygen toxicity).
- Note: high-flow oxygen via nasal cannulae (HFNC) or other positive pressure ventilation should **not** be used as it may worsen the pneumothorax.
- Surgical intervention may be required for a persistent air leak (>7–10 days), ipsilateral recurrence or contralateral pneumothorax. A CT scan is not routinely required.

Chronic neonatal lung disease (CNLD)

- See also Chapter 27, Neonatal medicine.
- CNLD most commonly occurs in infants born <32 weeks gestation and is defined as the need for respiratory support or supplementary oxygen for >4 weeks or at 36 weeks corrected gestation.
- CNLD is a result of premature birth, lung injury from ventilation, oxygen supplementation, pulmonary infection and may be accompanied by patent ductus arteriosus with pulmonary hypertension in more severe cases.

Clinical and radiological features

- Tachypnoea and increased work of breathing
- Persistent oxygen (or respiratory support) requirement
- CXR: Varied, bronchial wall thickening, hyperinflation and increased interstitial markings.

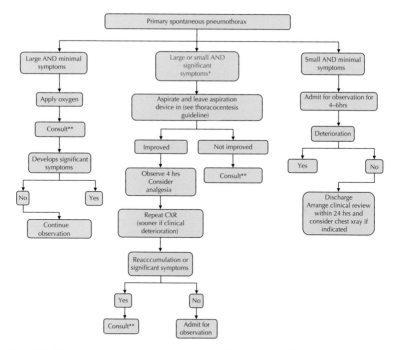

Figure 38.5 Primary spontaneous pneumothorax management algorithm. *Source*: Royal Children's Hospital Clinical Practice Guidelines – Primary spontaneous pneumothorax. Reproduced with permission from the Royal Children's Hospital.
Notes:
* Significant symptoms: Significant breathlessness, Hypoxia, Pain
** For the following groups of patients, consult for further advice.
- Age <12yrs: may have less reliable reporting of symptoms and size calculations may not be applicable
- Secondary pneumothorax
  ○ Underlying lung disease e.g. Cystic Fibrosis, chronic neonatal lung disease, asthma
  ○ Trauma or thoracic surgery
  ○ Positive pressure ventilation
  ○ Foreign body inhalation
  ○ Evidence of tension pneumothorax

Management
- Supplementary oxygen to maintain SaO2 >93%.
- Air test:
  ○ To determine safety for discharge home.
  ○ Monthly air tests once home to determine timing for recordable overnight oximetry in room air.
  Timing of ceasing supplementary oxygen is based on clinical assessment and when overnight SaO2 in room air are maintained >93%.
- Nutritional support to promote growth.
- Avoid tobacco smoke exposure.
- Influenza vaccine from 6 months.
- Recommendations about RSV immunoglobulin vary between centres (at RCH it is indicated for those with CNLD complicated by pulmonary hypertension or cardiac disease).

Tracheostomy management

- For comprehensive overview refer to RCH clinical practice guidelines (see useful resources below).
- Consult respiratory physician for tracheostomy advice.

USEFUL RESOURCES

- National Asthma Council – Australian Asthma Handbook website https://www.asthmahandbook.org. au/; National asthma guidelinse for professionals and other resources including patient resources.
- Bronchiolitis PREDICT guidelines https://www.predict.org.au; up to date information on Australasian bronchiolitis diagnostic and treatment recommendations.
- Australian Therapeutic guidelines – https://www.tg.org.au; Respiratory up to date medication treatment information.
- Royal Children's Hospital nursing tracheostomy guidelines https://www.rch.org.au/rchcpg/hospital_clinical_guideline_index/Tracheostomy_management/; extensive tracheostomy care information.

CHAPTER 39

Rheumatology

Jane Munro
Georgina Tiller

> ## Key Points
> - Acute onset monoarticular arthritis with fever is septic until proven otherwise.
> - Most acute non-septic arthritis is not Juvenile Idiopathic Arthritis (JIA).
> - Macrophage activation syndrome (MAS) is a multisystem inflammatory emergency and should be considered in an unexplained persistently febrile child with cytopenias.

Musculoskeletal assessment
History
- Nature of onset: acute or insidious? Single or multiple episodes?
- Timing and pattern of symptoms during the day?
  - Inflammatory = Early morning stiffness, improves with activity.
  - Mechanical = Post-activity pain, worsens with activity.
- Duration of illness >6 weeks is less likely to be reactive/post-viral arthritis.
- Consider triggers:
  - Intercurrent infections (respiratory, enteric or skin)
  - Post-viral arthritis is the commonest cause of transient arthritis
  - Immunisation or trauma
  - Medications (e.g. cefaclor)
- What does the child or parent consider to be the most symptomatic site; the joint, muscle, adjacent bone or a more diffuse area?
- Have they had previous therapy, what was the response?
- Extra-articular symptoms, particularly those relevant to rheumatic disease;
  - Lethargy, weight loss, mouth ulcers, alopecia or frontal hair breaking
  - Recurrent fevers
  - Raynaud phenomenon, rashes or photosensitivity
  - Ophthalmological symptoms: red sore eyes, change in vision or dry eyes
  - Weakness
  - Gastrointestinal symptoms
- While completing the systems review keep the following diagnoses in mind:
  - Systemic lupus erythematosus (SLE).
  - Acute lymphoblastic leukaemia (ALL).
  - Inflammatory bowel disease (IBD).
- Have normal physical activities or interests been interrupted?
- Assess the functional milieu of the patient; e.g. school progress, family and peer relationships, stress experiences.
- Check family history for other types of inflammatory arthritis, particularly the spondyloarthropathies, autoimmune disorders and pain syndromes (e.g. fibromyalgia or other models for pain behaviour).

Paediatric Handbook, Tenth Edition. Edited by Kate Harding, Daniel S. Mason and Daryl Efron.
© 2021 John Wiley & Sons Ltd. Published 2021 by John Wiley & Sons Ltd.

Examination

Observe the patient as they move about the room, looking for limitations or alterations in function, and be opportunistic when examining them.

- Examine all joints, not only the site of the presenting complaint. *There may be inflammation without symptoms in juvenile idiopathic arthritis (JIA).*
- Aim to localise the site of maximal discomfort (e.g. the joint capsule, adjacent bone or muscle belly, tendon or ligament attachments?).
- Examine for signs of systemic diseases with an articular component, and extra-articular features of JIA, in particular the skin, eyes, abdomen, nails and lymph nodes.

Clinical examination should include

- *Joints*: signs of inflammation such as swelling or tenderness, pain at the end of range, range of movement and deformity. Is there hypermobility?
- *Entheses*: bone attachment sites of ligaments/tendons (e.g. Achilles tendon).
- *Tendon sheaths* of fingers and toes (e.g. dactylitis in psoriasis).
- *Gait*: antalgic (pain) or limp, Trendelenburg sign.
- *Muscles*: tenderness, wasting or weakness, for example inability to toe or crouch walk (walking in a full squat position).
- *Patellar tracking pattern* – does the patella move vertically on walking?
- *Shoe sole* and heel-wearing pattern.
- *Leg length* measurement.
- *Spinal flexion*, including Schober test (the measurement of the lumbosacral range should increase by at least 6 cm on maximal flexion; the starting range is between the lumbosacral junction and a point 10 cm above).
- *Growth parameters.*

The pGALS is an excellent screening tool for joint examination (Table 39.1).

Table 39.1 The components of paediatric Gait, Arms, Legs, Spine screen (pGALS).

Screening questions
- Do you have any pain or stiffness in your joints, muscles or your back?
- Do you have any difficulty getting yourself dressed without any help?
- Do you have any difficulty going up-and downstairs?

Gait
- Observe the child walking
- 'Walk on your tip-toes/walk on your heels'

Arms
- 'Put your hands out in front of you'
- 'Turn your hands over and make a fist'
- 'Pinch your index finger and thumb together'
- 'Touch the tips of your fingers with your thumb'
- Squeeze the metacarpophalangeal joints
- 'Put your hands together/put your hands back to back'
- 'Reach up and touch the sky'
- 'Look at the ceiling'
- 'Put your hands behind your neck'

Legs
- Feel for effusion at the knee
- 'Bend and then straighten your knee'(active movement of knees and examiner feels for crepitus)
- Passive flexion (90°) with internal rotation of hip

Spine
- 'Open your mouth and put three of your (child's own) fingers in your mouth'
- Lateral flexion of cervical spine – 'Try and touch your shoulder with your ear'
- Observe the spine from behind
- 'Can you bend and touch your toes?' Observe curve of the spine from side and behind

Source: Foster et al. (2006). Musculoskeletal screening examination (pGALS) for school-age children based on the adult GALS screen. *Arthritis Care Research* 2006; 55(5): 709–716. Reproduced with permission from John Wiley & Sons Ltd.

Rheumatologic conditions
Juvenile idiopathic arthritis (JIA)
Assessment
- Age of onset <16 years of age
- Minimum duration of arthritis – 6 weeks
- Multiple disease subtypes (Table 39.2).

Investigations
There is no single diagnostic test for JIA. Imaging will be determined by site of pain and possible diagnosis.

Often useful
- Full blood examination (FBE), erythrocyte sedimentation rate (ESR) and C-reactive protein (CRP). Normal inflammatory markers do not exclude the diagnosis.

Occasionally useful
- Synovial fluid culture – if sepsis is considered.
- ANA for stratifying risk of uveitis in a patient with a diagnosis of JIA – beware of over-interpretation as up to 20% of normal children may have a low positive ANA.
- Rheumatoid factor (RF) – in polyarticular patients, older children or if the pattern of disease appears unusual.
- HLA-B27 genetic marker – if spondyloarthropathy is suspected. Remember almost 9% of the caucasian population are positive.
- Imaging – consider plain radiograph, bone scan and ultrasound.
  - In early arthritis, plain films usually give no more information than a careful examination (may be useful for difficult sites such as the hip, or if long history of arthritis).
  - Ultrasound can be a useful tool to look for effusion and synovitis.
  - MRI can be occasionally useful but is not usually an appropriate initial investigation.
- Diagnostic aspirate – indicated if sepsis or haemarthrosis is considered, but will not necessarily differentiate between other inflammatory arthritides.
- Specific bacterial/viral studies if the clinical picture is suggestive (e.g. ASOT, anti-DNase B, Yersinia and parvovirus serology), see post-infectious arthritis (below).

Not useful
- Serum uric acid

Table 39.2 JIA Subtypes.

| | Autoimmune/adaptive immunity | | | | Auto inflammatory/ innate immunity |
| | | | Spondyloarthropathy | | |
Oligoarticular	Polyarticular (pJIA)	Enthesitis related (ERA)	Psoriatic		Systemic (sJIA)
Young	≥ 5 joints	>6 years	Personal or		2 weeks of fever
F>M	Symmetrical small	Males	family history		Salmon pink
≤ 4 joints	& large joints	Acute symptomatic	of psoriasis		evanescent rash
Large joints	RF positive disease	uveitis	Nail pits		Lymphadenopathy
Hip disease uncommon	like adult RA	Raised inflammatory	Scalp rash		Hepatosplenomegaly
Risk of asymptomatic uveitis if	RF negative better	markers			Serositis
ANA positive	prognosis	Enthesitis			Joint involvement
Requires 3 monthly eye screening		Sacroilitis			can be absent at
					diagnosis
					Differentials infection
					or malignancy
ANA positive 60-80%	Only 5% of JIA is RF+	HLAB27 positive 80%	Risk of uveitis if ANA+		Risk of MAS

Management
Depends on the clinical picture of disease severity and subtype.

Principles
- Preserve joint function
- Control pain
- Manage complications
- Multidisciplinary approach: including physiotherapy, occupational therapy, and psychosocial support. Physical therapy is essential to maintain joint range and function. Splinting should be considered where appropriate.

Medications
- Initially NSAIDs, e.g. naproxen, indomethacin, diclofenac, piroxicam or ibuprofen.
- Second line disease modifying therapy, commonly methotrexate to minimise joint destruction.
- Oral steroid as initial treatment of systemic JIA or can be used short term as a bridge to disease modifying therapy in other JIA subtypes
- Intra-articular corticosteroid injections (used early in oligoarticular arthritis). Joint injections are usually performed with procedural sedation and analgesia (e.g. nitrous oxide).
- For children with severe or persistent arthritis and/or persistent systemic features (fever and/or uveitis) biological therapies including injectable TNF blockers may be required.

Clinical Pearl: Autoimmune antibody testing
ANA and antibody panels should not be ordered for non-specific symptoms such as musculoskeletal pain. There is no evidence that antibody testing enhances the diagnosis of musculoskeletal pain in children without clinical suspicion of a rheumatic disease established by careful history and examination.

Henoch–Schönlein purpura (HSP)
- Most common vasculitis in children.
- Predominant small vessel vasculitis with IgA deposition and leukocytoclastic vasculitis.

Clinical features
- Most common age of onset 3-15 years (M:F; 1.5:1)
- Often presents post an infection
- May present with one or more of the following:
  - Evolving crops of palpable purpura – predominantly buttocks and lower limbs
  - Abdominal pain, diffuse and colicky (may be associated with gastrointestinal (GI) bleeding or intussusception)
  - Arthralgia or arthritis of variable duration and severity
  - Nephritis (both nephritic and nephrotic presentations)
  - Other; oedema dorsum of the feet and hands, acute scrotal swelling and 'bruising', fever and fatigue
- Exclude other causes of purpura (see Chapter 17, Dermatologic conditions)

Investigations
- Urinalysis – screen for haematuria, quantify proteinuria
- Investigations other than urinalysis required only in atypical cases or when renal involvement is suspected
- FBE - exclude thrombocytopenia (platelets should be normal or increased)
- Coagulation studies – exclude bleeding diathesis / disseminated intravascular coagulation
- Renal function – urea, creatinine

Management
- Supportive – bed rest and analgesia.
- NSAIDs for joint pain
- Corticosteroids
  - Consider in the case of GI hemorrhage or severe orchitis
  - May reduce the duration and severity of joint and abdominal pain, but impact on risk of renal disease or HSP recurrence is unclear
  - Suggested dose prednisolone 1–2mg/kg/day (max 60mg) while symptomatic then wean

- Most have a self-limited disease within 4 weeks
- Recurrence occurs in 1/3 of patients; most within 6 weeks; can occur up to 2 years
- End stage renal disease in 1–3% of patients; urinalysis and blood pressure should be monitored post diagnosis. (Suggested protocol www.rch.org.au/clinicalguide/guideline_index/HenochSchonlein_Purpura)

Kawasaki disease
See Chapter 25, Infectious diseases.

Post-infectious arthritis
Acute rheumatic fever
See Chapter 25, Infectious diseases.

Post-streptococcal reactive arthritis
- Afebrile symmetrical non-migratory poly- or pauciarticular arthritis.
- Arthritis responds slowly to NSAIDs compared to response in rheumatic fever.
- Carditis may occur.
- Penicillin prophylaxis if carditis is present.

Post-enteric reactive arthritis
- Mainly *Salmonella*, *Shigella* and *Yersinia* (also reported with *Campylobacter and Giardia*).
- Clinically similar to the spondyloarthropathies; that is predominantly lower limb arthritis (including sacroiliitis), enthesitis is common and positive family history (especially if HLA-B27 positive). However, it may not present with all the classic clinical features.
- Consider Crohn's disease or ulcerative colitis.
- Associated features – acute anterior uveitis and sterile pyuria.
- Treatment – NSAIDs.

Post-viral arthritis
- Many viral illnesses are associated with arthritis.
- It is uncertain in most situations whether it is the primary (infective) or secondary (reactive) event; for example Epstein–Barr virus, rubella, adenovirus, varicella (beware of septic arthritis secondary to infected skin lesion), parvovirus B19 and hepatitis B.
- A transient arthritis often follows a non-specific 'viral' illness, the confirmation of which may be difficult and unnecessary.
- Treatment: NSAIDs probably shorten the duration.

Non-inflammatory causes of joint pain
Benign nocturnal limb pains ('growing pains')
- Onset at 3–7 years, often occurs in the evenings and at night.
- Well between attacks.
- Recurrent pain mainly involving the knee, calf and shin.
- No symptoms or signs of inflammation either on history or examination.
- Investigations (if undertaken) normal.
- Management involves analgesia (usually paracetamol), ibuprofen and reassurance; heat and massage/rubbing often help.

Joint Hypermobility syndromes
- Common, particularly in the older child/adolescent (<7 years of age all the features are normal variants).
- Spectrum of disease from benign joint hypermobility syndrome to Ehlers Danlos syndrome.
- The Beighton score is simple to use and is helpful to objectively measure hypermobility
- There can be a wide range of associated symptoms including fatigue, easy bruising, gastrointestinal symptoms, and sometimes the evolution of pain sensitization.
- Always thoroughly examine the joints of young people who present with widespread pain and fatigue and consider hypermobility.

Typical sites
- Hyperextension of the fingers parallel to the forearm
- Apposition of the thumb to the anterior forearm
- Hyperextension of the elbows, knees or both >10 degrees
- Excessive dorsiflexion of the ankles
- Hip flexion allowing the palms to be placed flat on ground

Clinical features
- Pain occurs typically in the afternoon or after exercise and occurs mostly in the lower limbs.
- The child may have features of patello-femoral dysfunction (anterior knee pain).
- The child may have transient joint effusions.
- Management: supportive treatment, physical therapy to strengthen muscles around the joints and reassurance if limited to the joints without significant symptoms.
- For young people with more complex presentations specialised allied health involvement is important.

Complex regional pain syndrome
See Chapter 6, Pain management.

Recurrent fever
- Prolonged fever defined as daily fever >14 days duration with wide differential including infection, inflammatory disease, malignancy and other (see chapter 25 Infectious diseases).
- Recurrent fever defined as 3 or more episodes of fever within a 6-month period occurring at least 7 days apart.
- Associated symptoms may include oral ulcers, rashes, gastrointestinal symptoms, musculoskeletal, ocular and neurologic manifestations.
- Interval between attacks of fever may be irregular or regular .
- Regular; consider cyclic neutropenia or periodic fevers with apthous stomatitis, pharyngitis and adenitis (PFAPA).
  - Irregular; consider auto-inflammatory syndrome or sequential self-limiting illnesses
- Patients typically feel well between episodes, and are often quite unwell during attacks of fever.
- Assessment should include:
- Clinical review during an episode of fever and when well
  - Fever diary including pattern of fever and associated symptoms
  - Laboratory tests during an episode and when well
    - FBC, ESR, CRP, ferritin, liver enzymes, albumin, LDH, immunoglobulins
  - Urinalysis
  - Consider, if indicated:
    - Infectious testing
    - Autoimmune serology (e.g. ANA)
    - Genetic testing

Macrophage activation syndrome (MAS)
- Macrophage activation syndrome (MAS) is multisystem inflammatory emergency
- Primary HLH (see chapter 24 Immunology) is an inherited inflammatory disease caused by abnormalities of natural killer cells, macrophages and T cells and usually occurs in infants and younger children
- Secondary HLH is often associated with infection (particularly EBV), malignancy or systemic inflammation
- MAS is a form of secondary HLH, and may complicate rheumatic diseases including sJIA, systemic lupus and Kawasaki disease

Consider MAS in a child who is persistently febrile in the context of the following clinical and laboratory features:
- Elevated ferritin
- Cytopenias; anemia, thrombocytopenia, neutropenia, (in systemic JIA, may see normalisation of previously elevated cell counts)
- Hepato- splenomegaly and lymphadenopathy

- Elevated triglycerides
- Decreased fibrinogen
- Elevated d-dimer
  Other important clinical and laboratory features:
- Coagulopathy
- Abnormal LFT's
- Persistently raised CRP but decreasing ESR (due to consumption of fibrinogen)
- Hemophagocytosis may be present on bone marrow, lymph node, liver or spleen biopsy
- CNS dysfunction, including headache, confusion, seizures, and coma

Treatment
- All patients require close monitoring and supportive management
- Consider involving intensive care unit early
- Where infection is suspected, antibiotic treatment concurrently may be appropriate
- High dose intravenous steroids, IVIG and plasmapheresis for life-threatening disease

USEFUL RESOURCES
- Paediatric Musculoskeletal Matters International: www.pmmonline.org/; resources and information on paediatric musculoskeletal disorders for clinicians.

CHAPTER 40

Sleep medicine

Amanda Griffiths
Harriet Hiscock

Key Points

- Sleep is made up of cycles of light (Rapid Eye Movement (REM)) and deep (non-REM) sleep with usually brief wakings in between.
- Most sleep problems are behavioural and are often due to a baby or child not learning how to fall asleep by themselves at the start of the night, resulting in difficulties re-settling between sleep cycles overnight.
- Several behavioural sleep strategies have good evidence for effectiveness.
- Melatonin may be used for behavioural insomnia, either as an adjunct to behavioural strategies, or when behavioural strategies have failed, but typically melatonin only helps children get to sleep, not stay asleep overnight.
- Obstructive sleep apnoea is the most common medical sleep problem and can be managed with watchful waiting (only if mild), a trial of nasal steroids (mild to moderate, especially if allergic rhinitis is present) or adenotonsillectomy (moderate-severe).

Normal sleep
Sleep stages
The two sleep states are rapid eye movements (REMs) and non-rapid eye movement (NREM) sleep.
- NREM sleep is further divided into three stages, NREM1 (light sleep) through to NREM3 (deep sleep) via EEG changes.
- REM/NREM cycles occur at intervals of 40-60 minutes in the infant and lengthen to 90 minutes in the preschooler.

Sleep patterns
The amount of sleep children have is highly variable. Table 40.1 shows percentiles for 24 hours sleep duration in Australian children aged 1–9 years.
- Around 3 months of age, the infant's circadian rhythm is emerging, with sleeping patterns becoming more predictable and most sleep occurring at night.
- By 6 months of age, most full-term healthy infants have the capacity to go through the night without a feed.
- Towards the end of the first year of life, the child's sleep architecture becomes like that of an adult, with most of the NREM3 occurring in the first third of the night and REM sleep concentrated in the second half of the night.
- The way an infant/child falls asleep at the start of the night is crucial for learning how to fall back to sleep at the end of each sleep cycle throughout the night.
- Infants who develop the ability to transition from sleep cycle to sleep cycle without parental assistance appear to sleep through the night.
- Most children stop regular naps by 5 years, providing they receive sufficient good quality sleep overnight. Those under 3 years may only nap for one sleep cycle at a time during the day. They are known as 'cat nappers" and typically sleep well overnight.

Paediatric Handbook, Tenth Edition. Edited by Kate Harding, Daniel S. Mason and Daryl Efron.

Table 40.1 Percentiles for total sleep duration per day, by age.

Age (years)	50th Percentile (hr/24hr)	2nd-98th percentile (hr/24hr)
1	14	10-18
3	12	9-15
5	11	8-14
7	10-11	7-14
9	10	6-14

Assessment

One-third of families will complain of difficulties with their child's sleeping patterns. Assessment should include:
- Detailed sleep history over 24 hours, including how (sleep associations e.g. rocking, feeding, use of dummy, falling asleep in car) and where the child goes to sleep, frequency and character of wakings, snoring and daytime functioning.
- Sleep patterns during weekends/holidays and with different caregivers.
- A sleep diary may help clarify the situation (Figure 40.1).
- Family and social history to examine the presence of contributing problems, such as parental depression and relationship problems.
- Exclusion of medical conditions contributing to disrupted sleep patterns such as obstructive sleep apnoea (OSA), asthma, eczema, cow's milk protein allergy (especially in infants), nocturnal seizures, gastro-oesophageal reflux disease, otitis media with effusion, and nasal obstruction.

Bedtime struggles and night-time waking

For infants <6 months of age, no interventions other than schedule manipulation (ensuring the infant is not overtired and that sleep times are adequately spaced) and anticipatory guidance are used.
- If parents want their infant to learn to settle by him/herself, they can try to settle their infant in their cot, leaving before they are asleep.
- In the first 3 months of life, some infants sleep better swaddled.

For older children, treatment plans must be tailored to the child and family.

Contributing factors
- Sleep associations occur when a child learns to fall asleep in a particular way, so that every time the child rouses from a sleep cycle (which is normal), they wake up fully and are unable to put themself back to sleep unless those particular associations are replicated.
- Frequent feeding can cause wakings both by sleep associations and by the child developing a 'learned hunger' response. Some children can develop patterns that lead to drinking large amounts of milk which affects not only their sleep patterns but eating during the day. Most healthy full-term babies can go without a night-time feed by 6 months.
- Erratic routines can contribute to sleep disturbance by inappropriate timing of naps and lack of a regular bedtime routine.
- Sometimes toddlers and preschoolers 'run the house' and parental inconsistent limit setting can exacerbate their bedtime struggles and night-time wakings.

Management
Detailed explanation about normal sleep and sleep cycles and sleep associations is the first step in management. Other management strategies include:
- Regular day–night routine needs to be established. An age-appropriate, enjoyable bedtime routine should be introduced to help the child learn to anticipate going to bed.
- Strategies to deal with inappropriate sleep associations all aim to provide the child with the opportunity to learn to fall asleep without parental assistance. Recommended interventions range from graduated extinction or controlled crying/comforting (i.e. checking the child at increasing periods of time until they fall asleep by

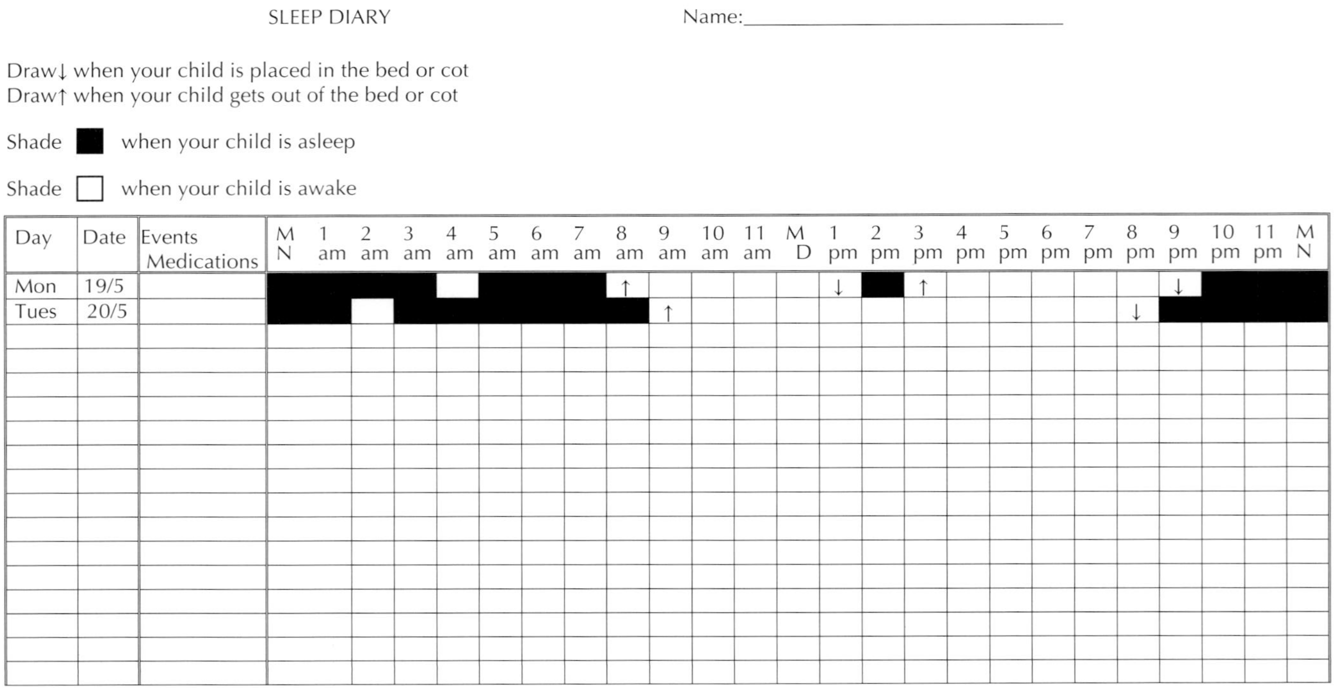

SLEEP DIARY

Name:_____

Draw↓ when your child is placed in the bed or cot
Draw↑ when your child gets out of the bed or cot

Shade ■ when your child is asleep

Shade ☐ when your child is awake

Day	Date	Events Medications	M N	1 am	2 am	3 am	4 am	5 am	6 am	7 am	8 am	9 am	10 am	11 am	M D	1 pm	2 pm	3 pm	4 pm	5 pm	6 pm	7 pm	8 pm	9 pm	10 pm	11 pm	M N
Mon	19/5									↑					↓			↑						↑			
Tues	20/5										↑											↑				

Figure 40.1 Sleep diary.

themselves) to a more gradual approach (including camping out with the gradual withdrawal of the presence of a caregiver over days to weeks). More anxious babies (and parents!) may respond better to the latter.

- If frequent night feeding is a problem, discuss reducing the amount of fluid over 3–10 nights and allowing the child to develop other ways to settle. You can do this by reducing duration of breast feeds (e.g. by 2 mins every 1-2 nights) or volume in the bottle (e.g. 20-40 mL every 1-2 nights). Make sure the last feed before bedtime is outside the bedroom and finishes 20 mins before bedtime. Reassure parents that daytime feeding will increase after 3 days.
- For children who come in and out of the bedroom at the start of the night, you can use a gate to keep them in the room and use a bedtime pass out (www.raisingchildren.net.au) for 1 exit only.
- Melatonin may be used for behavioural insomnia, either as an adjunct to behavioural management, or when behavioural interventions have failed. In this scenario, melatonin is being used for its hypnotic properties rather than its circadian rhythm effects. Melatonin has been found to be helpful in children with developmental disorders, ADHD and autism, but evidence is lacking for use in younger, typically developing children. Best practice supports behavioural interventions as first-line management in all children.
- Sedative medication is not recommended for children <2 years. Promethazine as single night-time dose – 0.5 mg/kg (max 10 mg) – may be used in conjunction with behavioural techniques over a short time period or for blocks of parental respite.

Clinical Conundrums: Does controlled comforting harm infants?

There is no evidence for this and in fact, evidence from randomized controlled trials suggests otherwise. Follow up of infants who have undergone controlled comforting shows lasting improvements in sleep and maternal mental health at child age 2 years and no adverse impacts on child behavior, parenting or the parent-child relationship 1 and 5 years later. Child cortisol levels (a marker of stress) are unaffected.

Night-time fears and anxiety

Night-time fears may present in the preschool and school-age child with bedtime struggles and refusal to sleep by themselves. There may be a precipitant (frightening movie, bullying at school) or it may be a manifestation of an anxiety disorder.

Management

- Address separation issues for the child, which may include the introduction of a transitional object.
- Camper bed technique: a camper bed and a parent are moved into the child's room. The parent spends the entire night in the child's bedroom for 2 weeks helping them overcome their fears and gaining confidence in their own bed and room. This is often used in conjunction with a reward/sticker chart. Once the child is sleeping through the night in their own bed and room, attention can be directed at encouraging the child to fall asleep by themselves at the beginning of the night. Once a child has gained that skill, the parent can gradually move out of the child's bedroom.
- Self-control techniques including relaxation, guided imagery and positive self-statements may also be used, again often in conjunction with reward/sticker chart.
- Make sure that the child is not in bed too early, allowing them the opportunity to further fuss and worry, which will interfere with sleep onset.

Night-time arousal phenomena and differentials

Sleepwalking and night terrors are disorders of partial arousal from NREM3 and therefore occur in the first third of the night. They share common characteristics such as the child is confused and unresponsive to the environment, they have retrograde amnesia and varying degrees of autonomic activation (dilated pupils, sweating, tachycardia). See Table 40.2.

- **Sleepwalking** occurs at least once in 15–30% of healthy children and is most common between 8 and 12 years. It can range from quiet walking, performance of simple tasks such as rearranging furniture or setting tables, to more frenetic and agitated behaviour. At times children open doors/windows and walk outside the home.

Table 40.2 Characteristics of night terrors, seizures and nightmares.

Characteristic	Night terrors	Nightmares	Epilepsy
Sleep stage	NREM 3	REM	NREM2 but can occur all stages
Time of night	First 1/3	Last 1/2	Any time
Wakefulness	Unrousable	Easily aroused	Usually unrousable
Amnesia	Yes	No	Yes, or may have some recall
Return to sleep	Easy	Difficult	Easy
Family history	Yes	No	Possibly

- **Night terrors** are most common between 4 and 8 years of age and have a prevalence of 3–5%. They usually begin with a terrified scream and the child may either thrash around in bed or get up and run around the house. Efforts to calm or contain the child often make the episode worse.

Differentials
- **Nightmares** generally occur during REM sleep and are thus more common in the second half of the night. They are vivid dreams accompanied by feelings of fear which wake the child up from sleep. They are most common in 3–6 year olds.
- **Nocturnal frontal lobe epilepsy (NFLE).** This can present with brief repetitive stereotypical movements ± vocalizations throughout the night which can be associated with awareness by the child. Alternatively, NFLE can present with bizarre complex stereotypic dystonic movements which typically last <2 minutes.

Management
Obtain detailed history including the timing and duration of events, and the exact nature of movements (rhythmic or stereotypical) and behaviours.
- Completion of a sleep diary.
- A home video may be useful to aid diagnosis.
- All but NFLE are generally self-limiting. Explain, reassure and discuss safety issues.
- Avoid sleep deprivation as this can precipitate events. Ensure regular bedtime routines and sleep patterns. If children are having difficulties settling due to night-time fears and worries, techniques discussed in previous section maybe applicable.
- If events occur at a consistent time, then scheduled awakening (waking the child 30 minutes before an event) may be useful.
- Sleep studies are required only if the history is unclear; if the nocturnal events are very frequent, violent or atypical; or if there is impaired sleep quality. The latter may be a clue to unrecognised OSA.
- Medication is rarely needed. In situations where no aetiology has been found and there are very frequent and disruptive events, low-dose clonazepam before bedtime may be useful for 4–6 weeks.
- If NFLE is suspected, then a sleep-deprived EEG or prolonged video EEG may be required. Most NFLE responds to carbamazepine.

Snoring and sleep-disordered breathing
Sleep provides a physiological stress to breathing which can unmask respiratory difficulties that may not be apparent during wakefulness.
- Snoring is the most common symptom of sleep-disordered breathing in children and can be associated with primary snoring (PS) through to OSA.
- PS refers to snoring not associated with sleep or ventilatory disturbances and occurs in up to 20% of children.

Obstructive sleep apnoea
OSA is defined as repeated episodes of partial or complete upper airway obstruction that disrupt normal ventilation and sleep.
- Incidence is 3% of children with peak incidence at 2–6 years due to adenotonsillar hypertrophy.

- Complications of severe OSA include growth failure and cor pulmonale, with the most common morbidity being impairment of behaviour and neurocognitive functioning.
- Symptoms include snoring, difficult or laboured breathing, apnoeas, mouth breathing, excessive sweating and restless or disturbed sleep. Children less commonly present with tiredness and lethargy. In older children, daytime symptoms may include behavioural and learning difficulties.
- Increased risk of OSA is associated with
  - Adenotonsillar hypertrophy
  - Obesity
  - Syndromes (e.g. Down syndrome, Prader–Willi)
  - Craniofacial abnormalities (e.g. Pierre-Robin, Crouzons)
  - Mucopolysaccharidoses
  - Achondroplasia and skeletal abnormalities
  - Neuromuscular weakness (e.g. Duchenne)
  - Hypotonia, hypertonia (e.g. cerebral palsy)
  - Prematurity
  - Previous palatal surgery (repaired cleft palate)
- Examination involves assessment of predisposing conditions and complications of OSA:
  - Growth: either failure to thrive or obesity
  - Craniofacial structure (retro/micrognathia, midface hypoplasia)
  - Mouth breathing
  - Nasal patency, septum, turbinates, allergic rhinitis
  - Tongue, pharynx, palate, uvula, tonsils
  - Pectus excavatum
  - Right ventricular hypertrophy, pulmonary hypertension.

Clinical Pearl: OSA and Down Syndrome

Infants/Children with Down Syndrome have a high prevalence of OSA due to small crowded upper airways, lymphoid hyperplasia and pharyngeal hypotonia – these children often need adeno-tonsillectomy as well as other treatments for OSA (tongue reduction surgery, CPAP) to improve.

Investigation

- Overnight oximetry is the most useful screening tool, with positive oximetry being diagnostic of OSA. Positive oximetry is defined as >3 clusters of SpO_2 desaturations, with at least 3 desaturations to <90%. It is important that the averaging time of the oximeter is short (i.e. 2–3 seconds). Negative or normal oximetry does not exclude OSA, although it may provide reassurance that the child is unlikely to have severe OSA while awaiting further assessment.
- Oximetry is limited in that it does not provide any information on the type of events associated with oxygen desaturations, CO_2 retention or sleep disruption. Oximetry should not be used to diagnose OSA in children less than 12 months,
- Overnight polysomnography (sleep study) continues to be the gold standard for diagnosis of OSA and should be performed if uncertainty persists in high-risk children, children <2 years of age, or those with co-morbid conditions where there is a risk of central sleep-disordered breathing in addition to OSA.
- Investigation by nasal endoscopy or lateral neck radiograph may have a place in assessing adenoidal size.

Management

- Adeno-tonsillectomy is first-line treatment for moderate to severe OSA, being effective in the majority of children. The role of adenoidectomy alone is unclear.
- Adenotonsillectomy is associated with a 2-week recovery period and there is a 2–3% risk of secondary haemorrhage especially 5–10 days post-operatively.
- Medical treatment is appropriate in mild to moderate OSA and includes:
  - Intranasal steroids for either reduction in adenoid size (short term: 6-8 weeks) or allergic rhinitis (long term) – the dose is 1 puff each nostril nocte for those under 12 yrs and 2 puffs each nostril nocte after 12 yrs and/or

○ Montelukast (Singulair) in certain situations e.g. Atopy (noting the 1:10 chance of significant anxiety/depression/behavioural disturbance on this medication) – the dose is 4 mg nocte up to 5 yrs, 5 mg nocte 5–14 yrs and 10 mg nocte after 14 yrs

- Management of obesity is important where this is the likely underlying cause, see Chapter 11, Growth.
- Non-invasive ventilation (usually continuous positive airway pressure CPAP) may be used for residual OSA, if there is a delay in surgery, or if surgery is contraindicated.

Latest Evidence: OSA treatment

CHAT is the only randomised controlled trial of treatment in children with obstructive sleep apnoea (New England Journal of Medicine, 2013, Marcus et al.)

- School aged children were randomised to adeno-tonsillectomy or watchful waiting with cognitive function assessed after 7 months
- 46% of those with watchful waiting and 79% of those post T&A resolved their OSA as detected by sleep study
- There was no difference in the results of the cognitive tool between the two groups

---

Polysomnography (sleep study)

Polysomnography involves the continuous and simultaneous recording of multiple physiological parameters related to sleep and breathing. Sleep studies are indicated for:

- OSA; primary snoring versus sleep-disordered breathing.
- Central sleep disordered breathing.
- Monitoring non-invasive ventilation requirements.
- Excessive daytime sleepiness (include multiple sleep latency testing if narcolepsy suspected).
- Atypical night-time disruptions including very frequent or violent awakenings.
- A full EEG montage is required if seizures are suspected.
- Periodic limb movement disorder.

USEFUL RESOURCES

- The Raising children network www.raisingchildren.net.au: evidence-based parenting website with step-by-step instructions for behavioural techniques including graduated extinction, adult fading, phasing out dummies and overnight feeding. Parent handouts for sleepwalking, night terrors, bedtime struggles and separation anxiety.
- Sleep for kids www.sleepforkids.org: launched by National Sleep Foundation aimed to provide information to children aged 7–12 years.
- Sleep podcast www.mcri.edu.au/sleeppodcast: for parents and clinicians advice on common sleep problems and their management from birth to adolescence, including ADHD and autism, from two Australian sleep experts.

CHAPTER 41

Surgery

Michael Nightingale
Aurore Bouty

Key Points

- Effective first aid limits the damage of a burn, use cool running water for 20 mins within 3 hours of the time of the burn.
- A child with an acute scrotum requires urgent surgical review and should not have a US performed as an initial investigation.
- Neonates and infants with inguinal hernias requires surgical attention whereas hydroceles will usually resolve without intervention.
- Pyloric stenosis requires careful fluid resuscitation but is not a surgical emergency.
- Physiological phimosis is a normal finding in young children and does not require treatment in the absence of symptoms.

Emergency surgical conditions

Major trauma

Trauma is a condition that involves many specialties in a Paediatric unit. Rather than a thorough plan for managing all major trauma, this section is an overview of the issues and problems that need consideration.

Major trauma is the most common cause of death in children over the age of one year. There is a trimodal distribution in timing of mortality (Table 41.1). Public health and safety measures such as seat belts and bike helmets may reduce immediate mortality, the vast majority of which are not amenable to medical intervention. Quality trauma care can reduce mortality in the early period and ameliorate potential late deaths.

Trauma ideally requires management by a team experienced in resuscitation, and the procedures that might be required for managing trauma. A trauma team may consist of the following:

- Team leader (a clinician experienced in resuscitation).
- Airway doctor and nurse (consider an anaesthetist, intensivist or emergency physician confident with managing a child's airway).
- Procedure doctor and nurse.
- Surgeon (ideally paediatric surgeon) to facilitate theatre when needed and as an expert in some procedures.
- Social worker or nurse to manage the family and the psychological needs of the child.
- Access to, or advice from, a neurosurgeon and orthopaedic surgeon is desirable.

Major trauma is ideally initially managed at a trauma centre, but if managed at another site early discussion with, and appropriate transfer to, the trauma centre are indicated.

Paediatric Handbook, Tenth Edition. Edited by Kate Harding, Daniel S. Mason and Daryl Efron.
© 2021 John Wiley & Sons Ltd. Published 2021 by John Wiley & Sons Ltd.

Table 41.1 Trimodal distribution in timing of mortality due to trauma.

Time	Cause
Immediate	Major neurological or vascular insult
Early (Golden Hour)	Brain, chest or abdominal injury
Late	Multiorgan failure or sepsis

Initial assessment

In major trauma several initial steps should be undertaken rapidly – often simultaneously. The history and events relating to the injury should be clarified. A rapid assessment of the respiratory, circulatory and neurological systems should be undertaken. The child should be reassured in simple appropriate language and the primary carer engaged where appropriate. Particular attention should be paid to keep the child warm with early and generous use of analgesia to provide comfort.

Management should follow the principles of the Early Management of Severe trauma (EMST) course of the Royal Australian College of Surgeons.

Primary survey

The aim of the primary survey is to identify and treat immediate life-threatening problems. Ensuring adequate oxygenation and blood pressure to perfuse the injured brain is of particular importance:.

- A – Airway maintenance with cervical spine control.
- B – Breathing and ventilation.
- C – Circulation with haemorrhage control.
- D – Disability: Neurological status. Do not ever forget the glucose.

Life-threatening problems should be rapidly identified and corrected. These include:

- Obstructed or inadequate airway.
- Inadequate breathing.
- Evidence of blood loss (tachycardia, poor perfusion, hypotension).
- Evidence of other complications such as pneumothorax/tension pneumothorax; haemothorax; pericardial tamponade; open wounds with active bleeding.

Management

The primary survey should be performed in a rapid but ordered fashion.

- Airway compromise may require an adjunct such as a guedel airway or intubation.
- Impaired ventilation can require finger thoracostomy and drain placement.
- Fluid resuscitation should begin with 0.9% NaCl or Hartmann's solution.
- If more than 40 mL/kg is needed, or there is obvious massive blood loss, blood should be immediately administered (initially O-negative, then crossmatched blood once available).
- Monitoring should at a minimum include continuous heart rate, pulse oximetry, frequent intermittent non-invasive BP, and intermittent measurement of temperature.
- All children involved in trauma must be considered to have injury to the spinal column until this can be assessed and cleared. Therefore, spinal alignment and neck immobilisation in a cervical collar is necessary until full assessment can be performed.

Trauma radiology should be performed as appropriate with a CXR, lateral c-spine and pelvic XR.

Laboratory investigations which may be considered include:

- Crossmatch of blood (mandatory for all major trauma)
- Blood gas analysis to assist with assessment of ventilation (maintenance of a normal PCO_2 in a child with a head injury)
- Electrolytes
- Coagulation tests (in prolonged resuscitation or massive transfusion)

Secondary survey

The secondary survey begins after the primary survey is completed and after management of immediate life-threatening conditions has begun.

- Full but modest exposure of all parts of the body is necessary to ensure no injuries are missed.
- Adequate analgesia and temperature control are very important in this phase of care.
- A secondary survey involves a top to toe (including log roll) comprehensive examination to document all obvious injuries and to institute management.
- Rectal and vaginal examination should be performed rarely and only by the most appropriate member of the trauma team.

Management

Imaging tests that may be considered in this phase include:
- FAST ultrasound scanning to identify intra-abdominal bleeding, pericardial effusion, and haemothorax or pneumothorax may be useful.
- CT scan (of brain, chest, abdomen, pelvis or spine may be indicated).
- Angiography.

Definitive management of injuries identified in a secondary survey should be undertaken by the appropriate specialist surgical teams.

Tertiary survey

A tertiary survey is performed to identify and catalogue all injuries. It is usually initiated within 24 hours of admission after the initial resuscitative phase. This should be completed prior to discharge.

Burns

Burns can be a devastating injury for children and their families. The majority of burns in children are caused by scalds from hot liquids, but other common causes include contact with hot surfaces and flame burns. The severity of a burn depends on its size, depth and the anatomical area involved.

The treatment of a burn aims to:
- Prevent and treat shock
- Provide adequate analgesia
- Prevent infection
- Obtain early skin cover
- Prevent hypertrophic scar formation
- Restore function and correct cosmetic defect
- Prevent recurrence of injury and promote accident prevention

First aid

First aid aims to limit the damage caused by a burn.
- Stop the burning process.
- Remove any source of heat such as affected clothing.
- Commence cooling as soon as possible (within 3 hours from time of burn), with cool, running water for 20 minutes total duration. Cooling should be targeted to the affected area only.
- Do NOT apply ice or ice slush as this may cause additional tissue damage.
- Do NOT apply hydrogel burn products (e.g. Burnaid®) as a first aid measure UNLESS there is no access to a water source.
- Cold water compresses are less effective than running water to cool a burn wound and must be changed frequently.
- Applying plastic (cling) wrap to burn wound after cooling, aids analgesia and limits heat loss and evaporation.
- Irrigate any chemical burns with copious volumes of water.
- Burns to the eyes require early irrigation with copious volumes of normal saline or water.

Assessment

The management of a burn should follow the principles of trauma management as described above. The initial assessment of a burn should include its extent and its depth.

Extent of burn

The usual adult formula (rule of nines) is not applicable to children. In infancy, the head is relatively large and contributes proportionally more to the total surface area. As the child grows, the lower limbs contribute more

Table 41.2 Depth of burns.

Depth	Cause	Surface/Colour	Pain	Treatment
Superficial	Sun, flash, minor scald	Dry, minor blisters, erythema	Painful	Expose Non adherent dressing
Superficial Partial	Scald	Moist, reddened with broken blisters	Painful	Nanocrystalline silver dressing, e.g. Acticoat
Deep Partial	Scald, minor flame, contact	Moist, white slough, red mottled	Painless	Nanocrystalline silver dressing, e.g. Acticoat
Deep	Flame, severe scald, or contact	Dry, white, charred	Painless	Nanocrystalline silver dressing, e.g. Acticoat or SSD cream until split skin graft

to the total surface area. The burned areas should be plotted accurately on the body chart and the area calculated with the aid of the Lund–Browder chart. The extent of the burn is commonly overestimated, leading to excessive fluid administration.

Depth of burn
See Table 41.2.

Management
Pain relief
- Immediate, effective analgesia should be provided, with the route and choice of analgesia determined by the condition of child and potency of analgesia required.
- Rapid options include intranasal fentanyl (1.5 mcg/kg) or IV morphine (0.1mg/kg given in titrated boluses).
- Dressing changes should be accompanied by appropriate analgesia and sedation.
Infection
- Once the extent and depth of the burn have been assessed the tetanus immunisation status should be checked.
- A booster with tetanus toxoid ± tetanus immunoglobulin given as appropriate (see The RCH Clinical practice guideline, Managing tetanus prone wounds available at www.rch.org.au/clinicalguide/guideline_index/Management_of_tetanusprone_wounds/).
Minor burns
- Superficial burns <5% of the BSA are suitable for outpatient treatment, unless they occur on the face, neck, hands, feet or perineum. Infants <12 months are more likely to require admission.
- Blisters should be left intact.
- Gently cleanse and remove loose skin.
- If burns are definitely superficial, dress with tulle gras and an absorbent dressing (e.g. gauze). Do not use Hypafix-type dressing directly on the burn.
- Immobilise with a crepe bandage, plaster slab or sling, if indicated.
- In partial thickness burns of indeterminate depth, the use of nanocrystalline dressing is recommended, for example Acticoat. These dressings should be left in place for 3 or 7 days depending on the product used.

Major burns
Superficial burns >5% of the BSA and deep burns, may require admission to hospital. Any child with burns >10% of the BSA, consider transfer to a specialist paediatric burns centre. Older children with more extensive superficial burns, such as sunburn, may be managed as outpatients.
- It is important to document the time, causative agent, circumstances of the burn, treatment initiated including first aid and the child's general health. If the history is inconsistent with the injury, consider child abuse.
- Carefully chart the extent and depth of the burn and the child should be weighed if possible. Observations of general condition, pulse, respiration rate, temperature, BP and fluid balance (including hourly urine output estimations) are necessary.
- Severe burns to the face consider early endotracheal intubation, as the face swells, airway obstruction may occur, making intubation difficult.

- Smoke inhalation may lead to acute respiratory distress syndrome (ARDS) where ventilation perfusion defects result in hypoxemia, alveolar collapse, shunting and decreased lung compliance.
- Carboxyhaemoglobin (COHb) and cyanide concentration should be measured in all children with burns/ smoke inhalation. Symptoms of hypoxemia manifest at levels >30% COHb. Treatment is supplemental oxygen, as CO binding to Hb is reversible.

The management of burns >10% of BSA requires venous access.

- Blood for baseline laboratory studies, including haemoglobin, haematocrit and serum electrolytes should be taken.
- In severe burns include blood group and a crossmatch.
- Fluid resuscitation should be commenced (see below).
- In burns >15% of BSA, insert a silastic urethral catheter for hourly urine volume and a nasogastric tube.
- Analgesia or sedation should be administered as necessary.

Care should be taken in ward management to guard against cross-infection.

- Antibiotics should not be prescribed routinely.
- On admission, swabs should be taken of the burn area, nose, throat and rectum.
- In major burns, multiple 3 mL punch biopsy specimens are the most reliable method of detecting infection.
- Antibiotics are usually only given for proven infection and on the basis of sensitivity tests.
- If septicaemia is suspected clinically, blood culture should be performed and empiric antibiotics commenced.

Fluid management

- Children with burns >10% TBSA require both resuscitation and maintenance fluids.
- Resuscitation fluids are given at a volume/rate estimated using the Modified Parkland's Formula: 3-4 mL x kg x % TBSA (24-hour total volume) with Hartmann's solution.
  - Commence rate to give 50% of this volume in first 8 hours from time of injury (not time of presentation); if >8 hours since injury discuss fluids with a burns service.
  - Ongoing resuscitation fluid rates are guided by urine output, and vital signs.
  - Aim for urine output 1 mL/kg/hr, with resuscitation fluid rate increased or decreased accordingly.
- Maintenance fluid requirements should not be neglected.
  - Initially these are given intravenously.
  - Most children will tolerate small amounts of feeds (30–60 mL/h) after 4–8 hours.
  - If this is tolerated, increase the quantity to 4 hourly.
  - In minor burns, oral fluids may be commenced earlier.
  - After 48 hours, most fluid intake is usually oral. Children who refuse to drink, or who have burns to the face and mouth, may require nasogastric feeding.

Escharotomies should be considered if the peripheral circulation to a limb is jeopardised. Before commencing this procedure contact a paediatric burns unit. Respiratory difficulties require particular attention; intensive care or escharotomy to the trunk may be required.

Nutrition

- All children with burns should receive a high-calorie diet containing adequate protein, vitamin and iron supplements.
- In severe burns there is a marked increase in metabolic rate and gastric tube feeding with a complete fluid diet (e.g. Isocal or Ensure) should be instituted early and adjusted to maintain or increase body weight.
- The involvement of a dietician is recommended.

Physiotherapy and occupational therapy should be commenced early and continued throughout the course of burn care. Splints and pressure dressings are necessary to control hypertrophic scar formation. The play therapist also has an important role.

The acute scrotum

The term 'acute scrotum' describes a red, swollen and tender scrotum. There are many possible causes for this presentation, many of which do not require surgical management. The most important cause is ischaemia due to torsion of the testis. This condition is difficult to distinguish from more benign causes and is regarded as a surgical emergency to avert complete infarction. For these reasons, all boys with an acute scrotum should have an urgent surgical review.

Torsion of the testicular appendage

The testicular appendage is the remnant of the cranial end of the Mullerian duct. It is shaped like an inverted tear drop. The larger the remnant is the more likely it is able to twist and cut off its blood supply. As embryologically it is related to the female genital tract, it will enlarge in response to the increased oestrogen stimulation that occurs at the onset of puberty in boys, so it most commonly presents in peripubertal boys, but it can occur at any age.

- It is the most common cause of the acute scrotum.
- Typically, boys will present with gradual onset of a dull persistent pain in their hemi scrotum without systemic symptoms. The pain may be present for some time before scrotal signs evolve. Examination is less painful than in testicular torsion and testis is maximally tender at the upper pole. A torted appendage may be palpated.
- The diagnosis can only be made if the infarcted appendage can be seen through the scrotal skin. This is known as the "Blue Dot" sign and is pathognomonic of the condition (Figure 41.1). If this is not present other causes cannot be excluded.
- Once diagnosed the condition can be managed conservatively or with a semi-elective surgical procedure to remove the appendage.

Testicular torsion

Torsion of the testis can occur at any age but is most common in infants and adolescents.

- In infants the entire scrotal contents twist as they have not fully adhered to the scrotal fascia.
- In adolescents an abnormally high fixation of the tunica vaginalis to the spermatic cord can predispose an enlarging testis to a torsion event.
- It is generally accepted that the testis will infarct after 6 hours of complete ischaemia.

Ischaemia causes sudden onset of severe pain.

- Autonomic symptoms such as nausea and vomiting are often present, due to the generous sympathetic supply to the testis.
- The testis will often lie horizontally high in the scrotum, feeling hard and exquisitely tender.

The diagnosis can only be excluded by definitive diagnosis of another condition.

- Once suspected an emergency surgical procedure is required to confirm the diagnosis, detort the testis and determine if it is salvageable.
- An orchidectomy may be required but fixation of both testes, or the sole remaining testis, to minimize the risk of recurrence is mandatory.

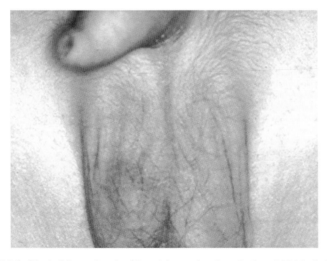

Figure 41.1 The "Blue Dot" sign seen in torsion of the testicular appendage. *Source*: Beasley et al. 2018. Paediatric Surgical Diagnosis 2nd edition. CRC Press. Reprinted with permission from CRC Press.

Epididymo-Orchitis

Infection of the testis and/or the epididymis is an uncommon cause of an acute scrotum in boys. It is caused by the reflux of infected urine into the vas deferens. In a young child this may be due to an anatomically abnormal urinary tract, and in an adolescent due to sexual activity. The cause is rarely haematological spread. The symptoms are usually gradual in onset, mild and associated with fever, tachycardia and dysuria. The diagnosis can be confirmed with an abnormal urine microscopy and subsequent culture.

Idiopathic scrotal oedema

The exact cause of idiopathic scrotal oedema remains unknown, but it causes an allergic type reaction in the scrotal skin with redness, swelling and tenderness. The symptoms start gradually and are mild. The scrotal skin is tender but on careful examination the testes are not tender. Unlike the other causes of scrotal pain, the condition involves both sides of the scrotum and the inflammation can spread onto the abdominal wall and femoral are. When this is found the diagnosis is confirmed.

Clinical Pearl: Testicular assessment
- Examination of the testes is a vital part of the assessment of abdominal pain in boys and should never be forgotten or excluded.
- Boys will commonly relate the onset of symptoms to minor trauma, but traumatic testicular injury is a very rare event.
- Ultrasound cannot definitively exclude testicular torsion and will delay management – it should never be performed in the initial assessment of the acute scrotum.

Common surgical conditions

Appendicitis

Appendicitis is the most common abdominal condition requiring surgery in childhood and must be considered in any child presenting with significant abdominal pain. The appendix is a vestigial organ in the right lower quadrant of the abdomen. Obstruction of the lumen causes appendicitis, usually by impacted faeces called a faecolith, though other causes such as lymphoid hyperplasia, parasites and rarely tumours can occur.

The symptoms and signs of appendicitis are related to the degree of peritoneal irritation and the position of the appendix.
- The classical description is of colicky periumbilical pain migrating to a continuous pain in the right iliac fossa with associated anorexia, fever, nausea.
- Mild vomiting and loose stools are frequently seen.
- Examination shows localised peritonitis with guarding in the right iliac fossa.
- Peritonitis may not occur in retrocaecal appendicitis.
- In pelvic appendicitis there may be only vague suprapubic tenderness.
- Repeated clinical examination is the most sensitive test for appendicitis.
- Routine blood tests should not be performed.
- An abdominal ultrasound may be helpful in difficult cases to exclude other causes of abdominal pain.

Surgery to remove the inflamed appendix through a laparoscopic approach is the gold standard for management. The use of anitbiotics as primary management for simple appendicitis is a management strategy being investigated in clinical trials.

Clinical Pearl: Appendicitis
Any child admitted with a diagnosis of gastroenteritis that does not respond to fluid resuscitation over a 24 hour period must have a surgical review to exclude conditions such as appendicitis.

Intussusception

Ileocolic intussusception occurs one segment of ileum telescopes inside the adjacent distal bowel causing intestinal obstruction. The bowel invaginates because a lead point is pushed through into the distal bowel by peristalsis. In the vast majority of cases the lead point is due to lymphoid tissue within the ileal wall becoming enlarged due to a viral infection and is most common in children aged 3 months to 2 years. This is known as idiopathic intussusception. Intussusception can also occur when a pathological lead point is present such as a Meckel's diverticulum, duplication cysts, polyps or conditions such as cystic fibrosis and is more common when intussusception occurs outside the normal age range. Intussusception can progress to cause ischaemic infarction of the involved bowel with perforation and peritonitis.

Clinical presentation of ileocolic intussusception

- Small bowel obstruction with presenting with intermittent colicky abdominal pain, progressive vomiting becoming bile stained and lethargy/pallor.
- The classic 'red currant jelly stool' is a late feature due to mucosal infarction.
- The mass of invaginated bowel can sometimes be palpated in the right abdomen before small bowel distension occurs.

Transient small bowel-small bowel intussusception is sometimes seen in gastrointestinal illness due to disordered peristalsis. It is self limiting, does not cause clinical obstruction and requires no particular management.

Management

- Initial management is aimed at resuscitation.
- An AXR can show bowel obstruction in advanced cases and rarely free intraperitoneal air.
- Ultrasound is the key investigation to confirm the diagnosis and is highly sensitive and specific.
- Treatment consists of an air enema performed by an experienced radiologist in order to push the intussusceptum back into the proximal bowel to relieve the obstruction. This may take several attempts to be successful and may be augmented by the use of steroids.
- If free air or peritonitis are present or if multiple attempts fail, surgery may be required for correction.

Pyloric stenosis

Pyloric stenosis is an acquired thickening of the gastric outlet which results in obstruction. The aetiology is unclear but includes a genetic component and is much more common in boys.

- It usually presents between 2 and 6 weeks of age; that is chronological age, regardless of prematurity.
- The classical symptoms are of progressive milky vomits becoming projectile, with associated weight loss and continual hunger.
- Left untreated there will be progression to severe dehydration.
- Prominent gastric peristalsis can occur in an enlarged stomach occurs due to pyloric obstruction, and if the stomach is collapsed experienced hands can palpate the pyloric thickening knows as the tumour.
- Ultrasound is a valuable adjunct to diagnosis.

Management

Early surgical consultation is recommended but pyloric stenosis is not a surgical emergency.

- Careful fluid resuscitation is essential prior to surgery.
- Vomiting in these infants results in loss of gastric fluid (water and HCl). The kidneys initially conserve H+ but once the baby becomes dehydrated, water and Na+ are conserved in exchange for K+ and H+.
- The resulting condition is hypovolaemia with alkalosis, low chloride and potassium.
- Even if serum K+ is normal, there is total body potassium deficiency.
- Inappropriate rapid rehydration can result in cerebral oedema.
- Fluid resuscitation should follow principles of deficit replacement in addition to ongoing maintenance.
- The deficit should be replaced slowly over 12–24 hours.
- Normal saline with the addition of potassium when the infant is passing urine is an appropriate fluid.

Clinical Pearl: Pyloric stenosis

Gastric peristalsis is an easier sign to observe than palpation of the pyloric tumour for inexperienced practitioners. Open the curtains and expose the abdomen and observe for waves of contraction moving from left to right across the upper abdomen whilst taking the history from the parents.

Umbilical hernia

Shortly after birth the fibromuscular umbilical ring, which has allowed passage of the cord vessels into the abdomen, starts to contract. If this process is delayed, then the peritoneum and abdominal contents may bulge through forming a hernia.

- This is a common finding in newborn children.
- It often increases in size in the first few months of life and can be a bluish colour when tense during crying as a consequence of increased abdominal pressure rather than the cause of discomfort.
- Strangulation is extremely rare.
- For most infants parental reassurance is all that is required.
- If a hernia persists beyond the age of 2 years, an operation as a day case is recommended before starting school. The operation is primarily cosmetic, although strangulation can occur during adult life (particularly during pregnancy).

Inguinal hernia

In males the testis descends into the scrotum through the inguinal canal during the final trimester of pregnancy. In females the inguinal canal transmits the round ligament of the uterus. A diverticulum of the peritoneum descends with the testis or ligament and subsequently obliterates late in pregnancy or in the first few months of life. In both cases if the diverticulum persists then an inguinal hernia may develop.

- The vast majority of inguinal hernias are indirect i.e. they follow the path of the inguinal canal.
- They are more common in males.
- 60% will be on the right side.
- The greatest incidence is in the first year of life.
- They may contain omentum, small bowel, the appendix or the ovary in girls.

Hernias typically present with an incidental bulge noted in the area overlying the external ring.

- It becomes more prominent at times when the infant is crying or straining.
- Clinical examination will occasionally not reveal an abnormality with the diagnosis based on the history alone.
- A thickening in the cord may be felt which is described as a 'silk glove' sign which describes the sensation of the layers of the hernial sac gliding over each other.
- A hernial sac with content may be able to be felt and reduced to confirm the diagnosis.
- Both sides of the groin should always be checked, as should the position of the testes.

Complications can occur as a result of an inguinal hernia. Incarceration occurs when the hernial contents cannot be returned to the abdomen. If the blood supply to the contents becomes impaired the hernial contents become strangulated which can result in infarction of both the contents and the testis from compression of the testicular vessels.

Inguinal hernia requires surgical correction. The younger the infant, is the more urgent repair becomes as the risk of incarceration and strangulation are higher.

Urological conditions
Antenatal urinary tract dilatation

Antenatal urinary tract dilatation (also known as hydronephrosis), is the most common abnormal finding on antenatal ultrasound. However, a vast majority of them will resolve spontaneously. It is important to obtain a detailed antenatal scan to allow for risk stratification and appropriate post-natal management. Table 41.3 summarises the incidence and characteristics of the most common underlying diagnoses for antenatal dilatation of the urinary tract.

Antenatal dilatation of the urinary tract is graded according the antero-posterior diameter of the renal pelvis in a transverse plan (APD) and association of calyceal and parenchymal changes according to the Society for Foetal Urology (SFU) grading system (Tables 41.4 and 41.5). It is important that progress is evaluated at two time points during pregnancy, ideally in the second and third trimester.

A minimum number of parameters need to be reported on the ultrasound to allow for appropriate management. These include:

- Sex of the foetus
- Presence of two kidneys or solitary kidney
- Quality of the renal parenchyma on each side (degree of cortico-medullary differentiation, echogenicity, thinning, presence of cortical cysts)
- Collecting system (single or duplex, degree of pelvic and calyceal dilatation, APD)
- Association with a ureteric dilatation
- Bladder (megacystis, bladder wall thickening, ureterocele, key-hole sign (dilated posterior urethra suspicious of PUV))
- Amniotic fluid volume

Table 41.3 Incidence and characteristics of the most common diagnoses underlying antenatal urinary tract dilatation.

Underlying diagnosis	Incidence in ANH	F:M ratio	Kidneys	Ureters	Bladder	Amniotic fluid
Transient hydronephrosis	41–88%	1:1	Transiently abnormal	Not seen	Normal	Normal
Pelviureteric junction (PUJ) obstruction	10–30%	1:3-4	Hydronephrosis	Not seen	Normal	Normal
Vesicoureteric reflux (VUR)	10–20%	5:1	Hydronephrosis if high-grade	Variable	Normal	Normal
Vesicoureteric junction (VUJ) obstruction	5–10%	1:3	Hydronephrosis	Dilated	Normal	Normal
Ureterocele/ectopic ureter/duplex system	5–7%	6:1	Large cyst, possible duplex kidney	Dilated	Normal or enlarged	Normal
Multicystic dysplastic kidney	4–6%	1:1	Large cysts of variable size	Not seen	Normal	Normal
Posterior urethral valves	1–2%	Male only	Bilateral hydronephrosis +/- parenchymal changes	Dilated	Enlarged, thick-walled	Variable; diminished or absent in severe obstruction

Table 41.4 Definition of antenatal dilatation of the urinary tract according to APD and post-natal likelihood of pathological diagnosis.

Degree of ANH	Second trimester	Third trimester	Risk of post-natal pathological diagnosis
Mild	4 to <7 mm	7 to <9 mm	12%
Moderate	7 to ≤10 mm	9 to ≤15 mm	45%
Severe	>10 mm	>15 mm	88%

Table 41.5 Definition of antenatal dilatation of the urinary tract according to SFU.

Grade	Pattern of renal sinus splitting
0	No splitting
I	Urine in pelvis barely splits sinus
II	Urine fills intrarenal pelvis
III	SFU Grade 2 and minor calyces uniformly dilated and parenchyma preserved
IV	SFU Grade 3 and parenchyma thin

Source: Chen et al. (2010). Antenatal Hydronephrosis. Urological Science 21. 109–112. Reproduced with permission from Elsevier.

The most important diagnosis to rule out is lower urinary tract obstruction (LUTO) (also known as bladder outlet obstruction (BOO)), particularly posterior urethral valve in a male.
- PUV carries a high risk of chronic kidney disease.
- Ideally parents of foetuses with suspicion of such a diagnosis should be referred antenatally to a Paediatric Urologist and/or a Paediatric Nephrologist for counselling.

- Suspicious signs of PUV include male sex, megacystis, bilateral ureteric and pelvi-calyceal dilatation, key-hole sign, urinoma or foetal ascites, oligohydramnios.
- These findings warrant close monitoring throughout pregnancy.

Post-natal management

Urgent post-natal ultrasound scan prior to discharge of the newborn and discussion of the results with the Urology or Nephrology team is warranted for any infant with antenatal pelvi-calyceal dilatation associated with any of the following signs:

- Bilateral or unilateral on a solitary kidney
- Severe dilatation with APD >15mm in the third trimester
- Renal parenchyma abnormality
- Oligohydramnios
- Evidence of lower urinary tract abnormality (megacystis, thick-walled bladder, ureterocele)

The need for catheter insertion should be discussed with Urology. In all these cases, except for isolated pelvi-calyceal dilatation, antibiotic prophylaxis should be started.

In all other cases, USS should be performed between 3 and 7 days of life to avoid underestimating the degree of dilatation during the period of physiological oliguria of the newborn.

- In the absence of worrying features, a repeat USS at 4-6 weeks of life and referral to Urology and/or Nephrology outpatient should be organised.
- Antibiotic prophylaxis is not recommended in isolated pelvi-calyceal dilatation.

Hydroceles

If the peritoneal diverticulum partially obliterates a small amount of fluid may track into the scrotum through the patent processus vaginalis. The fluid accumulates within the tunica vaginalis in boys or in the canal of nuck in girls forming a cystic swelling.

It can be diagnosed clinically by

1. Being able to palpate the cord completely above the swelling i.e. it does not extend into the inguinal canal
2. Not being able to reduce the swelling (the processus acts as a flap valve)
3. Glowing brightly when transilluminated

Hydroceles will usually resolve without treatment before the age of 2. If they persist after this time, surgical repair is required.

Varicocele

A varicocele is caused by enlargement of veins in the pampiniform plexus. It feels like 'a bag of worms' in the scrotum, best detected with the child standing. It is almost always on the left side and is associated with a dragging ache in the scrotum, though some cases are noticed incidentally. Varicoceles can cause impairment of testicular growth and relative infertility and should have a surgical assessment. Varicoceles can be treated with interventional radiological techniques or through laparoscopic surgery.

Undescended testis

The testis descends into the scrotum on the spermatic cord in the final trimester of pregnancy. Normal positioning of the testis in the scrotum is important for testicular development.

- The cord contains the cremasteric muscle which will pull the testis close to the abdomen as part of the flight/fright response.
- This normal reflex develops in the first few months of life and is maximal between the ages of 2 and 8.
- It is a frequent cause of concern to parents during childhood but requires no management.
- A retractile testis occurs when the cremasteric reflex is overactive. The testis is rarely seen in the scrotum by parents but can be comfortably placed there during clinical exam.
- Truly retractile testes merit a surgical review as a small number will represent the onset of acquired maldescent.

When the testis cannot be brought to the bottom of the scrotum at birth, it is a congenital undescended testis.

- This is caused by incomplete migration of the gubernaculum to the scrotum.
- An assessment should be made by a paediatric surgeon between 3–6 months of life (as the testis may descend further in the first few months of life) and
- An orchidopexy is performed at 6–12 months of age.

Some boys present with undescended testis later in childhood (4–10 years).
- This is the result of failure of elongation of the spermatic cord with age, caused by persistence of a fibrous remnant of the processus vaginalis.
- Surgery is recommended if the testis does not remain in the bottom of the scrotum, to optimise fertility.

In some boys no testis is palpable. This may be because the testis is held in the abdomen or muscle wall, or it can represent testicular atrophy as a result of a torsion event antenatally.

Penile conditions
See Figure 41.2.

Smegma deposits
Smegma may build up under a non retractile foreskin. They present as doughy yellow lumps and can be confused with tumours and cysts. They are a normal variant and will resolve as the foreskin becomes more retractile.

Balanoposthitis
Posthitis is an infection of the foreskin which often occurs with infection of the glans penis called Balanitis. The infection causes redness, inflammation, swelling and sometimes a white exudate. Treatment with local antiseptic ointment (e.g. neomycin eye ointment) beneath the foreskin and topical hydrocortisone 1% are used in mild cases. Oral antibiotics (e.g. co-trimoxazole) may also be added. If the whole penile shaft skin is red and swollen to the pubis, IV antibiotics may be required.

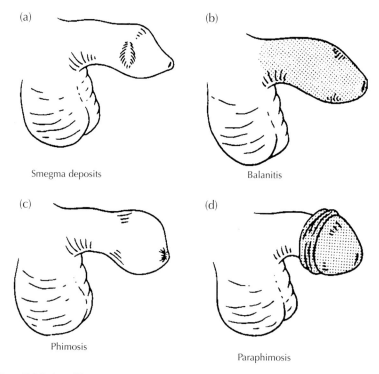

(a) Smegma deposits

(b) Balanitis

(c) Phimosis

(d) Paraphimosis

Figure 41.2 Penile conditions.

Phimosis

The foreskin in a newborn is not retractile due to tightness of the preputial opening. This is known as physiological phimosis.

- This naturally loosens during childhood till the foreskin is retractile over the glans and in the absence of symptoms requires no treatment.
- Phimosis may result in urine and smegma accumulating under the foreskin causing chemical irritation as it is converted to ammonia.
- Episodes of secondary infection can also occur.
- In this situation treatment with topical steroid for 2–4 weeks is used loosen and relax the foreskin.

Pathological phimosis is scarring of the preputial opening.

- This can be caused by attempts at forceful retraction of the foreskin or by an inflammatory process such as balanitis xerotica obliterans (BXO).
- This can be identified by white scar tissue at the preputial opening.
- Pathological phimosis requires surgical review for the consideration of circumcision or preputioplasty.

Paraphimosis

This is an acutely painful condition, which results from a retracted foreskin trapped behind the glans, forming an oedematous ring constricting the exposed and swollen glans penis.

- Manual reduction should be attempted in all cases.
- To facilitate the procedure, use topical local anaesthetic cream (e.g. EMLA cream) 5 minutes before reduction, and consider the use of nitrous oxide.
- Ice and adrenaline-containing creams should not be applied.
- Failure to reduce the paraphimosis requires urgent surgical consultation.

Hypospadias

Hypospadias is caused by the impaired development of the tissues forming the urethra on the ventral aspect of the penis. It is the most common congenital abnormality of the penis and affects 1 in 350 boys.

The clinical features of hypospadias are

- The urethral orifice (meatus) opens on the ventral surface of the penis and does not reach the end of the glans.
- There is deficiency of the ventral foreskin known as a 'dorsal hood'.
- There is ventral bending of the penis known as chordee.

These features cause several functional problems and in severe cases can result in ambiguous genitalia (see Chapter 19, Endocrinology). Surgical correction is performed between 6 and 12 months of age.

CHAPTER 42

Trans and gender diverse health

Michelle Telfer
Ken Pang

Key Points
- In Australia, 1.2–2.3% of the population identify as trans or gender diverse (TGD).
- Establish with the child or adolescent whether they have a preferred name and pronouns (he/she, him/her, they/them) and respectfully use these to address them at all times.
- Recognise the vulnerability of TGD children and adolescents due to their experiences of stigma, discrimination, social isolation, bullying and family rejection.
- Provide support and treatment for depression, anxiety, self-harm and suicidal ideation.
- Refer to available gender services, should treatment for gender dysphoria be desired.

Increased visibility and societal acceptance of gender diversity has led to a rise in children and adolescents presenting to primary care and specialist medical services seeking advice, support and gender affirming psychological and medical care. Two large population-based studies undertaken in New Zealand (Clarke et al. 2014) and Australia (Sixth National Survey of Secondary Students and Sexual Health 2018) estimate that 1.2–2.3% of adolescents identify as trans or gender diverse (TGD).

TGD identities are widely considered to be part of the natural spectrum of human diversity. Frequently however, being TGD is accompanied by gender dysphoria, which is the distress that arises due to incongruence between a person's gender identity and their sex assigned at birth. TGD individuals remain at high risk of harm due to stigma, discrimination, social exclusion and isolation, family rejection, bullying and physical assault. This is associated with serious mental health issues, with high rates of depression, anxiety, self-harming and ever attempting suicide, seen in Australian TGD young people.

Increasing evidence demonstrates that mental health outcomes can be improved with a supportive and gender affirming approach to the care and treatment of TGD children and adolescents. In contrast, withholding gender affirming treatment can exacerbate distress and psychiatric morbidity, including increasing the risk of self harm and suicide. Similarly, past practices aiming to align one's gender identity with birth assigned sex, known as conversion or reparative therapies, are now considered unethical. This is due to a lack of treatment efficacy and evidence demonstrating harm to the health and well-being of children and adolescents subjected to such practices. See Table 42.1 for terminology.

Clinical Pearl: Using respectful and affirming language
Creating an environment that demonstrates inclusiveness and respect for diversity is essential when providing care to TGD children and adolescents. Even an act as simple as displaying a rainbow flag on your ID badge can send a positive message of support and assist young people to feel more comfortable. Asking a young person at their first appointment if they have a preferred name and pronouns, then using these consistently to address them across all care aspects, is vital. Some young people without the benefit of supportive parents or carers may request use of a preferred name or pronoun only when being seen on their own. It is important to respect and enact this to enable optimal therapeutic engagement as well as ensuring patient confidentiality and safety.

Paediatric Handbook, Tenth Edition. Edited by Kate Harding, Daniel S. Mason and Daryl Efron.
© 2021 John Wiley & Sons Ltd. Published 2021 by John Wiley & Sons Ltd.

Table 42.1 Terminology.

Terminology	
Gender identity	A person's innermost concept of self as male, female, a blend of both or neither. One's gender identity can be the same or different from their sex assigned at birth.
Gender expression	The external presentation of one's gender, as expressed through one's name, clothing, behaviour, hairstyle or voice, and which may or may not conform to socially defined behaviours and characteristics typically associated with being either masculine or feminine.
Gender diverse	A term to describe people who do not conform to their society or culture's expectations for males and females. Being transgender is one way of being gender diverse, but not all gender diverse people are transgender.
Assigned male at birth	A person who was thought to be male when born and initially raised as a boy.
Assigned female at birth	A person who was thought to be female when born and initially raised as a girl.
Trans or transgender	A term for someone whose gender identity is not congruent with their sex assigned at birth.
Cisgender	A term for someone whose gender identity aligns with their sex assigned at birth.
Trans boy/male/man	A term to describe someone who was assigned female at birth and identifies as a boy/male/man.
Trans girl/female/woman	A term to describe someone who was assigned male at birth and identifies as a girl/female/woman.
Non-binary	A term to describe someone who doesn't identify exclusively as male or female.
Gender fluid	A person whose gender identity varies over time.
Agender	A term to describe someone who does not identify with any gender.
Brotherboy and Sistergirl	Aboriginal and Torres Strait Islander people may use these terms in a number of different contexts, however they can be used to refer to trans and gender diverse people. Brotherboy typically refers to masculine spirited people who were assigned female at birth. Sistergirl typically refers to feminine spirited people who were assigned male at birth.

Supporting trans and gender diverse children and adolescents

Expression of gender diversity may commence from very early in childhood, during adolescence or any time throughout adulthood. The clinical needs of each individual will differ significantly depending on the person's age, developmental stage, their current circumstances and desire for intervention. The options for treatment that may be considered in the best interest for one person, may not be helpful for another, necessitating individualised care. In practice this may involve a combination of psychological, medical, surgical, nursing and allied health interventions. In this way, optimal care is delivered via a coordinated, integrated multidisciplinary approach.

Mental health support

A non-judgemental, safe and supportive gender affirming approach is required, and may involve working not only with the young person but also their family and school. Individual support for the child might involve helping them to explore, understand and affirm their gender identity, as well as optimising any co-existing mental health difficulties. Family support is associated with optimal mental health outcomes and working with family members to help develop a shared understanding of the child or adolescent's experience may be necessary. Support within the educational environment can reduce bullying and harassment, a common experience for TGD young people which can result in depression, anxiety, increased suicide risk, school refusal and compromised academic potential.

Social transition

Social transition should be child-led and involves the outward expression of one's gender identity through the adoption of a preferred name, pronouns, hairstyle or clothing that is stereotypically associated with the gender the person identifies as. Social transition is associated with a reduction in distress and improved emotional functioning, with evidence demonstrating that trans children who have socially transitioned have rates of depression, anxiety and self-worth comparable to their cis-gender peers. For adolescents with a masculine identity, social transition may include masculinisation of the chest via breast binding, while for adolescents with a feminine identity it may include feminisation through chest padding, genital tucking and hair removal.

Voice and communication training

Voice is an important aspect of gender expression and speech therapy can assist in the development of skills to enable communication in a manner consistent with a TGD adolescent's gender identity.

Menses suppression

TGD adolescents assigned female at birth frequently report significant distress with menstruation. Menses suppression can be readily managed with the use of oral norethisterone. Other available methods include continuous use of a combined oral contraceptive or insertion of a levonorgestrel-releasing intrauterine device.

Pubertal suppression

Pubertal suppression is undertaken after puberty has begun, to reduce the distress associated with development of secondary sexual characteristics resulting from the adolescent's endogenous oestrogen or testosterone production. Use of gonadotrophin releasing hormone analogues (GnRHa) stops physical changes such as breast growth in TGD adolescents assigned female at birth and voice deepening and facial hair development in TGD adolescents assigned male at birth. If GnRHa are ceased, puberty will resume normally. In addition to reducing distress, pubertal suppression also provides the adolescent time to develop emotionally and cognitively prior to consideration of gender affirming hormone treatment whose effects are partially irreversible. Puberty is normally a time when bone strength increases substantially, and monitoring of bone mineral density is necessary with pubertal suppression.

Gender affirming hormones

Oestrogen and testosterone are used to affirm a young person's gender identity by feminising or masculinising their physical appearance. Physical changes following commencement of oestrogen or testosterone occur over months to years and show varying degrees of reversibility (Table 42.2 and Table 42.3).

Fertility counselling

Fertility counselling is an important component of obtaining informed consent for hormonal intervention. Pubertal suppression will inhibit reproductive capacity, although this should be fully reversible. Testosterone also impairs reproductive function. This too appears reversible given multiple documented cases of successful pregnancies in trans males previously treated with testosterone. Oestrogen has an adverse effect on sperm production in most trans females, and the reversibility of this process is unknown. It is therefore recommended that TGD adolescents be informed of these likely effects, and different fertility preservation options discussed, including gamete cryopreservation.

Table 42.2 Physical effects of oestrogen.

Effect of oestrogen	Onset	Maximum	Reversibility
Redistribution of body fat	3-6 months	2-3 years	Likely
Decrease in muscle mass and strength	3-6 months	1-2 years	Likely
Softening of skin and decreased oiliness	3-6 months	unknown	Likely
Decreased libido	1-3 months	3-6 months	Likely
Decreased spontaneous erections	1-3 months	3-6 months	Likely
Breast growth	3-6 months	2-3 years	Not possible
Decreased testicular volume	3-6 months	2-3 years	Unknown
Decreased sperm production	Unknown	> 3 years	Unknown
Decreased terminal hair growth	6-12 months	>3 years	Possible
Scalp hair	Variable		
Voice changes	None		

Table 42.3 Physical effects of testosterone.

Effect of testosterone	Onset	Maximum	Reversibility
Skin oiliness and acne	1-6 months	1-2 years	Likely
Facial and body hair growth	6-12 months	4-5 years	Unlikely
Scalp hair loss	6-12 months		Unlikely
Increased muscle mass and strength	6-12 months	2-5 years	Likely
Fat redistribution	1-6 months	2-5 years	Likely
Cessation of menses	1-6 months		Likely
Clitoral enlargement	1-6 months	1-2 years	Unlikely
Vaginal atrophy	1-6 months	1-2 years	Unlikely
Deepening of voice	6-12 months	1-2 years	Not possible

Clinical Controversies: Transgender health care for children and adolescents

Transgender health care for children and adolescents remains a relatively new field, with current treatment guidelines based on available evidence and expert consensus. The field is evolving, and there is an ongoing need for more research to help inform clinical practice.

Consent to medical treatment

Until November 2017, consent for hormone treatment in trans adolescents required authorisation by the Family Court of Australia. This situation changed, following a court case known as Re: Kelvin (2017).

Timing of commencement of hormone treatment

The age at which adolescents become competent to consent to their own medical treatment is varied, especially for interventions with complex risk-benefit ratios such as gender affirming hormone treatment. Decisions should be individualised and made in the best interest of the adolescent involved, ideally with the clinicians working together with the young person and their family. Whilst later commencement of hormone treatment provides time for progression of emotional maturation of the adolescent, this must be balanced with the biological, psychological and social cost of delaying intervention, with increased self harm and suicide being a significant risk.

Surgical interventions for adolescents

Chest reconstructive surgery is an integral part of the transition process for many TGD individuals assigned female at birth. Undertaking this procedure during adolescence can be beneficial in terms of the young person's mental health.

Treatment interventions in adolescents with a non-binary gender identity

Some adolescents have a non-binary gender identity, and do not identify exclusively as male or female. Although many of these individuals do not desire medical interventions, some request hormone or surgical treatment to produce a physical appearance that aligns with their non-binary identity. An adolescent who was assigned female at birth may, for example, request no hormone treatment at all but desire chest reconstructive surgery to masculinise their chest. Alternatively, reduced doses of testosterone or testosterone taken for a limited period, may be sufficient to induce desired irreversible masculinising effects such as voice deepening without requiring long term hormone treatment. Whilst this may present challenges for clinicians, individualised patient-centred care that balances the risks and benefits to the young person and allows for autonomy and agency, can be beneficial to the mental health outcomes of these young people.

Antimicrobial guidelines

Nigel Curtis
Mike Starr

Infection	Likely organisms	Initial antimicrobials[1] (maximum dose)	Duration of treatment[2] and other comments
CENTRAL NERVOUS SYSTEM / EYE			
Brain abscess	Often polymicrobial *S. milleri* and other streptococci Anaerobes Gram-negatives *S. aureus*	Flucloxacillin[3] 50 mg/kg (2 g) IV 6H *and* 3rd gen cephalosporin[4] *and* Metronidazole 15 mg/kg (1 g) IV stat, then 7.5 mg/kg (500 mg) IV 8H	3 weeks minimum Penicillin hypersensitivity or risk of MRSA[3]: substitute Flucloxacillin with Vancomycin 15 mg/kg (500 mg) IV 6H
Post-neurosurgery	As above plus *S. epidermidis*	As above but substitute Flucloxacillin with Vancomycin 15 mg/kg (500 mg) IV 6H	Uncomplicated 10 days minimum Complicated 3 weeks minimum
Encephalitis	Herpes simplex virus Enteroviruses Arboviruses *M. pneumoniae*	Aciclovir 20 mg/kg IV 12H (<30 weeks gestation), 8H (>30 weeks gestation to <3 months corrected age) 500 mg/m² IV 8H (3 months – 12 years) 10 mg/kg IV 8H (>12 years)	3 weeks minimum Consider adding Azithromycin if *M. pneumoniae* suspected
Meningitis Over 2 months of age	*S. pneumoniae*[5] *N. meningitidis* *H. influenzae* type b[6]	3rd gen cephalosporin[4]	*S. pneumoniae* 10 days *N. meningitidis* 5–7 days *H. influenzae* type b 7–10 days
Over 2 months of age and possibility of penicillin-resistant pneumococci[5]	As above	3rd gen cephalosporin[4] *and* Vancomycin 15 mg/kg (500 mg) IV 6H	Consider addition of Dexamethasone 0.15 mg/kg (10 mg) IV 6H for 4 days
Under 2 months of age	As above plus Group B streptococci *E. coli* and other Gram-negative coliforms *L. monocytogenes*	Benzylpenicillin 60 mg/kg (2 g) IV 12H (week 1 of life) 6H (week 2–4 of life) 4H (>week 4 of life) *and* Cefotaxime[3]	Gram-negative 3 weeks GBS/Listeria 2–3 weeks Substitute Benzylpenicillin with Vancomycin if possibility of penicillin-resistant pneumococci[5]
With shunt infection, post- neurosurgery, head trauma or CSF leak	As for over 2 months of age plus *S. epidermidis* *S. aureus* Gram-negative coliforms incl. *P. aeruginosa*	Vancomycin 15 mg/kg (500 mg) IV 6H *and* Ceftazidime 50 mg/kg (2 g) IV 8H	10 days minimum

(continued)

Infection	Likely organisms	Initial antimicrobials[1] (maximum dose)	Duration of treatment[2] and other comments
Contact prophylaxis	N. meningitidis	Ciprofloxacin 250 mg (5–12 years) 500 mg (≥12 years) oral single dose Unable to take tablets: Rifampicin 5 mg/kg (<1 month) or 10 mg/kg (≥1 month) (max 600 mg) oral bd for 2 days	2 days
Contact prophylaxis	H. influenzae type b	Rifampicin 20 mg/kg (600 mg) oral daily	4 days
Postseptal (orbital) cellulitis	S. aureus H. influenzae spp. S. pneumoniae M. catarrhalis Gram-negatives Anaerobes	Flucloxacillin[3] 50 mg/kg (2 g) IV 6H **and** 3rd gen cephalosporin (dose for severe infection)[4]	IV duration based on severity and improvement (usually 3–4 days) Switch to Amoxicillin/clavulanate (400/57 mg per 5 mL) 22.5 mg/kg (875 mg) (Amoxicillin component) = 0.3 mL/kg (11 mL) oral bd 10 days minimum total duration Consider adding Metronidazole if not responding
Preseptal (periorbital) cellulitis Mild	Group A streptococci S. aureus	Cefalexin 33 mg/kg (500 mg) oral tds	7–10 days
Moderate	H. influenzae spp.	Flucloxacillin[3] 50 mg/kg (2 g) IV 6H **or** Ceftriaxone 50 mg/kg (2 g) daily (for hospital-in-the-home)	Bilateral findings and/or painless or non-tender swelling in a well looking child is more likely to be an allergic reaction
Severe, or not responding, or under 5 years of age and non-Hib immunised	As above plus H. influenzae type b[6]	Flucloxacillin[3] 50 mg/kg (2 g) IV 6H **and** 3rd gen cephalosporin[4]	IV duration based on severity and improvement (usually 34 days) 10 days minimum total duration
CARDIOVASCULAR			
Endocarditis Native valve or homograft	Viridans streptococci Other streptococci Enterococcus spp. S. aureus	Benzylpenicillin 60 mg/kg (2 g) IV 6H **and** Flucloxacillin[3] 50 mg/kg (2 g) IV 6H **and** Gentamicin 7.5 mg/kg (360 mg) IV daily (<10 years) 6 mg/kg (360 mg) IV daily (≥10 years)	4–6 weeks Gentamicin 1 mg/kg (80 mg) IV 8H for 1–2 weeks when used only for synergy (Gentamicin monitoring is generally not required with low dose in this setting)
Artificial valve, post-surgery or suspected MRSA[4]	As above plus S. epidermidis	Vancomycin 15 mg/kg (500 mg) IV 6H **and** Flucloxacillin[3] 50 mg/kg (2 g) IV 6H **and** Gentamicin 7.5 mg/kg (360 mg) IV daily (<10 years) 6 mg/kg (360 mg) IV daily (≥10 years)	

Endocarditis prophylaxis For dental procedures only	Viridans streptococci S. aureus S. pneumoniae Other Gram-positive cocci Enterococcus spp.	Amoxicillin 50 mg/kg (2 g) Local anaesthetic: give orally 1 hour before procedure General anaesthetic: give IV with induction	Penicillin hypersensitivity: substitute Amoxicillin with Cefalexin 50 mg/kg (2 g) oral Immediate or severe penicillin hypersensitivity: substitute with Clindamycin 20 mg/kg (600 mg) oral or IV
GASTROINTESTINAL			
Diarrhoea Salmonella spp. isolated in infant under 3 months of age or in immunocompromised	Salmonella spp.	3rd gen cephalosporin[4]	5–7 days Antibiotic treatment is generally unnecessary for most other organisms Consider adding Azithromycin in returned travellers from regions with high prevalence of cephalosporin resistance
Antibiotic-associated	C. difficile	Metronidazole 7.5 mg/kg (400 mg) oral tds	7–10 days
Giardiasis	G. lamblia	Metronidazole 30 mg/kg (2 g) oral daily or Tinidazole 50 mg/kg (2 g) oral stat	3 days Single dose
Peritonitis or ascending cholangitis	Gram-negative coliforms Anaerobes Enterococcus spp.	Ampicillin or Amoxicillin 50 mg/kg (2 g) IV 6H **and** Gentamicin 7.5 mg/kg (360 mg) IV daily (<10 years) 6 mg/kg (360 mg) IV daily (≥10 years) **and** Metronidazole 15 mg/kg (1 g) IV stat, then 7.5 mg/kg (500 mg) IV 8H	Up to 14 days See footnote 7 re Gentamicin dosing/monitoring
Threadworm (Pinworm)	Enterobius vermicularis	Mebendazole 50 mg oral (<10 kg) 100 mg oral (≥10 kg) or Pyrantel 10 mg/kg (1 g) oral	Single dose; may need to repeat after 14 days Treat whole family
GENITOURINARY			
Urinary tract infection Over 6 months of age and not sick	E. coli P. mirabilis K. oxytoca Other Gram-negatives	Cefalexin 33 mg/kg (500 mg) oral bd or Trimethoprim 4 mg/kg (150 mg) oral bd or Trimethoprim/Sulfamethoxazole (8/40 mg/mL) 0.5 mL/kg (20 mL) oral bd	5 days

(continued)

563

Infection	Likely organisms	Initial antimicrobials' (maximum dose)	Duration of treatment² and other comments
Under 6 months of age or sick or acute pyelonephritis	As above plus *Enterococcus* spp.	Benzylpenicilin 60 mg/kg (2 g) IV 6H *and* Gentamicin 7.5 mg/kg (360 mg) IV daily (<10 years) 6 mg/kg (360 mg) IV daily (≥10 years) 5 mg/kg (360 mg) IV daily (week 1 of life)	5–7 days for UTI 10–14 days for pyelonephritis See footnote 6 re Gentamicin dosing/monitoring
UTI prophylaxis	As above	Trimethoprim 2 mg/kg (150 mg) oral daily *or* Trimethoprim/Sulfamethoxazole (8/40 mg/mL) 0.25 mL/kg (20 mL) oral daily	Routine prophylaxis is not recommended
RESPIRATORY			
Epiglottitis	*H. influenzae* type b⁶	Ceftriaxone 50 mg/kg (1 g) IV daily	5 days Consider addition of Dexamethasone
Gingivostomatitis In immunocompromised Ir immunocompetent (only if within 72 hours of onset with severe pain and dehydration)	Herpes simplex virus	Aciclovir 500 mg/m² IV 8H (3 months–12 years) 10 mg/kg IV 8H (>12 years) Consider Aciclovir 10 mg/kg (400 mg) oral five times daily	7 days Until no new lesions Newer
Influenza	Influenza A, B	Oseltamivir 3 mg/kg oral bd (Birth – 12 months) 30 mg oral bd (>12 months and <15 kg) 45 mg oral bd (15–23 kg) 60 mg oral bd (23–40 kg) 75 mg oral bd (>40 kg)	5 days
Otitis externa Acute diffuse	*S. aureus* *S. epidermidis* *P. aeruginosa* *Proteus* spp. *Klebsiella* spp.	Topical steroid/antibiotic drops	7 days Clean ear canal (± insertion of wick soaked in drops if ear canal oedematous)
Acute localised (furuncle) ± cellulitis	*S. aureus* Group A streptococci	Flucloxacillin³ 50 mg/kg (2 g) IV 6H	5 days
Failure of first-line treatment, high fever or severe persistent pain	As above plus *P. aeruginosa*	Piperacillin/Tazobactam 100 mg/kg (4 g) (Piperacillin component) IV 8H	14 days minimum Consider fungal infection

Condition	Organisms	Treatment	Duration/Notes
Otitis media	Viruses S. pneumoniae M. catarrhalis H. influenzae spp. Group A streptococci	Consider no antibiotics for 48 hours if over 6 months of age **If treatment indicated** Amoxicillin 30 mg/kg (1 g) oral bd	5 days Treatment indicated if infection in one hearing ear or associated with cochlear implant
Pertussis	B. pertussis	Azithromycin 10 mg/kg (500 mg) oral daily (Birth – 6 months), 10 mg/kg oral on Day 1, then 5 mg/kg (250 mg) daily (≥6 months) *or* Clarithromycin 7.5 mg/kg (500 mg) oral bd	5 days 7 days Can be given up to 3 weeks after contact with index case or if symptoms <3 weeks
Pneumonia Mild (outpatient)	Viruses S. pneumoniae H. influenzae spp.	Amoxicillin 30 mg/kg (1 g) oral tds	3–5 days
Moderate (inpatient)	As above	Amoxicillin 30 mg/kg (1 g) oral tds	5 days Consider Benzylpenicillin 60 mg/kg (1.2 g) IV 6 H if unable to tolerate oral intake or vomiting
Severe (≥2 of: severe respiratory distress, severe hypoxaemia or cyanosis, marked tachycardia, altered mental state OR empyema	As above plus S. aureus Group A streptococci Gram-negatives	Flucloxacillin[3] 50 mg/kg (2 g) IV 6H **and** 3rd gen cephalosporin[4]	10 days minimum[2] Consider adding Azithromycin 10 mg/kg (500 mg) IV daily to cover M. pneumoniae and other atypical pathogens and Oseltamivir to cover influenza virus
Tonsillitis	Viruses Group A streptococci (GAS)	Features of GAS infection in child ≥4 years AND high-risk group **or** suppurative complications: Phenoxymethylpenicillin (Penicillin V) 250 mg oral bd (<20 kg) 500 mg oral bd (≥20 kg) *or* Benzathine benzylpenicillin 450mg (600 000 units) IM (<20 kg), 900 mg (1.2 million units) IM (>20 kg) as a single dose	10 days oral treatment High-risk groups: • Indigenous Australians • Maori and Pacific Islander • Personal history of rheumatic fever or rheumatic heart disease • Family history of rheumatic fever or rheumatic heart disease • Immunosuppressed

(continued)

565

Infection	Likely organisms	Initial antimicrobials[1] (maximum dose)	Duration of treatment[2] and other comments
Quinsy (peritonsillar abscess)		Amoxicillin/Clavulanate 25 mg/kg (1 g) (Amoxicillin component) IV 8H (≥3 months and ≥4 kg)	10 days
Retropharyngeal abscess		Amoxicillin/Clavulanate 25 mg/kg (1 g) (Amoxicillin component) IV 8H (≥3 months and ≥4 kg)	10–14 days
SKIN/SOFT TISSUE/BONE			
Bites (animal/human)	Viridans streptococci S. aureus Group A streptococci Oral anaerobes E. corrodens Pasteurella spp. (cat and dog) C. canimorsus (dog)	Amoxicillin/Clavulanate (400/57 mg/5 mL) 22.5 mg/kg (875 mg) (Amoxicillin component) 0.3 mL/kg (11 mL) oral bd	5 days Treat established infection Prophylaxis generally not required, except: • Presentation delayed >8 hours • Puncture wound unable to be adequately debrided • Bite on hands, feet, face • Bite involves deep tissues (e.g. bones, joints, tendons) • Bite involves an open fracture • Immunocompromised patient • Cat bites Check tetanus immunisation status
If severe, penetrating injuries, esp. involving joints or tendons	As above	Amoxicillin/Clavulanate 25 mg/kg (1 g) (Amoxicillin component) IV 12H (Birth – 3 months or <4 kg), 8H (≥3 months and ≥4 kg)	14 days Increase to 6H in severe infections (≥3 months and ≥4 kg)
Cellulitis Mild/moderate (outpatient)	Group A streptococci S. aureus	Cefalexin 33 mg/kg (500 mg) oral tds (1 g max for moderate cellulitis)	5–10 days If rapidly progressive consider adding Clindamycin 10 mg/kg (600 mg) IV 6H

	Organisms	Antimicrobial	Notes
Moderate/severe (inpatient)		Flucloxacillin[3] 50 mg/kg (2 g) IV 6H or Ceftriaxone 50 mg/kg (2 g) IV daily (for hospital-in-the-home)	
Facial cellulitis in child under 5 years of age and non-Hib immunised	As above plus S. pneumoniae H. influenzae spp.[6]	Flucloxacillin[3] 50 mg/kg (2 g) IV 6H and 3rd gen cephalosporin[4]	
Necrotising fasciitis	As above	Vancomycin 15 mg/kg (500 mg) IV 6H and Meropenem 20 mg/kg (1 g) IV 8H and Clindamycin 15 mg/kg (600 mg) IV 8H	Consider IVIg
Dental abscess	Often polymicrobial Viridans and anginosus group streptococci Oral anaerobes S. aureus	Amoxicillin 25 mg/kg (500 mg) oral tds or Benzylpenicillin 50 mg/kg (1.2g) IV 6H	7 days Dental/surgical management required
Head lice	Pediculus humanus var. capitis	1% permethrin liquid or cream rinse	Repeat after one week
Impetigo	Group A streptococci S. aureus	Mupirocin 2% ointment top 8H if localised or Cefalexin 33 mg/kg (500 mg) oral bd	5 days
Lymphadenitis (cervical) Mild	S. aureus Group A streptococci Oral anaerobes	Cefalexin 33 mg/kg (500 mg) oral tds	7 days
Severe	As above	Flucloxacillin[3] 50 mg/kg (2 g) IV 6H	May require longer than 7 days
Osteomyelitis Uncomplicated	S. aureus Group A streptococci S. pneumoniae	Flucloxacillin[3] 50 mg/kg (2 g) IV 6H	Switch to oral Cefalexin 45 mg/kg (1.5 g) oral tds once afebrile plus clinical improvement plus inflammatory markers decreasing 3 weeks for uncomplicated cases[2]
If under 5 years of age and non-Hib immunised	As above plus H. influenzae type b[6]	Flucloxacillin[3] 50 mg/kg (2 g) IV 6H and 3rd gen cephalosporin[4]	
In patient with sickle cell anaemia	As above plus Salmonella spp.	Flucloxacillin[3] 50 mg/kg (2 g) IV 6H and 3rd gen cephalosporin[4]	3 weeks minimum

(continued)

Infection	Likely organisms	Initial antimicrobials[1] (maximum dose)	Duration of treatment[2] and other comments
With penetrating foot injury	As above plus *P. aeruginosa*	Piperacillin/Tazobactam 100 mg/kg (4 g) (Piperacillin component) IV 8H	Surgical intervention important
Scabies	*Sarcoptes scabiei*	Permethrin 5% cream top	One application from neck down; leave on for minimum of 8H (usually overnight) May need to repeat after 7 days Treat whole family
Septic arthritis	As for osteomyelitis	As for osteomyelitis	3 weeks for uncomplicated cases[2] Always consider surgical drainage
Chickenpox In immunocompromised or neonate **Shingles** In immunocompromised Involving eye	Varicella zoster virus	Aciclovir 20 mg/kg IV 12H (<30 weeks gestation), 8H (>30 weeks gestation – <3 months corrected age) 500 mg/m² IV 8H (3 months – 12 years) 10 mg/kg IV 8H (>12 years) Oral treatment (above) **and** Aciclovir ointment to eye 5 times per day	7 days Consider zoster immunoglobulin for neonates or immunocompromised exposed to chickenpox Shingles in immunocompetent children does not generally require treatment

SEPTICAEMIA (UNDER 2 MONTHS OF AGE)

Infection	Likely organisms	Initial antimicrobials[1] (maximum dose)	Duration of treatment[2] and other comments
Septicaemia Community-acquired infection	Group B streptococci *E. coli* and other Gram-negative coliforms *L. monocytogenes* *H. influenzae* spp.[6] plus those listed below for 'Septicaemia with unknown CSF'	Benzylpenicillin 60 mg/kg IV 12H (week 1 of life) 6H (week 2–4 of life) 4H (>week 4 of life) **and** Cefotaxime[3]	Duration depends on culture results Premature neonates require special dosing consideration Also consider disseminated HSV infection, particularly under 2 weeks of age
If abdominal source suspected	As above plus Anaerobes	Amoxicillin or Ampicillin 50 mg/kg (2 g) IV 6H **and** Gentamicin 5 mg/kg IV 24H (week 1 of life) 7.5 mg/kg IV daily thereafter **and** Metronidazole 15 mg/kg IV stat, then 7.5 mg/kg IV 8H	
If *S. aureus* suspected (e.g. umbilical infection)	As above plus *S. aureus*	Add Flucloxacillin[3] 50 mg/kg IV 12H (week 1 of life) 8H (week 1–4 of life) 6H (>week 4 of life)	

SEPTICAEMIA (OVER 2 MONTHS OF AGE)

Condition	Organisms	Treatment	Notes
Septicaemia with unknown CSF	S. pneumoniae[5] N. meningitidis S. aureus Group A streptococci Gram-negatives	Flucloxacillin[3] 50 mg/kg (2 g) IV 6H **and** 3rd gen cephalosporin[4]	Duration depends on culture results
If central line in situ (non-oncology) or suspected MRSA infection	As above plus S. epidermidis	Substitute Flucloxacillin with Vancomycin 15 mg/kg (500 mg) IV 6H	
Septicaemia with normal CSF	As above	Flucloxacillin[3] 50 mg/kg (2 g) IV 6H **and** Gentamicin 7.5 mg/kg (360 mg) IV daily (<10 years) 6 mg/kg (360 mg) IV daily (≥10 years)	Duration depends on culture results
In non-Hib immunised	As above plus H. influenzae type b[6]	Flucloxacillin[3] 50 mg/kg (2 g) IV 6H **and** 3rd gen cephalosporin[4]	
In neutropenic patient	As above plus Enterococcus spp. P. aeruginosa	Piperacillin/Tazobactam 100 mg/kg (4 g) (Piperacillin component) IV 6H (8H if <6 months) If systemic compromise **or** high-risk cancer treatment **or** inpatient onset of symptoms **add** Amikacin 22.5 mg/kg (1.5 g) IV daily (<10 years) 18 mg/kg (1.5 g) IV daily (≥10 years)	Local protocols for fever and neutropenia may differ Target trough (<2 mg/L pre 3rd dose) If suspected C. difficile colitis add Metronidazole 7.5 mg/kg IV/oral 8H
In neutropenic patient with potential line infection (or with severe sepsis or suspected resistant Gram-positive infection)	As above plus Gram-positive cocci incl. S. epidermidis	Piperacillin/Tazobactam as above **and** Amikacin as above **and** Vancomycin 15 mg/kg (500 mg) IV 6H	
Toxic shock syndrome	S. aureus Group A streptococci	As for Septicaemia above (give Flucloxacillin dose IV 4H) **and** Clindamycin 15 mg/kg (600 mg) IV 8H **and** Intravenous immunoglobulin 2g/kg IV	GAS contact prophylaxis: Cefalexin 25 mg/kg (1 g) oral bd for 10 days

Notes to antimicrobial guidelines

- These guidelines have been developed to assist doctors with their choice of initial empiric treatment.
- Except where specified, they **do not apply to neonates or immunocompromised patients.**
- Always ask about previous hypersensitivity reactions to antibiotic.
- The choice of antimicrobial, dose and frequency of administration for continuing treatment may require adjustment according to the clinical situation.
- The recommendations are not intended to be prescriptive and alternative regimens may also be appropriate.
- Antimicrobial recommendations may vary according to local antimicrobial susceptibility patterns; please refer to local guidelines.

1. Antimicrobial choice and dose

- Antibiotics should be changed to narrow spectrum agents once sensitivities are known.
- Dose adjustments may be necessary for neonates, and for children with renal or hepatic impairment.
- Alternative antimicrobial regimens may be more appropriate for neonates, immunocompromised patients or others with a special infection risk (e.g. cystic fibrosis, sickle cell anaemia).
- Resistance to antimicrobials is an increasing problem worldwide. Of particular concern is the increasing incidence of penicillin-resistant pneumococci (see footnote 5). It is important to take into account local resistance patterns when using these guidelines.

2. Duration of treatment

- Duration of treatment is given as a guide only and may vary with the clinical situation.
- 'Step down' from intravenous to oral treatment is appropriate in many cases.
- **Durations given generally refer to the minimum total intravenous plus oral treatment** (*See McMullan et al. Lancet Infect Dis. 2016;16:e139–52*).

3. Methicillin-resistant *Staphylococcus aureus* (MRSA)

- If penicillin hypersensitivity or risk of MRSA: substitute Flucloxacillin with Vancomycin 15 mg/kg (500 mg) IV 6H *or* Clindamycin 15mg/kg (600mg) oral tds *or* Trimethoprim with sulfamethoxazole (8/40 mg/mL) 4/20 mg/kg bd (320/1600mg) oral bd.
- Risk factors for infection with MRSA:
  - Residence in an area with high prevalence of MRSA, e.g. Northern Territory, remote communities in northern Queensland.
  - Previous colonisation or infection with MRSA (particularly recent).
  - Aboriginal and Torres Strait Islander or Pacific Islander child.

4. Third-generation cephalosporins

- Cefotaxime: 50 mg/kg (2 g) IV 12H (week 1 of life), 6–8H (week 2–4 of life), 6H (>week 4 of life).
- Ceftriaxone: usual 50 mg/kg (2 g) IV daily;
  - severe (including meningitis and brain abscess) 100 mg/kg (2 g) IV daily or 50 mg/kg (1 g) IV 12H.
  - Where possible, ceftriaxone should be avoided in neonates <41 weeks gestation, particularly if jaundiced or receiving calcium containing solutions, including TPN.

5. Pneumococci with reduced susceptibility to penicillin

- The prevalence of invasive strains that are highly resistant to penicillin or cephalosporins in Melbourne remains low.
- A third-generation cephalosporin remains the drug of first choice for the empiric treatment of meningitis, however Vancomycin should be added if *S. pneumoniae* is suspected (e.g. Gram-positive cocci on CSF microscopy). This should be stopped if *S. pneumoniae* sensitivity to a third-generation cephalosporin is confirmed, as will be the case with most isolates, or once an alternative aetiology is confirmed.
- Penicillin remains the drug of first choice for the empiric treatment of non-CNS infections, such as suspected pneumococcal pneumonia, regardless of susceptibility. High doses of penicillin overcome resistance in this setting and should be used for confirmed non-CNS infection caused by penicillin-resistant pneumococci.

(continued)

6. Invasive *H. influenzae* type b disease

- Since the introduction of *H. influenzae* type b (Hib) immunisation, there has been a dramatic decline in the incidence of invasive disease.
- However, in children with potential invasive disease who are not fully immunised against Hib, therapy should include cover against Hib.

Therapeutic dose monitoring

Gentamicin once-daily dosing

- Once-daily administration of gentamicin is safe and effective for most patients. Certain patients, such as neonates and those with cystic fibrosis, endocarditis or renal failure, may require special dosing consideration.
- The regimen for monitoring Gentamicin levels is different for once-daily and 8, 12 or 18H dosing, and depends on renal function:
  - Normal renal function – if more than 3 doses required, the trough level (pre-dose) should be checked before the third dose and then every 3 days (target level <1 mg/L).
  - Abnormal renal function – trough levels may need to be checked earlier and more frequently (target level <1 mg/L).
  - Renal failure – levels should be checked prior to each dose and the results should be discussed with a specialist familiar with therapeutic drug monitoring before the next dose is given.

Vancomycin

- Target trough level 10–15 mg/L for cellulitis, 15–20 mg/L for severe infection (bacteraemia, endocarditis, pneumonia, osteomyelitis, meningitis) or known high MIC.

Index

Page locators in **bold** indicate tables. Page locators in *italics* indicate figures. This index uses letter-by-letter alphabetization.

Paediatric Handbook, Tenth Edition. Edited by Kate Harding, Daniel S. Mason and Daryl Efron.
© 2021 John Wiley & Sons Ltd. Published 2021 by John Wiley & Sons Ltd.